Sports Nutrition, Exercise and Medicine

Sports Nutrition, Exercise and Medicine

Edited by **Pablo De Souza**

Callisto Reference
New York

Published by Callisto Reference,
106 Park Avenue, Suite 200,
New York, NY 10016, USA
www.callistoreference.com

Sports Nutrition, Exercise and Medicine
Edited by Pablo De Souza

International Standard Book Number: 978-1-63239-699-0 (Hardback)

Printed in China.

Contents

Preface

Sports Nutrition, Exercise and Medicine are rapidly growing fields of study. Nutrition and exercise play a significant role in sports. They directly affect the performance of athletes; thereby making it necessary for them to follow a healthy diet and exercise regularly. This book covers in detail some existent theories and innovative concepts revolving around these fields. It strives to provide a fair idea about these disciplines and to help develop a better understanding of this field. As these branches of study are constantly evolving, this book will help the readers to gain thorough knowledge about the concepts of sports nutrition, exercise and medicine.

All of the data presented henceforth, was collaborated in the wake of recent advancements in the field. The aim of this book is to present the diversified developments from across the globe in a comprehensible manner. The opinions expressed in each chapter belong solely to the contributing authors. Their interpretations of the topics are the integral part of this book, which I have carefully compiled for a better understanding of the readers.

At the end, I would like to thank all those who dedicated their time and efforts for the successful completion of this book. I also wish to convey my gratitude towards my friends and family who supported me at every step.

Editor

Comparison of coconut water and a carbohydrate-electrolyte sport drink on measures of hydration and physical performance in exercise-trained men

Douglas S Kalman[1], Samantha Feldman[1], Diane R Krieger[1] and Richard J Bloomer[2*]

Abstract

Background: Sport drinks are ubiquitous within the recreational and competitive fitness and sporting world. Most are manufactured and artificially flavored carbohydrate-electrolyte beverages. Recently, attention has been given to coconut water, a natural alternative to manufactured sport drinks, with initial evidence indicating efficacy with regard to maintaining hydration. We compared coconut water and a carbohydrate-electrolyte sport drink on measures of hydration and physical performance in exercise-trained men.

Methods: Following a 60-minute bout of dehydrating treadmill exercise, 12 exercise-trained men (26.6 ± 5.7 yrs) received bottled water (BW), pure coconut water (VitaCoco®: CW), coconut water from concentrate (CWC), or a carbohydrate-electrolyte sport drink (SD) [a fluid amount based on body mass loss during the dehydrating exercise] on four occasions (separated by at least 5 days) in a random order, single blind (subject and not investigators), cross-over design. Hydration status (body mass, fluid retention, plasma osmolality, urine specific gravity) and performance (treadmill time to exhaustion; assessed after rehydration) were determined during the recovery period. Subjective measures of thirst, bloatedness, refreshed, stomach upset, and tiredness were also determined using a 5-point visual analog scale.

Results: Subjects lost approximately 1.7 kg (~2% of body mass) during the dehydrating exercise and regained this amount in a relatively similar manner following consumption of all conditions. No differences were noted between coconut water (CW or CWC) and SD for any measures of fluid retention ($p > 0.05$). Regarding exercise performance, no significant difference ($p > 0.05$) was noted between BW (11.9 ± 5.9 min), CW (12.3 ± 5.8 min), CWC (11.9 ± 6.0 min), and SD (12.8 ± 4.9 min). In general, subjects reported feeling more bloated and experienced greater stomach upset with the CW and CWC conditions.

Conclusion: All tested beverages are capable of promoting rehydration and supporting subsequent exercise. Little difference is noted between the four tested conditions with regard to markers of hydration or exercise performance in a sample of young, healthy men. Additional study inclusive of a more demanding dehydration protocol, as well as a time trial test as the measure of exercise performance, may more specifically determine the efficacy of these beverages on enhancing hydration and performance following dehydrating exercise.

Keywords: Hydration, Coconut Water, Sport Drink, Exercise

* Correspondence: rbloomer@memphis.edu
[2]The University of Memphis, Cardiorespiratory/Metabolic Laboratory, Department of Health and Sport Sciences, 106 Roane Fieldhouse, Memphis, TN 38152
Full list of author information is available at the end of the article

Background

Fluid loss during strenuous, long duration exercise is commonplace and can result in thermal stress, impaired cognition and cardiovascular function, accelerated fatigue, and impaired exercise performance [1,2]. Recommendations for fluid intake before, during, and following exercise are well described [3,4] and are typically followed by most athletes seeking enhanced physical performance. Abiding by such recommendations appears particularly important when exercising in hot and humid environmental conditions, where fluid loss may be high [5].

Although water is often suggested to many general fitness enthusiasts who may exercise for relatively short periods of time (< 75 minutes), carbohydrate-electrolyte sport drinks are highly recommended and appear to be the beverage of choice for most serious athletes–aerobic athletes in particular [2]. This is partly fueled by scientific recommendations for the consumption of such beverages [6,7], and partly by the widespread marketing campaigns of large sport nutrition and beverage companies. Regardless, carbohydrate-electrolyte beverages are widely consumed and represent a multi-billion dollar segment of the food and beverage industry [8].

Some individuals prefer natural alternatives to the manufactured sport drinks. For example, many sport drinks contain fructose and/or maltodextrin, artificial flavors and sweeteners, and added electrolytes (e.g., sodium, potassium). With more emphasis recently within the sport nutrition industry on "natural" beverages, some athletes and recreationally active fitness enthusiasts seek alternatives to the manufactured sport drink. While water is indeed a reasonable solution for some, those involved in longer duration exercise bouts often require and demand carbohydrate and electrolytes within their beverage of choice. For these individuals, coconut water may be considered as one viable alternative.

Coconut water is naturally occurring, is very rich in potassium, contains sodium, chloride, and carbohydrate [9], and is viewed as the hydrating beverage of choice in certain parts of the world [10]. Clinically, coconut water may be used as an oral rehydration aid to replace fluid loss from the gastrointestinal tract in patients suffering severe dehydration due to diarrhea [11,12]. It has also been used intravenously with success [13]. Although not linked specifically to hydration, coconut water has been reported to have antioxidant properties [14], which may aid in neutralizing reactive oxygen species production resulting from long duration exercise [15].

In relation to sport nutrition, coconut water has been reported to provide hydrating effects similar to those of carbohydrate-electrolyte sport drinks [16-18]. Unfortunately, these studies have focused exclusively on hydration measures as primary outcome variables (following a period of dehydrating exercise and consumption of the assigned beverage), while not emphasizing actual exercise performance during the rehydrating period. Hence, while the rehydrating effects of coconut water may be similar to those of carbohydrate-electrolyte sport drinks, an equally important question for most athletes and coaches is whether or not the hydration status equates to actual physical performance. Considering the above, we investigated the effects of two different forms of coconut water (concentrated and not from concentrate) and a carbohydrate-electrolyte sport drink on measures of hydration status and physical performance in exercise-trained men.

Methods

Subjects and Screening

Exercise-trained men were recruited to participate. Eligibility was determined by completion of a health history form (Physical Activity Readiness Questionnaire [PAR-Q]) and physical examination. Prior to the start of the study, subjects were engaged in a program of regular exercise for a minimum of the past six months, without difficulty in walking or running on a treadmill. All subjects were instructed to maintain their pre-study exercise program throughout the course of the study, with the exception of refraining from exercise during the 24 hours prior to each test day. Subjects were nonsmokers, did not report any history of cardiovascular, metabolic, neurological, or orthopedic disorders that may have impacted their ability to participate in the study, and did not start the use of any new nutritional supplement over the course of the study; however, they were allowed to continue using nutritional supplements they had been using prior to beginning the study (e.g., multivitamins). Prior to participation, each subject was informed of all procedures, potential risks, and benefits associated with the study through both verbal and written form in accordance with the approved procedures of the Aspire Institutional Review Board for Human Subjects Research (La Mesa, CA; approval date of December 23, 2010). Subjects signed an informed consent form prior to being admitted into the study.

At the initial screening visits, subjects' height via stadiometer (Holtain Limited; Britain) and body mass via digital scale (Detecto; Webb City, MO) were measured and recorded. Body mass was obtained with subjects wearing only a gown and their underwear. Body mass measures following exercise were obtained only after subjects were thoroughly towel dried. Heart rate and blood pressure (using subjects' left arm) were recorded following a minimum of five minutes of quiet rest, while subjects were seated in a chair. A 12-lead

Table 1 Characteristics of 12 exercise-trained men

Variable	Value
Age at Screening (years)	26.6 ± 5.7 24.0 (21.0 - 35.0)
Ethnicity	
Hispanic	12 (100%)
Total	12 (100%)
Race	12 (100%)
Caucasian	12 (100%)
Total	12 (100%)
Height (cm)	175.4 ± 4.1 175.0 (168.6 - 181.2)
Body Mass at Screening (kg)	77.2 ± 6.3 78.4 (66 - 85.8)
Body Mass Index ($kg \cdot m^{-2}$)	25.1 ± 1.8 26.1 (21.5 - 26.9)
Systolic Blood Pressure (mm Hg)	118.4 ± 13.2 120.5 (97.0 - 145.0)
Diastolic Blood Pressure (mm Hg)	73.9 ± 6.7 74.0 (64.0 - 87.0)
Heart Rate ($beats \cdot minute^{-1}$)	68.8 ± 14.4 66.5 (48.0 - 99.0)
Glucose ($mg \cdot dL^{-1}$)	92.5 ± 4.0 91.5 (87.0 - 99.0)
Blood Urea Nitrogen ($mg \cdot dL^{-1}$)	15.2 ± 3.0 16.0 (9.0 - 19.0)
Creatinine ($mg \cdot dL^{-1}$)	1.0 ± 0.2 1.0 (0.7 - 1.2)
Alkaline Phosphatase ($Units \cdot L^{-1}$)	82.0 ± 41.0 73.0 (32.0 - 177.0)
Aspartate Amino Transaminase ($Units \cdot L^{-1}$)	21.4 ± 4.4 20.5 (16.0 - 29.0)
Alanine Amino Transferase ($Units \cdot L^{-1}$)	20.8 ± 5.8 21.0 (11.0 - 30.0)
White Blood Cell count ($thousands \cdot \mu L^{-1}$)	6.9 ± 1.7 6.7 (4.2 - 9.8)
Red Blood Cell count ($millions \cdot \mu L^{-1}$)	5.3 ± 0.4 5.3 (4.5 - 6.1)
Hemoglobin ($g \cdot dL^{-1}$)	15.0 ± 1.0 15.3 (13.1 - 16.0)
Hematocrit (%)	47.7 ± 3.0 47.9 (42.8 - 52.2)

Data are mean ± SD (top row); median and (range) provided in bottom row

electrocardiogram was obtained and analyzed for normality, to ensure subject suitability for participation. Blood samples were collected from subjects for routine assessment of clinical chemistry parameters (e.g., metabolic panel and complete blood count). Please see Table 1 for subject descriptive characteristics. A familiarization trial of the exercise performance test was also conducted during the initial laboratory visit. A description of this test is provided below.

Test Days

On each of the four test days, subjects reported to the lab in the morning following an overnight fast (no food or beverages other than water were allowed after midnight). The time of day for testing each subject was matched for all subsequent test days (± 60 minutes). Subjects were instructed not to exercise or to consume alcohol during the 24 hours prior to each test day, but to consume water liberally up to the time they reported to the lab for testing. Adherence to study instructions was confirmed with all subjects on each day of testing. Following all baseline assessments, subjects were provided with a standardized breakfast consisting of a bagel and one tablespoon of cream cheese. They were also provided with up to 470 mL of water.

Dehydrating Exercise Test

Sixty minutes following the conclusion of the standardized breakfast, subjects performed the dehydrating exercise test. It should be noted that of the total of 48 test visits (12 subjects × 4 visits), slight deviations in the time from food intake to the start of the dehydrating exercise test were noted for 14 of the tests (i.e., started before or after the set 60 minute time). Specifically, nine tests were conducted within 15 minutes of this time, two tests were conducted within 30 minutes of this time, and three tests were conducted within 45 minutes of this time. We do not believe these deviations significantly influenced the findings; in particular considering that these were equally dispersed among the four conditions.

The dehydrating exercise consisted of two, 30-minute bouts of walking/jogging, interspersed with a 10 minute rest period. Specifically, subjects walked/jogged at 2, 3, 4, 5, 6 and 7 miles per hour on a motorized treadmill, using a grade of 0%. Five minutes of exercise was performed at each speed. Following the initial 30 minutes of exercise, a 10-minute break was allowed, during which time subjects walked around and/or remained seated. Subjects then repeated the above sequence of speeds for an additional 30 minutes of exercise. Hence, a total of 60 minutes of exercise was performed within the 70 minute period. All exercise was performed in a climate controlled room, with an average temperature of 36° Celsius and an average relative humidity of 48%. This dehydrating exercise protocol has been reported to induce a 2 to 3% reduction in body weight [19]. During the three hour period from the end of the dehydrating exercise test to the start of the performance exercise test, subjects were required to rest quietly without food or beverage intake (with the exception of the assigned condition). During this time, as well as during the performance exercise test, subjects remained in a thermoneutral environment (i.e., 22 degrees Celsius).

Conditions

Within minutes following the conclusion of the dehydrating exercise test (after all measurements were obtained–see Table 2), subjects received their assigned condition (beverage). The study design involved a random order, single blind (subject and not investigators), cross-over assignment to one of the following four conditions: Supermarket brand bottled water, pure coconut water (VitaCoco®; New York, NY), coconut water from concentrate, or a carbohydrate-electrolyte sport drink (5-6% carbohydrate solution). The amount of each beverage was determined based on the total amount of body mass lost during the dehydrating exercise protocol using the equation: $1300\ mL \cdot kg^{-1} \times kg\ loss$ = amount of beverage consumed (mL). This provided a weighted volume amount of beverage equal to approximately 125% of the actual body mass lost. Based on this, the amount of beverage consumed equated to 2159 ± 249 mL for bottled water, 2220 ± 367 mL for VitaCoco®, 2253 ± 358 mL for coconut water from concentrate, and 2184 ± 358 mL for the sport drink, with no differences noted between conditions ($p > 0.05$). Subjects were allowed 60 minutes to consume the entire volume of beverage. Each condition was consumed on a different test day, with a minimum of five days separating test visits.

Performance Exercise Test

Three hours after the completion of the dehydrating exercise test (and two hours after subjects consumed their assigned condition), a test of physical performance was conducted using a treadmill as previously done [20]. Specifically, subjects began walking on a motorized treadmill at a self-selected comfortable speed (0% grade) for five minutes. At the conclusion of the five-minute period, the actual performance test began. The protocol involved an increase in intensity every three minutes. While the speed of the treadmill remained constant at 4.2 miles per hour throughout the test, the grade increase in the following manner: min 1-3, 0%; min 4-6, 2.5%; min 7-9, 5%; min 10-12, 7.5%; min 13-15, 10%; min 16-18, 12.5%; min 19-21, 15%. Subjects exercised until volitional exhaustion and the total exercise time was recorded. This identical protocol was administered at the screening visit (for familiarization) and on each of the four test day visits. Therefore, we do not believe that there was any significant degree of "learning" involved with this test.

Outcome Measures

In addition to the measure of total exercise time obtained in the performance test described above, the following variables were used as outcome measures; some of which have been discussed previously [21]. With regard to hydration status, body mass, fluid retention (based on body mass), plasma osmolality, and urine specific gravity were measured. Specifically, for fluid retention based on body mass, it was expected that the administration of test product at the amount prescribed would bring the subject's body mass back to very near its pre-exercise level. The rehydrating efficacy of the test product was indicated by how well this volume of fluid was retained over the two hours following consumption. Therefore, the body mass immediately post beverage consumption (which occurred at 1 hour post dehydrating exercise) was considered the "baseline"; this was subtracted from the body mass values at 2 and 3 hours post dehydrating exercise, and this difference was divided by the mass of beverage that had been consumed, then multiplied by 100 to yield the "percent of rehydrating fluid retained" at 2 and 3 hours. It should be noted that

Table 2 Study timeline and outcome measures

Time → Variable ↓	Pre Dehydrating Exercise Test	Immediately Post Dehydrating Exercise Test	1 Hour Post Dehydrating Exercise Test	2 Hours Post Dehydrating Exercise Test	3 Hours Post Dehydrating Exercise Test†	Immediately Post Performance Exercise Test
Body Mass††	X	X*	X**	X	X	
Plasma Osmolality	X	X			X	
Urine Specific Gravity	X	X			X	
Subjective Measures (VAS)		X	X	X	X	
Heart Rate	X	X			X	X
Blood Pressure	X	X			X	X

† The Performance Exercise Test began following this measurement time (total exercise time was recorded)

†† Body Mass was used to calculate fluid retention (as described in the Methods section)

* For determination of fluid volume to consume

** For determination of "baseline" body mass

body mass was accurately determined using an electronic scale with subjects dry and wearing only a gown and underwear. In additional, all fluid volumes delivered to subjects were meticulously measured. Our use of body mass was used as a surrogate efficacy indicator of hydration as done previously [22].

Plasma osmolality and urine specific gravity were determined using standard procedures. Osmolality was determined by freezing point depression. Specific gravity was determined using reagent test strips. Although we did not measure urine osmolality, it has been concluded by Armstrong and colleagues that "urine osmolality and urine specific gravity may be used interchangeably to determine hydration status" [23]. Both plasma osmolality and urine specific gravity have been used previously as indicators of hydration status [24], and were obtained prior to the dehydrating exercise test, immediately following the dehydrating exercise test, and prior to the performance exercise test.

With regard to subjective measures, thirst, bloatedness, refreshed, stomach upset, and tiredness were determined using a 5-point visual analog scale. Answers were scaled from 1 to 5 where 1 was the lowest and 5 was the highest score. These were assessed immediately, 60 minutes, 120 minutes, and 180 minutes following the dehydrating exercise test.

Heart rate and blood pressure were measured at the following times: Prior to the dehydrating exercise test, immediately following the dehydrating exercise test, prior to the performance exercise test, and immediately following the performance exercise test. A schematic of the study timeline for all outcome measures is provided in Table 2.

Physical Activity and Dietary Intake

Subjects were instructed to maintain their normal physical activity throughout the study period, with the exception of refraining from strenuous physical activity during the 24 hours preceding each test day. They were also given specific instructions regarding abstinence from alcohol consumption during the 24 hours immediately preceding the test days. Dietary intake was to be maintained through the study period, with the exception of reporting to the lab in a fasted state on each of the four test days. No food records were maintained in this study, which may be considered by some to be a limitation of this work.

Statistical Analysis

The sample size was determined based on convenience and a power analysis was carried out to determine the effect sizes that would provide an 80% chance of obtaining a significant result of $p \leq 0.05$, when testing the outcome measures using the paired Student t test. Using a sample of 12 subjects, an 18% difference in fluid retention between products would be needed to detect statistical significance. All numerical variables were tested for normality by the Anderson-Darling test. Outcome measures as described within the text above for each variable, at each time point, were analyzed by the paired Student t test. All analyses were performed using "*R*" statistical software (version 2.13.1; *R* Foundation for Statistical Computing). Statistical significance was set at $p \leq 0.05$. The data are presented as mean ± SD.

Results

Overview and Adverse Effects

All subjects successfully completed all aspects of this study, with the exception of one subject who was unable to consume the volume of coconut water from concentrate in the allotted time. Therefore, the trial for this subject was not included in the analysis (n = 11 for coconut water from concentrate). Very few adverse events were noted and all were characterized as mild (e.g., stomach upset), likely due to the consumption of a high volume of fluid (> 2 liters) in a relatively short period of time (≤ 60 minutes).

Performance Data

Regarding treadmill performance, no significant difference ($p > 0.05$) was noted in total exercise time between bottled water (11.9 ± 5.9 minutes), VitaCoco® (12.3 ± 5.8 minutes), coconut water from concentrate (11.9 ± 6.0 minutes), and sport drink (12.8 ± 4.9 minutes).

Hydration Data

In regard to body mass, subjects lost approximately 1.7 kg during the dehydrating exercise (~2% of starting body mass), regained this amount in a similar manner following consumption of all conditions, and slowly lost approximately 1 kg over the subsequent two hours (Table 3). However, body mass ($p = 0.023$) was slightly greater with coconut water from concentrate compared only to bottled water (when expressed as change from pre dehydrating exercise at 3 hours post dehydrating exercise). No other differences were noted between conditions for body mass ($p > 0.05$). In regard to fluid retention (based on body mass), similar findings were observed (as this measure is influenced by body mass), with greater values for coconut water from concentrate compared only to bottled water ($p = 0.041$) at 3 hours post dehydrating exercise. At 3 hours post dehydrating exercise (2 hours after rehydration) values were numerically highest for coconut water from concentrate (~52%), lowest for bottled water (~35%), and intermediate for VitaCoco® and sport drink (~40%); although these differences were not statistically significant ($p > 0.05$). No other differences were noted between

Table 3 Body mass of exercise-trained men before and after dehydrating exercise

Time	VitaCoco®	Sport Drink	Coconut Water From Concentrate	Bottled Water
Pre Dehydrating Exercise	78.5 ± 7.4 79.2 (65.2 - 89.0)	77.8 ± 7.1 78.2 (65.2 - 87.3)	77.5 ± 7.6 75.6 (64.9 - 88.4)	77.8 ± 7.6 78.2 (64.8 - 89.3)
Immediately Post Dehydrating Exercise	76.9 ± 7.2 77.4 (63.9 - 87.2)	76.1 ± 6.8 76.6 (63.8 - 85.3)	75.8 ± 7.5 73.7 (63.3 - 86.5)	76.2 ± 7.4 76.5 (63.5 - 87.4)
1 hour Post Dehydrating Exercise	78.4 ± 7.3 79.0 (65.5 - 88.9)	77.7 ± 7.2 77.8 (65.1 - 87.6)	77.6 ± 7.6 75.5 (65.0 - 88.6)	77.9 ± 7.6 78.1 (64.9 - 90.1)
2 hours Post Dehydrating Exercise	78.1 ± 7.2 78.3 (65.5 - 88.8)	77.4 ± 7.0 77.6 (65.1 - 87.0)	77.3 ± 7.5 75.2 (64.8 - 88)	77.4 ± 7.5 77.6 (64.7 - 88.9)
3 hours Post Dehydrating Exercise*	77.6 ± 6.9 78.0 (65.5 - 87.9)	77.0 ± 6.8 77.2 (64.9 - 86.3)	76.9 ± 7.4 75.0 (64.6 - 87.6)	76.9 ± 7.3 76.9 (64.5 - 88.0)

Data are mean ± SD (top row); median and (range) provided in bottom row

*Coconut water from concentrate greater than bottled water (p = 0.023); when expressed as change from Pre Dehydrating Exercise at 3 hours Post Dehydrating Exercise. No other differences noted (p > 0.05).

conditions for fluid retention ($p > 0.05$). Data are presented in Table 4. Plasma osmolality displayed similar results as noted for body mass and fluid retention, with greater values for coconut water from concentrate compared only to bottled water ($p = 0.049$; when expressed as change from pre dehydrating exercise at 3 hours post dehydrating exercise). In general, this measure increased after dehydrating exercise, indicating dehydration of the subjects, and returned toward baseline at 3 hours post dehydrating exercise, indicating rehydration of the subjects. No other differences were noted between conditions for plasma osmolality ($p > 0.05$). Data are presented in Table 5. No differences were noted between conditions for urine specific gravity, with this measure relatively constant and within the normal range over the measurement period ($p > 0.05$). Data are presented in Table 6.

Subjective Data

All four conditions quenched thirst with no significant differences between conditions ($p > 0.05$). Subjects reported feeling bloated with all four conditions, as per statistically significant increases at 1 hour post dehydrating exercise. Over the two hour rehydration period, the bloatedness decreased for all four conditions but remained statistically significant at 3 hours post dehydrating exercise for VitaCoco® ($p = 0.012$) and coconut water from concentrate ($p = 0.034$). Subjects generally felt refreshed after rehydration, with a statistically significant increase for bottled water over VitaCoco® at 1 hour post dehydrating exercise ($p = 0.036$). No other differences were noted ($p > 0.05$). The two coconut-based products tended to produce more stomach upset than bottled water or sport drink, with significant findings at 3 hours post dehydrating exercise for VitaCoco® and sport drink ($p = 0.034$), VitaCoco® and bottled water ($p = 0.046$), coconut water from concentrate and sport drink ($p = 0.020$) and coconut water from concentrate and bottled water ($p = 0.020$). Tiredness generally tended to decrease immediately post dehydrating exercise, with no significant differences between conditions ($p > 0.05$). All subjective data are presented in Table 7.

Heart Rate and Blood Pressure Data

No differences were noted between conditions for heart rate, systolic blood pressure, or diastolic blood pressure ($p > 0.05$). Data for these variables are presented in Table 8.

Table 4 Fluid retention of exercise-trained men before and after dehydrating exercise

Time	VitaCoco®	Sport Drink	Coconut Water From Concentrate	Bottled Water
1 hour Post Dehydrating Exercise	73.6 ± 22.1 76.0 (30.9 - 101.5	76.4 ± 21.1 77.9 (37.6 - 101.5)	83.5 ± 9.7 84.0 (67.2 - 101.5)	82.1 ± 22.3 88.0 (42.8 - 115.9)
2 hours Post Dehydrating Exercise	59.6 ± 31.7 71.4 (-3.8 - 99.0)	60.6 ± 19.5 66.8 (28.4 - 90.9)	67.6 ± 13.7 63.0 (37.8 - 85.5)	56.9 ± 26.6 62.1 (0.0 - 95.7)
3 hours Post Dehydrating Exercise*	39.0 ± 37.9 35.7 (-42.2 - 99.0)	40.3 ± 24.9 38.9 (-5.7 - 74.8)	51.7 ± 14.9 46.2 (29.4 - 75.6)	34.7 ± 23.9 32.9 (-10.7 - 65.5)

Data are mean ± SD (top row); median and (range) provided in bottom row

*Coconut water from concentrate greater than bottled water (p = 0.041) at 3 hours Post Dehydrating Exercise. No other differences noted (p > 0.05).

Table 5 Plasma osmolality of exercise-trained men before and after dehydrating exercise

Time	VitaCoco®	Sport Drink	Coconut Water From Concentrate	Bottled Water
Pre Dehydrating Exercise	289.3 ± 4.5 288.5 (282.0 - 300.0)	291.5 ± 6.0 290.0 (283.0 - 305.0)	293.0 ± 5.6 291.0 (287.0 - 305.0)	292.0 ± 5.0 291.0 (282.0 - 300.0)
Immediately Post Dehydrating Exercise	297.5 ± 5.6 297.5 (290.0 - 309.0)	297.7 ± 8.0 297.0 (289.0 - 320.0)	297.5 ± 6.1 296.0 (289.0 - 309.0)	297.6 ± 4.5 297.5 (290.0 - 305.0)
3 hours Post Dehydrating Exercise*	291.2 ± 6.6 290.0 (285.0 - 310.0)	289.6 ± 5.5 288.0 (283.0 - 304.0)	291.8 ± 5.7 289.0 (286.0 - 306.0)	290.3 ± 5.1 289.5 (284.0 - 302.0)

Data are mean ± SD (top row); median and (range) provided in bottom row

*Coconut water from concentrate greater than bottled water ($p = 0.049$); when expressed as change from Pre Dehydrating Exercise at 3 hours Post Dehydrating Exercise. No other differences noted ($p > 0.05$).

Discussion

Findings from the present investigation indicate that all of the tested beverages are capable of promoting rehydration after one hour of dehydrating exercise. With few exceptions at selected time points, findings for all rehydration variables were essentially the same when comparing the carbohydrate-electrolyte sport drink, coconut water (concentrated and not from concentrate), and bottled water. Moreover, no differences were noted in treadmill performance during the rehydration period. These data are specific to a sample of young, exercise-trained, healthy men.

Maintaining hydration status is vital for athletes and can directly impact exercise performance [25]. As such, many studies have been conducted to determine the optimal rehydration strategies. While water intake is likely an adequate rehydration approach for many individuals, others (e.g., athletes involved in vigorous training) may require intake of water-carbohydrate or carbohydrate-electrolyte mixtures [2], in addition to other nutrients [26]. Such an approach has been reported to be superior to water alone and is generally considered the ideal recommendation for individuals engaged in long duration, strenuous bouts of acute exercise [2,4].

Related to the above, the use of coconut water has been considered by many, as this beverage provides a natural source of carbohydrate and electrolytes [9]. Specifically, coconut water has been reported to provide sugar (~1 g · dL^{-1}), potassium (~51 mEq · L^{-1}), sodium (~33 mEq · L^{-1}), and chloride (~52 mEq · L^{-1}) [9]; however, this may vary depending on species of coconut palm. Coconut water has been reported to provide hydrating effects similar to those of carbohydrate-electrolyte sport drinks [16-18].

Saat and colleagues used a cross-over study to assess the effectiveness of fresh young coconut water and a carbohydrate-electrolyte beverage, compared to water on measures of whole body rehydration and blood volume restoration during a two hour rehydration period following a bout of dehydrating exercise [16]. A sample of eight young men participated and consumed the assigned beverage at a volume equal to 120% of the fluid loss during exercise. No statistically significant differences were noted between conditions for any outcome measure; however, blood volume restoration was noted to be slightly greater for coconut water. This same group reported similar findings in a follow-up study published in 2007 [17], using the same volume of beverages (120% of fluid loss during exercise). More recently, Idárraga and Aragón-Vargas studied the rehydrating effect of coconut water following exercise [18]. On three different days, six men and five women were dehydrated to approximately 2% body mass by exercising in a climate-controlled laboratory. On each day and in random order, subjects were rehydrated with fresh coconut water, a sport drink, or plain water using a volume equal to 120% of body weight lost during exercise. Subjects were then monitored for three hours, with urine collection every 30 minutes. No differences were

Table 6 Urine specific gravity of exercise-trained men before and after dehydrating exercise

Time	VitaCoco®	Sport Drink	Coconut Water From Concentrate	Bottled Water
Pre Dehydrating Exercise	1.0204 ± 0.0087 1.02 (1.01 - 1.03)	1.0218 ± 0.0096 1.03 (1.00 - 1.032)	1.0217 ± 0.0106 1.03 (1.01 - 1.03)	1.0231 ± 0.0068 1.03 (1.01 - 1.03)
Immediately Post Dehydrating Exercise	1.0158 ± 0.0102 1.02 (1.01 - 1.03)	1.0165 ± 0.0112 1.018 (1.00 - 1.03)	1.0153 ± 0.0098 1.02 (1.00 - 1.03)	1.0161 ± 0.0077 1.02 (1.00 - 1.03)
3 hours Post Dehydrating Exercise	1.0200 ± 0.0098 1.03 (1.01 - 1.03)	1.0060 ± 0.0037 1.01 (1.00 - 1.02)	1.0139 ± 0.0066 1.02 (1.00 - 1.03)	1.0055 ± 0.0022 1.01 (1.00 - 1.01)

Data are mean ± SD (top row); median and (range) provided in bottom row

No differences noted ($p > 0.05$).

Table 7 Subjective ratings of exercise-trained men before and after dehydrating exercise

Time	VitaCoco®	Sport Drink	Coconut Water From Concentrate	Bottled Water
Thirst				
Immediately Post DHE	4.08 ± 1.16	4.42 ± 0.67	4.45 ± 0.69	4.67 ± 0.65
1 hour Post DHE	1.17 ± 0.58	1.33 ± 0.89	1.36 ± 0.67	1.08 ± 0.29
2 hours Post DHE	1.50 ± 0.52	1.58 ± 0.67	1.45 ± 0.52	1.50 ± 0.67
3 hours Post DHE	1.67 ± 0.65	1.83 ± 0.94	1.45 ± 0.82	1.92 ± 1.00
Bloatedness				
Immediately Post DHE	1.33 ± 0.49	1.33 ± 0.65	1.55 ± 1.04	1.33 ± 0.49
1 hour Post DHE	3.58 ± 1.00	3.42 ± 1.24	4.00 ± 1.34	3.08 ± 1.24
2 hours Post DHE	2.75 ± 0.97	1.67 ± 0.65	2.82 ± 1.17	1.50 ± 0.67
3 hours Post DHE	2.33 ± 1.23	1.42 ± 0.67	2.45 ± 1.21	1.25 ± 0.62
Refreshed				
Immediately Post DHE	1.92 ± 1.00	2.08 ± 1.24	2.09 ± 1.22	1.67 ± 0.89
1 hour Post DHE	3.25 ± 1.36	3.83 ± 1.27	3.82 ± 1.08	4.17 ± 1.19
2 hours Post DHE	3.33 ± 1.23	3.67 ± 1.23	3.64 ± 1.50	3.58 ± 1.16
3 hours Post DHE	3.17 ± 1.19	3.33 ± 1.15	3.55 ± 1.51	3.50 ± 1.09
Stomach Upset				
Immediately Post DHE	1.58 ± 0.79	1.25 ± 0.45	1.00 ± 0.00	1.00 ± 0.00
1 hour Post DHE	2.75 ± 1.29	2.00 ± 1.35	3.18 ± 1.66	1.67 ± 0.89
2 hours Post DHE	3.33 ± 1.23	1.25 ± 0.62	3.09 ± 1.51	1.25 ± 0.45
3 hours Post DHE	2.92 ± 1.31	1.17 ± 0.39	2.55 ± 1.44	1.08 ± 0.29
Tiredness				
Immediately Post DHE	3.58 ± 1.00	3.92 ± 0.79	3.82 ± 0.98	4.08 ± 0.79
1 hour Post DHE	2.83 ± 0.83	3.08 ± 0.90	2.64 ± 0.92	2.92 ± 1.00
2 hours Post DHE	2.08 ± 0.90	2.58 ± 0.90	2.36 ± 0.81	2.33 ± 0.98
3 hours Post DHE	2.08 ± 0.90	2.50 ± 1.00	2.18 ± 0.98	2.33 ± 0.78

Data are mean ± SD

Thirst: No differences between conditions ($p > 0.05$).

Bloatedness: 3 hours Post DHE > Immediately Post DHE for VitaCoco® ($p = 0.012$) and coconut water from concentrate ($p = 0.034$)

Refreshed: 1 hour Post DHE > Immediately Post DHE for bottled water compared to VitaCoco® ($p = 0.036$).

Stomach Upset: Greater stomach upset at 3 hours Post DHE for VitaCoco® compared to sport drink ($p = 0.034$), VitaCoco® compared to bottled water ($p = 0.046$), coconut water from concentrate compared to sport drink ($p = 0.020$) and coconut water from concentrate compared to bottled water ($p = 0.020$).

Tiredness: No differences between conditions ($p > 0.05$).

DHE = Dehydrating Exercise

noted between coconut water and sport drink for urine volume or fluid retention (both were better than plain water).

These above studies focused exclusively on hydration measures, following a period of dehydrating exercise and consumption of the assigned beverage, while not emphasizing exercise performance during the rehydrating period. The present study, using a similar fluid volume as used previously, extends these findings by noting similar exercise performance results for natural coconut water (concentrated and not from concentrate) and a carbohydrate-electrolyte sport drink. For most athletes and coaches, this finding is likely of most importance. Our data indicate that coconut water can provide similar benefits as compared to a typical sport drink in terms of exercise performance (as measured based on treadmill time to exhaustion), in addition to measures of hydration. That being said, one potential concern is subject tolerance to coconut water in such high volumes. Subjects reported feeling somewhat bloated and experienced mild stomach upset with the two forms of coconut water used in the present investigation (Table 7), which is likely due to the high volume of fluid required to be consumed in such a short period of time. As with most beverages, individual tolerance to coconut water should be determined prior to use.

It should be noted that this study explored many end-points at many time-points, each being compared between four products. Consequently, many hundreds of separate pairwise comparisons were carried out, each generating a p value, raising the issue of multiplicity and inflated Type-1 error. No multiple-test adjustments (Bonferroni or other) were applied - it would have been unrealistic and unproductive to try to establish a study-

Table 8 Heart rate and blood pressure of exercise-trained men before and after dehydrating exercise

Time	VitaCoco®	Sport Drink	Coconut Water From Concentrate	Bottled Water
Heart Rate				
Pre DHE	63.6 ± 8.7	63.3 ± 6.7	64.6 ± 11.6	62.7 ± 6.5
Immediately Post DHE	102.1 ± 19.9	101.8 ± 12.8	103.4 ± 13.0	102.0 ± 18.1
Pre PE	70.2 ± 11.2	71.2 ± 9.8	68.5 ± 9.1	64.2 ± 7.6
Immediately Post PE	86.8 ± 15.0	88.0 ± 17.5	96.1 ± 35.7	84.6 ± 15.2
Systolic Blood Pressure				
Pre DHE	122.8 ± 9.6	119.6 ± 9.5	121.0 ± 9.4	122.3 ± 8.4
Immediately Post DHE	109.2 ± 9.6	116.8 ± 12.1	113.6 ± 11.7	112.7 ± 4.3
Pre PE	122.1 ± 9.4	116.7 ± 8.4	120.9 ± 9.3	117.6 ± 8.7
Immediately Post PE	120.8 ± 11.9	121.6 ± 9.6	117.7 ± 9.9	115.7 ± 10.3
Diastolic Blood Pressure				
Pre DHE	77.8 ± 5.2	75.0 ± 7.5	78.3 ± 7.3	76.7 ± 3.9
Immediately Post DHE	66.8 ± 7.1	73.1 ± 7.0	71.1 ± 7.3	72.2 ± 5.9
Pre PE	76.3 ± 4.3	74.1 ± 5.6	74.8 ± 5.8	73.5 ± 5.2
Immediately Post PE	77.6 ± 6.6	76.6 ± 6.4	74.5 ± 6.6	74.3 ± 7.5

Data are mean ± SD
No differences noted ($p > 0.05$).
DHE = Dehydrating Exercise
PE = Performance Exercise

wide 0.05 alpha level, which would have required impossibly small p-values on individual tests. So it should be kept in mind that each individual p value has a one-in-twenty chance of being nominally significant ($p < 0.05$) purely from random fluctuations. Conclusions of relative efficacy among the different products should not be based simply on isolated p values, but rather on a consideration of the complete set of data for each endpoint. Likewise, observed values were not simply put into a repeated-measures ANOVA to test for overall changes over time - most endpoints displayed very significant changes at certain time points (such as from baseline to immediately post-dehydrating exercise). It was much more appropriate to examination the changes (and differences in mean changes between products) only over certain physiologically-meaningful intervals, and individual t-tests were much more directly interpretable, and therefore more useful, in assessing these specific changes.

Conclusion

Considering the above, our data indicate that both coconut water (natural, concentrated and not from concentrate) and bottled water provide similar rehydrating effects as compared to a carbohydrate-electrolyte sport drink. Moreover, none of the beverages impacted treadmill exercise performance differently during the rehydration period. Additional study is needed with consideration for the inclusion of a more demanding dehydration protocol, aimed at reducing body mass beyond the 2% mark obtained in the present investigation may be warranted. Finally, while treadmill time to exhaustion is routinely used in laboratory studies, the use of a time trial test as the measure of exercise performance may be more appropriate. Investigators may consider these suggestions when designing future studies focused on the potential rehydrating ability of coconut water and other beverages.

Acknowledgements
Funding for this work was provided by VitaCoco® Company (New York, NY).

Author details
[1]Miami Research Associates, Nutrition/Endocrinology Department, 6141 Sunset Drive, Suite 301, Miami, FL 33143. [2]The University of Memphis, Cardiorespiratory/Metabolic Laboratory, Department of Health and Sport Sciences, 106 Roane Fieldhouse, Memphis, TN 38152.

Authors' contributions
DSK, SF, and DRK were responsible for the study design, coordination of the study, and oversight of data collection and analysis. RJB assisted in manuscript preparation. All authors read and approved of the final manuscript.

Competing interests
Financial support for this work was provided by VitaCoco® Company (New York, NY). The investigators have no direct or indirect interest in VitaCoco®. RJB has received research funding or has acted as a consultant to nutraceutical and dietary supplement companies.

References

1. Rodriguez NR, DiMarco NM, Langley S, American Dietetic Association, Dietetians of Canada, American College of Sports Medicine: **Position of the American Dietetic Association, Dietitians of Canada, and the American**

College of Sports Medicine: **Nutrition and athletic performance.** *J Am Diet Assoc* 2009, **109(3)**:509-27.
2. von Duvillard SP, Arciero PJ, Tietjen-Smith T, Alford K: **Sports drinks, exercise training, and competition.** *Curr Sports Med Rep* 2008, **7(4)**:202-8.
3. American College of Sports Medicine, Sawka MN, Burke LM, Eichner ER, Maughan RJ, Montain SJ, Stachenfeld NS: **American College of Sports Medicine position stand. Exercise and fluid replacement.** *Med Sci Sports Exerc* 2007, **39(2)**:377-90.
4. Von Duvillard SP, Braun WA, Markofski M, Beneke R, Leithäuser R: **Fluids and hydration in prolonged endurance performance.** *Nutrition* 2004, **20(7-8)**:651-6.
5. Convertino VA, Armstrong LE, Coyle EF, Mack GW, Sawka MN, Senay LC Jr, Sherman WM: **American College of Sports Medicine position stand. Exercise and fluid replacement.** *Med Sci Sports Exerc* 1996, **28(1)**:i-vii.
6. Rehrer NJ: **Fluid and electrolyte balance in ultra-endurance sport.** *Sports Med* 2001, **31(10)**:701-15.
7. Kreider RB, Wilborn CD, Taylor L, Campbell B, Almada AL, Collins R, Cooke M, Earnest CP, Greenwood M, Kalman DS, Kerksick CM, Kleiner SM, Leutholtz B, Lopez H, Lowery LM, Mendel R, Smith A, Spano M, Wildman R, Willoughby DS, Ziegenfuss TN, Antonio J: **ISSN exercise & sport nutrition review: research & recommendations.** *J Int Soc Sports Nutr* 2010, **7**:7.
8. , http://researchwikis.com/Sports_Drink_Market: Accessed 10/18/11.
9. Chavalittamrong B, Pidatcha P, Thavisri U: **Electrolytes, sugar, calories, osmolarity and pH of beverages and coconut water.** *Southeast Asian J Trop Med Public Health* 1982, **13(3)**:427-31.
10. Kuberski T, Roberts A, Linehan B, Bryden RN, Teburae M: **Coconut water as a rehydration fluid.** *N Z Med J* 1979, **90(641)**:98-100.
11. Chavalittamrong B, Pidatcha P, Thavisri U: **Electrolytes, sugar, calories, osmolarity and pH of beverages and coconut water.** *Southeast Asian J Trop Med Public Health* 1982, **13(3)**:427-31.
12. Adams W, Bratt DE: **Young coconut water for home rehydration in children with mild gastroenteritis.** *Trop Geogr Med* 1992, **44(1-2)**:149-53.
13. Campbell-Falck D, Thomas T, Falck TM, Tutuo N, Clem K: **The intravenous use of coconut water.** *Am J Emerg Med* 2000, **18(1)**:108-11.
14. Mantena SK, Jagadish , Badduri SR, Siripurapu KB, Unnikrishnan MK: **In vitro evaluation of antioxidant properties of Cocos nucifera Linn. water.** *Nahrung* 2003, **47(2)**:126-31.
15. Fisher-Wellman K, Bloomer RJ: **Acute exercise and oxidative stress: a 30 year history.** *Dyn Med* 2009, **8**:1.
16. Saat M, Singh R, Sirisinghe RG, Nawawi M: **Rehydration after exercise with fresh young coconut water, carbohydrate-electrolyte beverage and plain water.** *J Physiol Anthropol Appl Human Sci* 2002, **21(2)**:93-104.
17. Ismail I, Singh R, Sirisinghe RG: **Rehydration with sodium-enriched coconut water after exercise-induced dehydration.** *Southeast Asian J Trop Med Public Health* 2007, **38(4)**:769-85.
18. Idárraga AP, Aragón-Vargas LF: **Post-exercise rehydration with coconut water [abstract].** *Med Sci Sports Exerc* 2010, **42(5)**:575.
19. Moran DS, Heled Margaliot M, Shani Y, Laor A, Margaliot S, Bickes E, Shapiro Y: **Hydration status measurement by radio frequency absorptiometry in young athletes - a new method and preliminary results.** *Physiol Meas* 2004, **25**:51-59.
20. Antonio J, Sanders MS, Ehler LA, Uelmen J, Raether JB, Stout JR: **Effects of exercise training and amino acid supplementation on body composition and physical performance in untrained women.** *Nutrition* 2000, **16**:1043-1046.
21. Cheuvront SN, Ely BR, Kenefick RW, Sawka MN: **Biological variation and diagnostic accuracy of dehydration assessment markers.** *Am J Clin Nutr* 2010, **92(3)**:565-73.
22. Wong SH, Chen Y: **Effect of a carbohydrate-electrolyte beverage, lemon tea, or water on rehydration during short-term recovery from exercise.** *Int J Sport Nutr Exerc Metab* 2011, **21(4)**:300-10.
23. Armstrong LE, Maresh CM, Castellani JW, Bergeron MF, Kenefick RW, LaGasse KE, Riebe D: **Urinary indices of hydration status.** *Int J Sport Nutr* 1994, **4(3)**:265-79.
24. Popowski LA, Oppliger RA, Patrick Lambert G, Johnson RF, Kim Johnson A, Gisolf CV: **Blood and urinary measures of hydration status during progressive acute dehydration.** *Med Sci Sports Exerc* 2001, **33(5)**:747-53.
25. Lopez RM, Casa DJ, Jensen KA, Demartini JK, Pagnotta KD, Ruiz RC, Roti MW, Stearns RL, Armstrong LE, Maresh CM: **Examining the influence of hydration status on physiological responses and running speed during trail running in the heat with controlled exercise intensity.** *J Strength Cond Res* 2011, **25(11)**:2944-54.
26. Spaccarotella KJ, Andzel WD: **Building a beverage for recovery from endurance activity: a review.** *J Strength Cond Res* 2011, **25(11)**:3198-204.

International Society of Sports Nutrition position stand: energy drinks

Bill Campbell[1†], Colin Wilborn[2†], Paul La Bounty[3], Lem Taylor[2†], Mike T Nelson[4], Mike Greenwood[5†], Tim N Ziegenfuss[6], Hector L Lopez[6], Jay R Hoffman[7], Jeffrey R Stout[7], Stephen Schmitz[8†], Rick Collins[9†], Doug S Kalman[10], Jose Antonio[11†] and Richard B Kreider[5*]

Abstract

Position Statement: The International Society of Sports Nutrition (ISSN) bases the following position stand on a critical analysis of the literature on the safety and efficacy of the use of energy drinks (ED) or energy shots (ES). The ISSN has concluded the following. 1. Although ED and ES contain a number of nutrients that are purported to affect mental and/or physical performance, the primary ergogenic nutrients in most ED and ES appear to be carbohydrate and/or caffeine. 2. The ergogenic value of caffeine on mental and physical performance has been well-established but the potential additive benefits of other nutrients contained in ED and ES remains to be determined. 3. Consuming ED 10-60 minutes before exercise can improve mental focus, alertness, anaerobic performance, and/or endurance performance. 4. Many ED and ES contain numerous ingredients; these products in particular merit further study to demonstrate their safety and potential effects on physical and mental performance. 5. There is some limited evidence that consumption of low-calorie ED during training and/or weight loss trials may provide ergogenic benefit and/or promote a small amount of additional fat loss. However, ingestion of higher calorie ED may promote weight gain if the energy intake from consumption of ED is not carefully considered as part of the total daily energy intake. 6. Athletes should consider the impact of ingesting high glycemic load carbohydrates on metabolic health, blood glucose and insulin levels, as well as the effects of caffeine and other stimulants on motor skill performance. 7. Children and adolescents should only consider use of ED or ES with parental approval after consideration of the amount of carbohydrate, caffeine, and other nutrients contained in the ED or ES and a thorough understanding of the potential side effects. 8. Indiscriminant use of ED or ES, especially if more than one serving per day is consumed, may lead to adverse events and harmful side effects. 9. Diabetics and individuals with pre-existing cardiovascular, metabolic, hepatorenal, and neurologic disease who are taking medications that may be affected by high glycemic load foods, caffeine, and/or other stimulants should avoid use of ED and/or ES unless approved by their physician.

Introduction

According to published research, energy drinks (ED) are the most popular dietary supplement besides multivitamins in the American adolescent and young adult population [1-3]. ED are also reported to be the most popular supplement among British athletes [4]. More recently, energy shots (ES) have also been purported to possess ergogenic value on mental focus and/or performance [5]. It is important to make a distinction between ED, ES, and sports drinks. Sports drinks are a unique category within the beverage industry and are marketed to consumers with the primary function of promoting hydration, replacing electrolytes and sustaining endurance performance capacity. They typically provide a small amount of carbohydrate (e.g., 6-8 grams/100 ml) and electrolytes (sodium, potassium, calcium, magnesium). ED, on the other hand, typically contain higher amounts of carbohydrate along with nutrients purported to improve perceptions of attention and/or mental alertness. Low calorie ED are also marketed to increase mental alertness, energy metabolism, and performance. Energy shots are typically 2-4 oz. servings of concentrated fluid

* Correspondence: rkreider@hlkn.tamu.edu
†Equal contributors
[5]Exercise & Sport Nutrition Lab, Department of Health & Kinesiology, Texas A&M University, College Station, Texas, TX 77843-4243, USA
Full list of author information is available at the end of the article

containing various purported ergogens. Since ED and ES contain carbohydrate, caffeine, and/or nutrients that may affect mental focus and concentration, they have the potential to affect exercise capacity and perceptions of energy and/or fatigue. The purpose of this position stand is to critically evaluate the scientific literature and make recommendations in regards to the role that ED and/or ES may have on exercise performance and energy expenditure/metabolism. Additionally, we will discuss safety considerations in regards to the use of ED and/or ES.

Methods

This analysis represents a systematic review of the literature on the effects of "energy drinks" on exercise and cognitive performance as well as primary ingredients contained in popular energy drinks. A comprehensive literature search was performed by searching the Medline database of the US National Library of Medicine of the National Institutes of Health. The search strategy involved entering "energy drinks" and commercial names of energy drinks and/or caffeinated beverages as well as a search of primary nutrients contained in popular energy drinks (e.g., caffeine, carbohydrate, taurine, glucoronolactone, Guarana, Yerba Mate, etc.). It is important to note, from a United States regulatory perspective, several of these ED are marketed as dietary supplements and not beverages, and the label on the product will indicate which category of Food and Drug Administration (FDA) authority the product falls under. Each category has its own set of governing laws and regulations. For example, depending on the category, the labels will include Supplement Facts (dietary supplements) or Nutrition Facts (beverages). A paper summarizing the literature related to ED was presented at the 2011 International Society of Sports Nutrition Annual meeting. Thereafter, a position stand writing team was organized to develop this paper. Drafts of this position stand were then reviewed by all authors as well as the Research Committee of the International Society of Sports Nutrition (ISSN). The final version of this paper was then adopted as the official position of the ISSN.

Ergogenic/performance considerations

The ingestion of nutrients prior to, during, and/or following exercise can affect exercise performance and/or training adaptations [6]. ED typically contain water, carbohydrates (e.g., glucose, maltodextrin), vitamins, minerals, and "proprietary blends" of various nutrients purported to increase energy, alertness, metabolism, and/or performance (e.g., caffeine, taurine, amino acids, glucoronolactone, Guarana, Ginkgo biloba, Carnitine, Panax ginseng, Green Tea, Yerba Mate, etc.). Therefore, ingestion of ED or ES prior to, during, and/or following exercise could have some ergogenic value. Tables 1 and 2 present a list of ingredients found in several ED/ES marketed in the United States. The next section provides an overview of the potential ergogenic value of some of the most commonly found nutrients in ED/ES.

Caffeine

Caffeine is the most common ingredient utilized in energy drinks. Caffeine is extracted from the raw fruit of over sixty species of coffee plants (*coffea Arabica*), all part of the methylxanthine family. Caffeine is also extracted from tea, kola nuts, and cocoa. After ingestion, caffeine is quickly absorbed and increases in plasma concentrations are generally observed between 30 – 60 minutes following ingestion [7]. The difference in absorption time is dependent on the physicochemical formulation properties of the product dose [8]. Caffeine is a strong cardiovascular stimulant that increases epinephrine output to a greater extent when ingested via its anhydrous formulation when compared to an equal amount of brewed or instant caffeinated coffee [9,10]. In addition, caffeine's half-life ranges from approximately 2 to 10 hours with 0.5% - 3.5% of its content excreted unchanged in urine and select amounts eliminated via perspiration [11]. A recent position stand from the Journal of the International Society of Sports Nutrition [7] summarized the effects of caffeine on exercise performance as follows:

1. Caffeine is effective for enhancing sport performance in trained athletes when consumed in low-to-moderate dosages (~3-6 $mg{\cdot}kgBM^{-1}$) and overall does not result in further enhancement in performance when consumed in higher dosages (≥ 9 $mg{\cdot}kgBM^{-1}$).
2. Caffeine exerts a greater ergogenic effect when consumed in an anhydrous state as compared to coffee.
3. It has been shown that caffeine can enhance vigilance during bouts of extended exhaustive exercise, as well as periods of sustained sleep deprivation.
4. Caffeine is ergogenic for sustained maximal endurance exercise, and has been shown to be highly effective for time-trial performance.
5. Caffeine supplementation is beneficial for high-intensity exercise, including team sports such as soccer and rugby, both of which are categorized by intermittent activity within a period of prolonged duration.
6. The literature is equivocal when considering the effects of caffeine supplementation on strength-power performance, and additional research in this area is warranted.
7. The scientific literature does not support caffeine-induced diuresis during exercise, or any harmful change in fluid balance that would negatively affect performance.

Table 1 List of ingredients described on nutrient panels found in some energy drinks

Ingredient	A	B	C	D	E
Calories	100	110	140	120	140
Carbohydrate	27	28	31	32	30
Calories from Fat	-	-	-	-	
Vitamin C	-	100 mg	-	100 mg	6.7mg
Thiamin	-	0.1 mg	-	-	0.2 mg
Riboflavin B2	1.7 mg	1.5 mg	3.4 mg	20%	0.2 mg
Niacin B3	20 mg	21.7 mg	20 mg	10%	2.2 mg
Vitamin B6	40 mg	2.1 mg	2 mg	10%	1.5 mg
Vitamin B12	6 mcg	4.5 mcg	6 mcg	10%	4.7 mcg
Pantothenic Acid	-	36 mg	-	10%	1.1 mg
Sodium	180 mg	200 mg	40 mg	75 mg	190 mg
Potassium	-	10 mg	10 mg	-	65 mg
Phosphorus	-	-	-	40 mg	90 mg
Taurine	1,000 mg	600 mg	1000 mg	-	-
Panax Ginseng	200 mg	-	25	-	-
Proprietary Blend	2,500 mg L-Carnitine, Glucose, Caffeine, Guarana, Inositol, Glucuronolactone, Maltodextrin	Caffeine (77 mg)	325 mg Ginko Biloba (150 mg), Caffeine (80 mg), Guarana (25 mg), Inositol (25 mg), L-Carnitine (25 mg), Milk Thistle (20 mg)	Guarana, maltodextrin, caffeine, taurine, panax ginseng, calcium	Citrulline Malate, L-Glutamine, L-Arginine, Quercetin, L-Leucine, L-Valine,

Table 2 List of ingredients described on nutrient panels found in some energy shots

Ingredient	A	B	C	D	E
Calories	4	4	20	9	0
Carbohydrate	-	-	4 g	1 g	0
Calories from Fat		-	-	-	
Vitamin C	-	100 mg	-	-	126%
Niacin	30 mg	33 mg	33 mg	-	
Vitamin B6	40 mg	40 mg	40 mg	-	
Folic Acid	400 mcg	400 mcg	400 mcg	-	
Vitamin B12	500 mcg	500 mcg	500 mcg	-	
Sodium	18 mg	0 mg	0 mg	-	10
Potassium	-	10 mg	10 mg	-	26
Proprietary	1,870 mg	2,300 mg	2,200 mg	910 mg	527 mg
Blend	Taurine, Glucuronolactone, Malic Acid, N-Acetyl L-Tyrosine, L-Phenylalanine, Caffeine, Citicoline	Glucouronolactone (425 mg), N-Acetyl L-Tyrosine (400 mg), L-Phenylalanine (375 mg), Taurine (350 mg), Malic Acid 300 mg), Caffeine (200 mg), Green Tea Extract (150 mg), Ginseng Extract (150 mg)	Glucouronolactone (420 mg), L-Phenylalanine (380 mg), D-Ribose (350 mg), N-Acetyl L-Tyrosine (325 mg), Malic Acid (300 mg), Caffeine (175 mg), Green Tea Extract (150 mg), Ginseng Extract (100 mg)	Caffeine Citrate, Caffeine Anhydrous, Evoburn, Octapomine, Gugulsterone E & Z, Yerbe Mate, Green Tea, Synephrine, cAMP, Vinpocetine, Yohimbe HCL	Beta-Alanine, Vitamin C, Caffeine Anhydrous (158 mg), Evoburn, N-Acetyl-L-Tyrosine, Hordinine, 5-Hydroxy-L-Trypotophan (5-HTP), Potassium, N-methyl Tyramine, Sulbutlamine, Vinpocetine, Yohimbine HCl, St. John's Wort Extract

As demonstrated below, several studies have reported significant improvements in both aerobic and resistance exercise with a relative dosage of approximately 2 $mg{\cdot}kgBM^{-1}$of caffeine. This is less than the amount recommended (3-6 $mg{\cdot}kgBM^{-1}$) to enhance performance [7], and may contribute to the hypothesis that the synergistic effects of the various ingredients contained in ED/ES are responsible for the reported improvements in exercise performance.

Carbohydrate

Another common ingredient in most ED is some type of carbohydrate source (e.g., glucose, sucrose, maltodextrin, etc.). Energy drinks also typically contain glucuronolactone, an ingredient which is involved in ascorbic acid synthesis and is metabolized into xylulose [12]. Evidence from numerous studies indicates that carbohydrate feeding during exercise of about 45 minutes or longer can improve endurance capacity and performance [13,14]. Mechanisms by which carbohydrate feeding prior to and during exercise improves endurance performance include maintaining blood glucose levels, maintaining high levels of carbohydrate oxidation, and the sparing of liver and possibly skeletal muscle glycogen [15]. Peak rates of carbohydrate oxidation are commonly around 1 g of carbohydrate per minute or 60 $g{\cdot}hr^{-1}$. Glucose, sucrose, maltodextrins and amylopectin are oxidized at high rates, while fructose, galactose and amylose are oxidized at lower rates (approximately 25-50% lower) [16]. Consequently, sports drinks typically contain a mixture of various types of carbohydrates designed to optimize exogenous carbohydrate oxidation [17].

ED's contain approximately 25-30 grams of carbohydrate per 240 mL (8 fluid ounces) serving. This amount nearly meets the lower value of 30 grams/hour recommended during endurance exercise, but falls short of the upper range of 60 $g{\cdot}hr^{-1}$. In order to meet this upper level of 60 grams of carbohydrate per hour during endurance exercise, approximately 530 mL (18 fluid ounces) of a typical ED per hour would need to be consumed. While the total carbohydrate content of typical ED is quite high, a shortcoming exists in regards to the concentration of commercially available energy drinks. The American College of Sports Medicine [18] and the ISSN [6,17] recommend ingesting carbohydrate in a 6-8% solution (6-8 grams per 100 ml of fluid) during endurance exercise. A typical ED provides carbohydrates at a greater concentration, typically around an 11-12% solution. Ingesting higher percentages (>10%) of carbohydrate in fluids has been reported to delay gastric emptying and increase gastrointestinal distress [19,20]. Consequently, athletes who want to use ED as sports drinks may need to dilute the beverage and/or alternate consumption of ED and water during exercise.

Other nutrients

Tables 3, 4, and 5 present a list of additional nutrients commonly found in ED or ES. Most ED and ES also contain a small amount of vitamins (e.g., thiamin, riboflavin, niacin, Vitamin B6, Vitamin B12, pantothenic acid, Vitamin C) and electrolytes (e.g., sodium, potassium, phosphorus, etc.). While the addition of these nutrients may add to the nutrient density of these products, there is little evidence that ingestion of these vitamins and minerals in the amounts found in ED and ES would provide any ergogenic benefit during exercise performance in well-nourished individuals [17,18]. Additionally, ED and ES typically contain nutrients purported to promote cognition and mental focus (e.g., Taurine, Ginkgo biloba, L-Tyrosine, Citocoline, 5-Hydroxy-L-Tryptophan [5-HTP], St. John's Wort, etc.), stimulants (e.g., caffeine, Guarana, Green Tea, Synephrine, Yerba mate, Yohimbine, Tyramine, Vinpocetine, etc.), and/or various purported ergogenic nutrients (e.g., Panax Ginseng, L-Carnitine, D-Ribose, β-Alanine, Inositol, Citrulline, Quercetin, etc.). While there are data to support the potential ergogenic value of some of these nutrients on cognitive function and/or exercise capacity [17,18]; the amounts found in ED and ES are generally much lower than the typical concentrations associated with an ergogenic effect. Consequently, it is unclear whether adding these nutrients to ED and/or ES provides a synergistic or additive effect to the carbohydrate and caffeine found in these products. In addition, adding these nutrients to the caffeine found in ED and/or ES may change the adverse effect profile of these finished products, and warrant further study.

Exercise performance

Several studies have investigated the effects of ED consumption prior to exercise. The types of exercise that were evaluated include resistance exercise [167,168], anaerobic exercise [169], and aerobic/endurance exercise [62,170-172].

Ingestion prior to anaerobic exercise

Many of the studies investigating the effects of ED ingestion on anaerobic performance measures have been conducted within the past several years. In a crossover study (separated by seven days), Forbes and colleagues [168] gave 15 physically active college-aged students a commercially available energy drink standardized with 2 $mg{\cdot}kgBM^{-1}$of caffeine or an isoenergetic, isovolumetric, non-caffeinated placebo 60-minutes prior to exercise. The exercise consisted of three sets of 70% one repetition maximum (1RM) bench press conducted to failure on each set with one minute of rest between each set. Following the resistance exercise bout, three x 30-second Wingate Anaerobic Capacity tests were also conducted with two minutes of rest between each test. The ED

Table 3 Potential ergogenic nutrients contained in energy drinks that may affect cognition and/or mental performance

Ingredient	Potential ergogenic value	Scientific support
Taurine	Improved mental focus, concentration, serve as antioxidant, glucose homeostasis [21-24]	Some supportive evidence with ED and fed animals [25-35]
Gingko Biloba	Improve memory and mental concentration	Some supportive evidence on memory (e.g., 120 mg/d) [36-39]. No known effects at dosages found in ED or ES.
L-Tyrosine	Prevents depletion of catecholamines, may ameliorate declines in cognition with acute stress [40-47]	Some supportive evidence on cognition (e.g., 2 g/d, 150 mg acute ingestion with cold exposure) [41,43,46,48,49]. No effects on performance capacity [42,50]. No known effects at dosages found in ED or ES.
Citicoline	Intermediate in the generation of phosphatidylcholine from choline. Increase dopamine receptor densities and delay memory impairment [51,52].	Some supportive evidence with large doses (8.5 g prior to and during exercise) and in fed animals [52]. No known effects at dosages found in ED or ES.
5-Hydroxy-L-Trypotophan (5-HTP)	Precursor to serotonin [53,54]. Purported antidepressant, appetite suppressant, & sleep aid [53,55-58].	Some evidence in treatment of depression [53,55-58] and 5-HT fed animals on muscle performance [54,59,60]. Role on exercise performance at dosages found in ED and ES is unknown.
St. John's Wort	Anti-depressant [56-58].	Some supportive evidence [56-58]. No known effects at dosages found in ED or ES.

significantly increased total bench press repetitions over three sets (approximately 6% more repetitions completed) but had no effect on Wingate peak or average power.

In a similarly designed study, a commercially available energy drink (providing an average of 2.1 mg of caffeine per kg of body mass) given to physically active male and female participants 45 minutes prior to exercise resulted in a significant increase in leg press total lifting volume (12% increase as compared to a carbohydrate placebo) but had no effect on bench press total lifting volume [167] or multiple 20-second Wingate-type cycle sprints [173]. Hoffman and colleagues [169] gave male strength/power athletes an ED containing an average of 1.8 $mg \cdot kgBM^{-1}$of caffeine or a placebo beverage that was similar in taste and appearance but contained only inert substances. Following the ingestion of the ED, three separate 20-second Wingate tests separated by about 15 minutes were performed. Results revealed that there were no significant differences between trials in any anaerobic power measure. In a recent publication, 12 healthy male and female non-resistance trained participants ingested a commercially available ED standardized at either 1 or 3 $mg \cdot kgBM^{-1}$of caffeine or a placebo beverage (containing no caffeine) in a randomized, repeated measures design [65]. Sixty minutes following beverage ingestion, each participant completed 10-to-100% 1RM

Table 4 Potential stimulants contained in energy drinks that may affect performance capacity

Ingredient	Potential ergogenic value	Scientific support
Caffeine	Stimulant. Increases metabolism and lipolysis [2,8,9,61].	Increases alertness, mood, cognitive function [2,8,9,61]. Increases fat oxidation, spares glycogen utilization, improves exercise [7,9-11,62-65].
Guarana	Natural source of caffeine. Similar properties to caffeine.	Similar to caffeine effects.
Green Tea Extract	Contains high amounts of caffeine and catechin polyphenols (e.g., epigallocatechin gallate or EGCG). Serves as antioxidant. Similar effects as caffeine [66,67]	Some supportive evidence of increased metabolism [68-76]. Specific role at dosages found in ED is unknown.
Synephrine	Alternative to ephedrine. Naturally derived from *Citrus aurantium*. Stimulant with less cardiovascular effects than ephedrine. Purported to increase metabolism and promote weight loss.	Evidence of a mild stimulant effect on metabolism and weight loss [77-82]. No known effects at dosages found in ED.
Yerba mate	Contains three xanthines (caffeine, theobromine, and theophylline). Similar properties to caffeine	Similar to caffeine effects. Some supportive evidence [83-85] No known effects at dosages found in ED and ES.
Yohimbine	Alkaloid with stimulant and aphrodisiac properties [86-90].	Similar to caffeine effects. Effects at dosages found in ED are unknown.
Tyramine	Naturally-occurring monoamine derived from tyrosine. Acts as a catecholamine (dopamine, NE, Epi) releasing agent. Degraded to octopine. Increases blood pressure and can serve as neurotransmitter [91-93].	Mild cardiovascular stimulant. Effects at dosages found in ED / ES are unknown.
Vinpocetine	Alkaloid of vincamine extracted from periwinkle plant (Vinca) minor. Vasodilatory and memory enhancing properties [94,95].	No known effects at dosages found in ED or ES.

Table 5 Other potential ergogenic nutrients contained in energy drinks that may affect performance

Ingredient	Potential ergogenic value	Scientific support
Panax Ginseng	Contains ginsenosides which are purported to have anti-inflammatory, antioxidant, and anticancer effects. Purported to enhance perceptions of energy, increase stamina and improve nitrogen balance [96].	Most well-controlled research does not support the ergogenic effects for ginseng [97-111]. No known effects at dosages found in ED and ES.
L-Carnitine	Involved in shuttling long chain fatty acids into mitochondria. Purported to promote lipolysis [112].	Limited supportive ergogenic value in athletes or on weight loss [112]. No known effects at dosages found in ED and ES.
D-Ribose	Involved in ATP synthesis. Theoretically, D-ribose supplementation can increase ATP availability.	Some evidence of improved exercise capacity in clinical populations [113] but limited evidence that high dose ribose supplementation affects exercise capacity [114-119]. No known effects at dosages found in ED and ES.
Beta Alanine	Increases muscle carnosine levels, increases muscle buffering, and attenuates fatigue during high intensity exercise [120-124].	Growing scientific evidence of improved anaerobic capacity (2-4 g/d) [125-138]. No known effects at dosages found in ED and ES.
Inositol	Carbohydrate that is not classified as sugar. Involved in insulin signaling, nerve transmission, serotonin modulation, and fat oxidation [139].	No known effects at dosages found in ED or ES.
Citrulline Malate	Optimizes blood flow via arginine-nitric oxide pathway; purported to reduce fatigue and buffer acidity during exercise [140,141].	Some evidence that high dosages (e.g., 6 – 8 g) can affect exercise capacity and/or anabolism [142-149]. No known effects at dosages found in ED and ES.
Quercetin	Reported to have antioxidant, anti-inflammatory, antiviral, and immune-modulatory effects [150].	Several studies indicate that Quercetin supplementation (e.g., 1 g/d for 7 d) increases maximal aerobic capacity and time to fatigue [151-166]. No known effects at dosages found in ED or ES.

power-load tests for the bench press and half-squat. Ingestion of the ED with 1 mg·kgBM^{-1}of caffeine was not enough to raise the power output during the power-load tests. However, the ingestion of an ED with 3 mg·kgBM^{-1}of caffeine increased maximal power output by 7% in both the half-squat and bench-press as compared to the ingestion of a placebo [65]. A recent study by Gonzalez and colleagues [174] indicated that an energy matrix consisting of caffeine, taurine and glucoronolactone consumed 10-min prior to a workout resulted in an 11.9% improvement ($p < 0.05$) in the number of repetitions performed during 4 sets of the squat or bench press exercise using 80% of the subject's 1-RM. In addition, the average power output for the workout was significantly higher for subjects consuming the energy drink compared to subjects consuming the placebo.

In addition to resistance and high intensity anaerobic exercise, the effects that ED exert on speed/agility performance has also been investigated. Collegiate female soccer players ingested an ED containing 1.3 mg·kgBM^{-1}of caffeine and 1 gram of taurine or a caffeine and taurine-free placebo 60 minutes prior to repeated agility t-tests [175]. No difference in agility *t*-test performance between the ED and placebo groups was reported. Specifically, the highest difference reported between the two groups was during the third set of eight agility t-tests, and the difference reached only 1.15% between the groups. It is unlikely that the carbohydrate content alone in ED is responsible for improvements in resistance exercise performance. In support of this view, the majority of studies in which supplemental carbohydrate was ingested prior to a resistance-training bout did not report improvements in resistance training performance [176-178].

Conclusion

ED (containing approximately 2 mg·kgBM^{-1}caffeine) consumed 45 to 60 minutes prior to anaerobic/resistance exercise may improve upper- and lower- body total lifting volume, but has no effect on repeated high intensity sprint exercise, or on agility performance.

Ingestion prior to endurance exercise

Several studies have investigated the effects of ED ingestion prior to aerobic exercise [62,170-172,179]. In the earliest of these studies, Alford and colleagues [172] investigated the effects of ingesting a commercial ED on aerobic endurance. In a repeated measures, crossover design, young healthy participants ingested 250 mL of a commercial ED (containing 80 mg of caffeine and 26 grams of carbohydrate), a carbonated water beverage, or no beverage at all 30 minutes prior to performing an endurance exercise bout. Test days for separate treatments were assessed within a week. Aerobic performance was analyzed by the amount of time that exercise could be maintained at 65-75% of maximum heart rate on a cycle ergometer. Significant improvements in aerobic performance were reported for the commercial ED treatment. Aerobic performance was 8% and 14% longer after ingesting the commercial ED as compared to the carbonated water and no beverage treatment, respectively.

In one of only two studies that have investigated the effects of ingesting a sugar/carbohydrate-free ED on performance capacity, Candow and colleagues [170] reported no improvements in high intensity run time-to-exhaustion performed at 80% of VO_2max on a treadmill in physically active college-aged participants. The sugar-free ED contained 2 mg·kgBM^{-1}caffeine and was ingested one-hour prior to the exercise bout [170]. In contrast, Walsh and colleagues [179] reported significant improvements in treadmill run time to exhaustion following ingestion of a carbohydrate-free ED. In this randomized cross-over investigation, 15 recreationally active participants ingested an ED 10-minutes prior to engaging in a treadmill run-to exhaustion test at 70% VO_2max [179]. The ED utilized in this study did not contain any carbohydrate, and unlike other ED products, contained nearly eight grams of the amino acids L-leucine, L-isoleucine, L-valine, L-arginine and L-glutamine. Unfortunately, the published study did not disclose the precise amount of caffeine contained in the ED, but instead referred to a ~2 g "proprietary blend" of caffeine, taurine, and glucoronolactone. The placebo used as a comparison was sweetened water that was similar in color and volume. It was reported that participants consuming the ED were able to run 12.5% longer than during the placebo treatment [179].

The two most common protocols used to assess aerobic performance are time to exhaustion at a given exercise intensity (e.g., exercise at 70% of maximum oxygen uptake until exhaustion) and time trial performance for a set distance (e.g., 40 km time trial). Time trials have greater validity than time to exhaustion because they provide a good physiological simulation of actual performance and correlate with actual performance [180,181]. Ivy and colleagues [62] were the first research group to utilize a time trial component in conjunction with ED consumption. In this investigation, trained male and female cyclists completed two trials in a repeated measures crossover design separated by one week. After a 12 hour fast, the cyclists ingested a commercially available ED providing approximately 2.3 mg·kgBM^{-1}caffeine or an artificially colored, flavored, and sweetened-water placebo 40-minute prior to the exercise bout. Performance during the exercise bout was measured as the time to complete a standardized amount of work equal to 1 hr of cycling at 70% of maximal power output. Results revealed a significant difference between the treatments in relation to performance with the ED treatment completing the time trial ~4.7% faster than the placebo treatment [62].

Conclusion

ED containing approximately 2 mg·kgBM^{-1}caffeine consumed 10 to 40 minutes prior to aerobic exercise improve cycling and running performance in both trained cyclists and recreationally active participants. In the one investigation in which no aerobic performance improvement was reported, the ED (containing 2 mg·kgBM^{-1}caffeine) was ingested 60-minutes prior to the performance assessment. In light of the other findings, ingestion of the caffeine-containing ED 60-minutes prior to the exercise bout may be too long of a period to realize improvements in aerobic exercise performance.

Mood/reaction time/alertness

Reaction time, concentration, alertness, and subjective feelings of energy/vitality are important in many competitive activities such as hitting a baseball, returning a serve in tennis, and dodging strikes and kicks in a mixed martial arts competition. Strategies to improve these attributes are often sought after by individuals competing in certain athletic endeavors. Over the past several years, research has investigated the effects that ED ingestion has on these (and other) variables.

Seidl and coworkers [31] conducted a study utilizing three common ingredients (i.e., caffeine, taurine, glucuronolactone) typically found in ED and compared it to a placebo group. Participants were evaluated at night to see if ingestion of these nutrients affected mood and motor function in fatigued participants. Interestingly, the investigators found that at the end of the experiment, reaction time was significantly longer in the placebo group, but remained unchanged in the group that consumed the ED ingredients. Similarly, vitality scores, feelings of well-being, and social extrovertedness were all significantly decreased in the placebo group, but did not change in the ED group [31].

Scholey and colleagues [182] investigated the effects of an ED (containing primarily caffeine, glucose, ginseng and ginkgo biloba drink) or a placebo beverage on five aspects of cognitive performance and mood. Thirty minutes after consuming ED, two of the five variables (i.e., "secondary memory" and "speed of attention") were significantly improved as compared to the placebo beverage [182]. Other investigators also reported that when caffeine was combined with carbohydrates in a carbonated beverage, performance and mood were improved and/or maintained during fatiguing and cognitively demanding tasks relative to placebo [183]. Similarly, ED containing caffeine and glucose have also been shown to enhance event related potentials (i.e., a measure of brain activity in real time obtained from an electroencephalogram), which may translate to improvements in reaction time [184].

Hoffman and colleagues [169] reported that when male strength/power athletes consumed 120 ml of a commercially available ED or a placebo, reaction time and subjective feelings of energy and focus were significantly improved in those consuming the ED. Furthermore, the investigators also noted a statistical trend (*p=0.06*) towards an increase in alertness. In a similar study, Walsh and colleagues [179] examined the effects of ingesting an "energy matrix" (2.05 g of caffeine, taurine, glucuronolactone), amino acids (7.9 g of L-leucine, L-isoleucine, L-valine, L-arginine and L-glutamine), di-creatine citrate (5 g), and β-alanine (2.5 g) mixed with 500 ml of water or a placebo) 10-minutes prior to exercise on aerobic performance and subjective measures of focus, energy, and fatigue in recreationally active male and females. Results revealed that participants ingesting the ED increased time to exhaustion while running at 70% of VO_2max by 12.5% ($p = 0.012$), they reported greater focus ($p = 0.031$), energy ($p = 0.016$), and less fatigue ($p = 0.005$) prior to exercise; and, that their ratings of focus ($p = 0.026$) and energy ($p = 0.004$) were greater 10 minutes into exercise [179]. However, no significant differences in energy, fatigue, and focus were observed between groups immediately post-exercise [179].

Howard and coworkers [185] evaluated the effects of acute ingestion of a glucose containing ED on behavioral control. In this study, 80 participants were randomly assigned to consume 1.8, 3.6, or 5.4 ml/kg of an ED, a placebo, or no drink in a counterbalanced manner. Participants completed a behavioral control task and subjective measures of stimulation, sedation, and mental fatigue before and 30-minutes after ingestion of the assigned drinks. Results revealed that those consuming the ED decreased reaction times on the behavioral control task, increased subjective ratings of stimulation and decreased ratings of mental fatigue. The greatest improvements in reaction times and subjective measures were observed with the lower dose and improvements diminished as the dose increased. Earlier research conducted by Alford and associates [172] supported these findings by demonstrating that individuals ingesting 250 ml of this same ED had significantly better reaction time, concentration, memory, and subjective alertness compared to a placebo. Smit and coworkers [183] suggested that caffeine is most likely the primary ingredient that improves mood and performance during fatiguing and cognitively demanding tasks, with carbohydrates playing a minor role. However, caffeine and carbohydrate may act in a synergistic manner [182]. To support this view, a recent paper by Pettitt et al [186] reported that while ingestion of an ED prior to exercise affected aerobic metabolism during and following cycling exercise, the secondary ingredients found in the ED had no additive effects.

Conclusion

To date, most studies on ED have reported improvements in mood, reaction time, and/or markers of alertness, even though the relative importance of the various ingredients is not fully understood. The primary ergogenic value appears to be due to the caffeine and/or carbohydrate contained in these drinks. Individuals looking to enhance reaction time, mental alertness, and/or focus may benefit from consuming an ED prior to exercise.

Energy drinks and their role in energy expenditure and weight loss

As shown in Table 4, ED and some commercial beverages designed to increase metabolism typically contain a number of stimulants (e.g., caffeine, Guarana, Green Tea, synephrine, Yerba mate, Yohimbine, Tyramine, Vinocetine, etc.). Several low-calorie ED and beverages have been marketed as "thermogenic blends" with a focus on increasing metabolism. Theoretically, ingestion of ED prior to exercise may increase energy expenditure which over time could help manage and/or promote weight loss. In support of this theory, studies have shown that ingestion of caffeine (e.g., 200-500 mg) can increase acute (1-24 hours) energy expenditure [187-193], chronic (28 days) energy expenditure [194], and elevate plasma free-fatty acid and glycerol levels [187,194,195]. Collectively, these findings suggest that the stimulant properties of caffeine contained in ED can elevate an individual's metabolic rate as well as elevate the rate of lipolysis in the body. However, these studies used various types of caffeine/stimulant/vitamin-enriched coffee [189-193], a caffeine/stimulant blend supplement [187,189,193], and various calorie-free thermogenic ED [190,194-197]. Additionally, the dosage of caffeine used in some of these beverages that are marketed as a thermogenic supplements is typically higher (e.g., 200-500 mg) than the concentrations found in ED and ES marketed for increasing athletic performance or alertness (i.e., about 80 – 200 mg). With this said, there is some data that indicates that acute ingestion of ED has been shown to enhance energy expenditure, metabolic rate, catecholamine secretion, and/or lipolysis [187,198]

In terms of weight loss, Roberts and colleagues [194] reported that 28 days of consumption of a calorie free ED (336 ml/day) promoted small (i.e., 18.9 ± 1.5 to 18.3 ± 1.5 kg) but statistically significant ($p<0.05$) reductions in fat mass compared to controls (i.e., 18.1 ± 1.3 to 18.4 3± 1.2 kg). Similarly, Stout and associates [199] evaluated the effects of consuming an ED or placebo 15-minutes prior to exercise training and ad-libitum on non-training days for 10-weeks on changes in body composition and fitness. Results revealed that those consuming the ED experienced greater changes in fat mass (-6.6% vs. -0.35%, $p<0.05$), peak aerobic capacity (+13.8% vs. 5.4%, $p<0.01$), and treadmill time to exhaustion (+19.7% vs. 14.0%, $p<0.01$). These findings suggest that consumption of ED during training and/or weight loss may provide some additive ergogenic benefits. However, it should be noted that recent review on ED by Higgins and associates [200] found that many of the commonly used additional ingredients (e.g., Ma Huang, willow bark, synephrine, calcium, cayenne/black pepper extracts) that are contained in the "thermogenic blends" of several of these products are not contained in some of the most commonly used ED. It is also important to note that daily consumption of high calorie ED could promote weight gain. Consequently, additional research is necessary to determine whether ingesting low-calorie ED or ES may affect training adaptations and/or weight loss.

Conclusion

Consumption of low calorie ED and thermogenic beverages have been reported to increase resting energy expenditure and fat metabolism on an acute basis. Preliminary studies suggest that ingesting some types of ED and thermogenic beverages prior to exercise during training could promote positive adaptations in body composition. However, more research is needed to determine whether daily use of ED would affect long-term energy balance and body composition.

Safety considerations

ED have had a negative connotation in the media and more recently medical community, mostly related to potential concerns about excessive caffeine intake [201,202] and/or potential deleterious effects of mixing ED with alcohol [203]. While safety concerns and use of alcohol go beyond the scope of this paper, the reader is referred to a recent viewpoint published in the Journal of the American Medical Association related to safety concerns of mixing ED with alcohol [203]. In terms of use of ED in the traditional sense, most concerns have been based on case studies or adverse event reports that have serve only to document a potential association, but does not establish causality. In reality, there are currently only a few studies (acute or long term) that have investigated the side effects of ED [204-209]. There appear to be two primary active nutrients in most ED and ES (i.e., carbohydrate and caffeine) that may possess safety concerns in some populations. Many ED contain 25 – 50 g of simple sugars, therefore, ingestion of ED prior to exercise are likely to rapidly increase insulin in order to maintain normal blood glucose levels. For this reason, diabetics and pre-diabetics should avoid high glycemic load ED or consider consuming low carbohydrate versions of ED [201,202].

Very often, ED also contain various stimulants with the most common being caffeine. Some concern has been raised about excessive caffeine intake that could be obtained from consuming too many ED and/or from a lack of knowledge that that some ingredients contained in ED may contain caffeine [201,202]. Currently in the United States, the FDA has regulated the limit of caffeine in soft drinks to 0.02 percent (10mg/oz.) of the product, but this is not currently enforced for ED or ES. As of December 2012, the US-FDA along with the US Congress has begun to study products marketed as ED or ES, however no formal new guidelines have been published. The Nutrition Facts Panel on food labels are not required to always list caffeine since it is not a nutrient. However, if caffeine is added to a food, it must then be listed [210]; therefore many individuals may consume more caffeine than they realize [201,202]. In Canada, caffeine levels are limited to 180 mg per drink [211]. The caffeine content of common ED and ES has been reported to range from about 100 to 286 mg [202]. As a comparison, the average cup of coffee or contains between 40 and 150 mg caffeine, while a 20 oz. cup of Starbucks regular drip coffee has been found to contain as much as 480 mg of caffeine [212].

The potential side effects of caffeine include: insomnia, nervousness, restlessness, gastric irritation, nausea, vomiting, tachycardia, tremors, and anxiety; which have been reported at doses as low as 250 to 300 mg [5,201-204,209]. Caffeine availability is ubiquitous and it is one of the most extensively studied substances in the food supply with a long history as generally regarded as safe when consumed in moderation [61]. However, all substances may be toxic under the right conditions, with toxicity being a function of the interaction of many physiologic variables that include the following: acute and chronic dosing, route of administration, genetics, age, sex, environment, and intrinsic health of the individual being exposed. Young adults have been found to have subclinical coronary atherosclerosis [213]. In addition, post-mortem assessment of sudden cardiac death in young persons (<35 years) reveals a variety of anatomic abnormalities of the coronary arteries, myocardium, valves and the conduction system [214]. Such unknown pre-existing risk factors may increase the risk of adverse events, particularly cardiovascular ones, in individuals consuming EDs, due to underlying disease. In fact, even water can be toxic given certain conditions with an LD_{50} (lethal acute dose for 50 percent in test species) of greater than 90 mL/kg in rats [215]. It is possible to overdose on caffeine and there are a handful of case reports in the literature [5,209,216-218]. A lethal dose of caffeine has been typically in excess of 5 g [217], which equates to about 42 cups of coffee at 120 mg of caffeine per cup. Sepkowitz [201] recently suggested that an intake of 3 grams of caffeine (equivalent to ingesting 12 or so highly caffeinated ED within a few hours) could elicit significant adverse effects. The average caffeine per serving in most ED and ES range between 75 and 200 mg, an amount similar to the caffeine found in a premium cup of coffee [202].

Nawrot and colleagues [219] stated that in a healthy adult population, up to 400 mg of caffeine daily was not associated with any adverse effects. In another review, Higdon et al. [220] presented data in children stating no adverse effects were seen with doses under 3 $mg{\cdot}kgBM^{-1}{\cdot}day^{-1}$. As with most drugs, the exact amount of caffeine where side effects will occur varies from person to person based on genetics, age, liver cytochrome P450-CYP1A2 isozyme function, concurrent medications or substances that may affect hepatic metabolism, body mass, and sensitivity. Additionally, it is unknown whether inclusion of other stimulants in ED and/or ES may increase or decrease the threshold for experiencing side effects. For this reason, some groups do not recommend ED or ES for athletes participating in exercise lasting less than 1 hour [200], despite the admission of inadequate long-term data. The longest duration studies on ED or ES we were able to find was 10 weeks and these studies did not report any change in clinical safety markers [199,206]. Nevertheless, since ED and ES often contain other stimulants that can have a synergistic effect with caffeine, more research is needed to determine the long-term effects of habitual intake of ED and ES before definitive conclusions can be drawn.

Several reports have expressed concern about the safety of ED [5,200,205,221]. For example, Worthley and associates [222] tested 50 young male and female adults one hour before and one hour after consuming 250 ml of a sugar-free ED containing approximately 80 mg of caffeine. The investigators found that mean arterial pressure increased by approximately 3.8 mmHg while resting heart rate was not affected. Additionally, platelet aggregation increased by 13.7% compared to only a 0.3% change in the control group while endothelial function decreased. The researchers noted that the component of the ED that was associated with these results was not clear. However, they suggested that since endothelial dysfunction and impaired platelet function are associated with elevated glucose levels, it is possible that glucuronolactone contained in the ED might have contributed to the observed detrimental effects of energy drinks [222]. More research is needed to corroborate these findings as well as to determine whether these acute changes would pose any long-term health risk.

Bichler and cohorts [26] investigated a combination of caffeine and taurine (two common ingredients in ED) in a double-blind study of college students. Subjects consumed either caffeine and taurine pills or a placebo and then completed a memory assessment while heart rate and blood pressure were monitored. The combination caused a significant **decline** in heart rate and an increase in mean arterial blood pressure. Steinke et al. [223] studied 15 healthy adults who abstained from caffeine for 48 hours prior to and during the study in addition to being fasted overnight. Baseline measurements of blood pressure and heart rate were measured. On day one of the study, each participant consumed 500 mL (2 cans) of an ED and measurements were repeated 30 minutes, 1 hour, 2 hours, 3 hours, and 4 hours later. Participants also drank 500 mL of the ED drink daily for the next 5 days. The experiment was then repeated after 7-days. The investigators found that maximum mean heart rate occurred at 4 hours with significant increases of 7.8% and 11.0% on days 1 and 7, respectively. Blood pressures were increased approximately 7% after acute ingestion of the ED on day 1 (significant increase) but no differences were seen on day 7. Finally, in a case report, Usman and coworkers [221] reported that a young boy presented with palpitations and high blood pressure after consumption of an ED containing carbohydrate (40 g), sodium citrate, taurine (124 mg), caffeine, inositol (17 mg), Panax ginseng (6.98 mg), and other nutrients. The tachycardia and hypertension returned to normal after discontinuation of ED consumption.

Conclusion

Individuals with certain medical conditions (e.g., metabolic syndrome or diabetes mellitus) should avoid consumption of high glycemic drinks and/or foods and therefore should not consume the high calorie versions of ED. It would be prudent for individuals with known cardiovascular disease to avoid altogether their use of ED and/or ES, or other products with known cardiostimulant effects. While ED containing caffeine and other stimulants may have negative effects upon health and cardiac parameters in individuals with such pre-existing health conditions, the current evidence (although small) suggests that consumption of ED and ES are safe in healthy populations and similar to ingesting other foods and beverages containing caffeine. Finally, although it is estimated that only 1% of all dietary supplement adverse events are reported to FDA [224], given the number of servings of these products that are consumed daily, the rate of adverse events appears low in the population of consumers. Nevertheless, it is acknowledged that additional short- and long-term studies are needed to better determine any factors that increase the risk for adverse events. Additionally, since ED often contain several nutrients that contain caffeine and/or other stimulants, care should be taken to make sure that an excessive number of ED are not consumed within a short period of time.

Conclusions and recommendations

Based on a review of the available scientific and medical literature related to the safety and efficacy of the use of ED or ES, the Research Committee of the Society makes the following conclusions and recommendations.

1. Although ED and ES contain a number of nutrients that are purported to affect mental and/or physical performance, the primary ergogenic nutrients in most ED and ES appear to be carbohydrate and/or caffeine.
2. The ergogenic value of caffeine on mental and physical performance has been well-established but

the potential additive benefits of other nutrients contained in ED and ES remains to be determined.

3. Consuming ED 10-60 minutes before exercise can improve mental focus, alertness, anaerobic performance, and/or endurance performance.
4. Many ED and ES contain numerous ingredients; these products in particular merit further study to demonstrate their safety and potential effects on physical and mental performance.
5. There is some limited evidence that consumption of low-calorie ED during training and/or weight loss trials may provide ergogenic benefit and/or promote a small amount of additional fat loss. However, ingestion of higher calorie ED may promote weight gain if the energy intake from consumption of ED is not carefully considered as part of the total daily energy intake.
6. Athletes should consider the impact of ingesting high glycemic load carbohydrates on metabolic health, blood glucose and insulin levels, as well as the effects of caffeine and other stimulants on motor skill performance.
7. Children and adolescents should only consider use of ED or ES with parental approval after consideration of the amount of carbohydrate, caffeine, and other nutrients contained in the ED or ES and a thorough understanding of the potential side effects.
8. Indiscriminant use of ED or ES, especially if more than one serving per day is consumed, may lead to adverse events and harmful side effects.
9. Diabetics and individuals with pre-existing cardiovascular, metabolic, hepatorenal, and neurologic disease who are taking medications that may be affected by high glycemic load foods, caffeine, and/or other stimulants should avoid use of ED and/or ES unless approved by their physician.

Competing interests

BC has received university and private sector funded grants to conduct research on several dietary supplements and has received compensation for speaking at conferences and writing lay articles/books about dietary supplements. PLB has received compensation for contributing to edited books in relation to sports nutrition. CW has received academic and industry funding related to dietary supplements and honoraria from speaking engagements on the topic. LT has received academic and industry funding related to dietary supplements and honoraria for speaking at conferences. MTN declares no competing interests. MG has received academic and industry funding related to dietary supplementation but declares no competing interests regarding the contents of this manuscript. TNZ has received funding from the dietary supplement industry to conduct clinical research through The Center for Applied Health Sciences, has consulted for several dietary supplement companies, and currently serves as a scientific advisor to Biotest Laboratories. HLL has received funding from industry to conduct clinical research through The Center for Applied Health Sciences, has consulted for multiple dietary supplement and medical food companies, and currently serves as scientific and medical advisor to Nordic Naturals, Inc. JRS serves as a science advisor for Abbott Nutrition. SS has not competing interest to declare. RC has no competing interests to declare. DSK works for a Contract Research Organization that receives funding for clinical trials from the pharmaceutical and nutritional industries, serves as a Nutrition Consultant currently to the United States Tennis Association (USTA), Boca Raton, Florida, and serves as the also as the Florida International University, Department of Athletics, Sports Nutritionist. JA is a Sports Science Advisor to VPX/Redline in Weston FL. RBK has received external funding from industry through the institutions he has been affiliated with to conduct exercise and nutrition research, has served as a legal expert on exercise and nutrition related cases, and currently serves as a scientific advisor for Woodbolt International.

Authors' contributions

RBK prepared and delivered the presentation on energy drinks at the 2011 International Society of Sports Nutrition (ISSN) National meeting. BC, CW, LT, MTN, and MG developed the presentation into a draft of a position stand for review and editing by RBK. The final draft was then reviewed and edited by TZ, HL, JRH, JRS, SS, RC, DSK and JA. RBK incorporated recommendations into a final draft which was then reviewed, approved, and adopted as the official position of the ISSN by the Research Committee. All authors read and approved the final manuscript.

Author details

[1]Exercise and Performance Nutrition Laboratory, Dept. of Physical Education and Exercise Science, University of South Florida, 4202 E. Fowler Avenue, PED 214, Tampa, FL 33620, USA. [2]Human Performance Laboratory, University of Mary Hardin-Baylor, Belton, TX 76513, USA. [3]Department of Health, Human Performance, and Recreation, Baylor University, Box 97313, Waco, TX 76798, USA. [4]Department of Health and Human Performance, University of St. Thomas, St. Paul, MN 55105, USA. [5]Exercise & Sport Nutrition Lab, Department of Health & Kinesiology, Texas A&M University, College Station, Texas, TX 77843-4243, USA. [6]The Center for Applied Health Sciences, Stow, OH 44224, USA. [7]Institute of Exercise Physiology and Wellness, Department of Sport and Exercise Science, University of Central Florida, Orlando, FL 32816, USA. [8]Medical Surveillance and Risk Management, Shire HGT, 300 Shire Way, Lexington, MA 02421, USA. [9]Collins, McDonald & Gann, PC, Mineola, NY, USA. [10]Miami Research Associates, Endocrinology & Nutrition Department, 6141 Sunset Drive - Suite 301, Miami, FL 33143, USA. [11]Farquhar College of Arts and Sciences, Nova Southeastern University, Fort Lauderdale, FL, USA.

References

1. Froiland K, Koszewski W, Hingst J, Kopecky L: **Nutritional supplement use among college athletes and their sources of information.** *Int J Sport Nutr Exerc Metab* 2004, **14**:104–120.
2. Hoffman: **Caffeine and Energy Drinks.** *Strength Cond J* 2010, **32**:15–20.
3. Hoffman JR, Faigenbaum AD, Ratamess NA, Ross R, Kang J, Tenenbaum G: **Nutritional supplementation and anabolic steroid use in adolescents.** *Med Sci Sports Exerc* 2008, **40**:15–24
4. Petroczi A, Naughton DP, Pearce G, Bailey R, Bloodworth A, McNamee M: **Nutritional supplement use by elite young UK athletes: fallacies of advice regarding efficacy.** *J Int Soc Sports Nutr* 2008, **5**:22.
5. Wolk BJ, Ganetsky M, Babu KM: **Toxicity of energy drinks.** *Curr Opin Pediatr* 2012, **24**:243–251.
6. Kerksick C, Harvey T, Stout J, Campbell B, Wilborn C, Kreider R, Kalman D, Ziegenfuss T, Lopez H, Landis J, *et al*: **International Society of Sports Nutrition position stand: nutrient timing.** *J Int Soc Sports Nutr* 2008, **5**:17.
7. Goldstein ER, Ziegenfuss T, Kalman D, Kreider R, Campbell B, Wilborn C, Taylor L, Willoughby D, Stout J, Graves BS, *et al*: **International society of sports nutrition position stand: caffeine and performance.** *J Int Soc Sports Nutr* 2010, **7**:5.
8. Bonati M, Latini R, Galletti F, Young JF, Tognoni G, Garattini S: **Caffeine disposition after oral doses.** *Clin Pharmacol Ther* 1982, **32**:98–106.
9. Graham TE, Hibbert E, Sathasivam P: **Metabolic and exercise endurance effects of coffee and caffeine ingestion.** *J Appl Physiol* 1998, **85**:883–889.
10. McLellan TM, Bell DG: **The impact of prior coffee consumption on the subsequent ergogenic effect of anhydrous caffeine.** *Int J Sport Nutr Exerc Metab* 2004, **14**:698–708.
11. Kovacs EM, Stegen J, Brouns F: **Effect of caffeinated drinks on substrate metabolism, caffeine excretion, and performance.** *J Appl Physiol* 1998, **85**:709–715.

12. Oka H, Suzuki S, Suzuki H, Oda T: **Increased urinary excretion of L-xylulose in patients with liver cirrhosis.** *Clin Chim Acta* 1976, **67**:131–136.
13. Jeukendrup A, Brouns F, Wagenmakers AJ, Saris WH: **Carbohydrate-electrolyte feedings improve 1 h time trial cycling performance.** *Int J Sports Med* 1997, **18**:125–129.
14. Jeukendrup AE: **Carbohydrate intake during exercise and performance.** *Nutrition* 2004, **20**:669–677.
15. Coyle EF, Coggan AR, Hemmert MK, Ivy JL: **Muscle glycogen utilization during prolonged strenuous exercise when fed carbohydrate.** *J Appl Physiol* 1986, **61**:165–172.
16. Jeukendrup AE, Jentjens R: **Oxidation of carbohydrate feedings during prolonged exercise: current thoughts, guidelines and directions for future research.** *Sports Med* 2000, **29**:407–424.
17. Kreider RB, Wilborn CD, Taylor L, Campbell B, Almada AL, Collins R, Cooke M, Earnest CP, Greenwood M, Kalman DS, *et al*: **ISSN exercise & sport nutrition review: research & recommendations.** *J Int Soc Sports Nutr* 2010, **7**:7.
18. Rodriguez NR, Di Marco NM, Langley S: **American College of Sports Medicine position stand. Nutrition and athletic performance.** *Med Sci Sports Exerc* 2009, **41**:709–731.
19. Murray R, Bartoli W, Stofan J, Horn M, Eddy D: **A comparison of the gastric emptying characteristics of selected sports drinks.** *Int J Sport Nutr* 1999, **9**:263–274.
20. Maughan RJ, Leiper JB: **Limitations to fluid replacement during exercise.** *Can J Appl Physiol* 1999, **24**:173–187.
21. Franconi F, Loizzo A, Ghirlanda G, Seghieri G: **Taurine supplementation and diabetes mellitus.** *Curr Opin Clin Nutr Metab Care* 2006, **9**:32–36.
22. Dawson R Jr, Biasetti M, Messina S, Dominy J: **The cytoprotective role of taurine in exercise-induced muscle injury.** *Amino Acids* 2002, **22**:309–324.
23. Zhang M, Izumi I, Kagamimori S, Sokejima S, Yamagami T, Liu Z, Qi B: **Role of taurine supplementation to prevent exercise-induced oxidative stress in healthy young men.** *Amino Acids* 2004, **26**:203–207.
24. Obrosova IG, Stevens MJ: **Effect of dietary taurine supplementation on GSH and NAD(P)-redox status, lipid peroxidation, and energy metabolism in diabetic precataractous lens.** *Invest Ophthalmol Vis Sci* 1999, **40**:680–688.
25. Bakker AJ, Berg HM: **Effect of taurine on sarcoplasmic reticulum function and force in skinned fast-twitch skeletal muscle fibres of the rat.** *J Physiol* 2002, **538**:185–194.
26. Bichler A, Swenson A, Harris MA: **A combination of caffeine and taurine has no effect on short term memory but induces changes in heart rate and mean arterial blood pressure.** *Amino Acids* 2006, **31**:471–476.
27. Galloway SD, Talanian JL, Shoveller AK, Heigenhauser GJ, Spriet LL: **Seven days of oral taurine supplementation does not increase muscle taurine content or alter substrate metabolism during prolonged exercise in humans.** *J Appl Physiol* 2008, **105**:643–651.
28. Matsuzaki Y, Miyazaki T, Miyakawa S, Bouscarel B, Ikegami T, Tanaka N: **Decreased taurine concentration in skeletal muscles after exercise for various durations.** *Med Sci Sports Exerc* 2002, **34**:793–797.
29. Rutherford JA, Spriet LL, Stellingwerff T: **The effect of acute taurine ingestion on endurance performance and metabolism in well-trained cyclists.** *Int J Sport Nutr Exerc Metab* 2010, **20**:322–329.
30. Ward RJ, Francaux M, Cuisinier C, Sturbois X, De Witte P: **Changes in plasma taurine levels after different endurance events.** *Amino Acids* 1999, **16**:71–77.
31. Seidl R, Peyrl A, Nicham R, Hauser E: **A taurine and caffeine-containing drink stimulates cognitive performance and well-being.** *Amino Acids* 2000, **19**:635–642.
32. Goodman CA, Horvath D, Stathis C, Mori T, Croft K, Murphy RM, Hayes A: **Taurine supplementation increases skeletal muscle force production and protects muscle function during and after high-frequency in vitro stimulation.** *J Appl Physiol* 2009, **107**:144–154.
33. Wang FR, Dong XF, Tong JM, Zhang XM, Zhang Q, Wu YY: **Effects of dietary taurine supplementation on growth performance and immune status in growing Japanese quail (Coturnix coturnix japonica).** *Poult Sci* 2009, **88**:1394–1398.
34. Pierno S, De Luca A, Camerino C, Huxtable RJ, Camerino DC: **Chronic administration of taurine to aged rats improves the electrical and contractile properties of skeletal muscle fibers.** *J Pharmacol Exp Ther* 1998, **286**:1183–1190.
35. Warburton DM, Bersellini E, Sweeney E: **An evaluation of a caffeinated taurine drink on mood, memory and information processing in healthy volunteers without caffeine abstinence.** *Psychopharmacology (Berl)* 2001, **158**:322–328.
36. Jorm AF, Rodgers B, Christensen H: **Use of medications to enhance memory in a large community sample of 60-64 year olds.** *Int Psychogeriatr* 2004, **16**:209–217.
37. Elsabagh S, Hartley DE, File SE: **Limited cognitive benefits in Stage +2 postmenopausal women after 6 weeks of treatment with Ginkgo biloba.** *J Psychopharmacol* 2005, **19**:173–181.
38. Walesiuk A, Trofimiuk E, Braszko JJ: **Gingko biloba extract diminishes stress-induced memory deficits in rats.** *Pharmacol Rep* 2005, **57**:176–187.
39. Stoll S, Scheuer K, Pohl O, Muller WE: **Ginkgo biloba extract (EGb 761) independently improves changes in passive avoidance learning and brain membrane fluidity in the aging mouse.** *Pharmacopsychiatry* 1996, **29**:144–149.
40. Grevet EH, Tietzmann MR, Shansis FM, Hastenpflugl C, Santana LC, Forster L, Kapczinskil F, Izquierdo I: **Behavioural effects of acute phenylalanine and tyrosine depletion in healthy male volunteers.** *J Psychopharmacol* 2002, **16**:51–55.
41. Mahoney CR, Castellani J, Kramer FM, Young A, Lieberman HR: **Tyrosine supplementation mitigates working memory decrements during cold exposure.** *Physiol Behav* 2007, **92**:575–582.
42. Chinevere TD, Sawyer RD, Creer AR, Conlee RK, Parcell AC: **Effects of L-tyrosine and carbohydrate ingestion on endurance exercise performance.** *J Appl Physiol* 2002, **93**:1590–1597.
43. Deijen JB, Wientjes CJ, Vullinghs HF, Cloin PA, Langefeld JJ: **Tyrosine improves cognitive performance and reduces blood pressure in cadets after one week of a combat training course.** *Brain Res Bull* 1999, **48**:203–209.
44. Salter CA: **Dietary tyrosine as an aid to stress resistance among troops.** *Mil Med* 1989, **154**:144–146.
45. Smith ML, Hanley WB, Clarke JT, Klim P, Schoonheyt W, Austin V, Lehotay DC: **Randomised controlled trial of tyrosine supplementation on neuropsychological performance in phenylketonuria.** *Arch Dis Child* 1998, **78**:116–121.
46. Magill RA, Waters WF, Bray GA, Volaufova J, Smith SR, Lieberman HR, McNevin N, Ryan DH: **Effects of tyrosine, phentermine, caffeine D-amphetamine, and placebo on cognitive and motor performance deficits during sleep deprivation.** *Nutr Neurosci* 2003, **6**:237–246.
47. Waters WF, Magill RA, Bray GA, Volaufova J, Smith SR, Lieberman HR, Rood J, Hurry M, Anderson T, Ryan DH: **A comparison of tyrosine against placebo, phentermine, caffeine, and D-amphetamine during sleep deprivation.** *Nutr Neurosci* 2003, **6**:221–235.
48. O'Brien C, Mahoney C, Tharion WJ, Sils IV, Castellani JW: **Dietary tyrosine benefits cognitive and psychomotor performance during body cooling.** *Physiol Behav* 2007, **90**:301–307.
49. Wiesel FA, Edman G, Flyckt L, Eriksson A, Nyman H, Venizelos N, Bjerkenstedt L: **Kinetics of tyrosine transport and cognitive functioning in schizophrenia.** *Schizophr Res* 2005, **74**:81–89.
50. Struder HK, Hollmann W, Platen P, Donike M, Gotzmann A, Weber K: **Influence of paroxetine, branched-chain amino acids and tyrosine on neuroendocrine system responses and fatigue in humans.** *Horm Metab Res* 1998, **30**:188–194.
51. Jager R, Purpura M, Kingsley M: **Phospholipids and sports performance.** *J Int Soc Sports Nutr* 2007, **4**:5.
52. Warber JP, Patton JF, Tharion WJ, Zeisel SH, Mello RP, Kemnitz CP, Lieberman HR: **The effects of choline supplementation on physical performance.** *Int J Sport Nutr Exerc Metab* 2000, **10**:170–181.
53. Turner EH, Loftis JM, Blackwell AD: **Serotonin a la carte: supplementation with the serotonin precursor 5-hydroxytryptophan.** *Pharmacol Ther* 2006, **109**:325–338.
54. Chaouloff F, Laude D, Elghozi JL: **Physical exercise: evidence for differential consequences of tryptophan on 5-HT synthesis and metabolism in central serotonergic cell bodies and terminals.** *J Neural Transm* 1989, **78**:121–130.
55. Leu-Semenescu S, Arnulf I, Decaix C, Moussa F, Clot F, Boniol C, Touitou Y, Levy R, Vidailhet M, Roze E: **Sleep and rhythm consequences of a genetically induced loss of serotonin.** *Sleep* 2010, **33**:307–314.
56. Freeman MP, Helgason C, Hill RA: **Selected integrative medicine treatments for depression: considerations for women.** *J Am Med Womens Assoc* 2004, **59**:216–224.
57. Larzelere MM, Wiseman P: **Anxiety, depression, and insomnia.** *Prim Care* 2002, **29**:339–360. vii.
58. Thachil AF, Mohan R, Bhugra D: **The evidence base of complementary and alternative therapies in depression.** *J Affect Disord* 2007, **97**:23–35.

59. Hayashi Y, Jacob-Vadakot S, Dugan EA, McBride S, Olexa R, Simansky K, Murray M, Shumsky JS: **5-HT precursor loading, but not 5-HT receptor agonists, increases motor function after spinal cord contusion in adult rats.** *Exp Neurol* 2010, **221**:68–78.
60. Yamamoto T, Newsholme EA: **Diminished central fatigue by inhibition of the L-system transporter for the uptake of tryptophan.** *Brain Res Bull* 2000, **52**:35–38.
61. Heckman MA, Weil J, Gonzalez de Mejia E: **Caffeine (1, 3, 7-trimethylxanthine) in foods: a comprehensive review on consumption, functionality, safety, and regulatory matters.** *J Food Sci* 2010, **75**:R77–87.
62. Ivy JL, Kammer L, Ding Z, Wang B, Bernard JR, Liao YH, Hwang J: **Improved cycling time-trial performance after ingestion of a caffeine energy drink.** *Int J Sport Nutr Exerc Metab* 2009, **19**:61–78.
63. Goldstein E, Jacobs PL, Whitehurst M, Penhollow T, Antonio J: **Caffeine enhances upper body strength in resistance-trained women.** *J Int Soc Sports Nutr* 2010, **7**:18.
64. Del Coso J, Muñoz-Fernández VE, Muñoz G, Fernández-Elías VE, Ortega JF, Hamouti N, Barbero JC, Muñoz-Guerra J: **Effects of a Caffeine-Containing Energy Drink on Simulated Soccer Performance.** *PLoS One* 2012, **7**:e31380.
65. Del Coso J, Salinero JJ, Gonzalez-Millan C, Abian-Vicen J, Perez-Gonzalez B: **Dose response effects of a caffeine-containing energy drink on muscle performance: a repeated measures design.** *J Int Soc Sports Nutr* 2012, **9**:21.
66. Berube-Parent S, Pelletier C, Dore J, Tremblay A: **Effects of encapsulated green tea and Guarana extracts containing a mixture of epigallocatechin-3-gallate and caffeine on 24 h energy expenditure and fat oxidation in men.** *Br J Nutr* 2005, **94**:432–436.
67. Belza A, Toubro S, Astrup A: **The effect of caffeine, green tea and tyrosine on thermogenesis and energy intake.** *Eur J Clin Nutr* 2009, **63**:57–64.
68. Eichenberger P, Colombani PC, Mettler S: **Effects of 3-week consumption of green tea extracts on whole-body metabolism during cycling exercise in endurance-trained men.** *Int J Vitam Nutr Res* 2009, **79**:24–33.
69. Venables MC, Hulston CJ, Cox HR, Jeukendrup AE: **Green tea extract ingestion, fat oxidation, and glucose tolerance in healthy humans.** *Am J Clin Nutr* 2008, **87**:778–784.
70. Eichenberger P, Mettler S, Arnold M, Colombani PC: **No Effects of Three-week Consumption of a Green Tea Extract on Time Trial Performance in Endurance-trained Men.** *Int J Vitam Nutr Res* 2010, **80**:54–64.
71. Chen N, Bezzina R, Hinch E, Lewandowski PA, Cameron-Smith D, Mathai ML, Jois M, Sinclair AJ, Begg DP, Wark JD, *et al*: **Green tea, black tea, and epigallocatechin modify body composition, improve glucose tolerance, and differentially alter metabolic gene expression in rats fed a high-fat diet.** *Nutr Res* 2009, **29**:784–793.
72. Hursel R, Westerterp-Plantenga MS: **Green tea catechin plus caffeine supplementation to a high-protein diet has no additional effect on body weight maintenance after weight loss.** *Am J Clin Nutr* 2009, **89**:822–830.
73. Auvichayapat P, Prapochanung M, Tunkamnerdthai O, Sripanidkulchai BO, Auvichayapat N, Thinkhamrop B, Kunhasura S, Wongpratoom S, Sinawat S, Hongprapas P: **Effectiveness of green tea on weight reduction in obese Thais: A randomized, controlled trial.** *Physiol Behav* 2008, **93**:486–491.
74. Diepvens K, Kovacs EM, Nijs IM, Vogels N, Westerterp-Plantenga MS: **Effect of green tea on resting energy expenditure and substrate oxidation during weight loss in overweight females.** *Br J Nutr* 2005, **94**:1026–1034.
75. Diepvens K, Westerterp KR, Westerterp-Plantenga MS: **Obesity and thermogenesis related to the consumption of caffeine, ephedrine, capsaicin, and green tea.** *Am J Physiol Regul Integr Comp Physiol* 2007, **292**:R77–85.
76. Murase T, Haramizu S, Shimotoyodome A, Tokimitsu I, Hase T: **Green tea extract improves running endurance in mice by stimulating lipid utilization during exercise.** *Am J Physiol Regul Integr Comp Physiol* 2006, **290**:R1550–1556.
77. Fugh-Berman A, Myers A: **Citrus aurantium, an ingredient of dietary supplements marketed for weight loss: current status of clinical and basic research.** *Exp Biol Med (Maywood)* 2004, **229**:698–704.
78. Haller CA, Benowitz NL, Jacob P 3rd: **Hemodynamic effects of ephedra-free weight-loss supplements in humans.** *Am J Med* 2005, **118**:998–1003.
79. Kim GS, Park HJ, Woo JH, Kim MK, Koh PO, Min W, Ko YG, Kim CH, Won CK, Cho JH: **Citrus aurantium flavonoids inhibit adipogenesis through the Akt signaling pathway in 3T3-L1 cells.** *BMC Complement Altern Med* 2012, **12**:31.
80. Peixoto JS, Comar JF, Moreira CT, Soares AA, de Oliveira AL, Bracht A, Peralta RM: **Effects of Citrus aurantium (bitter orange) fruit extracts and p-synephrine on metabolic fluxes in the rat liver.** *Molecules* 2012, **17**:5854–5869.
81. Preuss HG, DiFerdinando D, Bagchi M, Bagchi D: **Citrus aurantium as a thermogenic, weight-reduction replacement for ephedra: an overview.** *J Med* 2002, **33**:247–264.
82. Stohs SJ, Preuss HG, Keith SC, Keith PL, Miller H, Kaats GR: **Effects of p-synephrine alone and in combination with selected bioflavonoids on resting metabolism, blood pressure, heart rate and self-reported mood changes.** *Int J Med Sci* 2011, **8**:295–301.
83. Pittler MH, Ernst E: **Dietary supplements for body-weight reduction: a systematic review.** *Am J Clin Nutr* 2004, **79**:529–536.
84. Pittler MH, Schmidt K, Ernst E: **Adverse events of herbal food supplements for body weight reduction: systematic review.** *Obes Rev* 2005, **6**:93–111.
85. Kang YR, Lee HY, Kim JH, Moon DI, Seo MY, Park SH, Choi KH, Kim CR, Kim SH, Oh JH, *et al*: **Anti-obesity and anti-diabetic effects of Yerba Mate (Ilex paraguariensis) in C57BL/6J mice fed a high-fat diet.** *Lab Anim Res* 2012, **28**:23–29.
86. Riley AJ: **Yohimbine in the treatment of erectile disorder.** *Br J Clin Pract* 1994, **48**:133–136.
87. Gupta RS, Sharma R, Sharma A, Bhatnager AK, Dobhal MP, Joshi YC, Sharma MC: **Effect of Alstonia scholaris bark extract on testicular function of Wistar rats.** *Asian J Androl* 2002, **4**:175–178.
88. Porst H: **The future of erectile dysfunction (ED).** *Arch Esp Urol* 2010, **63**:740–747.
89. Kucio C, Jonderko K, Piskorska D: **Does yohimbine act as a slimming drug?** *Isr J Med Sci* 1991, **27**:550–556.
90. Sax L: **Yohimbine does not affect fat distribution in men.** *Int J Obes* 1991, **15**:561–565.
91. deMarcaida JA, Schwid SR, White WB, Blindauer K, Fahn S, Kieburtz K, Stern M, Shoulson I: **Effects of tyramine administration in Parkinson's disease patients treated with selective MAO-B inhibitor rasagiline.** *Mov Disord* 2006, **21**:1716–1721.
92. Conlay LA, Maher TJ, Wurtman RJ: **Tyrosine's pressor effect in hypotensive rats is not mediated by tyramine.** *Life Sci* 1984, **35**:1207–1212.
93. Edwards DJ: **Possible role of octopamine and tyramine in the antihypertensive and antidepressant effects of tyrosine.** *Life Sci* 1982, **30**:1427–1434.
94. McDaniel MA, Maier SF, Einstein GO: **"Brain-specific" nutrients: a memory cure?** *Nutrition* 2003, **19**:957–975.
95. Polich J, Gloria R: **Cognitive effects of a Ginkgo biloba/vinpocetine compound in normal adults: systematic assessment of perception, attention and memory.** *Hum Psychopharmacol* 2001, **16**:409–416.
96. Bahrke MS, Morgan WP, Stegner A: **Is ginseng an ergogenic aid?** *Int J Sport Nutr Exerc Metab* 2009, **19**:298–322.
97. Engels HJ, Fahlman MM, Wirth JC: **Effects of ginseng on secretory IgA, performance, and recovery from interval exercise.** *Med Sci Sports Exerc* 2003, **35**:690–696.
98. Goulet ED, Dionne IJ: **Assessment of the effects of eleutherococcus senticosus on endurance performance.** *Int J Sport Nutr Exerc Metab* 2005, **15**:75–83.
99. Hsu CC, Ho MC, Lin LC, Su B, Hsu MC: **American ginseng supplementation attenuates creatine kinase level induced by submaximal exercise in human beings.** *World J Gastroenterol* 2005, **11**:5327–5331.
100. Hwang HJ, Kwak YS, Yoon GA, Kang MH, Park JH, Lee BK, Kim SJ, Um SY, Kim YM: **Combined effects of swim training and ginseng supplementation on exercise performance time, ROS, lymphocyte proliferation, and DNA damage following exhaustive exercise stress.** *Int J Vitam Nutr Res* 2007, **77**:289–296.
101. Kulaputana O, Thanakomsirichot S, Anomasiri W: **Ginseng supplementation does not change lactate threshold and physical performances in physically active Thai men.** *J Med Assoc Thai* 2007, **90**:1172–1179.
102. Liang MT, Podolka TD, Chuang WJ: **Panax notoginseng supplementation enhances physical performance during endurance exercise.** *J Strength Cond Res* 2005, **19**:108–114.
103. Reay JL, Scholey AB, Milne A, Fenwick J, Kennedy DO: **Panax ginseng has no effect on indices of glucose regulation following acute or chronic ingestion in healthy volunteers.** *Br J Nutr* 2009, **101**:1673–1678.
104. Engels HJ, Kolokouri I, Cieslak TJ 2nd, Wirth JC: **Effects of ginseng supplementation on supramaximal exercise performance and short-term recovery.** *J Strength Cond Res* 2001, **15**:290–295.
105. Eschbach LF, Webster MJ, Boyd JC, McArthur PD, Evetovich TK: **The effect of siberian ginseng (Eleutherococcus senticosus) on substrate utilization and performance.** *Int J Sport Nutr Exerc Metab* 2000, **10**:444–451.
106. Ferrando A, Vila L, Voces JA, Cabral AC, Alvarez AI, Prieto JG: **Effects of ginseng extract on various haematological parameters during aerobic exercise in the rat.** *Planta Med* 1999, **65**:288–290.

107. Ferrando A, Vila L, Voces JA, Cabral AC, Alvarez AI, Prieto JG: **Effects of a standardized Panax ginseng extract on the skeletal muscle of the rat: a comparative study in animals at rest and under exercise.** *Planta Med* 1999, **65**:239–244.
108. Ziemba AW, Chmura J, Kaciuba-Uscilko H, Nazar K, Wisnik P, Gawronski W: **Ginseng treatment improves psychomotor performance at rest and during graded exercise in young athletes.** *Int J Sport Nutr* 1999, **9**:371–377.
109. Allen JD, McLung J, Nelson AG, Welsch M: **Ginseng supplementation does not enhance healthy young adults' peak aerobic exercise performance.** *J Am Coll Nutr* 1998, **17**:462–466.
110. Engels HJ, Wirth JC: **No ergogenic effects of ginseng (Panax ginseng C.A. Meyer) during graded maximal aerobic exercise.** *J Am Diet Assoc* 1997, **97**:1110–1115.
111. Pieralisi G, Ripari P, Vecchiet L: **Effects of a standardized ginseng extract combined with dimethylaminoethanol bitartrate, vitamins, minerals, and trace elements on physical performance during exercise.** *Clin Ther* 1991, **13**:373–382.
112. Karlic H, Lohninger A: **Supplementation of L-carnitine in athletes: does it make sense?** *Nutrition* 2004, **20**:709–715.
113. Pauly DF, Pepine CJ: **D-Ribose as a supplement for cardiac energy metabolism.** *J Cardiovasc Pharmacol Ther* 2000, **5**:249–258.
114. Kerksick C, Rasmussen C, Bowden R, Leutholtz B, Harvey T, Earnest C, Greenwood M, Almada A, Kreider R: **Effects of ribose supplementation prior to and during intense exercise on anaerobic capacity and metabolic markers.** *Int J Sport Nutr Exerc Metab* 2005, **15**:653–664.
115. Kreider RB, Melton C, Greenwood M, Rasmussen C, Lundberg J, Earnest C, Almada A: **Effects of oral D-ribose supplementation on anaerobic capacity and selected metabolic markers in healthy males.** *Int J Sport Nutr Exerc Metab* 2003, **13**:76–86.
116. Berardi JM, Ziegenfuss TN: **Effects of ribose supplementation on repeated sprint performance in men.** *J Strength Cond Res* 2003, **17**:47–52.
117. Dunne L, Worley S, Macknin M: **Ribose versus dextrose supplementation, association with rowing performance: a double-blind study.** *Clin J Sport Med* 2006, **16**:68–71.
118. Eijnde BO, Van Leemputte M, Brouns F, Van Der Vusse GJ, Labarque V, Ramaekers M, Van Schuylenberg R, Verbessem P, Wijnen H, Hespel P: **No effects of oral ribose supplementation on repeated maximal exercise and de novo ATP resynthesis.** *J Appl Physiol* 2001, **91**:2275–2281.
119. Hellsten Y, Skadhauge L, Bangsbo J: **Effect of ribose supplementation on resynthesis of adenine nucleotides after intense intermittent training in humans.** *Am J Physiol Regul Integr Comp Physiol* 2004, **286**:R182–188.
120. Harris RC, Sale C: **Beta-alanine supplementation in high-intensity exercise.** *Med Sport Sci* 2013, **59**:1–17.
121. Hoffman JR, Emerson NS, Stout JR: **beta-Alanine supplementation.** *Curr Sports Med Rep* 2012, **11**:189–195.
122. Harris RC, Wise JA, Price KA, Kim HJ, Kim CK, Sale C: **Determinants of muscle carnosine content.** *Amino Acids* 2012, **43**:5–12.
123. Culbertson JY, Kreider RB, Greenwood M, Cooke M: **Effects of beta-alanine on muscle carnosine and exercise performance: a review of the current literature.** *Nutrients* 2010, **2**:75–98.
124. Hobson RM, Saunders B, Ball G, Harris RC, Sale C: **Effects of beta-alanine supplementation on exercise performance: a meta-analysis.** *Amino Acids* 2012, **43**:25–37.
125. Smith-Ryan AE, Fukuda DH, Stout JR, Kendall KL: **High-velocity intermittent running: effects of beta-alanine supplementation.** *J Strength Cond Res* 2012, **26**:2798–2805.
126. Saunders B, Sunderland C, Harris RC, Sale C: **beta-alanine supplementation improves YoYo intermittent recovery test performance.** *J Int Soc Sports Nutr* 2012, **9**:39.
127. Jagim AR, Wright GA, Brice AG, Doberstein ST: **Effects of beta-alanine supplementation on sprint endurance.** *J Strength Cond Res* 2012.
128. Sale C, Saunders B, Hudson S, Wise JA, Harris RC, Sunderland CD: **Effect of beta-alanine plus sodium bicarbonate on high-intensity cycling capacity.** *Med Sci Sports Exerc* 2011, **43**:1972–1978.
129. Kern BD, Robinson TL: **Effects of beta-alanine supplementation on performance and body composition in collegiate wrestlers and football players.** *J Strength Cond Res* 2011, **25**:1804–1815.
130. Walter AA, Smith AE, Kendall KL, Stout JR, Cramer JT: **Six weeks of high-intensity interval training with and without beta-alanine supplementation for improving cardiovascular fitness in women.** *J Strength Cond Res* 2010, **24**:1199–1207.
131. Sweeney KM, Wright GA, Glenn Brice A, Doberstein ST: **The effect of beta-alanine supplementation on power performance during repeated sprint activity.** *J Strength Cond Res* 2010, **24**:79–87.
132. Sale C, Saunders B, Harris RC: **Effect of beta-alanine supplementation on muscle carnosine concentrations and exercise performance.** *Amino Acids* 2010, **39**:321–333.
133. Van Thienen R, Van Proeyen K, Vanden Eynde B, Puype J, Lefere T, Hespel P: **Beta-alanine improves sprint performance in endurance cycling.** *Med Sci Sports Exerc* 2009, **41**:898–903.
134. Smith AE, Moon JR, Kendall KL, Graef JL, Lockwood CM, Walter AA, Beck TW, Cramer JT, Stout JR: **The effects of beta-alanine supplementation and high-intensity interval training on neuromuscular fatigue and muscle function.** *Eur J Appl Physiol* 2009, **105**:357–363.
135. Kendrick IP, Kim HJ, Harris RC, Kim CK, Dang VH, Lam TQ, Bui TT, Wise JA: **The effect of 4 weeks beta-alanine supplementation and isokinetic training on carnosine concentrations in type I and II human skeletal muscle fibres.** *Eur J Appl Physiol* 2009, **106**:131–138.
136. Stout JR, Graves BS, Smith AE, Hartman MJ, Cramer JT, Beck TW, Harris RC: **The effect of beta-alanine supplementation on neuromuscular fatigue in elderly (55-92 Years): a double-blind randomized study.** *J Int Soc Sports Nutr* 2008, **5**:21.
137. Hoffman JR, Ratamess NA, Faigenbaum AD, Ross R, Kang J, Stout JR, Wise JA: **Short-duration beta-alanine supplementation increases training volume and reduces subjective feelings of fatigue in college football players.** *Nutr Res* 2008, **28**:31–35.
138. Zoeller RF, Stout JR, O'Kroy JA, Torok DJ, Mielke M: **Effects of 28 days of beta-alanine and creatine monohydrate supplementation on aerobic power, ventilatory and lactate thresholds, and time to exhaustion.** *Amino Acids* 2007, **33**:505–510.
139. Einat H, Belmaker RH: **The effects of inositol treatment in animal models of psychiatric disorders.** *J Affect Disord* 2001, **62**:113–121.
140. Sureda A, Pons A: **Arginine and citrulline supplementation in sports and exercise: ergogenic nutrients?** *Med Sport Sci* 2013, **59**:18–28.
141. Bescos R, Sureda A, Tur JA, Pons A: **The effect of nitric-oxide-related supplements on human performance.** *Sports Med* 2012, **42**:99–117.
142. Bendahan D, Mattei JP, Ghattas B, Confort-Gouny S, Le Guern ME, Cozzone PJ: **Citrulline/malate promotes aerobic energy production in human exercising muscle.** *Br J Sports Med* 2002, **36**:282–289.
143. Figueroa A, Trivino JA, Sanchez-Gonzalez MA, Vicil F: **Oral L-citrulline supplementation attenuates blood pressure response to cold pressor test in young men.** *Am J Hypertens* 2010, **23**:12–16.
144. Hickner RC, Tanner CJ, Evans CA, Clark PD, Haddock A, Fortune C, Geddis H, Waugh W, McCammon M: **L-citrulline reduces time to exhaustion and insulin response to a graded exercise test.** *Med Sci Sports Exerc* 2006, **38**:660–666.
145. Meneguello MO, Mendonca JR, Lancha AH Jr, Costa Rosa LF: **Effect of arginine, ornithine and citrulline supplementation upon performance and metabolism of trained rats.** *Cell Biochem Funct* 2003, **21**:85–91.
146. Nagaya N, Uematsu M, Oya H, Sato N, Sakamaki F, Kyotani S, Ueno K, Nakanishi N, Yamagishi M, Miyatake K: **Short-term oral administration of L-arginine improves hemodynamics and exercise capacity in patients with precapillary pulmonary hypertension.** *Am J Respir Crit Care Med* 2001, **163**:887–891.
147. Perez-Guisado J, Jakeman PM: **Citrulline malate enhances athletic anaerobic performance and relieves muscle soreness.** *J Strength Cond Res* 2010, **24**:1215–1222.
148. Sureda A, Cordova A, Ferrer MD, Perez G, Tur JA, Pons A: **L-citrulline-malate influence over branched chain amino acid utilization during exercise.** *Eur J Appl Physiol* 2010, **110**:341–351.
149. Takeda K, Machida M, Kohara A, Omi N, Takemasa T: **Effects of citrulline supplementation on fatigue and exercise performance in mice.** *J Nutr Sci Vitaminol (Tokyo)* 2011, **57**:246–250.
150. Kressler J, Millard-Stafford M, Warren GL: **Quercetin and endurance exercise capacity: a systematic review and meta-analysis.** *Med Sci Sports Exerc* 2011, **43**:2396–2404.
151. Wu J, Gao W, Wei J, Yang J, Pu L, Guo C: **Quercetin alters energy metabolism in swimming mice.** *Appl Physiol Nutr Metab* 2012, **37**:912–922.
152. Sharp MA, Hendrickson NR, Staab JS, McClung HL, Nindl BC, Michniak-Kohn BB: **Effects of short-term quercetin supplementation on soldier performance.** *J Strength Cond Res* 2012, **26**(Suppl 2):S53–60.
153. O'Fallon KS, Kaushik D, Michniak-Kohn B, Dunne CP, Zambraski EJ, Clarkson PM: **Quercetin does not attenuate changes in markers of muscle**

function or inflammation after eccentric exercise. *Int J Sport Nutr Exerc Metab* 2012, .
154. Konrad M, Nieman DC, Henson DA, Kennerly KM, Jin F, Wallner-Liebmann SJ: The acute effect of ingesting a quercetin-based supplement on exercise-induced inflammation and immune changes in runners. *Int J Sport Nutr Exerc Metab* 2011, 21:338–346.
155. Abbey EL, Rankin JW: Effect of quercetin supplementation on repeated-sprint performance, xanthine oxidase activity, and inflammation. *Int J Sport Nutr Exerc Metab* 2011, 21:91–96.
156. Nieman DC, Williams AS, Shanely RA, Jin F, McAnulty SR, Triplett NT, Austin MD, Henson DA: Quercetin's influence on exercise performance and muscle mitochondrial biogenesis. *Med Sci Sports Exerc* 2010, 42:338–345.
157. Ganio MS, Armstrong LE, Johnson EC, Klau JF, Ballard KD, Michniak-Kohn B, Kaushik D, Maresh CM: Effect of quercetin supplementation on maximal oxygen uptake in men and women. *J Sports Sci* 2010, 28:201–208.
158. Bigelman KA, Fan EH, Chapman DP, Freese EC, Trilk JL, Cureton KJ: Effects of six weeks of quercetin supplementation on physical performance in ROTC cadets. *Mil Med* 2010, 175:791–798.
159. Utter AC, Nieman DC, Kang J, Dumke CL, Quindry JC, McAnulty SR, McAnulty LS: Quercetin does not affect rating of perceived exertion in athletes during the Western States endurance run. *Res Sports Med* 2009, 17:71–83.
160. Dumke CL, Nieman DC, Utter AC, Rigby MD, Quindry JC, Triplett NT, McAnulty SR, McAnulty LS: Quercetin's effect on cycling efficiency and substrate utilization. *Appl Physiol Nutr Metab* 2009, 34:993–1000.
161. Davis JM, Murphy EA, Carmichael MD, Davis B: Quercetin increases brain and muscle mitochondrial biogenesis and exercise tolerance. *Am J Physiol Regul Integr Comp Physiol* 2009, 296:R1071–1077.
162. Cureton KJ, Tomporowski PD, Singhal A, Pasley JD, Bigelman KA, Lambourne K, Trilk JL, McCully KK, Arnaud MJ, Zhao Q: Dietary quercetin supplementation is not ergogenic in untrained men. *J Appl Physiol* 2009, 107:1095–1104.
163. Quindry JC, McAnulty SR, Hudson MB, Hosick P, Dumke C, McAnulty LS, Henson D, Morrow JD, Nieman D: Oral quercetin supplementation and blood oxidative capacity in response to ultramarathon competition. *Int J Sport Nutr Exerc Metab* 2008, 18:601–616.
164. Henson D, Nieman D, Davis JM, Dumke C, Gross S, Murphy A, Carmichael M, Jenkins DP, Quindry J, McAnulty S, *et al*: Post-160-km race illness rates and decreases in granulocyte respiratory burst and salivary IgA output are not countered by quercetin ingestion. *Int J Sports Med* 2008, 29:856–863.
165. Nieman DC, Henson DA, Gross SJ, Jenkins DP, Davis JM, Murphy EA, Carmichael MD, Dumke CL, Utter AC, McAnulty SR, *et al*: Quercetin reduces illness but not immune perturbations after intensive exercise. *Med Sci Sports Exerc* 2007, 39:1561–1569.
166. Nieman DC, Henson DA, Davis JM, Angela Murphy E, Jenkins DP, Gross SJ, Carmichael MD, Quindry JC, Dumke CL, Utter AC, *et al*: Quercetin's influence on exercise-induced changes in plasma cytokines and muscle and leukocyte cytokine mRNA. *J Appl Physiol* 2007, 103:1728–1735.
167. Campbell B, Downing J, Kilpatrick M, La Bounty P, Elkins A, Williams S, dos Santos MG: The effects of a commercially available energy drink on resistance training and performance. *Med Sci Sports Exerc* 2010, 42:S315.
168. Forbes SC, Candow DG, Little JP, Magnus C, Chilibeck PD: Effect of Red Bull energy drink on repeated Wingate cycle performance and bench-press muscle endurance. *Int J Sport Nutr Exerc Metab* 2007, 17:433–444.
169. Hoffman JR, Kang J, Ratamess NA, Hoffman MW, Tranchina CP, Faigenbaum AD: Examination of a pre-exercise, high energy supplement on exercise performance. *J Int Soc Sports Nutr* 2009, 6:2.
170. Candow DG, Kleisinger AK, Grenier S, Dorsch KD: Effect of sugar-free Red Bull energy drink on high-intensity run time-to-exhaustion in young adults. *J Strength Cond Res* 2009, 23:1271–1275.
171. Cureton KJ, Warren GL, Millard-Stafford ML, Wingo JE, Trilk J, Buyckx M: Caffeinated sports drink: ergogenic effects and possible mechanisms. *Int J Sport Nutr Exerc Metab* 2007, 17:35–55.
172. Alford C, Cox H, Wescott R: The effects of red bull energy drink on human performance and mood. *Amino Acids* 2001, 21:139–150.
173. Campbell B, Kilpatrick M, Wilborn C, La Bounty P, Parker B, Gomez B, Elkins A, Williams S, Dos Santos JA: A commercially available energy drink does not improve peak power on multiple 20-second Wingate tests. *J Int Soc Sports Nutr* 2010, 7:P10.
174. Gonzalez AM, Walsh AL, Ratamess NA, Kang J, Hoffman JR: Effect of a pre-workout energy supplement on acute multi-joint resistance exercise. *J Sports Sci Med* 2011, 10:261–266.
175. Astorino TA, Matera AJ, Basinger J, Evans M, Schurman T, Marquez R: Effects of red bull energy drink on repeated sprint performance in women athletes. *Amino Acids* 2012, 42:1803–1808.
176. Haff GG, Koch AJ, Potteiger JA, Kuphal KE, Magee LM, Green SB, Jakicic JJ: Carbohydrate supplementation attenuates muscle glycogen loss during acute bouts of resistance exercise. *Int J Sport Nutr Exerc Metab* 2000, 10:326–339.
177. Kulik JR, Touchberry CD, Kawamori N, Blumert PA, Crum AJ, Haff GG: Supplemental carbohydrate ingestion does not improve performance of high-intensity resistance exercise. *J Strength Cond Res* 2008, 22:1101–1107.
178. Lambert CP, Flynn MG, Boone JB Jr, Michaud TJ, Rodriguez-Zayas J: Effects of carbohydrate feeding on multiple bout resistance exercised. *J Appl Sport Sci Res* 1991, 5:192–197.
179. Walsh AL, Gonzalez AM, Ratamess NA, Kang J, Hoffman JR: Improved time to exhaustion following ingestion of the energy drink Amino Impact. *J Int Soc Sports Nutr* 2010, 7:14.
180. Currell K, Jeukendrup AE: Validity, reliability and sensitivity of measures of sporting performance. *Sports Med* 2008, 38:297–316.
181. Laursen PB, Francis GT, Abbiss CR, Newton MJ, Nosaka K: Reliability of time-to-exhaustion versus time-trial running tests in runners. *Med Sci Sports Exerc* 2007, 39:1374–1379.
182. Scholey AB, Kennedy DO: Cognitive and physiological effects of an "energy drink": an evaluation of the whole drink and of glucose, caffeine and herbal flavouring fractions. *Psychopharmacology (Berl)* 2004, 176:320–330.
183. Smit HJ, Cotton JR, Hughes SC, Rogers PJ: Mood and cognitive performance effects of "energy" drink constituents: caffeine, glucose and carbonation. *Nutr Neurosci* 2004, 7:127–139.
184. Rao A, Hu H, Nobre AC: The effects of combined caffeine and glucose drinks on attention in the human brain. *Nutr Neurosci* 2005, 8:141–153.
185. Howard MA, Marczinski CA: Acute effects of a glucose energy drink on behavioral control. *Exp Clin Psychopharmacol* 2010, 18:553–561.
186. Pettitt RW, Niemeyer JD, Sexton PJ, Lipetzky A, Murray SR: Do the non-caffeine ingredients of energy drinks affect metabolic responses to heavy exercise? *J Strength Cond Res* 2012, [Epub ahead of print].
187. Bloomer RJ, Fisher-Wellman KH, Hammond KG, Schilling BK, Weber AA, Cole BJ: Dietary supplement increases plasma norepinephrine, lipolysis, and metabolic rate in resistance trained men. *J Int Soc Sports Nutr* 2009, 6:4.
188. Dulloo AG, Geissler CA, Horton T, Collins A, Miller DS: Normal caffeine consumption: influence on thermogenesis and daily energy expenditure in lean and postobese human volunteers. *Am J Clin Nutr* 1989, 49:44–50.
189. Jitomir J, Nassar E, Culbertson J, Moreillon J, Buford T, Hudson G, Cooke M, Kreider R, Willoughby DS: The acute effects of the thermogenic supplement Meltdown on energy expenditure, fat oxidation, and hemodynamic responses in young, healthy males. *J Int Soc Sports Nutr* 2008, 5:23.
190. Mendel RW, Hofheins JE: Metabolic responses to the acute ingestion of two commercially available carbonated beverages: a pilot study. *J Int Soc Sports Nutr* 2007, 4:7.
191. Rudelle S, Ferruzzi MG, Cristiani I, Moulin J, Mace K, Acheson KJ, Tappy L: Effect of a thermogenic beverage on 24-hour energy metabolism in humans. *Obesity (Silver Spring)* 2007, 15:349–355.
192. Taylor LW, Wilborn CD, Harvey T, Wismann J, Willoughby DS: Acute effects of ingesting Java Fittrade mark energy extreme functional coffee on resting energy expenditure and hemodynamic responses in male and female coffee drinkers. *J Int Soc Sports Nutr* 2007, 4:10.
193. Wilborn C, Taylor L, Poole C, Bushey B, Williams L, Foster C, Campbell B: Effects of ingesting a commercial thermogenic product on hemodynamic function and energy expenditure at rest in males and females. *Appl Physiol Nutr Metab* 2009, 34:1073–1078.
194. Roberts MD, Dalbo VJ, Hassell SE, Stout JR, Kerksick CM: Efficacy and safety of a popular thermogenic drink after 28 days of ingestion. *J Int Soc Sports Nutr* 2008, 5:19.
195. Dalbo VJ, Roberts MD, Stout JR, Kerksick CM: Acute effects of ingesting a commercial thermogenic drink on changes in energy expenditure and markers of lipolysis. *J Int Soc Sports Nutr* 2008, 5:6.
196. Dalbo VJ, Roberts MD, Stout JR, Kerksick CM: Effect of gender on the metabolic impact of a commercially available thermogenic drink. *J Strength Cond Res* 2010, 24:1633–1642.

197. Rashti SL, Ratamess NA, Kang J, Faigenbaum AD, Chilakos A, Hoffman JR: **Thermogenic effect of meltdown RTD energy drink in young healthy women: a double blind, cross-over design study.** *Lipids Health Dis* 2009, **8**:57.
198. Bloomer RJ, Canale RE, Blankenship MM, Hammond KG, Fisher-Wellman KH, Schilling BK: **Effect of the dietary supplement Meltdown on catecholamine secretion, markers of lipolysis, and metabolic rate in men and women: a randomized, placebo controlled, cross-over study.** *Lipids Health Dis* 2009, **8**:32.
199. Stout J, Moon J, Tobkin S, Lockwood C, Smith A, Graef J, Kendall K, Beck T, Cramer J: **Pre-workout consumption of Celsius(R) enhances the benefits of chronic exercise on body composition and cardiorespiratory fitness.** *J Int Soc Sports Nutr* 2008, **5**:P8.
200. Higgins JP, Tuttle TD, Higgins CL: **Energy beverages: content and safety.** *Mayo Clin Proc* 2010, **85**:1033–1041.
201. Sepkowitz KA: **Energy drinks and caffeine-related adverse effects.** *JAMA* 2012, :1–2 [Epub ahead of print].
202. Torpy JM, Livingston EH: **Energy drinks.** *JAMA* 2012, :1–1 [Epub ahead of print].
203. Howland JRDJ: **Risks of energy drinks mixed with alcohol.** *JAMA* 2012, :1–2 [Epub ahead of print].
204. Clauson KA, Shields KM, McQueen CE, Persad N: **Safety issues associated with commercially available energy drinks.** *J Am Pharm Assoc (2003)* 2008, **48**:e55–63. quiz e64-57.
205. Duchan E, Patel ND, Feucht C: **Energy drinks: a review of use and safety for athletes.** *Phys Sportsmed* 2010, **38**:171–179.
206. Lockwood CM, Moon JR, Smith AE, Tobkin SE, Kendall KL, Graef JL, Cramer JT, Stout JR: **Low-calorie energy drink improves physiological response to exercise in previously sedentary men: a placebo-controlled efficacy and safety study.** *J Strength Cond Res* 2010, **24**:2227–2238.
207. Pennington N, Johnson M, Delaney E, Blankenship MB: **Energy drinks: a new health hazard for adolescents.** *J Sch Nurs* 2010, **26**:352–359.
208. Weiss EP, Arif H, Villareal DT, Marzetti E, Holloszy JO: **Endothelial function after high-sugar-food ingestion improves with endurance exercise performed on the previous day.** *Am J Clin Nutr* 2008, **88**:51–57.
209. Petit A, Levy F, Lejoyeux M, Reynaud M, Karila L: **Energy drinks: an unknown risk.** *Rev Prat* 2012, **62**:673–678.
210. *Why isn't the amount of caffeine a product contains required of a food label?.* http://www.fda.gov/AboutFDA/Transparency/Basics/ucm194317.htm.
211. *Health Canada's proposed approach to managing caffeinated energy drinks.* http://www.hc-sc.gc.ca/fn-an/legislation/pol/energy-drinks-boissons-energisantes-eng.php.
212. McCusker RR, Goldberger BA, Cone EJ: **Caffeine content of specialty coffees.** *J Anal Toxicol* 2003, **27**:520–522.
213. Jin KN, Chun EJ, Lee CH, Kim JA, Lee MS, Choi SI: **Subclinical coronary atherosclerosis in young adults: prevalence, characteristics, predictors with coronary computed tomography angiography.** *Int J Cardiovasc Imaging* 2012, [Epub ahead of print].
214. Thiene G, Carturan E, Corrado D, Basso C: **Prevention of sudden cardiac death in the young and in athletes: dream or reality?** *Cardiovasc Pathol* 2010, **19**:207–217.
215. Radojevic N, Bjelogrlic B, Aleksic V, Rancic N, Samardzic M, Petkovic S, Savic S: **Forensic aspects of water intoxication: four case reports and review of relevant literature.** *Forensic Sci Int* 2012, **220**:1–5.
216. Holmgren P, Norden-Pettersson L, Ahlner J: **Caffeine fatalities–four case reports.** *Forensic Sci Int* 2004, **139**:71–73.
217. Kerrigan S, Lindsey T: **Fatal caffeine overdose: two case reports.** *Forensic Sci Int* 2005, **153**:67–69.
218. Rudolph T, Knudsen K: **A case of fatal caffeine poisoning.** *Acta Anaesthesiol Scand* 2010, **54**:521–523.
219. Nawrot P, Jordan S, Eastwood J, Rotstein J, Hugenholtz A, Feeley M: **Effects of caffeine on human health.** *Food Addit Contam* 2003, **20**:1–30.
220. Higdon JV, Frei B: **Coffee and health: a review of recent human research.** *Crit Rev Food Sci Nutr* 2006, **46**:101–123.
221. Usman A, Jawaid A: **Hypertension in a young boy: an energy drink effect.** *BMC Res Notes* 2012, **5**:591.
222. Worthley MI, Prabhu A, De Sciscio P, Schultz C, Sanders P, Willoughby SR: **Detrimental effects of energy drink consumption on platelet and endothelial function.** *Am J Med* 2010, **123**:184–187.
223. Steinke L, Lanfear DE, Dhanapal V, Kalus JS: **Effect of "energy drink" consumption on hemodynamic and electrocardiographic parameters in healthy young adults.** *Ann Pharmacother* 2009, **43**:596–602.
224. *Adverse event reporting for dietary supplements: an inadequate safety valve.* https://oig.hhs.gov/oei/reports/oei-01-00-00180.pdf.

3

The effectiveness of neuromuscular warm-up strategies, that require no additional equipment, for preventing lower limb injuries during sports participation: a systematic review

Katherine Herman, Christian Barton, Peter Malliaras and Dylan Morrissey*

Abstract

Background: Lower limb injuries in sport are increasingly prevalent and responsible for large economic as well as personal burdens. In this review we seek to determine which easily implemented functional neuromuscular warm-up strategies are effective in preventing lower limb injuries during sports participation and in which sporting groups they are effective.

Methods: Seven electronic databases were searched from inception to January 2012 for studies investigating neuromuscular warm-up strategies and injury prevention. The quality of each included study was evaluated using a modified version of the van Tulder scale. Data were extracted from each study and used to calculate the risk of injury following application of each evaluated strategy.

Results: Nine studies were identified including six randomized controlled trials (RCT) and three controlled clinical trials (CCT). Heterogeneity in study design and warm-up strategies prevented pooling of results. Two studies investigated male and female participants, while the remaining seven investigated women only. Risk Ratio (RR) statistics indicated 'The 11+' prevention strategy significantly reduces overall (RR 0.67, confidence interval (CI) 0.54 to 0.84) and overuse (RR 0.45, CI 0.28 to 0.71) lower limb injuries as well as knee (RR 0.48, CI 0.32 to 0.72) injuries among young amateur female footballers. The 'Knee Injury Prevention Program' (KIPP) significantly reduced the risk of noncontact lower limb (RR 0.5, CI 0.33 to 0.76) and overuse (RR 0.44, CI 0.22 to 0.86) injuries in young amateur female football and basketball players. The 'Prevent Injury and Enhance Performance' (PEP) strategy reduces the incidence of anterior cruciate ligament (ACL) injuries (RR 0.18, CI 0.08 to 0.42). The 'HarmoKnee' programme reduces the risk of knee injuries (RR 0.22, CI 0.06 to 0.76) in teenage female footballers. The 'Anterior Knee Pain Prevention Training Programme' (AKP PTP) significantly reduces the incidence of anterior knee pain (RR 0.27, CI 0.14 to 0.54) in military recruits.

Conclusions: Effective implementation of practical neuromuscular warm-up strategies can reduce lower extremity injury incidence in young, amateur, female athletes and male and female military recruits. This is typically a warm-up strategy that includes stretching, strengthening, balance exercises, sports-specific agility drills and landing techniques applied consistently for longer than three consecutive months. In order to optimize these strategies, the mechanisms for their effectiveness require further evaluation.

Keywords: neuromuscular training, lower limb, injuries, prevention

* Correspondence: d.morrissey@qmul.ac.uk
Centre for Sports and Exercise Medicine, William Harvey Research Institute, Bart's and the London School of Medicine and Dentistry, Queen Mary University of London, Mile End Hospital, Bancroft road, London, E1 4DG, UK

Background

Historically, stretching as part of a warm-up strategy before exercise has been strongly advocated to prevent injury [1]. However, current evidence suggests that stretching alone may confer no injury prevention benefit [2-5]. More recently, researchers and sports medicine practitioners have developed and investigated multi-factorial neuromuscular training strategies targeting injury prevention for a variety of sports and athletic levels. The importance of musculoskeletal injury prevention is highlighted by estimates that 22 million sports injuries occur in the UK each year [6]. Furthermore, sixty to seventy percent of the population in the UK are considered to be physically inactive. Physical inactivity is currently estimated to cost the UK economy £8.3 billion per annum and is more prevalent than obesity, alcohol misuse and smoking combined [7]. It is more important than ever to encourage people to engage in some form of physical activity [8] and the recent Chief Medical Officer report 2009 described physical activity as a 'wonder drug' or 'miracle cure' with huge potential benefits [6]. However, an inevitable consequence of increasing physical activity is an increased incidence of musculoskeletal injury. To reduce the resultant personal and economic burden, there is a need for practical, time efficient and cost-effective injury prevention strategies.

Neuromuscular training programmes are hypothesized to improve joint position sense, enhance joint stability and develop protective joint reflexes, ultimately preventing lower limb injuries. Hübscher *et al.* [9] recently completed a high quality systematic review on neuromuscular training programmes for sports injury prevention. A meta-analysis indicated that multi-intervention programmes may reduce lower limb, acute knee and ankle injuries and that balance programmes may reduce ankle injuries [9]. However, the practicality of these findings for many individuals, teams and clubs may be limited due to the need for equipment purchases (for example, balance boards) and the requirement of additional training sessions to normal practice and competition. In these cases, a more practical solution would be to encompass neuromuscular training programmes which do not require additional equipment and which can be incorporated into warm-up or current routines. A number of neuromuscular warm-up strategies which fit these criteria have been proposed, evaluated and published in the literature. Just two of these programmes were included by the Hübscher *et al.* [9] systematic review. Therefore, an up-to-date systematic review of the literature related to neuromuscular warm-up strategies which can be easily incorporated into warm-up or current routines and do not require the acquisition of additional equipment is needed to further guide recommendations for effective lower limb injury prevention.

The aims of this systematic review were: (1) to evaluate the efficacy of functional neuromuscular warm-up strategies which do not require additional equipment in preventing lower limb injury in order to guide clinical and sporting practice; and (2) to identify the common elements of successful strategies in order to guide future research.

Methods

Search and evaluation strategy

Embase, SPORTDiscus, Google Scholar, PubMed, ISI Web of Knowledge, Scirus and PEDro were searched for articles from inception to June 2011 and updated in January 2012. Search terms included (movement training OR neuromuscular OR proprioceptive OR proprioception OR plyometric) AND (training OR program OR programme) AND prevent* AND (injury OR injuries). Limits included English language (due to the cost of translation) and human studies. The reference list of retrieved articles was manually checked for potentially relevant studies.

Inclusion and exclusion criteria

Inclusion/exclusion criteria are shown in Table 1.

Quality Assessment

A modified version of the nine item van Tulder *et al.* [10] was used to assess the methodological quality of each study. The van Tulder *et al.* [10] criteria focus on the internal validity of clinical trials and recent evidence suggests it is reliable and has good face and content validity [11]. Two independent reviewers (KH and CB) scored each criterion. Any disagreement with scoring the methodological criteria was solved by consensus and a third reviewer (DM) was available if necessary, but was not needed.

Data extraction and analysis

Details of study design, participant characteristics, interventions, statistical analysis, results and study limitations were extracted and tabulated from each included study by one reviewer (KH). Additionally, two reviewers (KH and CB) extracted data related to participant numbers and injury incidence for the various types of lower limb injuries reported. Review Manager version 5.0 was used to calculate risk ratios (RR) and their 95% Confidence Intervals (CI) for all comparisons as well as to produce forest plots to represent this data visually. The number needed to treat (NNT) was calculated only for variables producing a statistically significant RR (that is, 95% confidence intervals did not cross 1.0). Sensitivity analysis was completed to identify if the use of equipment improved injury prevention. To complete this, the effectiveness of a selection of eight studies, five randomized controlled trials (RCTs) [12-16] and three cohort studies

Table 1 Study selection criteria.

Inclusion Criteria
Those studies:
• Which investigated neuromuscular warm-up strategies without the need for additional equipment other than that readily available at training or competition venues
• for the prevention of any lower limb injury (hip, thigh, knee, ankle, leg)
• using functional training
• could be performed anywhere (for example, on-pitch)
• without the use of specialist apparatus
• easily incorporated into regular activity
• Which are detailed enough for replication
• Where injury incidence was an outcome
Exclusion Criteria
Those studies:
• Where the intervention is not part of a warm-up program
• Using home-based exercises due to the poor uptake and regular commitment
• Using equipment (for example, wobble board training) due to cost and availability
• Where the intervention included training outside of sporting participation sessions
• Where participants had an ongoing injury
• Using no control or comparison group
• Which were non-peer reviewed articles
• Of single participant study design

[17-19] which utilized equipment in their programmes and, hence, were excluded from the primary review were evaluated using the same analytical approach.

Results

Literature search

The initial search identified 766 articles (Figure 1). Duplicates were excluded. Many studies were excluded because they involved use of additional equipment not readily available at training or competition venues (see Table 2). Relevant titles and abstracts were selected based on the inclusion criteria, yielding 15 articles. Application of inclusion/exclusion criteria to the full text left nine articles and excluded six articles; five studies because injury prevention was not the primary outcome [20-24] and one study because it lacked a control [25].

Methodological quality

Table 3 shows the results of the methodological quality assessment for the nine included studies. All nine studies scored a minimum of five points on the scale indicating they were of reasonable quality [10]. The following study weaknesses were noted: failure to blind participants to the intervention [26-33], unacceptable, inadequate or absent randomization [26,27,29], failure to blind researchers to the intervention [26-28,30], no intention to treat analysis [28,30], different group values at baseline [30], high drop-out rate [32] and poor compliance [32].

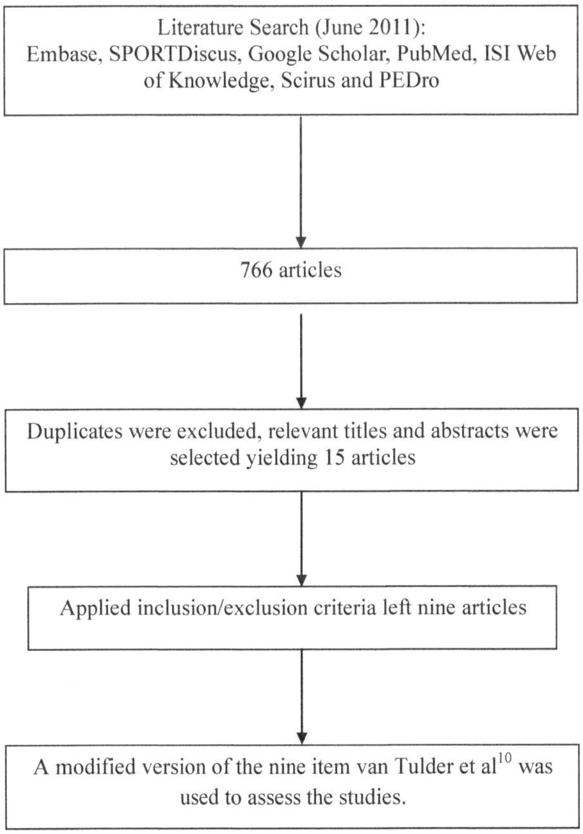

Figure 1 Flowchart to demonstrate the literature search.

Table 2 Reasons for exclusion of studies.

Study	Reason for study exclusion
Tropp *et al.* 1985	Ankle discs, orthoses used
Caraffa *et al.* 1996	Balance boards used
Bahr *et al.* 1997	Balance boards used
Hewett *et al.* 1999	Wobble boards used
Wedderkopp *et al.* 1999	Ankle discs used
Heidt *et al.* 2000	Treadmill sessions implemented
Söderman *et al.* 2000	Wobble boards used
Junge *et al.* 2002	Not detailed enough for replication
Kaminski et al. 2003	Injury prevention not the primary outcome
Stasinopoulos *et al.* 2004	Orthoses, balance boards used
Verhagen *et al.* 2004	Wobble boards used
Olsen *et al.* 2005	Wobble boards used
Garrick *et al.* 2005	Wobble boards used
Peterson *et al.* 2005	Balance boards used
Verhagen *et al.* 2005	Injury prevention not the primary outcome
McKuine *et al.* 2006	Wobble boards used
Mykleburst *et al.* 2007	Lack of control group, mats and balance boards used
Mohammadi *et al.* 2007	Orthoses, ankle weights, resistance bands, wobble boards used
McHugh *et al.* 2007	Foam stability pad used
Emery *et al.* 2007	Wobble boards used
Pasanen *et al.* 2008	Wobble boards used
Hupperets *et al.* 2008	Wobble boards used
Steffen *et al.* 2008	Injury prevention not the primary outcome
Hupperets *et al.* 2009	Balance boards used
Kraemer *et al.* 2009	Balance boards used
Lim *et al.* 2009	Injury prevention not the primary outcome
Eils *et al.* 2010	Wobble boards used
Eisen *et al.* 2010	Injury prevention not the primary outcome
Emery *et al.* 2010	Wobble boards used
Parkkari *et al.* 2011	Sticks used as part of a training approach

Description of Studies

Details of each study are summarized in Table 4 including study design, participants, neuromuscular warm-up strategy evaluated, control intervention, and outcomes evaluated. Studies included an average of 1,500 participants (range 1,020 to 2,020). Two studies [33,34] investigated male and female participants, while the remaining seven investigated females only [26-32]. The age range

Table 3 Assessment of methodological quality for each included study.

		Methodological Quality Criteria								
Study	Quality Score	A	B	C	D	E	F	G	H	I
Mandelbaum *et al.* [1]	5	N	N	Y	N	Y	Y	Y	Y	N
Pfeiffer *et al.* [1]	5	N	N	Y	N	Y	Y	Y	Y	NR
Gilchrist *et al.* [1]	5	NR	N	Y	N	Y	Y	Y	Y	N
Kiani *et al.* [1]	6	N	N	Y	Y	Y	Y	Y	Y	NR
LaBella *et al.* [1]	6	Y	N	N	N	Y	Y	Y	Y	Y
Soligard *et al.* [1]	7	NR	N	Y	Y	Y	Y	Y	Y	Y
Steffen *et al.* [1]	7	Y	N	Y	Y	Y	N	Y	Y	Y
Coppack *et al.* [1]	8	Y	N	Y	Y	Y	Y	Y	Y	Y
Brushøj *et al.* [1]	9	Y	Y	Y	Y	Y	Y	Y	Y	Y

A = acceptable method of randomization, B = concealed treatment allocation, C = similar group values at baseline, D = blinded assessor, E = no or similar co-interventions, F = acceptable compliance (≥75%), G = acceptable dropout rate (≤30%), H = similar timing of the outcome assessment in all groups, I = intention to treat analysis. Y, yes; N, no; NR, not reported.

Table 4 Summary of details regarding each included study.

Study	Design	Participants	Neuromuscular warm-up program	Control Group	Outcome
Mandelbaum *et al.* [26]	CCT	1,041 female soccer players, aged 14 to 18 years	Prevent Injury and Enhance Performance Programme: three basic warm-up exercises, five stretching exercises for the trunk and lower extremities, three strengthening exercises, five plyometric exercises and three soccer-specific agility drills. Performed before matches and training, 20 minutes, for two years	Normal warm-up strategy	ACL injuries
Pfeiffer *et al.* [27]	CCT	1,439 female soccer, basketball and volleyball players, aged 14 to 18 years	Knee Ligament Injury Prevention Programme: four progressive phases of jumping and landing forwards and backwards, two- and one-footed drills, plyometric and agility training. Performed either before or after training sessions twice a week, 20 minutes, for two consecutive seasons	Normal warm-up strategy	ACL injuries
Gilchrist *et al.* [28]	RCT	1,435 female football players, average age 19.9 years	Prevent Injury and Enhance Performance Program: Three basic warm-up exercises, five stretching exercises for the trunk and lower extremities, three strengthening exercises, five plyometric exercises and three soccer-specific agility drills. Before training, 20 minutes three times a week for 12 weeks	Normal warm-up strategy	Undefined knee and ACL injuries
Kiani *et al.* [29]	CCT	1,506 female football players, aged 13 to 19 years	The 'HarmoKnee' program: warm-up, muscle activation, balance, strength, core stability exercises. Performed twice a week preseason (three months), once a week during in-season training session (six months), total duration 20 to 25 minutes	Normal warm-up strategy	All new knee injuries
LaBella *et al.* [30]	RCT	1,558 female football and basketball players, average age 16 years	Knee Injury Prevention Program: combining progressive strengthening, plyometric, balance and agility exercises. In season for one year. Total duration 20 minutes before team practices, an abbreviated version with dynamic motion exercises only before games	Normal warm-up strategy	Gradual-onset lower extremity injuries, acute-onset non-contact lower extremity injuries, non-contact knee, ACL and ankle sprains
Soligard *et al.* [31]	RCT	1,982 female football players, aged 13 to 17 years	The '11+': 10 exercises including slow running, active stretching, controlled contact, exercises for strength, balance, jumping and soccer-specific agility drills. Before training, 20 minutes, only running exercises before match, for eight months	Normal warm-up strategy	Overall and overuse lower limb injuries, groin, posterior and anterior thigh injuries, undefined knee, MTSS and undefined ankle injuries
Steffen *et al.* [32]	RCT	2,020 female football players, aged 13 to 17 years	The '11': 10 exercises for core stability, balance, dynamic stabilization and eccentric hamstring strength. Two months preseason, six months in-season before training, 20 minutes for 15 consecutive training sessions then once a week thereafter	Normal warm-up strategy	Overall lower limb injuries, groin and thigh injuries, undefined knee and ACL injuries, and undefined ankle injuries
Coppack *et al.* [33]	RCT	1,502 male and female army recruits, aged 17 to 25 years	Anterior Knee Pain Prevention Training Programme: warm-up consisted of eight exercises closed chain strengthening exercises, 10 to 14 repetitions each; warm-down involved four stretching exercises, three repetitions. Performed at each training session (mean = seven per week), 15 minutes, for 14 weeks	Normal warm-up strategy (running, stretching, strengthening)	AKP
Brushøj *et al.* [34]	RCT	1,020 female and male army recruits aged 19 to 26 years	Prevention Training Programme: Five exercises for strengthening, balance, stretching performed in three sets of five to 25 repetitions. Before military training, 15 minutes, three times a week for 12 weeks	Strategy for the upper body	Overall and overuse lower limb injuries, AKP, patella tendinopathy, ITBFS, MTSS, ankle sprain and Achilles injuries.

ACL, anterior cruciate ligament; AKP, anterior knee pain; CCT, controlled clinical trial; ITBFS, iliotibial band friction syndrome; MTSS, medial tibial stress syndrome; RCT, randomized controlled trial.

of participants was 13 to 26 years. Five studies evaluated amateur football players [26,28,29,31,32], two studies evaluated army recruits [33,34], one study evaluated amateur football and basketball players [30] and one study evaluated amateur football, basketball and volleyball players [27]. Three studies evaluated primarily ACL injury [26-28], two studies assessed all lower extremity injury risk which included the foot, ankle, leg, knee, thigh, groin and hip [31,32], one study assessed lower extremity injuries which included knee and ankle [30], one study evaluated injuries to the knee including collateral ligament, ACL, meniscal and patella injuries [29], one study measured general overuse injuries [34] and one specifically anterior knee pain (AKP)[33]. Studies quantified injury incidence per 1,000 player hours [29,31,32], per 1,000 athlete exposures [26-28,30] and by cumulative incidence [33,34].

Undefined lower limb injuries

RRs for the effectiveness of neuromuscular warm-up strategies in preventing undefined lower limb injuries are shown in Figure 2. 'The 11+' [31] and 'KIPP' [30] were found to significantly reduce the risk of overall lower limb injuries (RR 0.67, CI 0.54 to 0.84, NNT 18; and RR 0.50, CI 0.33 to 0.76, NNT 24, respectively) and lower limb overuse injuries (RR 0.45, CI 0.28 to 0.71, NNT 31; and RR 0.44, CI 0.22 to 0.86, NNT 49, respectively). Similar to studies without equipment, the sensitivity analysis indicated a mixture of effective and ineffective warm-up programmes which used additional equipment.

Hip and thigh injuries

None of the strategies evaluated were able to produce significant reductions in hip or thigh injuries, with calculated risk ratios shown in Figure 3. A strong trend was indicated for the 'The 11' programme [32] to reduce groin injuries (RR 0.39, CI 0.15 to 1.02, NNT 77). Similarly, the sensitivity analysis failed to identify any warm-up programmes using equipment which were able to reduce the risk of hip and thigh injuries.

Knee injuries

RRs for the effectiveness of neuromuscular warm-up strategies in preventing knee injuries are shown in Figure 4. The 'HarmoKnee' [29] and 'The 11+' [31] programmes significantly reduced the risk of knee injuries (RR 0.22, CI 0.06 to 0.76, NNT 72; and RR 0.48, CI 0.32 to 0.72, NNT 28). Additionally, the PEP [26] strategy was the most effective at reducing ACL injuries (RR 0.18, CI 0.08 to 0.42, NNT 70). The PEP [28] also significantly reduced the risk of recurrence in those with previous non-contact ACL injuries ($P = 0.046$). The AKP PTP [33] was able to reduce the incidence of anterior knee pain (RR 0.27, CI 0.14 to 0.54, NNT 28). Similar to studies without equipment, the sensitivity analysis indicated a mixture of effective and ineffective warm-up programmes which used additional equipment to prevent knee injuries.

Lower leg and ankle injuries

RRs for the effectiveness of neuromuscular warm-up strategies in preventing lower leg and ankle injuries are shown in Figure 5. A strong trend was indicated for the 'KIPP' [30] strategy to reduce non-contact ankle sprains (RR 0.42, CI 0.18 to 1.01, NNT 77). However, none of the neuromuscular warm-up programmes evaluated produced a significant reduction in lower leg or ankle injuries. Contrary to this, five of the eight programmes using equipment which were evaluated in the sensitivity analysis significantly reduced the risk of ankle injury. Additional equipment used in successful studies included balance boards [13-15,17], sticks [16] and medicine balls [17].

	NM warm-up programme		Control		Risk Ratio
Study or Subgroup	Events	Total	Events	Total	M-H, Fixed, 95% CI
1.1.1 Overall					
'KIPP' (LaBella 2011)	32	737	65	755	0.50 [0.33, 0.76]
'The 11+' (Soligard 2008)	121	1055	143	837	0.67 [0.54, 0.84]
'The 11' (Steffen 2008)	181	1091	173	1001	0.96 [0.79, 1.16]
PTP (Brusøj 2008)	108	507	91	513	1.20 [0.93, 1.54]
1.1.2 Overuse					
'KIPP' (LaBella 2011)	12	737	28	755	0.44 [0.22, 0.86]
'The 11+' (Soligard 2008)	27	1055	48	837	0.45 [0.28, 0.71]

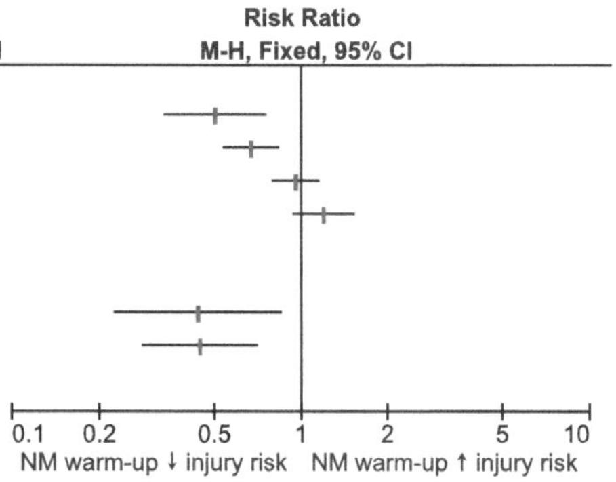

Figure 2 Forest plot graph demonstrating risk ratios for the effectiveness of neuromuscular warm-up strategies in preventing undefined lower limb injuries.

Study or Subgroup	NM warm-up programme Events	NM warm-up programme Total	Control Events	Control Total	Risk Ratio M-H, Fixed, 95% CI
1.2.1 Groin					
'The 11' (Steffen 2008)	6	1091	14	1001	0.39 [0.15, 1.02]
'The 11+' (Soligard 2008)	10	1055	9	837	0.88 [0.36, 2.16]
1.2.2 Thigh (undefined)					
'The 11' (Steffen 2008)	35	1091	28	1001	1.15 [0.70, 1.87]
1.2.3 Posterior thigh (hamstring)					
'The 11+' (Soligard 2008)	5	1055	8	837	0.50 [0.16, 1.51]
1.2.4 Anterior thigh					
'The 11+' (Soligard 2008)	9	1055	9	837	0.79 [0.32, 1.99]

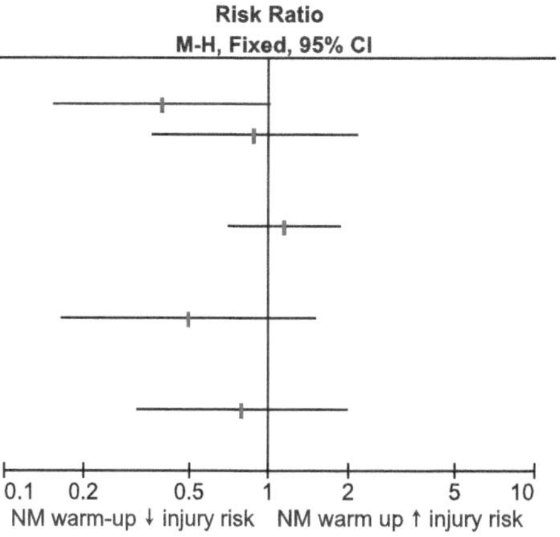

Figure 3 Forest plot graph demonstrating risk ratios for the effectiveness of neuromuscular warm-up strategies in preventing hip and thigh injuries.

Study or Subgroup	NM warm-up programme Events	NM warm-up programme Total	Control Events	Control Total	Risk Ratio M-H, Fixed, 95% CI
1.3.1 Knee (undefined)					
'HarmoKnee' (Kiani 2010)	3	777	13	729	0.22 [0.06, 0.76]
'The 11+' (Soligard 2008)	35	1055	58	837	0.48 [0.32, 0.72]
'KIPP' (LaBella 2011)	6	737	11	755	0.56 [0.21, 1.50]
'PEP' (Gilchrist 2008)	40	583	58	852	1.01 [0.68, 1.49]
'The 11' (Steffen 2008)	37	1091	30	1001	1.13 [0.70, 1.82]
1.3.2 Anterior cruciate ligament					
'HarmoKnee' (Kiani 2010)	0	777	5	729	0.09 [0.00, 1.54]
'PEP' (Mandelbaum 2005)	6	1885	67	3818	0.18 [0.08, 0.42]
'KIPP' (LaBella 2011)	2	737	6	755	0.34 [0.07, 1.69]
'PEP' (Gilchrist 2008)	7	583	18	852	0.57 [0.24, 1.35]
'The 11' (Steffen 2008)	4	1091	5	1001	0.73 [0.20, 2.73]
KLIPP (Peiffer 2006)	3	577	3	862	1.49 [0.30, 7.38]
1.3.3 Medial collateral ligament					
'HarmoKnee' (Kiani 2010)	0	777	1	729	0.31 [0.01, 7.67]
1.3.4 lateral collateral ligament					
'HarmoKnee' (Kiani 2010)	0	777	2	729	0.19 [0.01, 3.90]
1.3.5 Medial meniscus					
'HarmoKnee' (Kiani 2010)	0	777	3	729	0.13 [0.01, 2.59]
1.3.6 Anterior knee pain					
AKP PTP (Coppack 2011)	10	759	36	743	0.27 [0.14, 0.54]
PTP (Brusøj 2008)	27	507	23	513	1.19 [0.69, 2.04]
1.3.7 Patellar dislocation					
'HarmoKnee' (Kiani 2010)	1	777	3	729	0.31 [0.03, 3.00]
1.3.8 Patellar tendinopathy (jumper's knee)					
PTP (Brusøj 2008)	5	507	3	513	1.69 [0.41, 7.02]
1.3.9 Iliotibial band friction syndrome					
PTP (Brusøj 2008)	5	507	4	513	1.26 [0.34, 4.68]

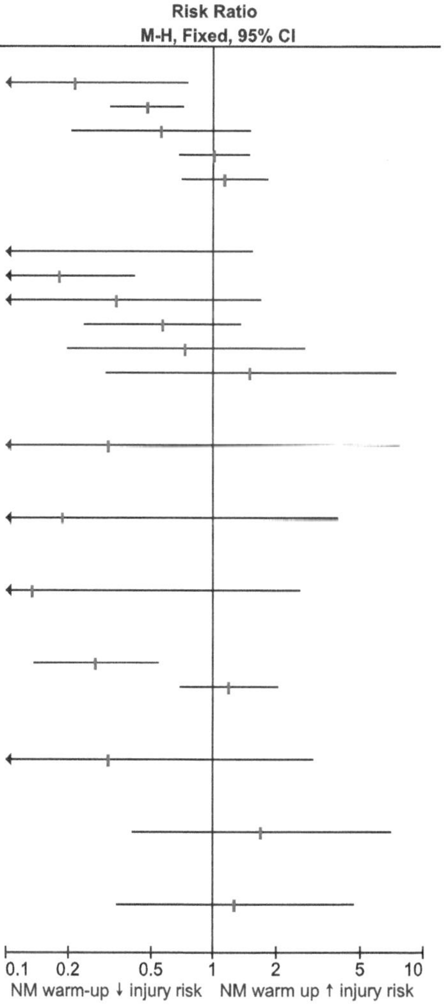

Figure 4 Forest plot graph demonstrating risk ratios for the effectiveness of neuromuscular warm-up strategies in preventing knee injuries.

Study or Subgroup	NM warm-up programme Events	NM warm-up programme Total	Control Events	Control Total	Risk Ratio M-H, Fixed, 95% CI
1.4.1 Medial tibial stress syndrome					
'The 11+' (Soligard 2008)	9	1055	12	837	0.60 [0.25, 1.41]
PTP (Brusøj 2008)	23	507	25	513	0.93 [0.54, 1.62]
1.4.2 Ankle (undefined)					
'The 11+' (Soligard 2008)	51	1055	52	837	0.78 [0.53, 1.13]
'The 11' (Steffen 2008)	79	1091	74	1001	0.98 [0.72, 1.33]
1.4.3 Ankle sprain					
'KIPP' (LaBella 2011)	7	737	17	755	0.42 [0.18, 1.01]
PTP (Brusøj 2008)	18	507	15	513	1.21 [0.62, 2.38]
1.4.4 Achilles					
PTP (Brusøj 2008)	9	507	3	513	3.04 [0.83, 11.15]

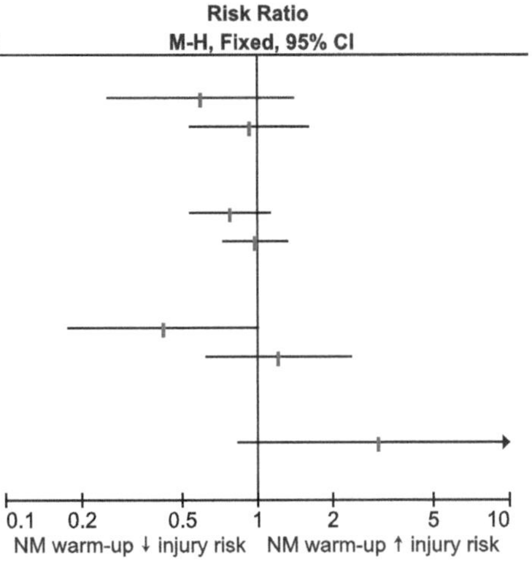

Figure 5 Forest plot graph demonstrating risk ratios for the effectiveness of neuromuscular warm-up strategies in preventing lower leg and knee injuries.

Discussion

This systematic review investigated the effectiveness of neuromuscular warm-up strategies for injury prevention. Based on available data a number of strategies appear to be effective in preventing lower limb injuries. Specifically, 'The 11+' [31] strategy may reduce overall and overuse lower limb injuries in young amateur female footballers; the 'KIPP' [30] strategy may reduce non-contact overall and overuse lower limb injuries in young amateur female basketball and volleyball players, the PEP strategy [26,28] may reduce ACL injuries in young amateur female footballers; and the AKP PTP [33] may reduce the incidence of overuse anterior knee pain in young male and female military recruits.

Study Analysis

The quality assessment criteria revealed that the studies had various methodological weaknesses affecting their internal validity. Firstly, sample sizes were often too low to evaluate specific injuries (for example, ankle sprains). If evaluating the effectiveness of neuromuscular warm-up programmes on more specific injuries, sample size calculations prior to commencement and recruitment of larger samples are recommended. Additionally, future studies should ensure blinding of assessors, concealment of treatment allocation, intention to treat analysis and more adequate randomization procedures to reduce the impact of issues relating to internal validity. External validity was also limited, in particular the applicability of the findings to age groups other than between 13 and 26 years.

There is also a need to determine the mechanism of effectiveness of neuromuscular warm-up strategies and determine whether injury reduction is the result of each individual component or due to a combination of exercises. No studies were identified which compared two different components or combinations of neuromuscular warm-up strategies and, in general, programmes targeted varying risk factors associated with a variety of specific injuries. Addressing this through further research will enable more emphasis on effective components of injury-specific interventions and facilitate the development of more successful neuromuscular warm-up strategies for injury prevention, specifically in reference to specific lower limb injuries.

There is limited homogeneity between the prevention strategies and the methods of recording injury incidence, making data pooling for meta-analysis inappropriate. Injury incidence was reported by a certified athletic trainer [28], a coach [26,27,30-32], an author [29,34] and participant self-reporting [33]. This may have led to a difference in the incidence of injury reporting due to the individuals' medical understanding of an injury. For example, the participants who are self-reporting may be less likely to complain of an injury perhaps due to a lack of medical insurance, compared to the author who, incidentally, is an orthopaedic consultant. The duration of the prevention strategies were 12 weeks [27,28,34], 14 weeks [33], eight months [31,32], nine months [29], and one [30] and two years [26]. Currently, it is unclear how these differences may have impacted outcomes. Further research is needed to determine the minimum participation period needed to provide protection against injury. The prevention strategies were not performed before every training session in the studies by Steffen *et al.* [32], Gilchrist *et al.* [28], LaBella *et al.* [30], Kiani *et al.* [29] and Brushøj *et al.* [34]. This potentially allowed other warm up strategies to confound any benefits of the neuromuscular training exercises and conversely for optimal effects not to be realized.

Adverse effects were only noted in four studies [26,28,31,33] and should be recorded more frequently in future studies. Those mentioned include muscle soreness at the introduction of the study [26], one minor hamstring strain [31] and one fractured tibia/fibula from falling over a ball while jumping over it [28]. It is important for studies to directly question participants about adverse effects so that safe, as well as effective, strategies are established.

Total incidence of lower limb injuries

The effectiveness of three neuromuscular warm-up strategies in preventing the total number of lower limb injuries was evaluated in studies included in this review. Of these, only 'The 11+' [31] and KIPP [30] were found to be effective, both reducing the risk of undefined lower limb and overuse lower limb injuries. The two strategies found to be ineffective were 'The 11' [32] and the PTP [34]. In the case of the 'The 11' [32] lack of effectiveness may be explained by poor compliance. 'The 11' [32] was only used in 52% of training sessions, most likely because of a seven-week summer break during the study. The training may have had an additive effect that was lost when detraining over this period and the number of teams using the strategy after this period dropped from 60% to 44%. The authors concluded that better compliance was needed for sufficient training effects to reduce injuries.

The PTP [34] may have been ineffective at reducing lower limb injuries in military recruits due to the sudden increase in intensity of participants' training, the low load of the participants' training and the lack of supervision/training of the soldiers. Additionally, the strategy was of a short duration (12 weeks) and used less technically demanding exercises (including no warm-up, agility or plyometric exercises).

Hip and thigh injuries

Hip and thigh injuries were recorded during the evaluation of two neuromuscular warm-up strategies, 'The 11 +' [31] and 'The 11' [32]. Neither strategy significantly reduced hip or thigh injury rates, most likely because they were not powered to do so. Highlighting this, 'The 11' [32] programme indicated a strong trend toward reduced risk of groin injuries. This would likely have been a significant finding had more participants been recruited. In addition to study power, the components of the strategies may not have been adequate to reveal protection against hip and thigh injuries. A recent review of hamstring injury prevention demonstrates that isometric warm-up exercises, hamstring flexibility and concentric and eccentric strength training may be protective against hamstring injuries [35]. Additionally, core strength is a recognized factor in reducing the risk of injury. Evidence suggests that core muscle weakness may increase the risk of groin strain injuries [36]. Both 'The 11+' [31] and 'The 11' [32] incorporated Nordic hamstring curls for hamstring strength training and plank exercises for core stability. However, the number of repetitions or the frequency of these exercises may have been inadequate to reduce injury rate.

Knee injuries

Knee injury rates were recorded in all of the nine studies, with six of these recording ACL injuries. Based on available data, four neuromuscular warm-up strategies were found to be effective in preventing knee injuries. These included individual studies showing 'The 11+' [31] and 'HarmoKnee' [29] programmes to reduce the risk of undefined knee injuries, the PEP to reduce significantly the risk of both ACL injuries [26] and their recurrence [28] and the AKP PTP [33] to reduce the risk of anterior knee pain development.

Success of the AKP PTP [33] may relate to strategy frequency as it was performed an average of seven times per week, totalling 105 minutes, a higher frequency compared to other studies. In comparison, the PTP [34] demonstrated no reductions in anterior knee pain, and this was used only three times a week totalling 45 minutes.

Despite investigating the same warm-up strategy (that is, the PEP strategy), Mandelbaum *et al.* [26] demonstrated a highly significant reduction in ACL injuries while Gilchrist *et al.* [28] showed only a trend toward risk reduction; a significant risk reduction in ACL injuries during practice, but the overall risk remaining unchanged. Reasons for this are likely to be the result of the study design and methodology. The study undertaken by Mandelbaum *et al.* [26] was a CCT with inherent methodological limitations, while Gilchrist *et al.* [28] performed a RCT providing gold standard evidence. In the study by Mandelbaum *et al.* [26] there was no blinding or randomization which introduced the potential for subject and allocation bias, respectively. Additionally, the authors in the study by Mandelbaum *et al.* [26] informed the intervention football clubs that they would be receiving a strategy to reduce injury and enhance performance. Participants and trainers were, therefore, not blinded and were likely to have been influenced by motivational bias. Of those remaining, one study informed participants of its purpose but did not disclose to which group they had been randomly allocated [27] while the others informed subjects of the purpose in a similar way to Mandelbaum *et al.* [26,28-34].

The PTP [34], and KLIPP [27] programmes did not convey any significant protection against knee injuries.

As previously discussed, this may relate to lack of advice, sudden increase in training and less demanding exercises in the PTP programme [34]. Additionally, the strategy components did not include any running or agility drills, which provide a comprehensive warm-up, and have been included in successful strategies such as 'The 11+' [31]. The KLIPP [27] did incorporate such exercises but their study had inherent methodological limitations. This strategy had the lowest frequency (two times per week) and this may partly explain its lack of effectiveness. The most successful strategies ('The 11+' [31], PEP [26,28] KIPP [30] and AKP PTP [33]) were performed at every training/match session suggesting that the effectiveness of neuromuscular warm-up strategies may depend on a dose-response relationship.

The 'HarmoKnee' [29] programme significantly reduced the risk of knee injuries. However, findings did not indicate a significant reduction in the risk of specific injuries including ACL, MCL, LCL or medial meniscus injuries, despite the intervention group injury numbers being zero for each. This is due to the very low number of injuries identified in the control group, with the number being five or below for each of these specific injuries and NNTs ranging from 146 (ACL injuries) to 729 (medial meniscus injuries). Until larger studies are completed evaluating the 'HarmoKnee' [29] programme, these results must be interpreted with caution. Considering the high costs associated with surgery and rehabilitation following injuries such as an ACL tear, these reduced rates may still be clinically meaningful.

Lower leg and ankle injuries

The effectiveness of four neuromuscular warm-up strategies which did not require additional equipment in preventing lower leg and ankle injuries were evaluated in studies from this review. Based on the results, no neuromuscular warm-up programme was able to reduce lower limb injury risk significantly. However, it should be considered that the KIPP [30] indicated a strong trend toward reduction of the incidence of ankle sprains, with an NNT of 77. Reasons for the prevention of ankle sprain injuries in the KIPP [30] strategy rather than the PTP [34] include the more comprehensive neuromuscular warm-up programme which took longer to perform and included lower repetitions of many more elements as well as dynamic exercises. Additionally, the study by Brushøj *et al.* [34] which evaluated the PTP programme had fundamental methodological flaws as mentioned earlier. No other strategies report significant reductions in lower leg or undefined ankle injuries. The '11+' [31] results showed a trend towards reduced risk of MTSS and undefined ankle injury; however, these were not convincing enough to conclude their effectiveness in injury prevention.

A previous systematic review comparing balance work (using balance boards) and neuromuscular exercises (without balance boards) revealed that ankle sprains were reduced by 36% and 50%, respectively [17]. Additionally, the sensitivity analysis completed in this review indicated that the addition of equipment, in particular balance boards, to warm-up programmes may be effective in reducing ankle injuries. This provides evidence that neuromuscular strategies can reduce ankle injuries. However, the practicality of these programmes may be questioned due to the need for acquisition of additional equipment requiring funding, maintenance and storage. Therefore, many sporting clubs and individuals, particularly in an amateur setting where most sports participation occurs, may consider that implementing such a programme is not worth the effort. In fact, this is the reason studies in our review were excluded if additional equipment were required. To impact on ankle injury prevention across all sports participation to a greater extent, design and evaluation of warm-up programmes which focus on dynamic balance and strengthening without the need for equipment such as balance boards is needed. If successful, this may provide a more practical and cost-effective alternative to using balance boards. Examples may include single leg balance exercises including throwing a ball with a partner and resisting a push from partners, hopping, and squat exercises including with heels raised and one leg squats.

Recommendations

According to the present systematic review, several practical neuromuscular warm-up strategies which do not require additional equipment that is not readily available at the usual amateur competition or training venues are effective to varying degrees at preventing lower limb injuries. However, in some instances a large number of participants would need to undertake a strategy before one injury is prevented. This is the case with the PEP [26] strategy requiring 70 participants to prevent one injury. 'The 11+' [31], 'KIPP' [30] and 'AKP PTP' [33] appear to provide more reasonable NNT values, requiring less than 35 participants to undertake the neuromuscular warm-up strategy to prevent one injury. Of these strategies, the KIPP [30] and '11+' [31] strategies prevent the most injuries with NNTs for overall lower limb injuries being just 18 and 24, respectively.

Importantly, this systematic review highlights several areas that may account for significantly better injury prevention when incorporating neuromuscular warm-up strategies. These include: (1) incorporation of stretching, strengthening and balance exercises, sports-specific agility drills and landing techniques; (2) completing the strategy for longer than three consecutive months; and (3) completing of the strategy at all training sessions. In addition to these programme specifics, further evaluation of the '11+' [31] programme has highlighted the importance of compliance, with high compliance being linked significantly to reduced lower limb injury risk [37].

Directions for Future Research

Further studies need to determine whether 'The 11+' [31], KIPP [30], 'HarmoKnee' [29], AKP PTP [33] and PEP [26,28] programmes are also effective in men, other age groups, and other sports as our review incorporated mainly women and involved only football, basketball, volleyball and military training. It is important to determine whether injury prevention programmes would also be effective if taught to older players who might possess more engrained poor motion patterns. In addition, healthcare professionals are encouraging middle-aged individuals to engage in sports and so research needs to include older individuals who are at a higher risk of sustaining an injury due to changed activity levels. It would also be beneficial to see if 'The 11+' [31], 'KIPP' [30], 'HarmoKnee' [29], PEP [26,28] strategy and AKP PTP [33] could be successfully combined to ultimately recommend a single injury prevention strategy. Finally, we need to know more about the mechanisms of injury prevention of neuromuscular warm-up strategies in order to optimize their effectiveness.

Conclusions

The current systematic review identified five practical neuromuscular warm-up strategies which do not require additional equipment and which may effectively reduce the risk of lower limb injuries. Specifically 'The 11+' reduced overall and overuse lower limb injuries and knee injuries in young amateur female football players, the 'KIPP' reduced non-contact overall and overuse lower limb injuries in young amateur female football and basketball players, the 'HarmoKnee'[29] programme reduced the risk of knee injuries, the 'PEP' strategy reduced the risk of non-contact ACL injury in young amateur female football players and the 'AKPPTP' reduced the risk of anterior knee pain in male and female military recruits. Further research evaluating the effectiveness of these strategies in more varied populations, particularly men and older individuals is now needed. To provide the greatest potential for reduced lower limb injury rates, it is recommended that neuromuscular warm-up strategies incorporate stretching, strengthening and balance exercises, sports-specific agility drills and landing techniques, and are completed for a duration of longer than three consecutive months at all training sessions. Identification of which neuromuscular warm-up strategy components are most beneficial and the mechanisms behind their effectiveness is needed to further reduce lower limb injury risks.

Authors' contributions

KH and CB were the primary initiators of the study while all authors made substantial contributions to data analysis and interpretation. All authors were involved in drafting and revising the manuscript and approved the penultimate version. The final version was approved and submitted by DM.

Competing interests

The authors declare that they have no competing interests.

References

1. Shehab R, Mirabelli M, Gorenflo D, Fetters MD: **Pre-exercise stretching and sports related injuries: knowledge, attitudes and practices.** *Clin J Sport Med* 2006, **16**:228-231.
2. Witvrouw E, Mahieu N, Danneels L: **Stretching and injury prevention: an obscure relationship.** *Sports Med* 2004, **34**:443-449.
3. Thacker SB, Gilchrist J, Stroup DF: **The impact of stretching on sports injury risk: a systematic review of the literature.** *Med Sci Sports Exerc* 2004, **36**:371-378.
4. Andersen JC: **Stretching before and after exercise: effect on muscle soreness and injury risk.** *J Athl Train* 2005, **40**:218-220.
5. Pope RP, Herbert RD, Kirwan JD: **A randomized trial of preexercise stretching for prevention of lower-limb injury.** *Med Sci Sports Exerc* 2000, **32**:271-277.
6. **Barclays survey reveals sports injury rate in the UK.** [http://www.personal.barclays.co.uk/BRC1/jsp/brccontrol?task=popup1group&value=11147&target=_blank&site=pfs].
7. Chief Medical Officer: **2009 Annual Report of the Chief Medical Officer.** London: Department of Health; 2010.
8. James PT, Rigby N, Leach R: **The obesity epidemic, metabolic syndrome and future prevention strategies.** *Eur J Cardiovasc Prev Rehabil* 2004, **11**:3-8.
9. Hübscher M, Zech A, Pfeifer K: **Neuromuscular training for sports injury prevention: a systematic review.** *Med Sci Sports Exerc* 2010, **42**:413-421.
10. van Tulder M, Furlan A, Bombardier C, Bouter L: **Editorial Board of the Cochrane Collaboration Back Review Group. Updated method guidelines for systematic reviews in the Cochrane collaboration back review group.** *Spine* 2003, **28**:1290-1299.
11. Olivo SA, Macedo LG, Gadotti IC, Fuentes J, Stanton T, Magee DJ: **Scales to assess the quality of randomized controlled trials: a systematic review.** *Phys Ther* 2008, **88**:156-175.
12. Olsen OE, Myklebust G, Engebretsen L, Holme I, Bahr R: **Exercises to prevent lower limb injuries in youth sports: cluster randomized controlled trial.** *BMJ* 2005, **330**:449-452.
13. Emery CA, Rose MS, McAllister JR, Meeuwisse WH: **A prevention strategy to reduce the incidence of injury in high school basketball: a cluster randomized controlled trial.** *Clin J Sport Med* 2007, **17**:17-24.
14. Pasanen K, Parkkari J, Pasanen M, Hiilloskorpi H, Mäkinen T, Järvinen M, Kannus P: **Neuromuscular training and the risk of leg injuries in female floorball players: cluster randomised controlled study.** *BMJ* 2008, **337**: a295.
15. Emery CA, Meeuwisse WH: **The effectiveness of a neuromuscular prevention strategy to reduce injuries in youth soccer: a cluster-randomised controlled trial.** *Br J Sports Med* 2010, **44**:555-562.
16. Parkkari J, Taanila H, Suni J, Mattila VM, Ohrankämmen O, Vuorinen P, Kannus P, Pihlajamäki H: **Neuromuscular training with injury prevention counselling to decrease the risk of acute musculoskeletal injury in young men during military service: a population-based, randomised study.** *BMC Med* 2011, **9**:35.
17. Wedderkopp N, Kaltoft M, Lundgaard B, Rosendahl M, Froberg K: **Prevention of injuries in young female players in European team handball. A prospective intervention study.** *Scand J Med Sci Sports* 1999, **9**:41-47.

18. Heidt RS, Sweeterman LM, Carlonas RL, Traub JA, Tekulve FX: **Avoidance of soccer injuries with preseason conditioning.** *Am J Sports Med* 2000, **28**:659-662.
19. McHugh MP, Tyler TF, Mirabella MR, Mullaney MJ, Nicholas SJ: **The effectiveness of a balance training intervention in reducing the incidence of noncontact ankle sprains in high school football players.** *Am J Sports Med* 2000, **35**:1289-1294.
20. Verhagen EA, van Tulder M, van der Beek AJ, Bouter L, van Mechelen W: **An economic evaluation of a proprioceptive balance board training programme for the prevention of ankle sprains in volleyball.** *Br J Sports Med* 2005, **39**:111-115.
21. Steffen K, Bakka HM, Myklebust G, Bahr R: **Performance aspects of an injury prevention program: a ten-week intervention in adolescent female football players.** *Scand J Med Sci Sports* 2008, **18**:596-604.
22. Eisen TC, Danoff JV, Leone JE, Miller TA: **The effects of multiaxial and uniaxial unstable surface balance training in college athletes.** *J Strength Cond Res* 2010, **24**:1740-1745.
23. Lim BO, Lee YS, Kim JG, An KO, Yoo J, Kwon YH: **Effects of sports injury prevention training on the biomechanical risk factors of anterior cruciate ligament injury in high school female basketball players.** *Am J Sports Med* 2009, **7**:1728-1734.
24. Kaminski TW, Buckley BD, Powers ME, Hubbard T, Ortiz C, Mattacola C: **Eff:ct of strength and proprioception training on eversion to inversion strength ratios in subjects with unilateral functional ankle instability.** *Br J Sports Med* 2003, **37**:410-415.
25. Myklebust G, Engebretsen L, Braekken IH, Skjølberg A, Olsen OE, Bahr R: **Prevention of anterior cruciate ligament injuries in female team handball players: a prospective intervention study over three seasons.** *Clin J Sport Med* 2003, **13**:71-78.
26. Mandelbaum BR, Silvers HJ, Watanabe DS, Knarr JF, Thomas SD, Griffin LY, Kirkendall DT, Garrett W: **Effectiveness of a Neuromuscular and Proprioceptive Training Program in Preventing Anterior Cruciate Ligament Injuries in Female Athletes: 2-Year Follow-up.** *Am J Sports Med* 2005, **33**:1003-1010.
27. Pfeiffer RP, Shea KG, Roberts D, Grandstrand S, Bond L: **Lack of effect of a knee ligament injury prevention program on the incidence of noncontact anterior cruciate ligament injury.** *J Bone Joint Surg Am* 2006, **88**:1769-74.
28. Gilchrist J, Mandelbaum BR, Melancon H, Ryan GW, Silvers HJ, Griffin LY, Watanabe DS, Randall WD, Dvorak J: **A randomized controlled trial to prevent noncontact anterior cruciate ligament injury in female collegiate soccer players.** *Am J Sports Med* 2008, **36**:1476-83.
29. Kiani A, Hellquist E, Ahlqvist K, Gedeborg R, Michaélsson K, Byberg L: **Prevention of soccer-related knee injuries in teenaged girls.** *Arch Intern Med* 2010, **170**:43-9.
30. LaBella CR, Huxford MR, Grissom J, Kim KY, Peng J, Christoffel KK: **Effect of neuromuscular warm-up on injuries in female soccer and basketball athletes in urban public high schools: cluster randomized controlled trial.** *Arch Pediatr Adolesc Med* 2011, **165**:1033-40.
31. Soligard T, Myklebust G, Steffen K, Holme I, Silvers H, Bizzini M, Junge A, Dvorak J, Bahr R, Anderson TE: **Comprehensive warm-up programme to prevent injuries in young female footballers: cluster randomised controlled trial.** *BMJ* 2008, **337**:a2469.
32. Steffen K, Myklebust G, Olsen OE, Holme I, Bahr R: **Preventing injuries in female youth football–a cluster-randomized controlled trial.** *Scand J Med Sci Sports* 2008, **18**:605-14.
33. Coppack RJ, Etherington J, Wills AK: **The effects of exercise for the prevention of overuse anterior knee pain: a randomized controlled trial.** *Am J Sports Med* 2011, **39**:940-8.
34. Brushøj C, Larsen K, Albrecht-Beste E, Nielsen MB, Løye F, Hölmich P: **Prevention of Overuse Injuries by a Concurrent Exercise Program in Subjects Exposed to an Increase in Training Load A Randomized Controlled Trial of 1020 Army Recruits.** *Am J Sports Med* 2008, **36**:663-670.
35. Petersen J, Holmich P: **Evidence based prevention of hamstring injuries in sport.** *Br J Sports Med* 2005, **39**:319-323.
36. Maffey L, Emery C: **What are the Risk Factors for Groin Strain Injury in Sport?: A Systematic Review of the Literature.** *Sports Medicine* 2007, **37**:881-894.
37. Soligard T, Nilstad A, Steffen K, Myklebust G, Holme I, Dvorak J, Bahr R, Andersen TE: **Compliance with a comprehensive warm-up programme to prevent injuries in youth football.** *Br J Sports Med* 2010, **44**:787-93.

4

Effect of betaine supplementation on cycling sprint performance

J Luke Pryor[1*], Stuart AS Craig[2] and Thomas Swensen[3]

Abstract

Purpose: To examine the effect of betaine supplementation on cycling sprint performance.

Methods: Sixteen recreationally active subjects (7 females and 9 males) completed three sprint tests, each consisting of four 12 sec efforts against a resistance equal to 5.5% of body weight; efforts were separated by 2.5 min of cycling at zero resistance. Test one established baseline; test two and three were preceded by seven days of daily consumption of 591 ml of a carbohydrate-electrolyte beverage as a placebo or a carbohydrate-electrolyte beverage containing 0.42% betaine (approximately 2.5 grams of betaine a day); half the beverage was consumed in the morning and the other half in the afternoon. We used a double blind random order cross-over design; there was a 3 wk washout between trials two and three. Average and maximum peak and mean power were analyzed with one-way repeated measures ANOVA and, where indicated, a Student Newman-Keuls.

Results: Compared to baseline, betaine ingestion increased average peak power (6.4%; $p < 0.001$), maximum peak power (5.7%; $p < 0.001$), average mean power (5.4%; $p = 0.004$), and maximum mean power (4.4%; $p = 0.004$) for all subjects combined. Compared to placebo, betaine ingestion significantly increased average peak power (3.4%; $p = 0.026$), maximum peak power max (3.8%; $p = 0.007$), average mean power (3.3%; $p = 0.034$), and maximum mean power (3.5%; $p = 0.011$) for all subjects combined. There were no differences between the placebo and baseline trials.

Conclusions: One week of betaine ingestion improved cycling sprint power in recreationally active males and females.

Keywords: Anaerobic power, Ergogenic aid, Creatine, Wingate

Background

Betaine is a nutrient found in a variety of animals, plants, and microorganisms [1]. It is a component of many foods, with whole grains (e.g., wheat, rye), spinach, shellfish and beets [2] being rich sources. As an organic osmolyte, betaine or trimethyl glycine, protects cells under stress, such as dehydration; it is also a source of methyl groups, via the methionine cycle, in many key biochemical pathways [1]. Betaine, therefore, plays an important role in several aspects of human health and nutrition and studies show that diets high in betaine decrease disease risk [1,3-5].

In addition to improving health, betaine may also improve sport performance. Since betaine is an osmolyte that protects cells under stress [6,7], initial studies on the potential ergogenicity focused on the acute effects of betaine ingestion on performance in the heat [8,9]. In one study, subjects ran in a heated environment (31.1°C) for 75 minutes at 65% of VO_2max followed by a performance run at 84% of VO_2max to volitional exhaustion [8]. Time to exhaustion was 16 to 21% (32 to 38 sec) greater when beverages with betaine or betaine and carbohydrate were consumed, respectively, but the changes were statistically insignificant ($p \geq 0.12$). In the other study, subjects completed a 15 min cycling time trial after riding for 2 hr at 60-75% VO_2max in the heat [9]; immediately after the time trial, isometric leg strength was also examined. Acute consumption of either a carbohydrate or a betaine and carbohydrate beverage before

* Correspondence: john.pryor@uconn.edu
[1]Department of Kinesiology, University of Connecticut, Storrs, CT 06269, U-1110, USA
Full list of author information is available at the end of the article

the test improved time trial performance by 10 and 14%, respectively, relative to a water control trial; there was no difference between the carbohydrate and carbohydrate and betaine trials. Isometric leg strength, however, was significantly greater after the betaine trials compared to the non-betaine trials.

This latter result catalyzed a series of inquires on the chronic effects of betaine ingestion (2 weeks) on various indices of strength and power [10,11]. The assumption being that since betaine is a methyl donor [1], it could theoretically boost creatine stores in the musculature, and therefore, improve strength and power [10]. Chronic betaine ingestion (at least 2.5 $g{\cdot}d^{-1}$ for 14 d) significantly improved bench press repetitions, volume load, throw power, isometric bench press force, vertical jump power, isometric squat force, and muscle endurance during a squat exercise [10-12]. Despite enhancing the aforementioned indices of lower extremity strength and power, chronic betaine ingestion did not improve Wingate anaerobic power [10]. The inability of betaine to enhance cycling sprint performance, as measured with the Wingate anaerobic power test, may be related to the duration of the test and the amount of recovery between trials. Perhaps the 30 sec Wingate test and the 5 min recovery period between trials were too long to fully assess betaine's putative ability to enhance sport specific strength and power, both of which contribute significantly to Wingate performance. A series of shorter work bouts interspersed with shorter periods of active recovery may be a more applicable test of betaine's potential to enhance anaerobic power while cycling. To that end, our purpose was to examine the effect of one week of betaine ingestion on anaerobic power as measured with a series of four, 12 sec work bouts on the cycle ergometer.

Methods

Subjects

Sixteen college-aged males (n = 9) and females (n = 7) volunteered to participate in this study; their mean ± SD for age, height, and weight were: 19 ± 0.8 y, 172 ± 12.0 cm, and 75 ± 14.9 kg and morphological data are present in Table 1. All subjects were free of lower body musculoskeletal injury and reported no limitations to exercise. Subjects were informed of the experimental procedures and known risks, and signed an informed consent approved by the Ithaca College Human Subjects Review Board prior to participation.

Table 1 Body Composition

Variable	Baseline	Placebo	Betaine
Body Weight (kg)	75.1 ± 14.9	74.9 ± 14.9	75.4 ± 14.9
Free Fat Mass (kg)	60.1 ± 14.6	59.8 ± 14.6	59.7 ± 14.5
Fat Mass (kg)	15.0 ± 0.3	15.1 ± 0.3	15.7 ± 0.4
Percent Fat Mass	20.1 ± 10.5	20.2 ± 10.4	20.9 ± 10.9
Total Body Water (kg)	44.0 ± 10.7	43.8 ± 10.7	43.7 ± 10.6

Data are mean ± SD

* $p < 0.05$ compared to corresponding baseline value

# $p < 0.05$ compared to corresponding placebo value

Experimental design

This investigation examined the effects of two drink solutions on cycling sprint performance with a double blind cross-over design. The placebo was a commercial carbohydrate-electrolyte beverage (Wegmans MVP), whereas the same carbohydrate-electrolyte beverage with 2.5 g of betaine (minimum purity is 99%; BetaPower™ DuPont Nutrition & Health, Tarrytown, NY) was the experimental drink. Since betaine is colorless and tasteless, subjects could not differentiate between the two solutions. Furthermore, to ensure drink anonymity, all cap ties were broken prior to consumption. Subjects completed three cycling sprint tests, the first of which served as a baseline measure. Subjects were match-paired based upon maximum peak power and assigned to consume either the placebo or betaine beverage. They were instructed to consume approximately half (295 mL) of their respective beverage twice a day for seven days, after which they were tested again. The last drink was consumed the morning of the test day and all testing sessions took place in the evening. Following a three-week washout phase, a second seven day supplementation period with the opposite beverage occurred followed by the third testing session. Prior to every laboratory session, we used the Tanita 350 bioimedance body fat analyzer to assess the subjects' weight, total body water, fat free mass, and percent body fat (BF 350; Tanita Corporation of America, Inc. Arlington Heights, IL). This unit is valid and reliable [13-16].

Performance testing

Prior to every sprint test, subjects pedaled at a self-selected pace against a light resistance for 5 min to warm up with two to three interspersed sprints of short duration. The sprint test followed which consisted of four, 12 sec work bouts on a Monark 834 E ergometer (Varberg, Sweden) against a resistance equal to 5.5% of body weight. Each work bout was separated by 2.5 min of cycling at zero resistance. At the completion of the test, subjects continued to pedal at zero resistance for 2.5 min to cool down. The ergometer was equipped with toe clips, seat height was standardized for each subject to allow for 10-15° of knee flexion, and vigorous verbal encouragement was provided for all tests. SMI Power software (Sports Medicine Industries, St. Cloud, MN) interfaced with the ergometer with an OptoSensor 2000 infrared sensor (Sports Medicine Industries, St. Cloud, MN) collected data every second. The sensor was calibrated before every testing session.

The following variables were measured during each sprint test: average peak power, maximum peak power, average mean power, and maximum mean power. Average peak and average mean power were calculated across the four work bouts in each sprint test; maximum peak and mean power were the highest values for the respective variables in any sprint test. Peak power was calculated as the highest power output over any five-second interval during a sprint test. The coefficient of variation for average peak power, maximum peak power, average mean power, and maximum mean power across two tests completed on separate days was assessed in a series of pilot studies (n = 6) and were 1.3, 1.8, 1.3, and 1.6%, respectively.

Statistical analyses

Data were analyzed using one-way repeated measures ANOVA. Where indicated, a Student Newman-Kuels test was used to identify specific differences (SigmaPlot v11, Systat Software Inc, San Jose, CA); alpha was set at 0.05 for all tests. Data are presented as mean ± SD.

Results

Based on the mean and SD for maximum peak power from the pilot study and an a priori assumption that a 4% change in power pre- to post-supplementation is meaningful, we used GPOWER software (Bonn, FRG) to determine that a sample size of 14 was needed to give us a power of 0.80 with an alpha of 0.05. Table 2 shows the mean and SD for average peak power, maximum peak power, average mean power and maximum mean power. Figures 1, 2, and 3 demonstrate mean and peak power across trials and gender. Compared to baseline, betaine ingestion increased average peak power (6.4%; $p < 0.001$), maximum peak power (5.7%; $p < 0.001$), average mean power (5.4%; $p = 0.004$), and maximum mean power (4.4%; $p = 0.004$) for all subjects combined. Compared to placebo, betaine ingestion significantly increased average peak power (3.4%; $p = 0.026$), maximum peak power (3.8%; $p = 0.007$), average mean power (3.3%; $p = 0.034$), and maximum mean power (3.5%; $p = 0.011$) for all subjects combined. There were no differences between the placebo and baseline trials. There were no differences across time or between conditions for any of the body composition variables.

Table 2 Combined power (watts) comparison for all subjects

Variable	Baseline	Placebo	Betaine
Peak Power			
Average	608 ± 140	626 ± 133	647 ± 144*#
Maximum	644 ± 144	656 ± 141	681 ± 145*#
Mean Power			
Average	560 ± 133	571 ± 126	590 ± 138*#
Maximum	596 ± 138	601 ± 131	622 ± 141*#

Data are mean ± SD

* $p < 0.05$ compared to corresponding baseline value

# $p < 0.05$ compared to corresponding placebo value

Discussion

Our purpose was to examine the effect of one week of betaine ingestion on anaerobic power as measured with a series of four, 12 sec work bouts. We found that one week of betaine ingestion (2.5 $g \cdot d^{-1}$) improved sprint performance by 5.5 ± 0.8% compared to baseline and 3.5 ± 0.2% compared to the carbohydrate placebo. These results contrast with data from Hoffman et al. [10], who reported daily consumption of 2.5 grams of betaine mixed with a commercially available carbohydrate beverage for 15 days did not enhance peak power, mean power, rate of fatigue, or total work across two Wingate trials separated by 5 min of active rest. One likely explanation for some of the difference in the results between the studies is the nature of the sprint test. Our subjects completed more sprints (4 vs. 2) of a shorter duration (12 vs. 30 sec) that were interspersed with shorter periods of active recovery (2.5 vs. 5 min) relative to the subjects in Hoffman et al. [10]. Experimental design may also account for some of the difference between the studies. Hoffman et al. [10] used a randomized repeated measures design, whereas we used a cross-over repeated measures design. Cross-over designs reduce the effects of confounding covariates and are more efficient statistically.

The likely mechanisms behind the increased power output we measured are related to methylation and osmolyte effects. Betaine supplementation may have elevated intramuscular creatine stores, increased muscle growth, or protected the muscle cells from stress-induced damage. The creatine hypothesis is attractive and supported by studies on betaine metabolism. In short, the liver enzyme betaine homocysteine methyltransferase transfers a methyl group from betaine to homocysteine, thereby producing dimethylglycine and methionine. The latter is then converted to S-adenosylmethionine (SAM), which subsequently acts as a methyl donor during creatine synthesis [17]. Studies show that betaine ingestion increases serum methionine, while betaine injection increases red blood cell SAM concentrations [18,19]. Our observed changes in sprint performance, moreover, are consistent with the performance effects of creatine supplementation, as shown in a meta-analysis [20]. Across 100 studies, creatine supplementation improved performance parameters by 5.7 ± 0.5% compared to baseline, whereas corresponding placebo effects were 2.4 ± 0.4%. More specifically, the meta-analysis showed that creatine supplementation improved lower extremity power by 5.6 ± 0.6% relative to baseline, which is similar to the 5.5 ± 0.8% increase we measured.

It is unlikely, however, that the amount of betaine consumed by our subjects (2.5 $g \cdot d^{-1}$ for 7 d) elicits the same

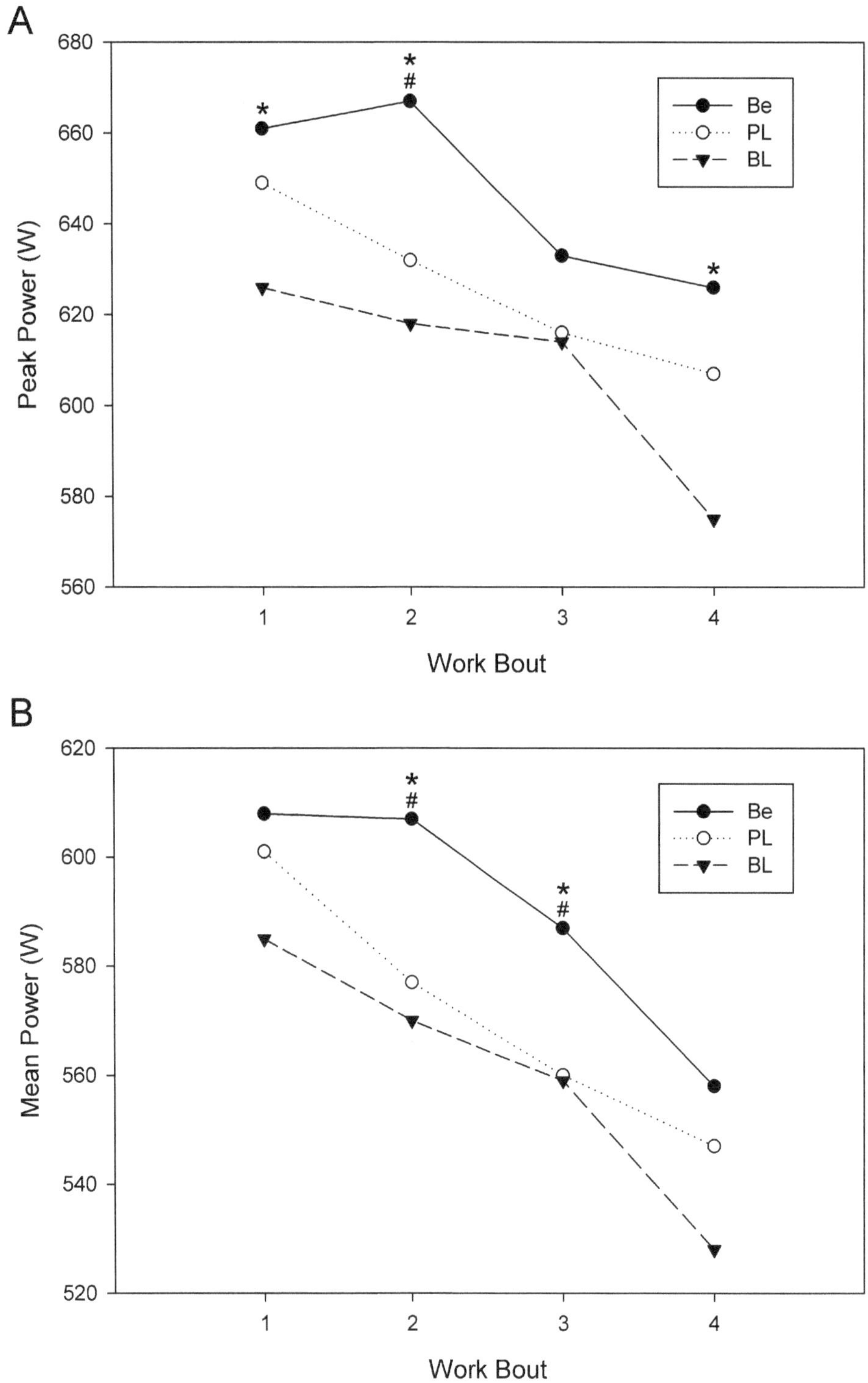

Figure 1 Individual cycle runs power comparison for all subjects. A: peak power; B: mean power. * $p < 0.05$ compared to corresponding baseline value. # $p < 0.05$ compared to corresponding placebo value. W = watts, BL = baseline, PL = placebo, Be = betaine.

effect as the typical daily dosage of creatine during the loading phase of approximately 25 grams. This conjecture is supported by recently published data showing that 2 $g{\cdot}d^{-1}$ of betaine for 10 day did not increase phosphorylcreatine levels compared to 20 $g{\cdot}d^{-1}$ of creatine for 10 day [21]. This study also showed that betaine supplementation did not increase squat and bench press 1 RM or bench and squat power, findings that are

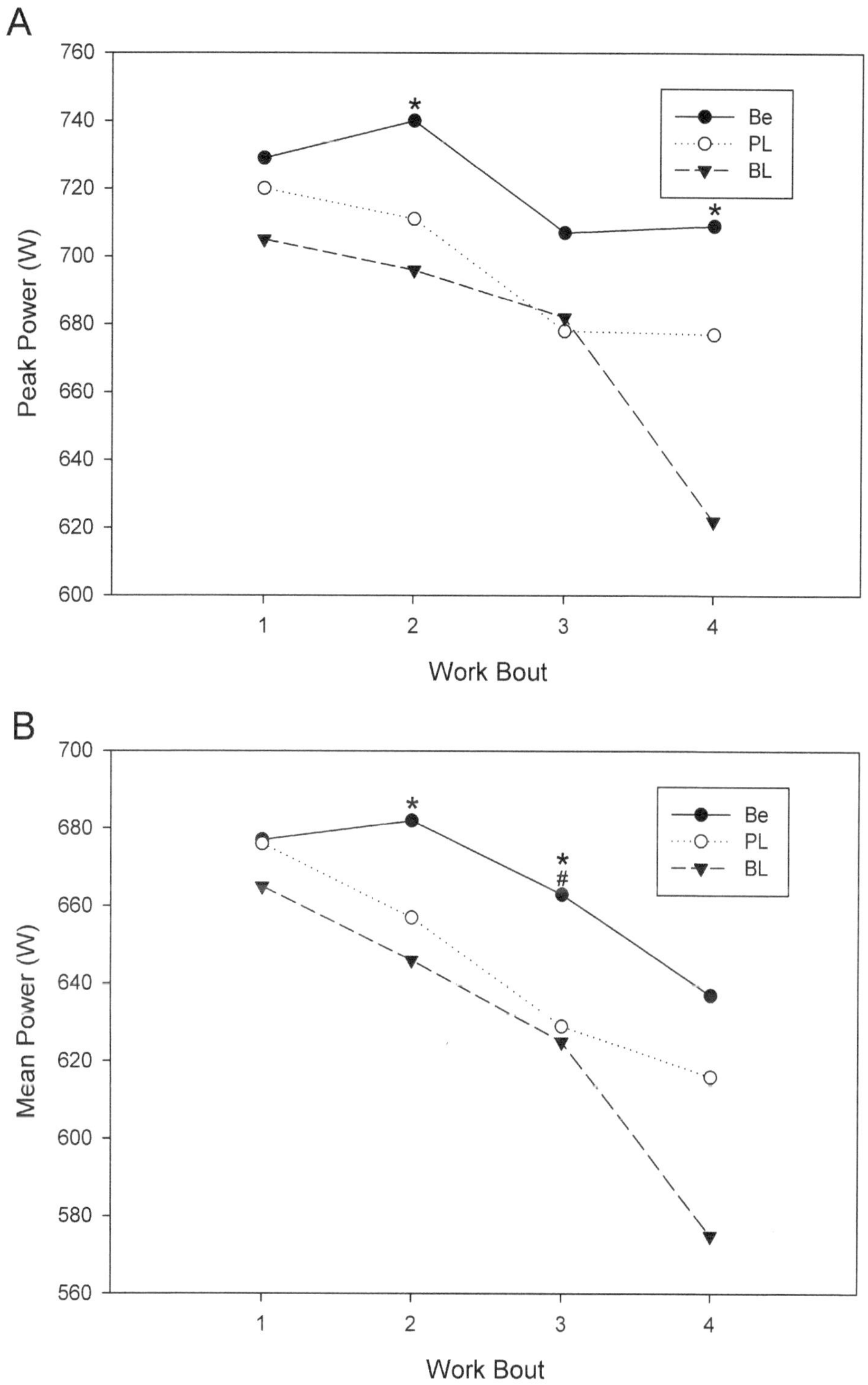

Figure 2 Individual cycle runs power comparison for males. A: peak power; B: mean power. * $p < 0.05$ compared to corresponding baseline value. # $p < 0.05$ compared to corresponding placebo value. W = watts, BL = baseline, PL = placebo, Be = betaine.

inconsistent with data from earlier studies [10-12]. Direct comparison among the studies is difficult. Betaine dosage was lower in the recent study (2 vs 2.5 $g \cdot d^{-1}$), supplementation time was shorter (10 vs 15 d) and power output was not assessed until 3-5 d after supplementation ended compared to immediately afterwards [10,11].

Last, betaine supplementation may have enhanced sprint performance by acting as an osmolyte to maintain

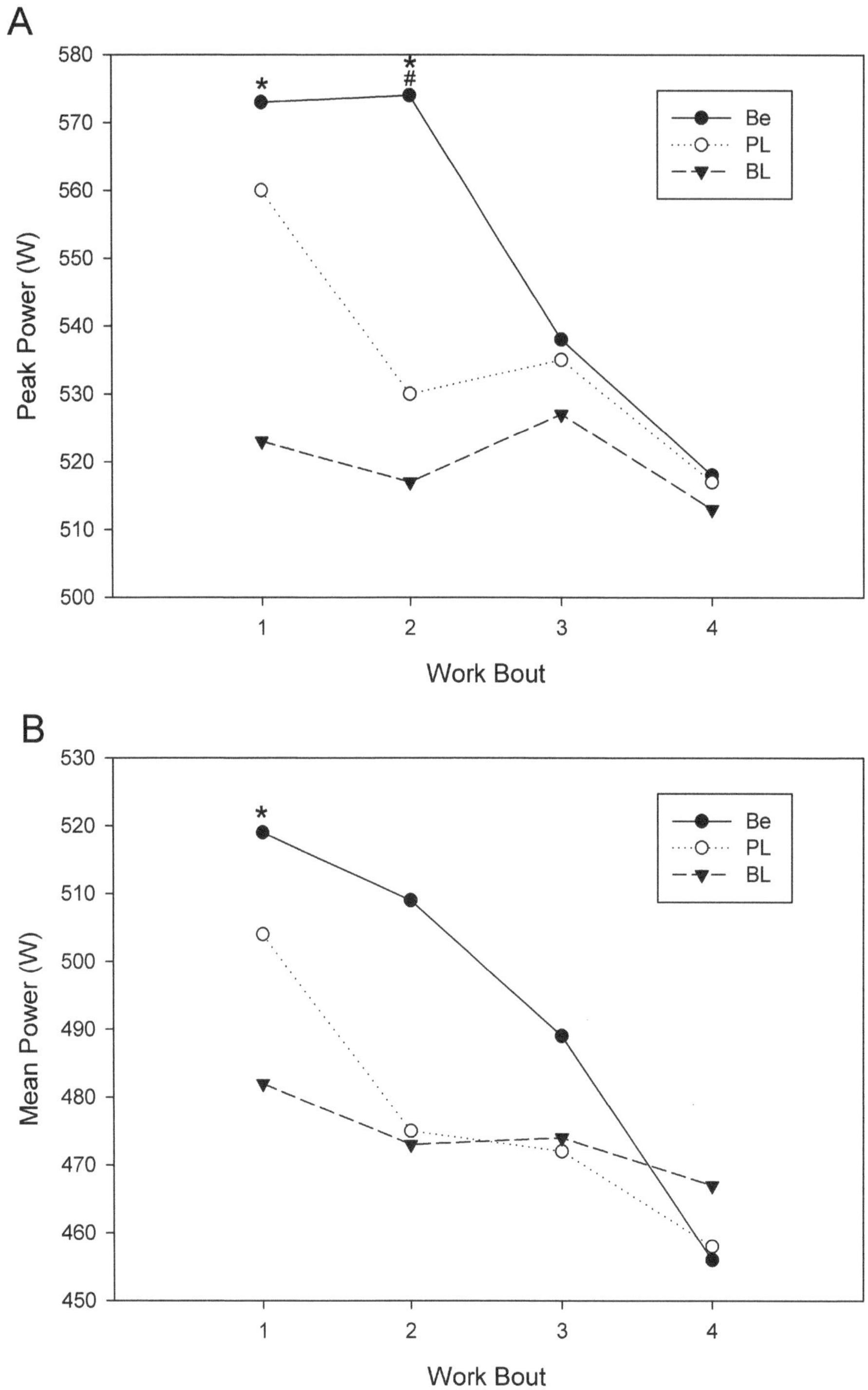

Figure 3 Individual cycle runs power comparison for females. A: peak power; B: mean power. * $p < 0.05$ compared to corresponding baseline value. # $p < 0.05$ compared to corresponding placebo value. W = watts, BL = baseline, PL = placebo, Be = betaine.

cell hydration and function under stress more effectively than placebo. Organic osmolytes are accumulated in cells when tissues are subjected to stress [6,22]. They help cells maintain optimal osmotic pressure, and allow proteins to maintain native folded conformation and stability without perturbing other cellular processes. Betaine helps maintain cell homeostasis by preventing formation of stress granules and keeping the mRNA associated machineries going under chronic hypertonicity [23]. Betaine is one of the most effective osmolytes, shown to facilitate a protective monolayer of water around biopolymers, enhance muscle cell survival and protein synthesis, and maintain myosin ATPase activity during periods of stress [24-26]. It may be that any or all of the aforementioned roles of betaine contributed to the 5.5% increase in power we observed.

Conclusion

We found that one week of betaine supplementation increased peak and mean anaerobic power by approximately 5.5% compared to baseline measures in recreationally active college age men and women. The magnitude of this change is similar to the change in anaerobic power following creatine supplementation. Future research should elucidate the mechanism of improved performance via betaine supplementation.

Acknowledgements

DuPont Nutrition & Health provided the BetaPower™ for the study. Authors would like to thank Michael Aoun for supplying the carbohydrate-electrolyte drink and Riana R. Pryor for her assistance with the study.

Author details

[1]Department of Kinesiology, University of Connecticut, Storrs, CT 06269, U-1110, USA. [2]DuPont Nutrition & Health, Tarrytown, NY, USA. [3]Ithaca College, Ithaca, NY, USA.

Authors' contributions

JLP participated in drafting, editing, and submitting the manuscript. SASC assisted with study design, statistical analysis and critically reviewed the manuscript for intellectual content. TS supervised the research group, ran the statistical analysis, interpreted data, and was involved with manuscript drafting. All authors read and approved the final manuscript.

Competing interests

JLP and TS declare that they have no competing interests and will not benefit from the results of the present study. SASC is an employee of DuPont Nutrition & Health. Publication of these findings should not be viewed as endorsement by the investigators, Ithaca College, the University of Connecticut, or the editorial board of the Journal of the International Society of Sport Nutrition.

References

1. Craig SAS: **Betaine in human nutrition.** *Am J Clin Nutr* 2004, **80**:539-549.
2. Zeisel SH, Mar MH, Howe JC, Holden JM: **Concentrations of choline-containing compounds and betaine in common foods.** *J Nutr* 2003, **133**:1302-1307.
3. Konstantinova SV, Tell GS, Vollset SE, Nygard O, Bleie O, Ueland PM: **Divergent associations of plasma choline and betaine with components of metabolic syndrome in middle age and elderly men and women.** *J Nutr* 2008, **138**:914-920.
4. Cho E, Willett WC, Colditz GA, Fuchs CS, Wu K, Chan AT, Zeisel SH, Giovannucci EL: **Dietary choline and betaine and the risk of distal colorectal adenoma in women.** *J Natl Cancer Inst* 2007, **99**:1224-1231.
5. Shaw GM, Carmichael SL, Yang W, Selvin S, Schaffer DM: **Periconceptional dietary intake of choline and betaine and neural tube defects in offspring.** *Am J Epidemiol* 2004, **160**:102-109.
6. Yancey PH, Clark ME, Hand SC, Bowlus RD, Somero GN: **Living with water stress: evolution of osmolyte systems.** *Science* 1982, **217**:1214-1222.
7. Cronje P: **Heat stress in livestock - role of the gut in its aetiology and a potential role for betaine in its alleviation.** *Recent Adv Anim Nutr Aust* 2005, **15**:107-122.
8. Armstrong LE, Casa DJ, Roti MW, Lee EC, Craig SAS, Sutherland JW, Fiala KA, Maresh CM: **Influence of betaine consumption on strenuous running and sprinting in a hot environment.** *J Strength Cond Res* 2008, **22**:851-860.
9. Millard-Stafford M, Warren GL, Hitchcock KM, Welling RL, Rosskopf LB, Snow TK: **Fluid replacement in the heat - effects of betaine.** *Med Sci Sports Exerc* 2005, **37**:S28.
10. Hoffman JR, Ratamess NA, Kang J, Rashti SL, Faigenbaum AD: **Effect of betaine supplementation on power performance and fatigue.** *J Int Soc Sports Nutr* 2009, **6**:7-17.
11. Lee EL, Maresh CM, Kraemer WJ, Yamamoto LM, Hatfield DL, Bailey BL, Armstrong LE, Volek JS, McDermott BP, Craig SAS: **Ergogenic effects of betaine supplementation on strength and power performance.** *J Int Soc Sports Nutr* 2010, **7**:27.
12. Trepanowski JF, Farney TM, McCarthy CG, Schilling BK, Craig SA, Bloomer RJ: **The effects of chronic betaine supplementation on exercise performance, skeletal muscle oxygen saturation, and associated biochemical parameters in resistance trained men.** *J Strength Cond Res* 2011, **25**:3461-3471.
13. Tyrrell VJ, Richards G, Hofman P, Gillies GF, Robinson E, Cutfield WS: **Foot-to-foot bioelectrical impedance analysis: a valuable tool for the measurement of body composition in children.** *Int J Obes* 2001, **25**:273-278.
14. Utter AC, Nieman DC, Ward AN, Butterworth DE: **Use of the leg-to-leg bioelectrical impedance method in assessing body composition change in obese women.** *Am J Clin Nutr* 1999, **69**:603-607.
15. Swartz AM, Evan MJ, King GA, Thompson DL: **Evaluation of a foot-to-foot bioelectrical impedance analyser in highly active, moderately active and less active young men.** *Br J Nutr* 2002, **88**:205-210.
16. Parker L, Reilly JJ, Christine S, Wells JCK, Pitsiladis Y: **Validity of six field and laboratory methods for measurement of body composition in boys.** *Obes Res* 2003, **11**:852-858.
17. du Vigneaud V, Simmonds S, Chandler JP, Cohn M: **A further investigation of the role of betaine in transmethylation reactions in vivo.** *J Biol Chem* 1946, **165**:639-648.
18. Storch KJ, Wagner DA, Young VR: **Methionine kinetics in adult men: effects of dietary betaine on L-[2H3-methyl-1-13C]methionine.** *Am J Clin Nutr* 1991, **54**:386-394.
19. Wise CK, Cooney CA, Ali SF, Poirier LA: **Measuring S-adenosylmethionine in whole blood, red blood cells and cultured cells using a fast preparation method and high-performance liquid chromatography.** *J Chromatogr B Biomed Sci Appl* 1997, **696**:145-152.
20. Branch JD: **Effect of creatine supplementation on body composition and performance: a meta-analysis.** *Int J Sport Nutr Exerc Metab* 2003, **13**:198-226.
21. Del Favero S, Roschel H, Artioli G, Ugrinowitsch C, Tricoli V, Costa A, Barroso R, Negrelli AL, Otaduy MC, da Costa Leite C, Lancha-Junior AH, Gualano B: **Creatine but not betaine supplementation increases muscle phosphorylcreatine content and strength performance.** *Amino Acids* 2011, doi: 10.1007/s00726-011-0972-5.
22. Kumar R: **Role of naturally occurring osmolytes in protein folding and stability.** *Arch Biochem Biophys* 2009, **491**:1-6.
23. Bounedjah O, Hamon L, Savarin P, Desdorges B, Curmi PA, Pastre D: **Macromolecular crowding regulates the assembly of mRNA stress granules after osmotic stress: a new role for compatible osmolytes.** *J Biol Chem* 2011, doi: 10.1074/jbc.M111.292748 jbc.M111.292748.
24. Ueland PM: **Choline and betaine in health and disease.** *J Inherit Metab Dis* 2011, **34**:3-15.
25. Kraemer WJ, Bailey BL, Clark JE, Apicella J, Lee EC, Comstock BE, Dunn-Lewis C, Volek J, Kupchak B, Anderson JM, Craig SAS, Mares CM: **The influence of betaine supplementation on work performance and endocrine function in men [abstract].** *J Strength Cond Res* 2011, **25**: s100-s101.
26. Brigotti M, Petronini P, Carnicelli D, Alfieri R, Bonelli M, Borghetti A, Wheeler K: **Effects of osmolarity, ions and compatible osmolytes on cell-free protein synthesis.** *Biochem J* 2003, **369**:369-374.

5

Substantial and reversible brain gray matter reduction but no acute brain lesions in ultramarathon runners: experience from the TransEurope-FootRace Project

Wolfgang Freund[1*†], Sonja Faust[1†], Frank Birklein[2], Christian Gaser[3], Arthur P Wunderlich[1], Marguerite Müller[1], Christian Billich[1], Markus S Juchems[1], Bernd L Schmitz[5], Georg Grön[4] and Uwe H Schütz[1,6]

Abstract

Background: During the extremely challenging 4,487 km ultramarathon TransEurope-FootRace 2009, runners showed considerable reduction of body weight. The effects of this endurance run on brain volume changes but also possible formation of brain edema or new lesions were explored by repeated magnetic resonance imaging (MRI) studies.

Methods: A total of 15 runners signed an informed consent to participate in this study of planned brain scans before, twice during, and about 8 months after the race. Because of dropouts, global gray matter volume analysis could only be performed in ten runners covering three timepoints, and in seven runners who also had a follow-up scan. Scanning was performed on three identical 1.5 T Siemens MAGNETOM Avanto scanners, two of them located at our university. The third MRI scanner with identical sequence parameters was a mobile MRI unit escorting the runners. Volumetric 3D datasets were acquired using a magnetization prepared rapid acquisition gradient echo (MPRAGE) sequence. Additionally, diffusion-weighted (DWI) and fluid attenuated inversion recovery (FLAIR) imaging was performed.

Results: Average global gray matter volume as well as body weight significantly decreased by 6% during the race. After 8 months, gray matter volume returned to baseline as well as body weight. No new brain lesions were detected by DWI or FLAIR imaging.

Conclusions: Physiological brain volume reduction during aging is less than 0.2% per year. Therefore a volume reduction of about 6% during the 2 months of extreme running appears to be substantial. The reconstitution in global volume measures after 8 months shows the process to be reversible. As possible mechanisms we discuss loss of protein, hypercortisolism and hyponatremia to account for both substantiality and reversibility of gray matter volume reductions. Reversible brain volume reduction during an ultramarathon suggests that extreme running might serve as a model to investigate possible mechanisms of transient brain volume changes. However, despite massive metabolic load, we found no new lesions in trained athletes participating in a multistage ultramarathon.

See related commentary http://www.biomedcentral.com/1741-7015/10/171

Keywords: body weight, brain volume, catabolism, DWI, lesion, MRI, ultramarathon

* Correspondence: freund-ulm@t-online.de
† Contributed equally
[1]Department of Diagnostic and Interventional Radiology, University Hospitals Ulm, Albert-Einstein-Allee 23, 89081 Ulm, Germany
Full list of author information is available at the end of the article

Background

In 2009 (19 April to 21 June) the TransEurope-FootRace 2009 (TEFR09) took place. It was the second European transcontinental multistage ultramarathon race and covered the distance from the south of Italy (Bari) to the North Cape [1,2]. A group of 67 endurance athletes with a mean age of 50.7 years ranging from 26 to 74 and encompassing 11 women and 56 men from 12 nations met the challenge. Their goal was to run 4,487 km (2,788 miles) in 64 days without a rest day. Therefore, they planned to complete an average distance of 70.1 km daily, that is, 1.7 marathon distances per day (minimum: 44 km/day, maximum: 95.1 km/day) for 64 consecutive days [1].

Brain lesions due to marathon running can be caused by many reasons. Some possible etiologies are facts, some are hypotheses derived from specific observations: exercise-associated hyponatremia in marathon runners is well known [3-5] and has been observed in a substantial fraction of long distance runners [6] and may lead to acute encephalopathy and brain edema [7]. Hyponatremia possibly arises from sodium loss caused by sweat and excessive drinking, inadequate suppression of antidiuretic hormone and inadequate mobilization of sodium from internal stores [5], sequestration of water during the run and sudden inflow of water after cessation of the run. This process can be accentuated by the widespread use of non-steroidal anti-inflammatory drugs among long distance runners [8]. Fatal cases of brain edema after a marathon run have been reported [6,7]. Edema in high altitude sickness has recently been reattributed to free radicals rather than hypoxic disruption of the brain barrier [9], so this form of edema might also arise in exhausting exercise in normal altitudes. Exertion can also lead to arterial hypertension, which has been linked to reversible posterior brain edema [10-12].

Disturbances of intravascular coagulation known to happen in marathon runners [13,14] may induce cerebral embolism. Also, brain lesions caused by prolonged asystoles due to 'athlete's heart' have been described [15].

Magnetic resonance imaging (MRI) is the most appropriate method for brain imaging. White matter changes detected by MRI are thought to be clinically relevant [16]. While visual rating scales have been widely used, lesion volume is thought to be more sensitive [17].

In contrast to brain lesions, brain atrophy is a normal physiological process, occurring mainly in the gray matter (GM) with rates from 0.11% [18] to 0.18% per year [19]. Brain atrophy is accelerated up to 2% per year in patients with Alzheimer's disease [20,21]. Also, brain atrophy is increased in patients with multiple sclerosis [22] or Huntington's disease [23], in which illness-related processes may cause brain atrophy. Patients with malnutrition syndromes such as anorexia nervosa [24], kwashiorkor [25] or alcoholism [26] have been shown to exhibit brain volume reduction, which is reversible by therapy [25-29]. The exact mechanism for the observed brain volume reduction is still not fully understood [24,25,28,30,31].

For exercise, no reports on accelerated brain atrophy exist. So far, moderate exercise has been reported to even prevent cognitive decline [32].

As expected from previous experiences from ultraendurance events [33-35] showing massive energy deficits with loss of fat and muscle mass, our TEFR09 participants also showed signs of a strong catabolic burden indicated by a considerable reduction of body weight (Figure 1).

Therefore, using repeated MRI measurements we investigated changes in global gray matter volumes, which were expected due to metabolic changes such as the energy deficit associated with long distance running. Furthermore, based on previous reports we performed lesion detection MRI to investigate the athletes' brains for edema or lesions.

Methods

Subjects

After approval of the local ethics committee (University of Ulm, decision 78/08-UBB/se) and in accordance with the Declaration of Helsinki, athletes without any contraindications to MRI were recruited after signing an informed consent. A total of 15 participants were initially enrolled into this natural study. We had planned to scan their brains before, twice during, and 8 months after the race. Due to the strong challenge and ensuing phenomena of fatigue, the compliance of runners to participate in MRI in the evening after a day of running was reduced and resulted in dropouts, such that the data of only a reduced number of runners could be included into the analysis. We carried out a global volumetric analysis with ten athletes covering three timepoints, and a second analysis with seven runners who also had the follow-up at timepoint 4, that is, 8 months after the end of the race.

All members of the ten-subject group (see Table 1) were men, with a mean age of 48.8 years (SD 12.7). Body weight was taken (always measured in the morning before breakfast) with a Tanita BC-545 BIA scale (Arlington Heights, IL, USA) to the nearest 0.1 kg. At the beginning of the race, their mean body weight was 73.6 kg (SD 6.6). Training data were collected with a custom-made questionnaire asking for training distances and times, races completed and results from these races. In the year preceding the race the ten runners had a mean training distance of 6,142 km (SD 2,367 km). Per week they performed a mean training distance of 118.3 km (SD 45.0 km) with a mean training duration of 12.9 hours/week (SD 3.4 h) and a mean training velocity of 8.8 km/h (SD 1.5 km/h).

The dropout of three runners from this group who were not able to participate in the follow-up did not substantially change the distribution of the above-mentioned

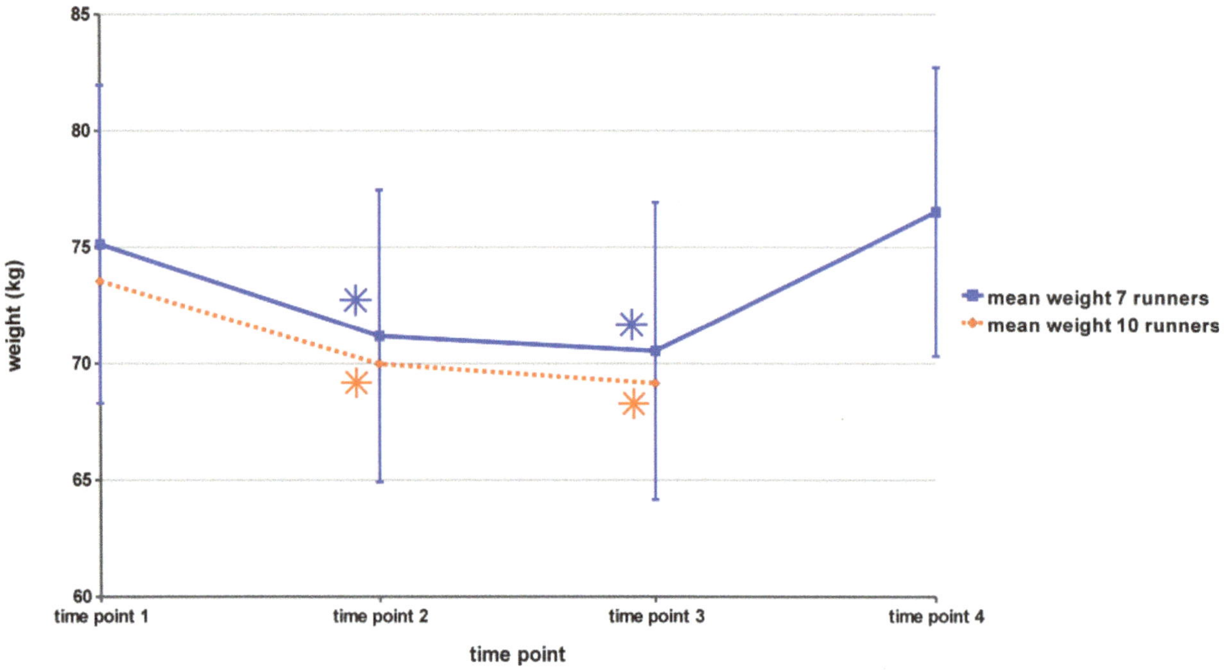

Figure 1 Mean body weight of the participating group of TransEurope-FootRace 2009 (TEFR09) athletes. Error bars denote standard deviation; asterisks show statistically significant differences from baseline (timepoint 1).

variables (see Table 1). Mean age, body weight and training parameters in the year before the race did not differ significantly.

As will be shown in the results section, both groups were representative for the majority of runners who were willing to provide these biological data.

MRI acquisition protocol

Scanning was performed on three identical 1.5 T Siemens (Erlangen, Germany) MAGNETOM Avanto MRI scanners with identical sequence parameters. Two scanners were located at our university. The third was a mobile MRI unit mounted on a truck escorting the runners [2]. The sequence parameters are given in Table 2, resulting in an isotropic resolution of 1 × 1 × 1 mm for the volumetric data.

Scanning was performed in the afternoon or evening after the completion of the daily stage, because the time schedules of the athletes would not permit other times (start in the early morning and running for 6 to 10 h). During this running time the scanner was moved to a new position at the new night quarters.

Study design

The first examination (timepoint 1) took place before the start of the race. Timepoints 2 and 3 were examined at 2,400 km and 4,000 km and the follow-up was performed at an average of 8 months after the end of race.

Table 1 Biometrical data of the study participants before the start of the TransEurope-FootRace 2009 (TEFR09)

Parameter	Seven-subject group	Ten-subject group	Non-study group (n = 34)	*P* value of difference (10 vs 34)	*P* value of difference (7 vs 34)
Age in years	51.1 (11.5)	48.8 (12.7)	50.4 (10.2)	0.693	0.867
Height, m	1.78 (0.04)	1.79 (0.04)	1.74 (0.08)	0.072	0.202
Weight at start, kg	75.1 (6.8)	73.6 (6.6)	69.9 (10.0)	0.285	0.196
Pre-race training, km/year	6,513 (2,689)	6,142 (2,367)	5,355 (1,620)	0.230	0.132
Pre-race training, km/week	125.8 (51.5)	118.3 (45.0)	103.0 (30.4)	0.214	0.117
Pre-race training, h/week	13.5 (3.8)	12.9 (3.4)	12.6 (3.2)	0.771	0.491
Pre-race mean velocity, km/h	8.8 (1.3)	8.8 (1.5)	8.2 (1.4)	0.207	0.266

Values are given as mean (SD).

Table 2 Magnetic resonance imaging (MRI) parameters of the sequences used in the study

Sequence parameters	MPRAGE	DWI EPI	FLAIR
TR (repetition time, ms)	2,100	3,700	9,000
TE (echo time, ms)	4.8	98	120
TI (inversion time, ms)	1,060	-	2,500
FA (flip angle, °)	15	90	150
NA (no. of acquisitions)	1	2	1
ETL (echo train length)	-	-	21
Bandwidth (Hz/voxel)	139	1,000	150
Slice thickness (mm)	1	5	5
Orientation	Sagittal	Transversal	Coronal
Matrix (interpolated from)	240 × 256	128 × 128	384 × 384 (187 × 187)
FOV (field of view, mm)	240 × 256	230 × 230	172 × 230
TA (time of acquisition)	8 min 25 s	1 min 4 s	2 min 24 s

Magnetization prepared rapid acquisition gradient echo (MPRAGE), diffusion-weighted echoplanar imaging (DWI EPI) and fluid attenuated inversion recovery (FLAIR) were used.

Image interpretation of the diffusion-weighted imaging (DWI) and fluid-attenuated inversion recovery (FLAIR) images

Two readers (experienced radiologists WF and UHS) independently interpreted the scans. To facilitate comparison between the scans, the images were read chronologically and new or old lesions were differentiated.

The DWI echoplanar imaging (EPI) sequence was read in the b1,000 weighting to search for focal or more diffuse diffusion restriction as a sign of intracellular edema. The FLAIR sequence was read to search for focal or diffuse signal alteration as a sign of edema or lesion.

The lesion volume of the three largest lesions was estimated by multiplication of the perpendicular diameters. If the lesion was only visible on one slice, the diameter perpendicular to the slice orientation was estimated by the mean of the two other diameters.

Statistical analysis of DWI and FLAIR image interpretation

Means and standard deviations and t tests (paired for the comparison of timepoints) were calculated using MS excel functions (Microsoft Office Excel 2003; Microsoft Corporation, Redmond, WA, USA). Results with $P < 0.05$ were considered as significant. Correlation tests were computed to look for significant correlation of the number of lesions and biometrical (weight, height or age) or sports-associated parameters (training intensity or participation in ultramarathons).

Inter-rater reliability

For rating of the number of lesions in DWI and FLAIR, the inter-rater reliability was analyzed.

Taking into account the critique of Bland and Altman [36] concerning the correlation coefficients to calculate the inter-rater reliability, we decided to use the parameter lambda as proposed by Jepsen *et al.* [37]. Lambda can be calculated as follows:

$$\lambda = \frac{2 \cdot VAR_X - VAR_D}{2 \cdot VAR_X}$$

Where VAR denotes the variance of the measurements X and D the difference between measurements of the two raters. The inter-rater reliability is rated as low for $\lambda < 0.25$. Values up to 0.5 are rated as fair, 0.5 to 0.75 as moderate to good and $\lambda > 0.75$ demonstrates good to excellent inter-rater reliability [38].

Data analysis of volumetric data from the magnetization prepared rapid acquisition gradient echo (MPRAGE) images

Analysis was performed with the software package SPM8 [39] including the VBM8 toolbox [40]. Preprocessing of imaging data before the statistical analysis was carried out using a specific batch for longitudinal data as implemented in VBM8. Individual T1 images were first aligned first to a T1 template in MNI-space (Montreal Neurological Institute) in order to bring them in a common reference frame with respect to translation and rotation. A mean image was calculated from these realigned images and a first realignment of raw data followed enclosing this mean image as a reference. At this stage individual images were bias corrected to account for signal inhomogeneities. The resulting images were segmented into GM, white matter (WM) and cerebrospinal fluid (CSF) using a Maximum-A-Posteriori technique and a partial volume estimation (PVE) [41].

In order to estimate global tissue volumes we estimated the sum of local tissue values across the whole brain. Global GM volumes across different timepoints were then tested on significant changes using an analysis of variance for repeated measurements. In case of a significant effect of factor 'time' global GM volume changes between timepoints were tested employing Newman-Keuls *post hoc* tests at the nominal level of α of P <0.05. To assess the stability of measurements among different scanners, total intracranial volume was measured in addition, computed as the sum of GM, WM, and total CSF volume. Ideally, this parameter should remain constant over time thereby indicating that measurements were not confounded by the necessary use of different scanners and that no systematic errors were imported into volume analysis.

Results

At the second timepoint runners had finished 2,475 km on average, and 4,001 km at timepoint 3. The average time between the follow-up measurement and the end of the race was 256 days. Due to constraints imposed by the demanding running as well as scanning schedules, not every runner was able to attend every session (see Tables 1 and 3), and thus the numbers scanned varied.

Biometrical data

As reference we had obtained biometrical data from a major sample of further 34 runners willing to provide these data (see Table 1). Comparing the group of ten participants included into the volumetric study to this major sample showed that biometrical data did not significantly differ, suggesting that the ten-subject group reflects a representative subsample of the entire runners group. Also the sample of 7 subjects who had participated in volumetric follow-up measurements was still representative for the major sample of 34 runners with respect to the same biometrical data (see Table 1).

Changes of body weight during and after the TEFR09

The mean body weight of the study subjects decreased during the run (see Table 4).

For both groups (N = 10 with timepoints 1 to 3 and out of these N = 7 who also attended follow-up) two different analyses of variance were computed to test on significant weight losses over time. For each group there was a significant main effect of 'time' (ten-subject (10s) group: F (2,18) = 34.19; P <0.0001; seven-subject (7s) group: F (3,18) = 28.42; P <0.0001). *Post hoc* tests in both groups showed significant weight losses and a regain of weight at follow-up (see Table 4 and Figure 1).

Changes of global gray matter volumes and total intracranial volume during and after the TEFR09

The mean global GM volume of the 10s group (see Table 4 and Figure 2) was 671.7 ml (SD 46.1) for timepoint 1, 645.5 ml (38.6) for timepoint 2 and 630.7 ml (49.4) for timepoint 3. The mean global GM volume of the 7s group runners (with follow-up) was 670.0 ml (SD 38.1) for timepoint 1, 642.9 ml (38.8) at timepoint 2, 630.5 ml (42.6) at timepoint 3 and 671.1 ml (19.5) at timepoint 4 (follow-up). For the 10s group and 7s group (with follow-up), two different analyses of variance were computed to test on significant global GM volume changes over time. Both analyses revealed a significant main effect of 'time' (10s group: F(2,18) = 18.76; P <0.0001; 7s group: F(3,18) = 10.70; P <0.001). For both the 10s group and the 7s group significant GM volume losses between timepoints and a regain at follow-up could be demonstrated (see Table 4 and Figure 2).

Total intracranial volume (TICV), however, showed no substantial changes over time. Absolute values for timepoints 1 to 3 for the 10s group were: 1,589.0 ml (SD 92.1), 1,586.6 ml (SD 93.7) and 1,584.4 ml (SD 93.1), respectively. At timepoint 4 TICV for the 7s group was 1,592.8 ml (SD 76.8). As for the analysis of GM volume changes, two different analyses of variance were computed to test on significant TICV changes over time. There were no significant effects of 'time' in the 10s group with three timepoints (F(2,18) = 2.29; P = 0.130) or in the 7s group with four timepoints (F(3,18) = 1.91; P = 0.165).

The TICV difference between timepoints 1 and 2 for the 10s group was -2.4 ml (SD 6.7), equaling 0.15% of the total intracranial volume. Between timepoint 1 and

Table 3 Lesion statistics from serial fluid-attenuated inversion recovery (FLAIR) imaging

Comparisons	No. of new lesions	No. of subjects	t Test	*P* value
t1 to t2	-0.08 (0.82)	12	-0.35	0.732
t2 to t3	-0.36 (0.64)	11	-1.90	0.087
t3 to t4	0.17 (0.52)	6	0.79	0.465
	Volume change of lesions			
t1 to t2	54.9 (247.4)	12	0.77	0.458
t2 to t3	38.3 (116.9)	11	1.09	0.302
t3 to t4	-100.42 (237.7)	6	-1.03	0.348

t1 = timepoint 1, start of the race; t2 = timepoint 2, after an average distance of 2,326 km; t3 = timepoint 3, after an average distance of 4,005 km from t1; t4 = timepoint 4, follow-up measurements around 8 months after finishing the race. No. of new lesions = across participants averaged number of new lesions (SD) observed between two consecutive timepoints. No. of subjects = number of subjects with two consecutive FLAIR measurements to enter a paired t test. Volume change of lesions = for calculation of lesion volumes see Methods section, shown is the difference between averaged sums of lesion volumes obtained at two consecutive timepoints, units are mm^3.

Table 4 Evolution of weight and gray matter (GM) brain volume during the TransEurope-FootRace 2009 (TEFR09)

Parameter	Weight in kg, 7s group	GM volume in ml, 7s group	Weight in kg, 10s group	GM volume in ml, 10s group
Timepoint 1, start	75.1 (6.8)	670.0 (38.1)	73.6 (6.6)	671.7 (46.1)
Timepoint 2, 2,400 km	71.2 (6.3)*	642.9 (38.8)**	70.0 (5.8)***	645.5 (38.6)****
Timepoint 3, 4,005 km	70.5 (6.4)*	630.5 (42.6)**	69.2 (5.9)***	630.7 (49.4)****
Timepoint 4, follow-up	76.5 (6.2)*	671.1 (19.5)**	NA	NA
Difference, timepoint 1-2	3.9 (*P* = 0.0002)	27.1 (*P* = 0.006)	3.6 (*P* = 0.0002)	26.2 (*P* = 0.0013)
Difference, timepoint 1-3	4.6 (*P* = 0.0002)	39.5 (*P* = 0.008)	4.4 (*P* = 0.0002)	40.6 (*P* = 0.0002)
Difference, timepoint 2-3	0.7 (0.419)	12.4 (*P* = 0.172)	0.8 (*P* = 0.159)	14.4 (*P* = 0.042)
Difference, timepoint 4-3	6.0 (*P* = 0.0002)	40.6 (*P* = 0.001)	NA	NA
Difference, timepoint 4-1	1.4 (*P* = 0.092)	1.1 (*P* = 0.898)	NA	NA

Values are mean (SD).

*P <0.0001 analysis of variance for effect of time with F(3,18) = 28.42; **P <0.001 analysis of variance for effect of time with F(3,18) = 10.70; ***P <0.0001 analysis of variance for effect of time with F(2,18) = 34.19; ****P <0.0001 analysis of variance for effect of time with F(2,18) = 18.76.

10s group = ten-subject group; 7s group = seven-subject group; NA = not applicable.

3 the difference was -4.6 ml (SD 7.4) or 0.29% of TICV. For the 7s group the difference between timepoint 1 and 4 was -4.6 ml (6.1) or 0.29%. All differences were non-significant.

Retrospectively, an exploratory analysis of putative white matter changes was computed in the 7s group with all four timepoints. An analysis of variance (ANOVA) revealed a significant effect of 'time' (F(3,18) = 4.34; *P* = 0.018), however it was much smaller than that observed for GM volume changes in this group (see above). *Post hoc* Newman-Keuls tests showed that this effect was merely due to an increase in WM volume of 3.9% from timepoint 1 to 3 (*P* = 0.041) while differences between timepoints 1 and 2 (*P* = 0.152) and between 2 and 3 (*P* = 0.261) were far from significant, as was the difference between timepoints 1 and 4 (*P* = 0.554).

Brain lesions

One FLAIR-weighted imaging dataset was lost, so that the number of subjects in the lesion analysis (last comparison) is smaller than in the volumetric analysis. With DWI, no=lesions were seen before, during or after the run (see Figure 3). With FLAIR imaging, there was a mean of three lesions visible before the start of the run (see Figure 4). However, no new lesions appeared during the run (see Table 3 and Additional file 1, Tables S1-3). Numerically, the mean number of lesions even seemed to decline during the run, whereas the volume of the lesions seemed to increase. However, this is partly due to the high number of lesions in subject 8, who did not attend follow-up. Observed differences were statistically not significant according to paired t tests.

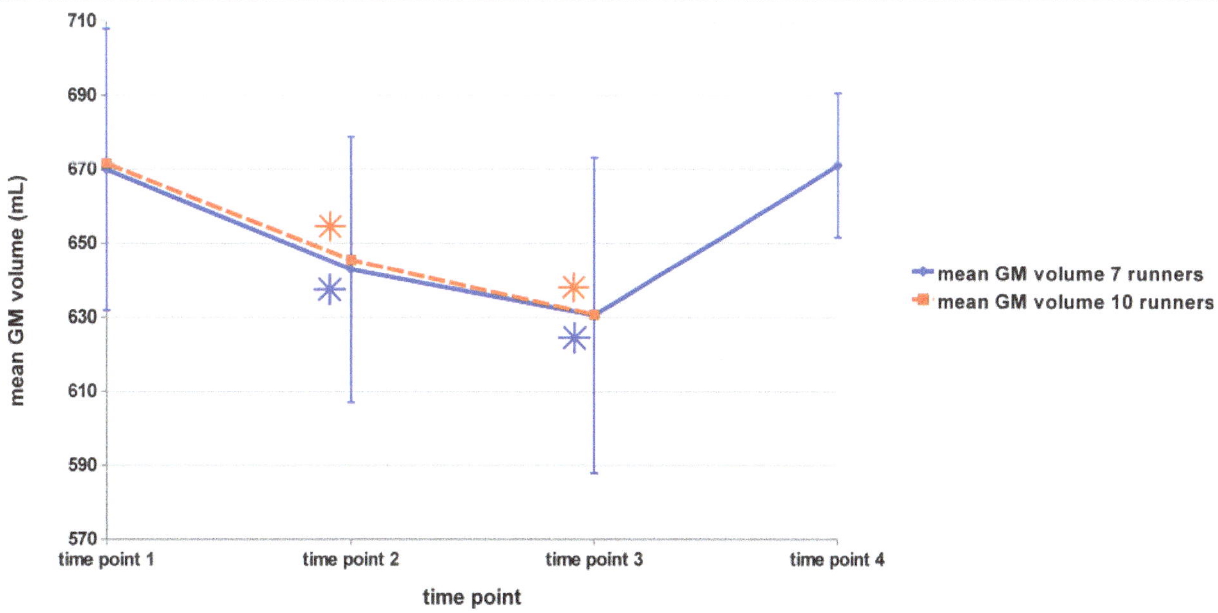

Figure 2 Mean global gray matter (GM) volume of the participating group of TransEurope-FootRace 2009 (TEFR09) athletes. Error bars denote standard deviation; asterisks show statistically significant differences from baseline (timepoint 1).

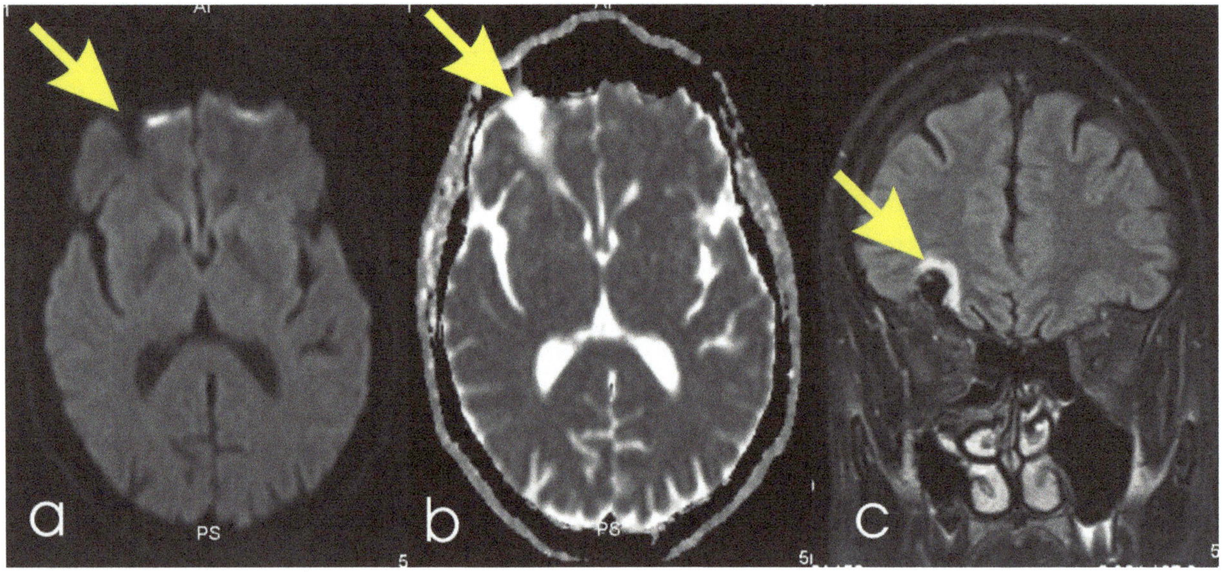

Figure 3 Exemplary slides of the sequences used to detect brain lesions. **(A)** Axial diffusion-weighted imaging, b1,000. The arrow points to an older postcontusional brain lesion. **(B)** Axial apparent diffusion coefficient map. The arrow points to the same lesion as in (A). **(C)** Coronal fluid attenuated inversion recovery (FLAIR) image. The arrow points to the same lesion as in (A).

There was no statistically significant correlation between the numbers of lesions observed and biometrical (weight, height or age) or sports-associated parameters (training intensity or participation in ultramarathons).

Inter-rater reliability

With diffusion-weighted imaging, there were no lesions recorded. Therefore, inter-rater reliability could not be calculated. For FLAIR, the numbers of lesions detected by both raters were nearly identical, so that calculated λ was 0.99.

Discussion

The main finding of our study was a global GM volume decrease during participation in an ultramarathon. This change was paralleled by a decreasing body weight. Both changes reversed to the baseline when measured about 8 months after the end of the race. DWI and FLAIR imaging revealed no new brain lesions during the race.

Observed loss in GM volume of about 6% during the 2 months of the race would equal (assuming linearity) an annual rate of 36%, and therefore appears substantial when compared with annual rates of volume losses associated

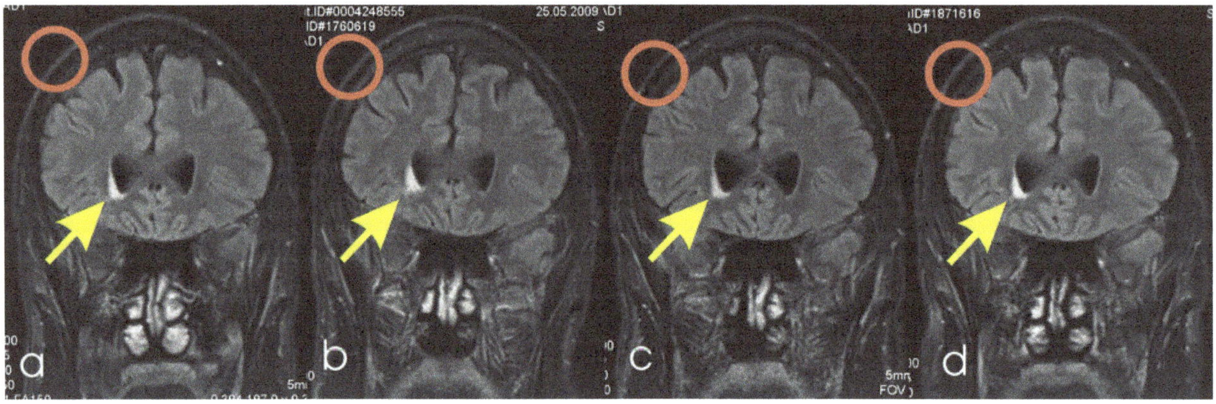

Figure 4 A lesion followed over time. Coronal fluid attenuated inversion recovery (FLAIR) image. The arrow points to a small periventricular lesion. The lesion shows no difference during the time course. However, the thickness of the subcutaneous fat layer (see red circle) shows a marked decrease from (A-C) and recovery at (D). **(A)** Timepoint 1 before the TransEurope-FootRace 2009 (TEFR09) in April 2009; **(B)** timepoint 2 during the race at 2,326 km; **(C)** timepoint 3 during the race at 4,005 km; **(D)** timepoint 4 at follow-up 8 months after the race.

with natural processes: aging leads to volume reductions of GM of less than 0.2% annually [18,19], Alzheimer's disease shows up to 2% loss per year [20], and multiple sclerosis leads to annual atrophy rates of about 0.5% [42]. At present, we can only speculate about the reasons that may be responsible for the observed loss in GM volume although the search for possible factors is constrained by two imminent characteristics: a substantial reduction during ultramarathon activity that was reversible upon follow-up. Therefore, possible factors should be consistent with this observation, especially reversibility of volume reduction.

Among the various factors causing brain volume changes [43], some major causes such as intake of alcohol or toxic substances can certainly be ruled out. Other factors such as inflammation and edema, changes in electrolyte balance, vascular permeability and dehydration, as well as protein catabolism cannot easily be discarded, and also systemic illnesses and corticosteroids must be taken into account [44]. For example, brain volume loss has been shown in illnesses such as kwashiorkor [25], Cushing's syndrome [45], and anorexia nervosa [29].

Body fat reduction due to the huge energy deficit incurred over the course of the race [46] has been shown in different multistage endurance events [34,35,47]. Besides fat loss, in one report on a multistage ultramarathon over 1,200 km a reduction of muscle mass was also noted [33]. Therefore, catabolism with reduction of fat and muscle mass has to be expected during a multistage ultramarathon and may represent a relevant factor for GM volume loss which is strongly supported by the apparently parallel loss of body weight (see Figure 4).

Under physiological conditions, the brain controls the calorie intake to secure a steady supply of necessary nutrients [48]. However, during phases of catabolism protein loss and hereby reduction of colloidal osmotic pressure and a shift of fluid to the subarachnoid spaces [43] can lead to a shrinkage of the whole brain, which may have contributed to a decrease of GM volume.

Recently it also has been suggested [29] that elevated cortisol levels might be responsible for GM reduction in patients with anorexia nervosa. The volume loss was seemingly reversible with reported recovery [27] after successful treatment. This has also been shown for hypercortisolism-induced brain atrophy [45] and for hippocampal atrophy that appeared reversible after hormone normalization [49]. Interestingly, some recent studies could show that endurance sports increase cortisol levels [50,51]. Hence, among those various conditions associated with GM volume reduction, hypercortisolism appears to be a likely candidate given that daily running with average distances of about 1.7 marathons activates the hypothalamic-pituitary-adrenal (HPA) axis.

Although dehydration has been shown to relate to a brain volume reduction of about 0.55%, which was reversible upon rehydration [52], the extent of these changes does not explain the changes of about 6% in our present study. Furthermore, our athletes were extremely well trained and were sufficiently provided with fluid throughout the entire race. Regardless, hyponatremia has been shown in marathon runners and has been linked to hypotonic encephalopathy [53] or brain edema [7]. However, hyponatremia among multistage ultramarathoners is rare according to a recent report [54], and our analysis of diffusion and T2-weighted MRI images did not show any new lesions or signs of edema in our sample. In presence of an excellent inter-rater reliability we detected only pre-race lesions in FLAIR imaging, representing older lesions (glial scars), which are expected to show up on each ensuing examination. Even though diminishing visibility of edema and glial scars during a phase of hypercortisolism might seem plausible, the numerical decrease of the average number of lesions on FLAIR imaging in our raw data was an artifact due to varying attendance of subjects (see Table 3 and Additional file 1, Tables S1-3 for paired t test comparisons). Therefore no statistically significant variations in the number of lesions were observed.

This absence of the formation of new brain edema also supports that hypoxic disruption of the brain barrier [9], or arterial hypertension (which has been linked to reversible posterior brain edema [10-12] in previous studies) are rather unlikely to have occurred during the race in our subjects included. Similarly, disturbances of intravascular coagulation known to happen in marathon runners [13,14] may produce focal lesions, but no new lesions were detected during the TEFR09 race.

What really distinguishes participants of TEFR09 from leisure athletes normally participating in marathon events is the amount of training they undertake: the TEFR09 participants had run a mean of 5,523 km (SD 1,874 km, range 2,500 km to 11,440 km) in the last year with a training volume of 106.3 km per week (SD 35.3 km/week, range 50 km to 200 km/week) [2]. This reflects a much more extensive training and pre-race running experience compared to participants of normal (half-) marathon distances (for example, average weekly workload of 14 km of a cohort in a previous study on (half-)marathon runners [55]). This difference in training volume has also been reported by others [56] who stated that the emphasis during leisure training is usually more on speed, whereas ultramarathoners focus on duration and thus on endurance. Given their training workload, TEFR09 participants were extremely adapted to the demands of ultramarathon running. This is also supported by the observation that the participants' ultimate goal was completion of the whole multistage race rather than winning single stages. Accordingly, a rather low incidence of exercise-associated hyponatremia in ultramarathoners is reported [33,57] and short term disturbances to the homeostasis of electrolytes or coagulation that may dominate during short race distances in less trained leisure athletes are rather unlikely to have contributed to the present results.

Given our above-mentioned criteria of substantiality and reversibility of present GM volume reductions only a subset of the discussed factors seem more likely than others to have contributed to present results. The loss of proteins as a likely relevant factor is further supported by the apparently strong common variation of body weight and GM volume which both returned to the baseline after 8 months. Furthermore, it is not unlikely that the return to baseline also aligned with hypercortisolism and possibly hyponatremia.

Therefore, further research is needed to find out each factor's contribution and their possible interaction leading to substantial and reversible GM volume loss during very long distance running.

Strengths and limits

The main strength of this study was its unique setting with a naturalistic and continuous observation of ultra-endurance athletes reaching the limits of physical endurance. However, this setup entailed its own limitation since the number of participating athletes was small and attendance varied. Nevertheless, this is the first study to report brain volume changes or possible brain lesions of multistage ultramarathon runners observed during the race with a mobile MRI scanner. Since this truck-mounted scanner was available only for the run, scanning before the race and on follow-up had to be performed on different scanners although these MRI scanners were identical models and used identical sequence parameters. Due to the scanning on different scanners this report is limited to the exploration of global brain volumes, which are thought to be much less sensitive to the problem of using different MRI scanners than voxel based morphometric analyses of regional volume differences. Furthermore, a calculation of total intracranial volume has shown that measurements were nearly identical across the different scanners. Variations of intracranial volumes were statistically insignificant and with 0.3% of the total more than a magnitude less than observed gray matter volume changes of 6%. Also, the results are deemed plausible, since the measurements during the race were performed on the same mobile scanner and the volume decrease continues from timepoint 1 over 2 to 3. This is expected because of the protracted metabolic load during the run. Systematic errors due to the change of the scanner between timepoint 1 and 2 would affect only the first comparison.

Therefore, present results on GM volumes changes over time are thought to be robust, although they had to be acquired on different scanners.

Conclusions

Whereas focal brain lesions and edema have been frequently reported in symptomatic athletes after single marathon runs, in the present study on prospectively observed participants of the multistage ultramarathon TEFR09, no new lesions were detected by serial MRI. It is thought that in well trained individuals, no short-term noxious brain events occur even after repeated loading in a multistage ultramarathon. However, reversible brain volume reduction during an ultramarathon could be shown. Possible mechanisms might be loss of proteins or hypercortisolism. On a larger scale, extreme running may serve as a model to better understand those mechanisms involved in transient brain volume reductions.

Further studies must not only address the exact mechanisms but also the behavioral consequences of these changes. It is possible that these findings might then be useful for the understanding of diseases characterized by (transient) brain volume changes.

Additional material

Additional file 1: Tables S1-3. Table S1: Fluid-attenuated inversion recovery (FLAIR) imaging of brain lesions. Observations from timepoint 1 (t1) to t2; only subjects with two consecutive measurements. The table contains single subject data for FLAIR lesion comparisons between timepoints 1 to 2. Table S2: FLAIR imaging of brain lesions. Observations from t2 to t3; only subjects with two consecutive measurements. The table contains single subject data for FLAIR lesion comparisons between timepoints 2 to 3. Table S3: FLAIR imaging of brain lesions. Observations from t3 to t4; only subjects with two consecutive measurements. The table contains single subject data for FLAIR lesion comparisons between timepoints 3 to 4.

Abbreviations

DWI EPI: diffusion-weighted echoplanar imaging; FLAIR: fluid-attenuated inversion recovery; GM: gray matter; MRI: magnetic resonance imaging; TEFR09: TransEurope-FootRace 2009; TICV: total intracranial volume; WM: white matter.

Authors' contributions

WF proposed and designed the study, read the images, worked on the statistical analysis and wrote the report. SF planned the statistical analysis of the volumetric data and performed it, and wrote parts of the report. FB helped to conceive and plan the study and wrote parts of the paper. CG revised the methodology of the statistical analysis and wrote parts of the paper. APW planned the study and the physical properties of the used sequences and wrote part of the manuscript. MM took part in the statistical analysis and revised the paper. MSJ participated in statistical analysis and wrote parts of the manuscript. BLS planned the study and wrote parts of the manuscript. CB planned the study and sampled data. GG contributed to the statistical analyses of the brain and non-brain data and wrote parts of the report. UHS planned the TEFR09 project and this study and sampled data and read the images. All authors critically revised and approved the final manuscript.

Competing interests

The authors declare that they have no competing interests.

Acknowledgements

This project was mainly supported by the German Research Association (DFG: 'Deutsche Forschungsgemeinschaft'), under grants SCHU 2514/1-1 and SCHU 2514/1-2. Other non-public funds were received from Siemens medical and the Medical Faculty of the University of Ulm. All funding was unrestricted. None of the funding bodies had any role in the study design, data collection, data analysis, data interpretation, manuscript preparation or decision to publish. Heike Wiedelbach and Martin Erhard participated in data acquisition.

Author details

[1]Department of Diagnostic and Interventional Radiology, University Hospitals Ulm, Albert-Einstein-Allee 23, 89081 Ulm, Germany. [2]Department of Neurology, University Medical Centre Mainz, Langenbeckstraße 1/503, 55131 Mainz, Germany. [3]Departments of Psychiatry and Neurology, Jena University Hospital, Jahnstraße 3, 07743 Jena, Germany. [4]Section Neuropsychology and Functional Imaging, University Hospitals Ulm, Leimgrubenweg 12-14, 89073 Ulm, Germany. [5]Section Neuroradiology, University Hospitals Ulm, Albert-Einstein-Allee 23, 89081 Ulm, Germany. [6]Outpatient Rehabilitation Centre at University Hospitals Ulm, Pfarrer-Weiß-Weg 10, 89077 Ulm, Germany.

References

1. Schulze I: *TransEurope-FootRace 2009. Bari-Nordkap - 4.487,7 km in 64 Tagesetappen* Leipzig, Germany: Engelsdorfer Verlag; 2010.
2. Schuetz UH, Schmidt-Trucksäss A, Knechtle B, Machann J, Wiedelbach H, Erhardt M, Freund W, Gröninger S, Brunner H, Schulze I, Brambs HJ, Billich C: **The Transeurope Footrace Project: longitudinal data acquisition in a cluster randomized mobile MRI observational cohort study on 44 endurance runners at a 64-stage 4,486km transcontinental ultramarathon.** *BMC Med* 2012, **10**:78.
3. Almond CS, Shin AY, Fortescue EB, Mannix RC, Wypij D, Binstadt BA, Duncan CN, Olson DP, Salerno AE, Newburger JW, Greenes DS: **Hyponatremia among runners in the Boston Marathon.** *N Engl J Med* 2005, **352**:1550-1556.
4. Levine BD, Thompson PD: **Marathon maladies.** *N Engl J Med* 2005, **352**:1516-1518.
5. Noakes TD, Sharwood K, Speedy D, Hew T, Reid S, Dugas J, Almond C, Wharam P, Weschler L: **Three independent biological mechanisms cause exercise-associated hyponatremia: evidence from 2,135 weighed competitive athletic performances.** *Proc Natl Acad Sci USA* 2005, **102**:18550-18555.
6. Kashyap AS, Anand KP, Kashyap S: **Sudden collapse of a young female cross country runner.** *Br J Sports Med* 2006, **40**:e11.
7. Ayus JC, Varon J, Arieff AI: **Hyponatremia, cerebral edema, and noncardiogenic pulmonary edema in marathon runners.** *Ann Intern Med* 2000, **132**:711-714.
8. Ayus JC: **Sodium and potassium disorders.** In *Textbook of critical care.* Edited by: Shoemaker WC. Philadelphia, PA: WB Saunders; 2000:853-861.
9. Bailey DM, Bartsch P, Knauth M, Baumgartner RW: **Emerging concepts in acute mountain sickness and high-altitude cerebral edema: from the molecular to the morphological.** *Cell Mol Life Sci* 2009, **66**:3583-3594.
10. Decker DA, Falchook AD, Yachnis AT, Waters MF: **Radiographic and pathologic findings in an atypical brainstem variant of reversible posterior leukoencephalopathy syndrome.** *Neurologist* 2009, **15**:364-366.
11. Bartynski WS: **Posterior reversible encephalopathy syndrome, part 1: fundamental imaging and clinical features.** *AJNR Am J Neuroradiol* 2008, **29**:1036-1042.
12. Bartynski WS: **Posterior reversible encephalopathy syndrome, part 2: controversies surrounding pathophysiology of vasogenic edema.** *AJNR Am J Neuroradiol* 2008, **29**:1043-1049.
13. Scobie BA: **Gastrointestinal emergencies with marathon-type running: omental infarction with pancreatitis and liver failure with portal vein thrombosis.** *N Z Med J* 1998, **111**:211-212.
14. Holman ND, Schneider AJ: **Multi-organ damage in exertional heat stroke.** *Neth J Med* 1989, **35**:38-43.
15. Slavich G, Poser S, Antonutto G, Fregolent R, Piccoli G, Enrico di Prampero P: **Prolonged nocturnal asystole and cerebral neurogliosis in a marathon runner.** *J Cardiovasc Med* 2011, **12**:901-903.
16. Pantoni L: **Leukoaraiosis: from an ancient term to an actual marker of poor prognosis.** *Stroke* 2008, **39**:1401-1403.
17. van Straaten EC, Fazekas F, Rostrup E, Scheltens P, Schmidt R, Pantoni L, Inzitari D, Waldemar G, Erkinjuntti T, Mantyla R, Wahlund LO, Barkhof F: **Impact of white matter hyperintensities scoring method on correlations with clinical data: the LADIS study.** *Stroke* 2006, **37**:836-840.
18. Good CD, Johnsrude IS, Ashburner J, Henson RN, Friston KJ, Frackowiak RS: **A voxel-based morphometric study of ageing in 465 normal adult human brains.** *Neuroimage* 2001, **14**:21-36.
19. Smith CD, Chebrolu H, Wekstein DR, Schmitt FA, Markesbery WR: **Age and gender effects on human brain anatomy: a voxel-based morphometric study in healthy elderly.** *Neurobiol Aging* 2007, **28**:1075-1087.
20. O'Brien JT, Paling S, Barber R, Williams ED, Ballard C, McKeith IG, Gholkar A, Crum WR, Rossor MN, Fox NC: **Progressive brain atrophy on serial MRI in dementia with Lewy bodies, AD, and vascular dementia.** *Neurology* 2001, **56**:1386-1388.
21. Fox NC, Crum WR, Scahill RI, Stevens JM, Janssen JC, Rossor MN: **Imaging of onset and progression of Alzheimer's disease with voxel-compression mapping of serial magnetic resonance images.** *Lancet* 2001, **358**:201-205.
22. Rudick RA, Fisher E, Lee JC, Simon J, Jacobs L: **Use of the brain parenchymal fraction to measure whole brain atrophy in relapsing-remitting MS. Multiple Sclerosis Collaborative Research Group.** *Neurology* 1999, **53**:1698-1704.
23. Tabrizi SJ, Scahill RI, Durr A, Roos RA, Leavitt BR, Jones R, Landwehrmeyer GB, Fox NC, Johnson H, Hicks SL, Kennard C, Craufurd D, Frost C, Langbehn DR, Reilmann R, Stout JC: **Biological and clinical changes in premanifest and early stage Huntington's disease in the TRACK-HD study: the 12-month longitudinal analysis.** *Lancet Neurol* 2011, **10**:31-42.
24. Katzman DK, Lambe EK, Mikulis DJ, Ridgley JN, Goldbloom DS, Zipursky RB: **Cerebral gray matter and white matter volume deficits in adolescent girls with anorexia nervosa.** *J Pediatr* 1996, **129**:794-803.
25. Gunston GD, Burkimsher D, Malan H, Sive AA: **Reversible cerebral shrinkage in kwashiorkor: an MRI study.** *Arch Dis Child* 1992, **67**:1030-1032.
26. Geibprasert S, Gallucci M, Krings T: **Alcohol-induced changes in the brain as assessed by MRI and CT.** *Eur Radiol* 2010, **20**:1492-1501.
27. Swayze VW, Andersen AE, Andreasen NC, Arndt S, Sato Y, Ziebell S: **Brain tissue volume segmentation in patients with anorexia nervosa before and after weight normalization.** *Int J Eat Disord* 2003, **33**:33-44.
28. Golden NH, Ashtari M, Kohn MR, Patel M, Jacobson MS, Fletcher A, Shenker IR: **Reversibility of cerebral ventricular enlargement in anorexia nervosa, demonstrated by quantitative magnetic resonance imaging.** *J Pediatr* 1996, **128**:296-301.
29. Castro-Fornieles J, Bargallo N, Lazaro L, Andres S, Falcon C, Plana MT, Junque C: **A cross-sectional and follow up voxel-based morphometric MRI study in adolescent anorexia nervosa.** *J Psychiatr Res* 2009, **43**:331-340.
30. Knudsen L, Drummond PD: **Cold-induced limb pain decreases sensitivity to pressure-pain sensations in the ipsilateral forehead.** *Eur J Pain* 2009, **13**:1023-1029.
31. Van den Eynde F, Treasure J: **Neuroimaging in eating disorders and obesity: implications for research.** *Child Adolesc Psychiatr Clin N Am* 2009, **18**:95-115.
32. Reimers CD, Knapp G, Tettenborn B: **Impact of Physical Activity on Cognition. Can Physical Activity Prevent Dementia?** *Aktuelle Neurologie* 2012, **39**:276-291.
33. Knechtle B, Duff B, Schulze I, Kohler G: **A multi-stage ultra-endurance run over 1,200 km leads to a continuous accumulation of total body water.** *J Sports Sci Med* 2008, **7**:356-364.
34. Knechtle B, Knechtle P, Schuck R, Andonie JL, Kohler G: **Effects of a Deca Iron Triathlon on body composition: a case study.** *Int J Sports Med* 2008, **29**:343-351.
35. Knechtle B, Salas Fraire O, Andonie JL, Kohler G: **Effect of a multistage ultra-endurance triathlon on body composition: World Challenge Deca Iron Triathlon 2006.** *Br J Sports Med* 2008, **42**:121-125.
36. Bland JM, Altman DG: **Statistical methods for assessing agreement between two methods of clinical measurement.** *Lancet* 1986, **1**:307-310.

37. Jepsen JR, Laursen LH, Hagert CG, Kreiner S, Larsen AI: **Diagnostic accuracy of the neurological upper limb examination I: inter-rater reproducibility of selected findings and patterns.** *BMC Neurol* 2006, **6**:8.
38. Portney LG, Watkins MP: **Correlations.** In *Foundations of Clinical Research: Applications to Practice. Volume 23.* Upper Saddle River, NJ: Prentice Hall Health; 2000:491-508.
39. FIL Methods Group: **SPM 8.** [http://www.fil.ion.ucl.ac.uk/spm/software/spm8/].
40. Structural Brain Mapping Group: **VBM8 Toolbox.** [http://dbm.neuro.uni-jena.de/vbm/download/].
41. Tohka J, Zijdenbos A, Evans A: **Fast and robust parameter estimation for statistical partial volume models in brain MRI.** *Neuroimage* 2004, **23**:84-97.
42. Kappos L, Traboulsee A, Constantinescu C, Eralinna JP, Forrestal F, Jongen P, Pollard J, Sandberg-Wollheim M, Sindic C, Stubinski B, Uitdehaag B, Li D: **Long-term subcutaneous interferon beta-1a therapy in patients with relapsing-remitting MS.** *Neurology* 2006, **67**:944-953.
43. Zivadinov R, Reder AT, Filippi M, Minagar A, Stuve O, Lassmann H, Racke MK, Dwyer MG, Frohman EM, Khan O: **Mechanisms of action of disease-modifying agents and brain volume changes in multiple sclerosis.** *Neurology* 2008, **71**:136-144.
44. Jagust WJ, Noseworthy JH: **Brain atrophy as a surrogate marker in MS: faster, simpler, better?** *Neurology* 2000, **54**:782-783.
45. Bourdeau I, Bard C, Noel B, Leclerc I, Cordeau MP, Belair M, Lesage J, Lafontaine L, Lacroix A: **Loss of brain volume in endogenous Cushing's syndrome and its reversibility after correction of hypercortisolism.** *J Clin Endocrinol Metabol* 2002, **87**:1949-1954.
46. Enqvist JK, Mattsson CM, Johansson PH, Brink-Elfegoun T, Bakkman L, Ekblom BT: **Energy turnover during 24 hours and 6 days of adventure racing.** *J Sports Sci* 2010, **28**:947-955.
47. Herbst L, Knechtle B, Lopez CL, Andonie JL, Fraire OS, Kohler G, Rust CA, Rosemann T: **Pacing strategy and change in body composition during a deca iron triathlon.** *Chinese J Physiol* 2011, **54**:255-263.
48. Peters A, Schweiger U, Pellerin L, Hubold C, Oltmanns KM, Conrad M, Schultes B, Born J, Fehm HL: **The selfish brain: competition for energy resources.** *Neurosci Biobehav Rev* 2004, **28**:143-180.
49. Starkman MN, Giordani B, Gebarski SS, Berent S, Schork MA, Schteingart DE: **Decrease in cortisol reverses human hippocampal atrophy following treatment of Cushing's disease.** *Biol Psychiatry* 1999, **46**:1595-1602.
50. Hew-Butler T, Noakes TD, Soldin SJ, Verbalis JG: **Acute changes in endocrine and fluid balance markers during high-intensity, steady-state, and prolonged endurance running: unexpected increases in oxytocin and brain natriuretic peptide during exercise.** *Eur J Endocrinol* 2008, **159**:729-737.
51. Kraemer WJ, Fragala MS, Watson G, Volek JS, Rubin MR, French DN, Maresh CM, Vingren JL, Hatfield DL, Spiering BA, Yu-Ho J, Hughes SL, Case HS, Stuempfle KJ, Lehmann DR, Bailey S, Evans DS: **Hormonal responses to a 160-km race across frozen Alaska.** *Br J Sports Med* 2008, **42**:116-120, discussion 120.
52. Duning T, Kloska S, Steinstrater O, Kugel H, Heindel W, Knecht S: **Dehydration confounds the assessment of brain atrophy.** *Neurology* 2005, **64**:548-550.
53. Siegel AJ, Verbalis JG, Clement S, Mendelson JH, Mello NK, Adner M, Shirey T, Glowacki J, Lee-Lewandrowski E, Lewandrowski KB: **Hyponatremia in marathon runners due to inappropriate arginine vasopressin secretion.** *Am J Med* 2007, **120**:461 e411-467.
54. Knechtle B, Knechtle P, Rust CA, Gnadinger M, Imoberdorf R, Kohler G, Rosemann T, Ballmer P: **Regulation of electrolyte and fluid metabolism in multi-stage ultra-marathoners.** *Horm Metab Res* 2012, **44**:919-926.
55. Freund W, Billich C, Brambs HJ, Weber F, Schuetz UH: **MRI changes of achilles tendon and hindfoot in experienced runners and beginners during training and after a (half)-marathon competition [in German].** *Zeitschrift fur Orthopadie und Unfallchirurgie* 2011, **149**:407-417.
56. Rüst CA, Knechtle B, Knechtle P, Rosemann T: **Similarities and differences in anthropometry and training between recreational male 100-km ultra-marathoners and marathoners.** *J Sports Sci* 2012, **30**:1249-1257.
57. Knechtle B, Knechtle P, Rosemann T: **Low prevalence of exercise-associated hyponatremia in male 100 km ultra-marathon runners in Switzerland.** *Eur J Appl Physiol* 2011, **111**:1007-1016.

6

Exercise therapy for bone and muscle health: an overview of systematic reviews

Kåre Birger Hagen*, Hanne Dagfinrud, Rikke Helene Moe, Nina Østerås, Ingvild Kjeken, Margreth Grotle and Geir Smedslund

Abstract

Background: Musculoskeletal conditions (MSCs) are widely prevalent in present-day society, with resultant high healthcare costs and substantial negative effects on patient health and quality of life. The main aim of this overview was to synthesize evidence from systematic reviews on the effects of exercise therapy (ET) on pain and physical function for patients with MSCs. In addition, the evidence for the effect of ET on disease pathogenesis, and whether particular components of exercise programs are associated with the size of the treatment effects, was also explored.

Methods: We included four common conditions: fibromyalgia (FM), low back pain (LBP), neck pain (NP), and shoulder pain (SP), and four specific musculoskeletal diseases: osteoarthritis (OA), rheumatoid arthritis (RA), ankylosing spondylitis (AS), and osteoporosis (OP). We first included Cochrane reviews with the most recent update being January 2007 or later, and then searched for non-Cochrane reviews published after this date. Pain and physical functioning were selected as primary outcomes.

Results: We identified 9 reviews, comprising a total of 224 trials and 24,059 patients. In addition, one review addressing the effect of exercise on pathogenesis was included. Overall, we found solid evidence supporting ET in the management of MSCs, but there were substantial differences in the level of research evidence between the included diagnostic groups. The standardized mean differences for knee OA, LBP, FM, and SP varied between 0.30 and 0.65 and were significantly in favor of exercise for both pain and function. For NP, hip OA, RA, and AS, the effect estimates were generally smaller and not always significant. There was little or no evidence that ET can influence disease pathogenesis. The only exception was for osteoporosis, where there was evidence that ET increases bone mineral density in postmenopausal women, but no significant effects were found for clinically relevant outcomes (fractures). For LBP and knee OA, there was evidence suggesting that the treatment effect increases with the number of exercise sessions.

Conclusions: There is empirical evidence that ET has beneficial clinical effects for most MSCs. Except for osteoporosis, there seems to be a gap in the understanding of the ways in which ET influences disease mechanisms.

Keywords: fibromyalgia, low back pain, neck pain, shoulder pain, osteoarthritis, rheumatoid arthritis, ankylosing spondylitis, osteoporosis, pain, physical function

Background

Musculoskeletal conditions (MSCs) are common, and have important consequences for the individual and for society. MSCs are the most common cause of severe long-term pain and physical disability, and in Europe, 20 to 30% of adults are affected at any one time [1-3]. It is estimated that MSCs represent nearly 25% of the total cost of illness in Sweden [4], and they are one of the most common causes of health problems limiting work ability [5]. About one in five consultations in primary care are for MSCs, and some of these patients are referred to other health professionals such as physiotherapists, occupational therapists, or chiropractors, to medical specialists such as rheumatologists, or to

* Correspondence: k.b.hagen@medisin.uio.no
National Resource Centre for Rehabilitation in Rheumatology, Department of Rheumatology, Diakonhjemmet Hospital, P.O. Box 23 Vinderen, 0319 Oslo, Norway

orthopedic surgeons. The burden that MSCs create has been recognized by the United Nations and WHO, with their endorsement of the Bone and Joint Decade 2000 to 2010 [6]. The prevalence of many of these conditions increases markedly with age, and many patients also have some common lifestyle factors (obesity, smoking, and physical inactivity). With the increasing number of older people and the ongoing changes in lifestyle, the burden of MSCs and other non-communicable diseases is predicted to increase [7].

MSCs form a heterogeneous group of over 200 different health problems that are linked anatomically and also linked by their association with pain and impaired physical function [8]. They range from conditions of acute onset and short duration to lifelong disorders. For many common MSCs such as regional pain syndromes, the underlying pathogenesis is poorly understood, and it is often not possible to produce a clear-cut diagnosis. Some, such as osteoarthritis (OA), are biologically well defined but clinically less well understood, whereas others, such as rheumatoid arthritis (RA) are both biologically and clinically well defined [9].

For decades, inactivity and bed rest were the mainstays of the management of many diseases, but there is now an increasing amount of evidence supporting the opposite view; that is, that physical activity and exercise are beneficial to health promotion and treatment. Although exercise and physical activity are closely related constructs, they have distinct meanings. The term 'physical activity' includes everyday activities that can contribute to well-being, whereas 'exercise' is physical activity that is planned, structured and repetitive [10]. The focus of this overview is exercise therapy (ET), which involves the prescription of a physical-activity program that involves the client undertaking voluntary muscle contraction and/or body movement with the aim of relieving symptoms or improving function, or of improving, retaining, or slowing deterioration of health [11].

Whereas systematic reviews of randomized trials usually summarize the evidence of one kind of intervention for a single condition, overviews of systematic reviews can summarize evidence from more than one systematic review of the same intervention for different conditions. There is, to our knowledge, only one published overview of systematic reviews that has focused on the effects of exercises for MSCs [12]. This overview was based on reviews published up to July 2007, and did not include specific diseases such as osteoporosis and inflammatory joint diseases. Thus, the most updated evidence may not be included in this overview. The main aim of the present overview was to synthesize evidence from systematic reviews on the effects of ET on pain and physical function for eight selected MSCs. In addition, we explored the evidence for the effect of ET on disease pathogenesis, and whether particular components of exercise programs are associated with the size of the treatment effects.

Methods

Criteria for considering reviews for inclusion

For this overview, we included systematic reviews on the effects of ET for four common conditions (FM, low back pain (LBP), neck pain (NP), and shoulder pain (SP)) and four specific musculoskeletal diseases (OA, RA, ankylosing spondylitis (AS), and osteoporosis). Other related conditions and musculoskeletal malformations and traumas were not included in this overview. All types of land-based ET interventions were considered.

Search methods for the identification of reviews

The first search, of the Cochrane database of systematic reviews, was performed in March 2012. All Cochrane reviews on exercises for the aforementioned MSCs were considered for inclusion. Two authors (GS and KBH) assessed the eligibility of reviews based on the inclusion criteria presented above. Cochrane reviews with the most recent update of January 2007 or before were not included, and we replaced these reviews by searching for non-Cochrane systematic reviews in MEDLINE, EMBASE, CINAHL, AMED, and PEDro, published after this date (for the electronic search strategy for MEDLINE, see Additional file 1). Two authors (GS and KBH) then screened these records for new reviews. If several reviews fulfilled the inclusion criteria, we included only one review per combination of disease, intervention, and outcome by choosing the newest review of high quality. If two or more reviews were equal for these criteria, we chose the review with the highest number of primary studies. We also searched in the same databases for reviews with the explicit aim of investigating the effect of exercise on the pathogenesis of MSCs, with no restrictions on publication date.

Outcome measures

ET. can have clinical effects by improving dominant symptoms, and we therefore chose to primarily focus on the core symptoms of MSCs: 1) any measure of pain, and 2) physical disability or physical function.

In addition, we collected data on the effect of ET on disease pathogenesis, and whether particular components of exercise programs are associated with the magnitude of treatment effects.

We did not focus on the general health benefits or complications of exercise because small to medium randomized controlled trials (RCTs) with short-term to intermediate follow-up may be inadequate to assess other health benefits such as the cardiovascular risk profile and the incidence of complications. Other potentially relevant outcomes, such as work participation and health-related quality of life, compliance, or costs, were not evaluated.

Data collection and analysis

One reviewer (GS) extracted data on population, intervention, comparison, and outcomes (inclusion criteria) and the methodological quality of included trials. The methodological quality was assessed using the AMSTAR (A Measurement Tool to Assess Systematic Reviews) checklist [13]. The 11 criteria shown in Table 1 were rated as 'met,' 'unclear/partly met,' or 'not met'. A second reviewer (KBH) independently verified the accuracy of the numeric results. Most reviews included several comparisons, and we included analyses that compared any exercise intervention with no or minimal exercise intervention. Because pain and function most often are continuous outcomes, data were summarized using the standardized mean difference (SMD) or weighted mean difference (WMD) with 95% confidence interval (95% CI) as reported in the included reviews. For dichotomous outcomes, odds ratio and 95% CI were presented. Pooled effect estimates were presented according to the model used in the reviews. For reviews that explored whether particular components of exercise programs were associated with the magnitude of treatment effects, we extracted the coefficients from meta-regression or sub-group analyses. Results from the review investigating the evidence for the effect of ET on disease pathogenesis were reported as in the original review.

Results

We identified 18 potentially relevant Cochrane systematic reviews. After reading the full text reviews, two were excluded because they did not focus on land-based ET, two because of irrelevant outcomes, four because of other diagnoses, and finally four because they had not been updated after January 2007 (for the excluded Cochrane reviews and reason for exclusion, see Additional file 2). The search for non-Cochrane reviews after 2007 resulted in 963 references (474 for LBP, 186 for SP, 303 for NP). Of these 963 references, 951 were excluded after screening of the title and abstract and, 12 were retrieved as full text; based on methodological quality and publication date 3 of the latter were included.

Description of included reviews

We included six Cochrane systematic reviews on patients with FM [14], OP [15], knee OA [16], hip OA [17], RA [18] and AS [19]. In addition, three non-Cochrane reviews comprising patients with SP [20], NP [21] and LBP [22] were included. The nine included reviews comprised at total of 224 trials with 24,059 patients. Characteristics of the included reviews are shown in Table 2.

Four reviews [14,15,18,19] were assessed to be of high methodological quality (all 11 criteria met), whereas in three reviews [16,17,22] eight to nine criteria were met. Finally, in two reviews [20,21] only three to four criteria were met. In addition, we included one review which investigated the evidence for the effect of ET on disease pathogenesis [23].

Effects of exercises

The effects on clinical outcomes are summarized in Table 3 (pain) and Table 4 (physical functioning).

Fibromyalgia

FM is characterized by persistent widespread musculoskeletal pain and tenderness. In clinical practice, chronic generalized musculoskeletal pain in all four quadrants of the body that cannot be traced to a specific structural or inflammatory cause is often diagnosed as FM. FM is also associated with other symptoms such as fatigue, stiffness, mood disturbance, abdominal pain, and headache. The 1990 American College of Rheumatology (ACR) diagnosis of FM was based on a history of widespread pain for a duration of longer than 3 months, and the presence of excessive tenderness on applying pressure to 11 of 18 specific muscle-tendon sites, whereas the preliminary

Table 1 The AMSTAR check list for methodological assessment.

No	Item
1	Was an 'a priori' design provided?
2	Was there duplicate study selection and data extraction?
3	Was a comprehensive literature search performed?
4	Was the status of publication (that is, 'gray' literature) used as an inclusion criterion?
5	Was a list of studies (included and excluded) provided?
6	Were the characteristics of the included studies provided?
7	Was the scientific quality of the included studies assessed and documented?
8	Was the scientific quality of the included studies used appropriately in formulating conclusions?
9	Were the methods used to combine the findings of studies appropriate?
10	Was the likelihood of publication bias assessed?
11	Were potential conflicts of interest included?

Table 2 Characteristics of included reviews.

Diagnosis [Reference]	Date assessed as up-to-date review	Patient inclusion criteria	Included trials/ patients	Methodological quality of included trials	Methodological quality of reviews [13]
Fibromyalgia [14]	August 2007	A confirmed diagnosis of fibromyalgia	34/2276	Mean van Tulder scores[a]: 7.33 for aerobic training; 4 for strength training)	Met: all
Low back pain [22]	August 2008	Non-specific low back pain (with or without leg pain) 12 weeks or longer	41/4485	Mean PEDro scores[b]: 6.33 for exercise versus no treatment), and 5.82 for exercise versus minimal intervention	Met: 2, 3, 4, 5, 6, 7, 8 and 9; not met: 10, 11; unclear: 1
Neck pain [21]	February 2008	Non-specific neck pain in adults	33/6218	Mean PEDro scores: 5.67	Met: 2, 6, 7, 11; not met: 3, 4, 5, 8, 9, 10; unclear: 1
Shoulder pain [20]	March 2011	Primary symptom of shoulder pain in adults	17/1436	Mean PEDro scores: 5.87	Met: 5, 7, 11; not met: 3, 4, 8, 10; unclear: 1, 2, 6, 9
Osteoporosis [15]	December 2010	Healthy postmenopausal aged women between 45 and 70 years	43/4320	Most trials were scored as 'unclear' for randomization, allocation concealment, attrition, selective reporting, and assessor blinding	Met: all
Osteoarthritis (knee) [16]	December 2007	Knee OA based on accepted criteria or self-reported knee OA on the basis of chronic joint pain	32/3616	Of 43 trials, 9 (28 %) studies had low risk of bias	Met: 1, 2, 4, 5, 6, 7, 8, 9, 11; not met: 3, 10
Osteoarthritis (hip) [17]	August 2008	Hip OA based on accepted criteria or self-reportedhip OA	5/267	Of 5 trials, 3 had low risk of bias and 2 trials had moderate risk of bias	Met: 1, 2, 4, 5, 6, 7, 8, 9, 11; not met: 3, 10
Rheumatoid Arthritis [18]	December 2008	Adults with classic or definite RA based on established criteria	8/575	4 of 8 trials fulfilled at least 8 of 10 methodological criteria	Met: all
Ankylosing spondylitis [19]	January 2007	AS based on the modified New York criteria	11/763	Of 11 trials, 3 had low risk of bias; 3 had moderate risk of bias, and 5 had high risk of bias	Met: all

[a]van Tulder quality scores for internal validity (0 to 11 scale).
[b]PEDro scale scores methodological quality with 11 items.

Table 3 Effect of exercise therapy on pain.

Diagnosis [Reference]	Intervention	Control	Included trials/patients	Treatment effect
Fibromyalgia [14]	Aerobic training	Various (wait list, control, no exercise, treatment as usual)	3/183	SMD[a] 0.65 (95% CI -0.09 to 1.39)
	Strength training	Control (not specified)	1/21	SMD 3.00 (95% CI 1.68 to 4.32)
Low back pain [22]	Exercise (many different types)	No treatment	5/NR[b]	WMD[c] -9.27 on a 100-point scale (95% CI-17.00 to -1.55)
		Minimal care	11/NR	WMD -4.83 on a 100-point scale (95% CI -9.36 to -0.30)
Neck pain [21]	General strength and conditioning exercises	Minimal or no intervention	3/76	WMD -12.00 on a 100-point scale (95% CI -22.00 to -2.00)
Shoulder pain [20]	Graded exercise therapy, progressive resistance, active range of motion	Active or no intervention	3/273	SMD -0.30 (95% CI -0.48 to -0.12)
Osteoporosis [15]	Static, dynamic, or non-weight-bearing exercise	Various	NR	NR
Osteoarthritis knee [16]	Any land-based therapeutic exercise regimens	Various (not specified)	32/3616	SMD -0.40 (95% CI -0.50 to -0.30)
Osteoarthritis hip [17]	Any land-based therapeutic exercise regimens	Various (not specified)	5/204	SMD -0.33 (95% CI -0.84 to 0.17)
Rheumatoid arthritis [18]	Short-term aerobic capacity and muscle-strength training	Various (not specified)	1/50	SMD -0.53 (95% CI -1.09 to 0.04)
	Short-term aerobic capacity training only	Various (not specified)	1/56	SMD -0.27 (95% CI -0.79 to 0.26)
Ankylosing spondylitis [19]	Supervised home exercise program	No intervention	1/155	SMD 0.49 (95% CI 0.17 to 0.81)

[a] Standardized mean difference.

[b]Not reported.

[c]Weighted mean difference.

Table 4 Effect of exercise therapy on physical functioning.

Diagnosis [Reference]	Intervention	Control	No trials/ patients in analyses	Treatment effect
Fibromyalgia [14]	Aerobic training	Various (wait list, control, no exercise, treatment as usual)	4/253	SMD[a] 0.66 (95% CI 0.41 to 0.92)
	Strength training	Control (not specified)	2/47	SMD 0.52 (95% CI -0.07 to 1.10)
Low back pain [22]	Exercise (many different types)	No treatment	9/NR[b]	WMD[c] -3.31 on a 100-point scale (95% CI -4.83 to -1.79)
		Minimal care	14/NR	WMD -6.41 on a 100-point scale (95% CI -9.76 to -3.05)
Neck pain [21]	General strength and conditioning exercises	Minimal or no intervention	2/141	WMD 1.00 on a 100-point scale (95% CI -3.00 to 5.00)
Shoulder pain [20]	Graded exercise therapy, progressive resistance, active range of motion	Active or no intervention	4/358	SMD 0.15 (95% CI 0.01 to 0.29)
Osteoporosis [15]	Static, dynamic, or non-weight-bearing exercise	Various	NR	NR
Osteoarthritis knee [16]	Any land-based therapeutic exercise regimen	Various (not specified)	32/3719	SMD -0.37 (95% CI -0.49 to -0.25)
Osteoarthritis hip [17]	Any land-based therapeutic exercise regimen	Various (not specified)	5/187	SMD -0.10 (95% CI -0.51 to 0.32)
Rheumatoid arthritis [18]	Short-term aerobic capacity and muscle-strength training	Various (not specified)	2/74	SMD -0.40 (95% CI -0.86 to 0.06)
	Short-term aerobic capacity training only	Various (not specified)	2/66	SMD -0.03 (95% CI -0.46 to 0.51)
Ankylosing spondylitis [19]	Supervised home exercise program	No intervention	1/155	SMD 0.12 (95% CI -0.20 to 0.43)

[a] Standardized mean difference.

[b] Not reported.

[c] Weighted mean difference.

2010 ACR criteria are based on a combination of widespread pain and multi-symptom severity, and do not require a physical or tender-point examination [24].

The Cochrane review of Busch *et al.* [14] compared first aerobic-only exercise interventions (only protocols of intensity recommended by the American College of Sports Medicine) with untreated control groups. Statistical pooling based on three trials with 183 patients indicated a positive non-significant effect on pain in favor of exercise (SMD = 0.65; 95% CI -0.09 to 1.39) and a significant effect in physical function (3 trials with 253 patients) (SMD 0.66; 95% CI 0.41 to 0.92). Later, meta-analyses from two low-quality trials compared strength-only exercise interventions with untreated control groups, and found a large and significant effect on pain (based on one trial with twenty-one patients) (SMD 3.00; 95% CI 1.68 to 4.32), and a non-significant effect in physical function: (SMD 0.52; 95% CI -0.07 to 1.10). Based on the number and quality of included trials, Bush *et al.* concluded that there was evidence of a moderate quality showing that short-term aerobic training at the intensity recommended for increases in cardiorespiratory fitness have beneficial effects on physical function and possibly pain. We were not able to identify any analyses exploring the effects of particular components of exercise. Pedersen and Saltin [23] found limited evidence for the effect of exercise on pathogenesis, that is, at least one relevant study of moderate quality is available.

Low back pain

LBP is generally defined as pain located between the lowest ribs and the inferior gluteal folds, with or without pain radiation to the legs [25]. Clinical guidelines classify LBP into 1) 'non-specific' LBP, 2) LBP affecting the nerve root, and 3) possible serious spinal pathology ('red flags') [26]. After 1 month with LBP symptoms, a specific cause can be identified for approximately 15% of patients [25]. Clinically, patients with LBP form a heterogeneous group presenting with pain of varying duration, and disability in terms of impairment of body function and structures, limitations on activity, and restrictions on participation in work and leisure.

The review by Ferreira *et al.* [22] sought to establish the effect of exercise on pain and disability in patients with chronic non-specific LBP, with the main aim of explaining heterogeneity between trials. For exercise versus minimal care (11 trials), they found a significant weighted mean difference (WMD) of -4.83 (on a 0 to 100 scale) favoring exercise for pain, (95% CI -9.36 to -0.30). For exercise versus no treatment (five trials) the WMD was also significantly in favor of exercise (-9.27, 95% CI -17.00 to -1.55). Further, they found positive and significant effects for disability. For exercise versus minimal care (14 trials), the WMD was -6.41 (95% CI -9.76 to -3.05), and for exercise versus no treatment (9 trials), the WMD was -3.31 (95% CI -4.83 to -1.79).

Ferreira *et al.* [22] also explored between-trial variability by meta-regression analyses, and found that only dosage was significantly associated with effect size in pain. 'Dosage' means number of exercise hours and sessions, and the results suggest that for each additional exercise session, the effect size would increase by 0.13 (95% CI 0.02 to 0.24) on a 100-point scale. There was no evidence for the effect of exercises on pathogenesis.

Neck pain

Although there is no general agreement on the classification of NP, the Task Force on Neck Pain and its Associated Disorders [27] suggested a classification of NP severity from grade 1 (no signs or symptoms suggestive of major structural pathology and no or minor interference with activities of daily living; will probably respond to minimal intervention such as reassurance and pain control; does not require intensive investigations or ongoing treatment) to grade IV (signs or symptoms of major structural pathology, such as fracture, myelopathy, neoplasm, or systemic disease; requires prompt investigation and treatment). Most people with NP do not recover completely, and between 50% and 85% of those who experience NP at some initial point will report it again 1 to 5 years later [28].

Leaver *et al.* [21] reported pooled outcomes from three trials showing significant reductions in pain (on a scale of 0 to 100) at the conclusion of a course of specific exercises (WMD -12.00, 95% CI -22.00 to -2.00). Pooled results from two trials that reported disability outcomes after general strength and conditioning exercise showed no significant difference compared with minimal intervention at the conclusion of treatment (WMD 1.00, 95% CI -3.00 to 5.00). We were not able to identify any reviews exploring between-trial heterogeneity or the effect of exercises on pathogenesis.

Shoulder pain

SP and shoulder disorders cover a broad spectrum of pain, symptoms, and diagnoses, including tendonitis, rotator-cuff disease, sub-acromial pain, impingement syndrome, and repetitive strain injury. As with NP, there is no general agreement on the classification of painful shoulder conditions [29]. Clinically, patients often present with SP together with stiffness, reduced range of motion, and/or with pain, or other symptoms radiating to the more proximal part of the arm.

Marinko *et al.* [20] included three studies on SP with pain as an outcome, and compared the effects of exercise versus other treatments on pain levels. Data were pooled by use of a random-effects model, which showed an overall SMD in favor of the exercise intervention

(SMD -0.30; 95% CI -0.48 to -0.12). Four studies included function as an outcome, and compared the effect of exercise versus an alternative intervention or no intervention. Data were pooled by use of a random-effects model, with an overall SMD of 0.15 (95% CI 0.01 to 0.29), indicating a minimal positive effect over no care or alternative interventions. We were not able to identify any reviews exploring between-trial heterogeneity or the effect of exercise on pathogenesis.

Osteoporosis

OP is characterized by a decrease in bone mineral density (BMD), resulting in an increased risk of fracture. The diagnostic criterion for OP is defined as BMD of more than 2.5 standard deviations below the mean bone density of young adult women, whereas the term 'established osteoporosis' includes the presence of a fragility fracture [30]. Clinically, OP is recognized by characteristic fractures after minimal traumas, most often in the hip, vertebrae, or distal forearm. Clinical consequences of OP fractures include pain and physical disability, with loss of independence and need for long-term care as a consequence. Increased mortality is also seen as a direct result of fracture.

In the Cochrane review 'Exercise for preventing and treating osteoporosis in postmenopausal women', Howe *et al.* [15] identified 43 RCTs with more than 4000 participants. None of the studies included pain or physical function as an outcome. Concerning disease pathogenesis in terms of BMD, meta-analyses from 24 RCTs with 1,441 participants showed significant differences in favor of exercise for percentage change in BMD at the spine (MD 0.85; 95% CI 0.62 to 1.07), and trochanter (10 RCTs with 815 participants; MD 1.03; 95% CI 0.56 to 1.49) for the comparison of any exercise to any non-exercise control. Thus, there is strong evidence for the effect of exercise on the pathogenesis of OP, which was also confirmed by Pedersen and Saltin [23]. When exploring the most effective intervention for BMD at the spine, Howe *et al.* [15] found a combination of exercise programs (MD 3.22; 95% CI 1.80 to 4.64) to be most effective, whereas non-weight-bearing high force exercise such as progressive resistance strength training for the legs was most effective for the neck of the femur (MD 1.03; 95% CI 0.24 to 1.82). Prevention of fractures is a main aim in management strategies for OP, and Howe *et al.* [15] reported that the risk of fracture in exercise groups was not significantly different from that in controls (OR 0.61; 95% CI 0.23 to 1.64 for four RCTs and 539 participants).

Osteoarthritis

OA is most frequently seen in the hands, hips, and knees, and is characterized by joint pain, stiffness, and functional limitations. From being thought of as a simple degenerative disease, there is now increasing evidence for the involvement of inflammation in OA [31]. The term 'symptomatic OA' is used when both joint-related symptoms and radiographic signs are present [32].

Although evidence-based recommendations for the treatment of OA consider exercise as a cornerstone of modern OA management, the research evidence from clinical trials in hand OA is very limited and conflicting [33]. For hip OA, Fransen *et al.* [17] included 5 RCTs with 204 patients, and reported a small, non-significant effect of exercise on pain in patients with hip OA (SMD -0.33, 95% CI -0.84 to 0.17). For physical function, the effect was also small and non-significant (SMD -0.10, 95% CI -0.51 to 0.32). The amount of research evidence for knee OA is substantially larger. Fransen *et al.* [16] pooled the results from 32 RCTs with more than 3,600 patients, and reported a beneficial effect of exercise with a SMD of -0.40 (95% CI -0.30 to -0.50) for pain; and SMD of -0.37 (95% CI -0.25 to -0.49) for physical function. Interestingly, sub-group analyses showed that studies evaluating programs providing at least 12 direct supervision occasions produced significantly greater effects than programs providing less than 12 supervised sessions for both pain ((SMD -0.46; 95% CI -0.60 to -0.32) versus SMD -0.28 (95% CI -0.40 to -0.16)) and function ((SMD -0.45; 95% CI -0.62 to -0.29) versus SMD -0.23 (95% CI -0.37 to -0.09)].

According to Pedersen and Saltin [23], there is no evidence for the effect of exercise on the pathogenesis of OA.

Rheumatoid arthritis

RA is the most common inflammatory rheumatic joint disease. The systemic inflammation leads to synovitis and bone erosion, primarily affecting the small joints of hands and feet, but the larger joints can also be involved. Further, RA is associated with extra-articular features and substantial co-morbidity, and a considerably increased risk of cardiovascular disease (CVD) has been reported [34]. The most typical clinical features of RA are joint pain, stiffness, and reduced physical functioning.

In their Cochrane review of dynamic exercises for RA, Hurkmans *et al.* [18] identified eight RCTs in total. For short-term aerobic capacity and muscle-strength training, statistical pooling of two trials (74 patients) showed a non-significant trend for a positive effect of exercise on functional ability (SMD -0.40, 95% CI -0.86 to 0.06), and data from one trial (50 patients) indicated a similar effect on pain (SMD -0.53, 95% CI -1.09 to 0.04). For short-term aerobic exercise only, the meta-analysis showed SMD of -0.27 (95% CI -0.79 to 0.26) for the effects of exercise on pain (1 trial with 56 patients), and SMD of -0.03 (95% CI -0.46 to 0.51) for functional ability (2 trials with 66 patients). We were not able to identify any analyses exploring the effects of particular components of exercise on the effect on clinical outcomes, and there is no evidence for the effect of exercise on the pathogenesis of RA [23].

Ankylosing spondylitis

AS is a chronic inflammatory rheumatic disease predominantly affecting the axial skeleton and the sacroiliac joints. The main clinical characteristics are pain, stiffness, and loss of spinal mobility, caused by inflammation and damage of spinal structures [35]. Other common features of AS are peripheral arthritis, enthesitis, and anterior uveitis, and recent research has also shown that AS is associated with an increased risk of CVD[36]. Radiographic sacroiliitis has traditionally been the diagnostic hallmark of AS, but the absence of definite radiographic sacroiliitis in the early disease stage has resulted in delays in diagnosis. Efforts have therefore been made to facilitate an early, pre-radiological diagnosis of axial spondyloarthritis [37].

When comparing home exercises with no intervention (1 trial with 155 patients), Dagfinrud *et al.* [19] found a significant positive effect of exercise on pain for patients with AS (SMD 0.49; 95% CI 0.17 to 0.81), and a non-significant effect on function (SMD 0.12; 95% CI -0.20 to 0.43). There is, to our knowledge, no evidence for the effect of exercise on the pathogenesis of AS, or whether particular components of exercise can improve clinical outcome.

Discussion

In this overview of systematic reviews on ET for muscle and bone health, we included 9 systematic reviews with a total of 224 trials and 24,059 patients. Overall, we found a substantial amount of empirical evidence supporting ET as a mainstay in the management of MSCs. However, there are differences in the number of included trials between the diagnostic groups included in the present overview. For common conditions such as chronic non-specific LBP and knee OA, there is a substantial number of trials with relatively consistent results showing that exercise has small to moderate beneficial effects on pain and function. For others, such as the inflammatory joint diseases (RA and AS), there are only one or two trials comparing exercises with non-exercise or minimal exercise interventions. When comparing the effect sizes on pain and physical functioning, there seems to be a trend towards larger effects of exercise on pain. The effect sizes were generally larger for pain than for physical function, with significant positive effects for pain in six conditions and for physical function in five conditions. This may indicate that there is no linear relationship between symptoms and functioning, and it may suggest that a relatively large reduction in symptoms is needed to improve physical function. There are also several other important components influencing function, such as environmental and personal factors.

We also intended to explore the evidence for the effect of ET on disease pathogenesis. However, we were not able to identify evidence for the influence of pathogenesis in MSCs, except for OP. Although the disease mechanisms for the common MSCs are largely unknown, there seems to be a gap in the understanding of why ET improves clinical outcome. From a clinical point of view, the most interesting question is 'which exercises for which patients?'. We therefore also explored whether particular components of exercise programs are associated with the size of the treatment effects. Because we did not include single trials comparing different exercise interventions, we could only identify indirect comparisons from the reviews. For LBP and knee OA, for which the substantial number of trials allowed explorative sub-group or meta-regression analyses, the results suggest that 'more is better'; that is, that the treatment effect increases with the number of exercise sessions. However, it is unclear whether the estimated increase is of clinical relevance.

One previous overview has addressed the effect of ET for MSCs [12]. Dziedzic *et al.* also concluded that ET is a beneficial component of the management of MSCs because it reduces pain and disability, and that there is limited evidence for the benefit of one particular approach to exercise over another. However, they also emphasized one important clinical caveat, namely that there is evidence that exercise should not be recommended for acute LBP [12], which was also supported by an updated systematic review [38].

There are several methodological challenges in summarizing evidence from systematic reviews only. There is a substantial number of new trials published in this field every year, and systematic reviews published some years ago may therefore not be based on the most up-to-date evidence. We therefore intended to include Cochrane reviews, because these should be regularly updated. However, this overview clearly shows that this is not the case. We excluded three out of nine eligible Cochrane reviews because they had not been updated after 2007. The decision to exclude Cochrane reviews that had not been updated during the previous five years was arbitrarily chosen and is open to debate. However, considering the substantial number of new trials that have been published on this topic in the past few years, we would suggest that including reviews that are more than 5 years old would not reflect the most up-to-date evidence. Although we performed extensive literature searches, the selection of the three non-Cochrane reviews can also be questioned. However, other systematic reviews on the effects of exercises for LBP, NP and SP also found more or less similar results. For LBP, Macedo *et al.* [39] systematically reviewed 14 RCTs on the effects of motor control exercises for persistent LBP. Their pooled estimates for the comparison between motor control exercise and minimal intervention in reducing pain and disability in both the short and long term were higher than those in the review of Ferreira *et al.* [21]. van Middelkoop *et al.* [40] provided an overview on the effects of ET in patients with chronic LBP; they included 37 RCTs that compared exercise with usual care and found that ET improved post-treatment pain intensity and disability. They also found no evidence that one particular type of ET was clearly more effective than others. In a review of nine trials on the effects of various types of exercise for prevention and cure of non-specific NP in office workers, Sihawong *et al.* [41] found strong evidence for the effects of muscle strengthening and endurance exercises in treating NP. Moderate evidence supported the use of muscle endurance exercise in reducing disability attributed to NP. Teasell *et al.* [42] reviewed the strength of evidence supporting various therapies for whiplash-associated disorder (WAD). They included 40 trials, and found that exercise and mobilization programs for acute and chronic WAD had the strongest supporting evidence, although many questions remain about the relative effects of various protocols. For SP, a recent systematic review of four RCTs examining the effects of exercise for rotator-cuff tendinopathy concluded that the available literature was supportive that exercise reduced pain and functional disability [43]. In a systematic review from 2011, Brudvig *et al.* [44] summarized the published research evidence on the effects of therapeutic exercise and joint mobilization compared with therapeutic exercise alone in patients with shoulder dysfunction. They found no evidence for the beneficial effects of the combination of therapeutic exercise and joint mobilization versus therapeutic exercise alone for reducing pain and increasing function.

An interesting finding of the present study is that Cochrane reviews seem to be of higher methodological quality than non-Cochrane reviews, which is also consistent with reviews specifically addressing this issue [45,46]. Because reviews provide limited information about included trials, the conclusions from tertiary research (overview of systematic reviews) may become too general to be considered as clinically relevant. However, we suggest that findings from overviews can be valuable as a 'compass' for the clinician, and that the decision on the type, dose, and timing of intervention should be shared between the clinician and patient at each clinical encounter. Another limitation related to clinical relevance is the magnitude of the estimated effect sizes. Using a traditional and very rough definition, SMDs between 0.30 and 0.65 can be considered as small to moderate. However, whether the effects are clinically worthwhile is a complex question that should also include the patient's perceptions of risks and costs with the actual treatment. The definition of relatively broad diagnostic groups used in the present overview might also be considered as a limitation from a clinician's point of view. For the regional pain syndromes (LBP, SP, and NP) it is obvious that one size does not fit all; that is, that the effect of ET might not be equal across diagnostic sub-groups. For example, for back pain a recent randomized trial compared stratification of the management based on the patient's prognosis with non-stratified current best practice, and found that stratified care produced disease-specific and general health benefits [47].

Although few reviews addressed potential adverse effects (AEs), exercise for people with MSCs is generally safe and well tolerated, but patients may report minor AEs of exercise such as pain and discomfort [48]. For OP, Howe *et al.* [15] found that fractures and falls were reported as AEs in some studies, but there was no significant effect on the numbers of fractures. By contrast, results from a systematic review showed that exercise can reduce falls, fall-related fractures, and several risk factors for falls in individuals with low BMD [49]. In general, there are few contraindications to prescription of exercise, but co-morbidities should be considered. When prescribing ET as part of the disease management, the exercise program must be individually adopted and targeted depending on the disease severity of the individual patient, and on their physical fitness and any co-morbid conditions. A number of co-morbidities may have an influence on the burden and prognosis of MSCs; in particular, inflammatory rheumatic diseases are associated with a considerably increased risk for CVD [36].

Conclusions

In conclusion, the present overview shows that ET can decrease pain and improve physical functioning, but there were substantial differences in the amount of research evidence across the included diagnostic groups. For example, the relevant comparison for knee OA included 32 trials with more than 3,600 patients, whereas the results for RA and AS are based on one or two trials with between 50 and 150 patients. Consequently, the pooled estimates for knee OA, LBP, FM, and SP showed consistently significant effects in favor of exercise for both outcomes, whereas for NP, hip OA, RA, and AS, the effect estimates were generally smaller and not always significant. However, for the management of all MSCs included in the present overview, ET is unanimously recommended.

There are, however, important limitations when it comes to implications for clinical practice and research. Firstly, for prescription of exercise programs with optimal health benefits for the individual patient, more knowledge is needed on which particular elements and modes of ET, as well as the doses and frequency of delivery, can improve the outcomes of interest. Secondly, knowledge of the potential influence of ET on disease parthenogenesis and the long-term effects on disease progression is currently very limited. Thirdly, it is still an open question whether the magnitude of the positive effects is clinically worthwhile and whether ET is a cost-effective intervention.

Note

* = included reviews

Authors' contributions

All authors contributed to the planning of this review, and all participated in the different phases of the trial-selection process. GS and KBH extracted data, and KBH wrote the first draft of the article. All authors read and provided feedback on the draft versions of the article. All the authors have read and approved the final version. KBH is the guarantor.

Competing interests

The authors declare that they have no competing interests.

Acknowledgements

We thank Hilde Iren Flaaten, librarian at the Diakonhjemmet Hospital, who performed the literature searches.

References

1. Woolf AD, Zeidler H, Haglund U, Carr AJ, Chaussade S, Cucinotta D, Veale DJ, Martin-Mola E: **Musculoskeletal pain in Europe: its impact and a comparison of population and medical perceptions of treatment in eight European countries.** *Ann Rheum Dis* 2004, **63**:342-347.
2. European Opinion Research Group EEIG: **Health, Food and Alcohol and Safety. Special Eurobarometer 186.** European Commission; 2003.
3. Picavet HS, Hazes JM: **Prevalence of self-reported musculoskeletal diseases is high.** *Ann Rheum Dis* 2003, **62**:644-650.
4. Jacobson L, Lindgren B: **Vad kostar sjukdomarna? (What are the costs of illness?).** Stockholm, Socialstyrelsen (National Board of Health and Welfare); 1996.
5. **National Board of Health and Welfare (Sweden).** Yearbook of Health and Medical Care; 2001.
6. **The burden of musculoskeletal diseases at the start of the new millennium. Report of a WHO scientific group.** *Technical Report Series* Geneva: World Health Organization; 2003, No. 919.
7. Hanson M, Gluckman P, Nutbeam D, Hearn J: **Priority actions for the non-communicable disease crisis.** *Lancet* 2011, **378**:566-577.
8. **European League Against Rheumatism.** [http://www.eular.org/myUploadData/files/Broschüre%20EULAR-OK.pdf], Accessed 19 October 2012.
9. **European Commission. Directorate – General Health and Consumer Protection. Indicators for monitoring musculoskeletal problems and conditions: Musculoskeletal problems and functional limitation. The great public challenge for the 21st century.** Oslo: University of Oslo; 2003.
10. Garber CE, Blissmer B, Deschenes MR, Franklin BA, LaMonte MJ, Lee IM, Nieman DC, Swain DP: **American College of Sports Medicine position stand. Quantity and quality of exercise for developing and maintaining cardiorespiratory, musculoskeletal, and neuromotor fitness in apparently healthy adults: guidance for prescribing exercise.** *Med Sci Sports Exerc* 2011, **43**:1334-59.
11. Taylor NF, Dodd KJ, Shields N, Bruder A: **Therapeutic exercise in physiotherapy practice is beneficial: a summary of systematic reviews 2002-2005.** *Aust J Physiother* 2007, **53**:7-16.
12. Dziedzic K, Jordan JL, Foster NE: **Land- and water-based exercise therapies for musculoskeletal conditions.** *Best Pract Res Clin Rheumatol* 2008, **22**:407-18.
13. Shea BJ, Hamel C, Wells GA, Bouter LM, Kristjansson E, Grimshaw J, Henry DA, Boers M: **AMSTAR is a reliable and valid measurement tool to assess the methodological quality of systematic reviews.** *J Clin Epidemiol* 2009, **62**:1013-20.
14. Busch AJ, Barber KA, Overend TJ, Peloso PMJ, Schachter CL: **Exercise for treating fibromyalgia syndrome.** *Cochrane Database Syst Rev* 2007, **4**: CD003786.
15. Howe TE, Shea B, Dawson LJ, Downie F, Murray A, Ross C, Harbour RT, Caldwell LM, Creed G: **Exercise for preventing and treating osteoporosis in postmenopausal women.** *Cochrane Database Syst Rev* 2011, **7**:CD000333.
16. Fransen M, McConnell S: **Exercise for osteoarthritis of the knee.** *Cochrane Database Syst Rev* 2008, **4**:CD004376.
17. Fransen M, McConnell S, Hernandez-Molina G, Reichenbach S: **Exercise for osteoarthritis of the hip.** *Cochrane Database Syst Rev* 2009, **3**:CD007912.
18. Hurkmans E, van der Giesen FJ, Vliet Vlieland TPM, Schoones J, Van den Ende ECHM: **Dynamic exercise programs (aerobic capacity and/or muscle strength training) in patients with rheumatoid arthritis.** *Cochrane Database Syst Rev* 2009, **4**:CD006853.
19. Dagfinrud H, Hagen KB, Kvien TK: **Physiotherapy interventions for ankylosing spondylitis.** *Cochrane Database Syst Rev* 2008, **1**:CD002822.
20. Marinko LN, Chacko JM, Dalton DA, Chacko CC: **The effectiveness of therapeutic exercise for painful shoulder conditions: a meta-analysis.** *J Shoulder Elbow Surg* 2011, **20**:1351-1359.
21. Leaver AM, Refshauge KM, Maher CG, McAuley JH: **Conservative interventions provide short-term relief for non-specific neck pain: a systematic review.** *J Physiother* 2010, **56**:73-85.
22. Ferreira ML, Smeets RJEM, Kamper SJ, Ferreira PH, Machado LAC: **Can we explain heterogeneity among randomized clinical trials of exercise for chronic back pain? A meta-regression analysis of randomized controlled trials.** *Phys Ther* 2010, **90**:1383-1403.
23. Pedersen BK, Saltin B: **The evidence for prescribing exercise as therapy in chronic disease.** *Scand J Med Sci Sports* 2006, **16(Suppl 1)**:3-63.
24. Wolfe F, Clauw DJ, Fitzcharles MA, Goldenberg DL, Katz RS, Mease P, Russell AS, Russell IJ, Winfield JB, Yunus MB: **The American College of Rheumatology preliminary diagnostic criteria for fibromyalgia and measurement of symptom severity.** *Arthritis Care Res* 2010, **62**:600-10.
25. Waddel G: **The Back Pain Revolution.** Edinburgh:Churchill Livingstone; 1998.
26. van Tulder M, Becker A, Bekkering GE, Breen A, del Real MT, Hutchinson A, Koes B, Laerum E, Malmivaara A, the COST B13 Working Group on Guidelines for the Management of Acute Low Back Pain in Primary Care: **European guidelines for the management of acute nonspecific low back pain in primary care.** *Eur Spine J* 2006, **15(Suppl2)**:169-191.
27. Guzman J, Hurwitz EL, Carroll LJ, Haldeman S, Cote P, Carragee EJ, Peloso PM, der van V, Holm LW, Hogg-Johnson S, Nordin M, Cassidy JD: **A new conceptual model of neck pain: linking onset, course, and care: the Bone and Joint Decade 2000-2010 Task Force on Neck Pain and Its Associated Disorders.** *Spine* 2008, **33(4 Suppl)**:14-23.
28. Côté P, van der Velde G, Cassidy JD, Carroll LJ, Hogg-Johnson S, Holm LW, Carragee EJ, Haldeman S, Nordin M, Hurwitz EL, Guzman J, Peloso PM: **The burden and determinants of neck pain in workers: results of the Bone and Joint Decade 2000-2010 Task Force on Neck Pain and Its Associated Disorders.** *Spine* 2008, **33(Suppl)**:60-74.

29. Eerd D, Beaton D, Cole D, Lucas J, Hogg-Johnson S, Bombardier C: **Classification systems for upper-limb musculoskeletal disorders in workers: a review of the literature.** *J Clin Epidemiol* 2003, **56**:925-36.
30. Kanis JA: **Assessment of fracture risk and its application to screening for postmenopausal osteoporosis: synopsis of a WHO report. WHO Study Group.** *Osteoporosis Int* 1994, **4**:368-381.
31. Dieppe P: **Developments in osteoarthritis.** *Rheumatology* 2011, **50**:245-7, (Oxford).
32. Kopec JA, Rahman MM, Berthelot JM, Le Petit C, Aghajanian J, Sayre EC, Cibere J, Anis AH, Badley EM: **Descriptive epidemiology of osteoarthritis in British Columbia, Canada.** *J Rheumatol* 2007, **34**:386-93.
33. Kjeken I, Smedslund G, Moe RH, Slatkowsky-Christensen B, Uhlig T, Hagen KB: **A Systematic Review of Design and Effects of Splints and Exercise Programs in Hand Osteoarthritis.** *Arthritis Care Res* 2011, **63**:834-48.
34. Avina-Zubieta JA, Thomas J, Sadatsafavi M, Lehman AJ, Lacaille D: **Risk of incident cardiovascular events in patients with rheumatoid arthritis: a meta-analysis of observational studies.** *Ann Rheum Dis* 2012, **71**:1524-9.
35. Braun J, Sieper J: **Ankylosing spondylitis.** *Lancet* 2007, **369**:1379-90.
36. Peters MJ, Symmons DP, McCarey D, Dijkmans BA, Nicola P, Kvien TK, McInnes IB, Haentzschel H, Gonzalez-Gay MA, Provan S, Semb A, Sidiropoulos P, Kitas G, Smulders YM, Soubrier M, Szekanecz Z, Sattar N, Nurmohamed MT: **EULAR evidence-based recommendations for cardiovascular risk management in patients with rheumatoid arthritis and other forms of inflammatory arthritis.** *Ann Rheum Dis* 2010, **69**:325-31.
37. Rudwaleit M, Taylor WJ: **Classification criteria for psoriatic arthritis and ankylosing spondylitis/axial spondyloarthritis.** *Best Pract Res Clin Rheumatol* 2010, **24**:589-604.
38. Dahm KT, Bruberg KG, Jamtvedt G, Hagen KB: **Advice to rest in bed versus advice to stay active for acute low back pain and sciatica.** *Cochrane Database Syst Rev* 2010, **6**:CD007612.
39. Macedo LG, Maher CG, Latimer J, McAuley JH: **Motor control exercise for persistent, nonspecific low back pain: a systematic review.** *Phys Ther* 2009, **89**:9-25.
40. van Middelkoop M, Rubinstein SM, Verhagen AP, Ostelo RW, Koes BW, van Tulder MW: **Exercise therapy for chronic nonspecific low-back pain.** *Best Pract Res Clin Rheumato* 2010, **24**:193-204.
41. Sihawong R, Janwantanakul P, Sitthipornvorakul E, Pensri P: **Exercise therapy for office workers with nonspecific neck pain: a systematic review.** *J Manipulative Physiol Ther* 2011, **34**:62-71.
42. Teasell RW, McClure JA, Walton D, Pretty J, Salter K, Meyer M, Sequeira K, Death B: **A research synthesis of therapeutic interventions for whiplash-associated disorder: part 1 - overview and summary.** *Pain Res Manag* 2010, **15**:287-94.
43. Littlewood C, Ashton J, Chance-Larsen K, May S, Sturrock B: **Exercise for rotator cuff tendinopathy: a systematic review.** *Physiotherapy* 2012, **98**:101-9.
44. Brudvig TJ, Kulkarni H, Shah S: **The effect of therapeutic exercise and mobilization on patients with shoulder dysfuction: a systematic review with meta-analysis.** *J Orthop Sports Phys Ther* 2011, **41**:734-48.
45. Jadad AR, Cook DJ, Jones A, Klassen TP, Tugwell P, Moher M, Moher D: **Methodology and reports of systematic reviews and meta-analyses: a comparison of Cochrane reviews with articles published in paper-based journals.** *JAMA* 1998, **280**:278-80.
46. Collier A, Heilig L, Schilling L, Williams H, Dellavalle RP: **Cochrane Skin Group systematic reviews are more methodologically rigorous than other systematic reviews in dermatology.** *Br J Dermatol* 2006, **155**:1230-5.
47. Hill JC, Whitehurst DG, Lewis M, Bryan S, Dunn KM, Foster NE, Konstantinou K, Main CJ, Mason E, Somerville S, Sowden G, Vohora K, Hay EM: **Comparison of stratified primary care management for low back pain with current best practice (STarT Back): a randomised controlled trial.** *Lancet* 2011, **378**:1560-71.
48. Bennell KL, Hinman RS: **A review of the clinical evidence for exercise in osteoarthritis of the hip and knee.** *J Sci Med Sport* 2011, **14**:4-9.
49. de Kam D, Smulders E, Weerdesteyn V, Smits-Engelsman BC: **Exercise interventions to reduce fall-related fractures and their risk factors in individuals with low bone density: a systematic review of randomized controlled trials.** *Osteoporosis Int* 2009, **20**:2111-25.

7

Pre-cooling for endurance exercise performance in the heat: a systematic review

Paul R Jones[1,2], Christian Barton[1], Dylan Morrissey[1], Nicola Maffulli[1*] and Stephanie Hemmings[1]

Abstract

Background: Endurance exercise capacity diminishes under hot environmental conditions. Time to exhaustion can be increased by lowering body temperature prior to exercise (pre-cooling). This systematic literature review synthesizes the current findings of the effects of pre-cooling on endurance exercise performance, providing guidance for clinical practice and further research.

Methods: The MEDLINE, EMBASE, CINAHL, Web of Science and SPORTDiscus databases were searched in May 2012 for studies evaluating the effectiveness of pre-cooling to enhance endurance exercise performance in hot environmental conditions (≥ 28°C). Studies involving participants with increased susceptibility to heat strain, cooling during or between bouts of exercise, and protocols where aerobic endurance was not the principle performance outcome were excluded. Potential publications were assessed by two independent reviewers for inclusion and quality. Means and standard deviations of exercise performance variables were extracted or sought from original authors to enable effect size calculations.

Results: In all, 13 studies were identified. The majority of studies contained low participant numbers and/or absence of sample size calculations. Six studies used cold water immersion, four crushed ice ingestion and three cooling garments. The remaining study utilized mixed methods. Large heterogeneity in methodological design and exercise protocols was identified. Effect size calculations indicated moderate evidence that cold water immersion effectively improved endurance performance, and limited evidence that ice slurry ingestion improved performance. Cooling garments were ineffective. Most studies failed to document or report adverse events. Low participant numbers in each study limited the statistical power of certain reported trends and lack of blinding could potentially have introduced either participant or researcher bias in some studies.

Conclusions: Current evidence indicates cold water immersion may be the most effective method of pre-cooling to improve endurance performance in hot conditions, although practicality must be considered. Ice slurry ingestion appears to be the most promising practical alternative. Interestingly, cooling garments appear of limited efficacy, despite their frequent use. Mechanisms behind effective pre-cooling remain uncertain, and optimal protocols have yet to be established. Future research should focus on standardizing exercise performance protocols, recruiting larger participant numbers to enable direct comparisons of effectiveness and practicality for each method, and ensuring potential adverse events are evaluated.

Keywords: Pacing, thermoregulation, internal cooling, cooling garment, cold water immersion, ice slurry ingestion

* Correspondence: n.maffulli@qmul.ac.uk
[1]Centre for Sports and Exercise Medicine, William Harvey Research Institute, Bart's and the London School of Medicine and Dentistry, Queen Mary University of London, Mile End Hospital, Bancroft Road, London E1 4DG, UK
Full list of author information is available at the end of the article

Background

Endurance exercise capacity has been reported to be diminished when exercising in hot environmental conditions, compared with normal and cold conditions [1-3]. A recent review evaluated the data of six International Association of Athletics Federations (IAAF) Gold Labeled Road Marathon races from 2001 to 2010 to determine which environmental factors have the largest impact on race performance [4]. The authors reported a median optimum environmental temperature of 6.2°C for men and 6.8°C for women. There was a consistent slowing of 0.03% for every 1°C increase in temperature above optimum and average performance decreases of -17.7% and -12.4% for men and women at +20°C above optimum. The authors concluded that temperature is the main environmental factor influencing marathon performance. Hot environmental temperatures also limit cycling performance. Peiffer and Abbiss [3] investigated cyclists performing a 40 km time trial in a heat chamber at different environmental temperatures. The authors reported a significantly lower mean power output for the participants at 37°C compared to at 17°C, 22°C and 27°C. A separate study reported that higher environmental temperatures reduce the time taken to reach volitional fatigue when cycling at a fixed intensity (70% maximal aerobic capacity (VO_2max)). Mean time to volitional fatigue decreased by 30 minutes between trials performed at 21°C (81.2 min) and 31°C (51.6 min) [1]. Although not all endurance events follow a linear model of performance decline with increasing environmental temperature [5], it is apparent that hot environmental temperatures above an optimum impair endurance exercise performance.

Understanding the physiological basis as to why the capacity to perform endurance exercise is reduced in hot (≥ 28°C) environments is needed to develop interventions that may improve performance. It was previously postulated that exhaustion in hot conditions was a result of circulatory failure (a reduction in cardiac output and muscle blood flow) diminishing the drive for further exercise [6]. However, Nielsen *et al.* [7] found evidence to challenge this. In this study athletes exercised at 60% VO_2max until exhaustion for 9 to 12 days in 40°C heat. The authors reported that exhaustion coincided with a core temperature of 39.7 ± 0.15°C. With acclimation, the athletes took progressively longer to reach this core temperature. No reduction in cardiac output was found at exhaustion and the authors concluded that high core temperature rather than circulatory failure was the limiting factor. However, thermoregulation and cardiovascular functioning are not separate entities and a number of physiological adaptations occurred with acclimation, such as earlier onset of the sweating response and improved cardiovascular efficiency, reducing cardiovascular strain and slowing the rate of rise of core body temperature, which likely contributed to the lower core body temperature at a given point of exercise reported in this study [7]. Another proposed hypothesis was that fatigue may arise from decreased substrate availability given that there is an observed increase in the rate of muscle glycogen utilization, and therefore depletion, when exercising in the heat, though this seems unlikely [3,8]. Febbraio *et al.* [8] reported that carbohydrate ingestion during cycling at 70% VO_2max in 33°C heat produced no ergogenic effect compared to a sweet placebo, nor did the athletes' blood glucose fall below resting levels during the trial. They concluded that fatigue was related to thermoregulatory factors as opposed to decreased substrate availability.

Current hypotheses propose that the critical limiting factor for exercise performance in the heat is an elevated core body temperature, at which an athlete will have to reduce their exercise intensity or risk heat-related injury [9]. It is thought that pre-cooling in hot environments will improve endurance exercise performance by lowering an athlete's preliminary core body temperature, thereby increasing the margin between the initial core temperature and temperatures at which athletic performance is affected. A lower core body temperature at a given point of exercise has a similar effect to that which occurs with acclimation [7] and enables athletes to exercise at higher intensities during self-paced exercise (or for a longer duration during constant pace exercise). A consistent core temperature at voluntary fatigue has also been observed across fitness groups [10]. The higher environmental heat load in hot conditions augments the rate of rise in core body temperature, reducing the time taken for an athlete to reach their limiting temperature [11].

The hypothesized link between increased core temperature and reduced endurance exercise performance has led to the proposal and evaluation of a number of cooling methods prior to sports participation (that is, pre-cooling). It is thought that pre-cooling in hot environments will improve endurance exercise performance by lowering an athlete's preliminary core body temperature and increasing the margin between the initial core temperature and critical limiting core temperature at which athletic performance declines [12]. An athlete would therefore have a lower core body temperature at a given point of exercise, similar to the effect that occurs with acclimation reported in the Nielsen *et al.* study [7], enabling athletes to exercise harder for longer. Early pre-cooling studies evaluated the effectiveness of methods such as cold water baths and cooling fans, with positive outcomes for endurance exercise performance reported [13,14]. However, clinical application of these methods is made difficult by the need for transportation and/or installation of equipment and facilities needed.

The potential of pre-cooling to improve sporting performance led scientists at the Australian Institute of Sport (AIS) to develop a cooling jacket for in-competition athletes, constructed from neoprene and designed to be packed with ice, prior to the Atlanta Games 1996, as a more practical and convenient alternative to the cold water baths and cooling fans used in laboratory studies. Of the 43 surveyed after Atlanta, all athletes felt that the jackets made a positive contribution to their performance at the Games [15]. Since this practical innovation, other novel pre-cooling strategies have been proposed and investigated, such as ice slurry ingestion [16-19].

Pre-cooling: theoretical mechanism of action

Different pre-cooling interventions are proposed to act via different mechanisms to reduce core body temperature and thus cool the body prior to exercise.

Cold water immersion

When immersed in water of an ambient temperature below the human thermoneutral zone in water (33 to 34°C), the human body will attempt to maintain its core temperature by reducing skin blood flow (vasoconstriction) [20]. Below this thermoneutral zone, vasoconstriction in isolation is not sufficient to maintain core temperature, so metabolic heat production is increased. However, if the cold stimulus is of a sufficiently low temperature and applied for long enough, heat loss will exceed heat production, causing a reduction in core temperature and increasing heat storage capacity [21].

Ice slurry ingestion

The phase change of solid ice (H_2O) to liquid water requires a large transfer of heat energy into the system, known as the 'enthalpy of fusion (melting)' of ice. Merrick *et al.* [22] reported that cold modalities that undergo phase change caused lower skin surface and intramuscular temperatures than modalities that do not undergo phase change. Therefore, when ice slurry is ingested, heat energy is transferred into the slurry mix from the surrounding tissues, rather than stored in the body, reducing the core temperature. A study investigating intravenous cooling in swine reported that ice slurry (-1°C to 0°C) cooled brain temperature more rapidly and effectively than chilled saline (0°C to 1°C) [23], which suggests that ice slurry may potentially be effective as a pre-exercise pre-cooling modality.

Cooling garment

Cooling garments primarily reduce skin temperature. Common strategies include wearing a vest that covers the torso with pockets for ice packs (ice vest) [24-26], or wearing a waist-length polyester blend shell with sleeves and a hood that has a phase change material sewn in (cooling jacket) [17,27]. Kay *et al.* [28] suggested that lowering skin temperature without a concomitant reduction in core body temperature prior to exercise, increasing the thermal gradient between core and skin, afforded participants a lower core temperature during exercise due to increased core to skin heat loss.

Although there is a significant body of work regarding pre-cooling and its effects on athletic performance, the literature concerning pre-cooling for endurance exercise performance has yet to be reviewed systematically and it is yet to be established which pre-cooling modality or mechanism of body cooling is the most effective. Two reviews provide comprehensive descriptions of pre-cooling and its application to sports performance [29,30]. However, neither combined available data to systematically analyze or compare different pre-cooling strategies. The conclusions drawn are therefore more open to bias than those of a systematic review and comparisons of methods subjective. Furthermore, both reviews were published before more recent pre-cooling strategies such as ice slurry ingestion had been investigated and reported on. Therefore, a more up-to-date evidence-based review, less open to bias is warranted.

Recently, Ranalli *et al.* [31], evaluating the effect of body cooling on aerobic and anaerobic exercise performance, concluded that pre-cooling conferred limited benefit to intermittent or anaerobic exercise performance. For the 'aerobic' section of the review, they included nine studies, yet only two of these studies evaluated cooling prior to exercise (pre-cooling). Considering practical limitations to cooling during competition for many sports, and the number of additional studies evaluating the effects of pre-cooling on endurance exercise performance in the literature, a systematic review of all studies where participants were cooled prior to exercise is required. Therefore, the aims of this systematic review were to (i) summarize the effectiveness of different pre-cooling procedures to improve endurance exercise performance by comparing, critiquing and combining results from each study; (ii) enable evidence-based decisions on appropriate pre-cooling athlete management to be made; and (iii) provide guidance for future research evaluating the efficacy of pre-cooling strategies which aim to enhance endurance exercise performance.

Methods

Inclusion and exclusion criteria

Repeated measures crossover studies and randomized controlled trials comparing a pre-cooling method(s) to control or no intervention in healthy adults were considered for inclusion. The pre-cooling method could be any that cooled a participant prior to commencing an endurance exercise protocol or event. A measure of aerobic endurance was required to be one of the outcome measures in each study. The ambient environmental temperature during the performance trials had to be at or above the human thermoneutral zone of environmental temperatures (≥ 28°C) [32,33].

Unpublished studies, case series studies, non-peer-reviewed publications, studies not involving humans, reviews, letters, opinion articles, articles and abstracts not in English were excluded. Studies that included participants with pathological conditions known to increase susceptibility to heat strain, such as spinal cord injury [34], were also excluded, as were studies that attempted to cool participants during exercise, those that used intermittent or team-based sport exercise protocols or protocols that primarily stressed the anaerobic energy pathway. Unpublished research was not sought. Although this may potentially lead to publication bias [35], it was deemed impractical to identify all unpublished work on pre-cooling and endurance exercise performance from all authors and institutions around the world.

Search strategy

The following databases were searched in May 2012 (week 4): MEDLINE (Ovid Web, 1948 to 2012 and Medline In-process and Other Non-Indexed Citations), EMBASE (1974 to 2012), CINAHL (1981 to 2012), Web of Science (1899 to 2012) and SPORTDiscus. Key terms used in the search strategy and results of the search are shown in Table 1. Reference lists and lists of citing articles were searched to ensure that no relevant studies had been missed by the search strategy. No additional papers were identified.

Review process

All titles and abstracts were downloaded into EndNote X4 (Thomson Reuters, Philadelphia, PA, USA) giving a set of 9922 citations. The set was crossreferenced and any duplicates were deleted, leaving a total of 4454 citations. Each title and abstract were evaluated for potential inclusion by two independent reviewers (PRJ and CB) using a checklist developed from the inclusion/exclusion criteria outlined above. If insufficient information was contained in the title and abstract to make a decision on a study, it was retained until the full text could be obtained for evaluation. Any disagreements regarding studies were resolved by a consensus meeting between the two reviewers, and a third reviewer (DM) was available if necessary.

Methodological quality assessment

Quality assessment was performed using the Physiotherapy Evidence Database (PEDro) Scale, which is a valid

Table 1 Search strategy and results from each included database

Search term/No.	MEDLINE	EMBASE	CINAHL	Web of Science	SPORTDiscus
1. Exercise	195,255	277,329	61,991	83,075	165,077
2. Exercising	6,474	7,981	1,441	224,807	3,909
3. Endurance	21,579	23,146	5,353	24,920	19,791
4. Performance	456,095	712,833	59,983	1,652,852	130,350
5. Pace	9,687	12,271	2,880	46,122	5,847
6. Pacing	30,907	35,549	6,433	174,740	12,163
7. Sport	12,294	58,671	4,820	56,118	650,712
8. Sports	45,270	41,390	17,268	As above	650,460
9. Sporting	2,332	3,711	2,719	As above	101,200
10. Aerobic	47,428	68,495	6,143	59,356	21,497
11. OR/terms 1 to 10	74,560	1,114,664	137,399	2,094,266	871,407
12. Pre-cool	7	10	1	47	3
13. Pre-cool	7	13	0	494	2
14. Pre-cooling	115	193	18	544	50
15. Pre-cooling	51	94	7	473	48
16. Pre-cooled	144	141	3	258	4
17. Pre-cooled	76	75	0	473	1
18. Cool	4,854	6,454	905	214,304	2,906
19. Cooled	7,789	9,630	231	204,690	200
20. Cooling	22,183	31,464	940	As above	1,145
21. OR/terms 12 to 20	31,903	43,280	1,919	214,676	4,022
22. 11 AND 21	2,489	3,606	326	25,367	2,233
23. Limit 22 to English language	2,373	3,358	322	1,089[a]	2,147

[a]Search also refined by appropriate categories: sports science; physiology; public, environmental and occupational health; cardiac cardiovascular systems, respiratory system.

measure of the methodological quality of clinical trials [36]. Each study is rated according to ten separate criteria on the PEDro scale that assess a study's internal validity and statistical reporting, then totaled to give a score out of 10. An additional criterion, 'sample size calculation', was included in the quality assessment as the authors felt it to be an important component of study methodology. This criterion did not contribute to the PEDro score. Two reviewers (PRJ and CB) applied the PEDro scale to each included study independently, and any scoring discrepancies were resolved through a consensus meeting, with a third reviewer (DM) available if necessary. Studies were considered high quality if PEDro scores were greater than 6, and low quality if 6 and below.

Statistical analysis and data synthesis

Means and standard deviations for all continuous data were extracted and effect sizes (Cohen's d) (with 95% CIs) calculated to allow comparison between the results of each study. Data were pooled using RevMan for Mac version 5.1.2 (The Nordic Cochrane Centre, Copenhagen, Denmark). If inadequate data were available from original studies to complete effect size calculations, attempts were made via email to contact the study's corresponding author for the required data. The presence of publication bias was determined by evaluating funnel plot asymmetry graphically [37,38].

Definitions for 'levels of evidence' were guided by recommendations made by van Tulder *et al.* [39] and are as given below:

'Strong evidence' = consistent findings among multiple high quality randomized controlled trials.

'Moderate evidence' = consistent findings among multiple low quality randomized controlled trials and/or non-randomized controlled trials, or one high quality randomized controlled trial.

'Limited evidence' = findings from one low quality randomized or non-randomized controlled trial.

'Conflicting evidence' = inconsistent findings among multiple trials.

Results

Following the search, 13 studies were deemed appropriate for inclusion (Figure 1). Table 2 shows the participant characteristics and investigation protocol for each included study.

Quality assessment of included studies

Of the 13 studies included in the review, 8 studies attained a PEDro score of 6/10 [16-19,26,27,40,41], 4 attained a score of 5/10 [24,25,42,43], and 1 study received a score of 4/10 (Table 3) [25]. Sample size calculations were not performed by any of the reviewed studies.

Additional data and publication bias

Corresponding authors of two additional studies eligible for review were contacted via email to request additional data necessary for inclusion in the review [44,45]. The required data had not been supplied at the time of going to press. A symmetrical funnel plot indicated the absence of publication bias [37,38].

Effectiveness of different pre-cooling modalities

Cold water immersion

Six studies evaluated the effectiveness of cold water immersion in enhancing endurance exercise performance compared to a control condition (see Figure 2) [19,28,40-43]. Performance measures evaluated included time to volitional fatigue exercising at a fixed exercise intensity [19,40,43], distance completed in a 30-minute self-controlled exercise test [28,42], and mean power output (MPO) over a 40-minute cycling time trial [41]. Three studies showed improved performance compared to a control condition (d = 2.01, 1.41 and 1.48 respectively) [19,40,43]. Consistent with significant findings, the remaining three studies showed a trend for cold water immersion to improve performance, though this was not statistically significant (d = 0.61, 0.42 and 0.74 respectively) [28,41,42]. Therefore, moderate evidence is indicated for the effectiveness of cold water immersion to improve endurance exercise performance in hot environments.

Ice slurry ingestion

Four studies evaluated the effectiveness of ingesting an ice slurry beverage in enhancing endurance exercise performance compared to a control condition (see Figure 3) [16-19]. The control condition was consumption of a volume of water equal to that of the ingested ice slurry in each study. Performance measures evaluated included time taken to cycle a set distance and MPO [16,17], and time to volitional fatigue at a fixed exercise intensity [18,19]. One study showed a statistically significant performance improvement in the pre-cooling condition (d = 1.16) [18]. All three remaining studies reported a trend towards improved performance in the pre-cooling condition for both time taken and MPO [16,17,19]. Therefore, limited evidence is indicated for the effectiveness of ice slurry ingestion to improve endurance exercise performance in hot environments.

Cooling garment

Three studies evaluated the effectiveness of a cooling garment in enhancing endurance exercise performance compared to a control condition (see Figure 4) [24,26,27]. Two studies [24,26] used an ice vest as their cooling

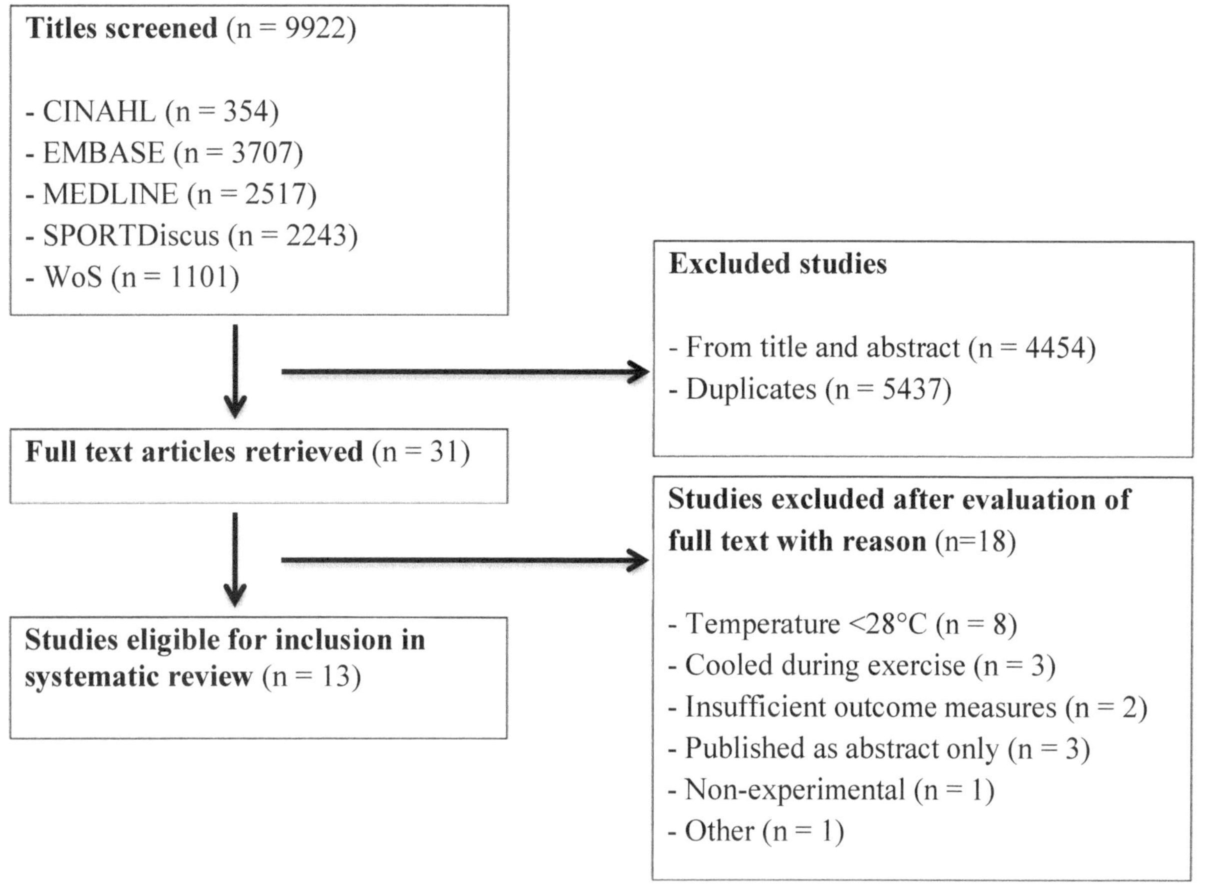

Figure 1 QUOROM (for 'Quality of Reporting of Meta-analyses' using standards developed by the QUOROM group) flow diagram, summarizing study selection for inclusion.

garment, and the other used a cooling jacket covering the torso, arms, and head with a hood [27]. Performance measures evaluated included time taken to complete a 5 km run [24], time to volitional fatigue on an incremental treadmill test [26], and time taken to complete a fixed amount of work (kJ) and MPO while cycling [27]. There were no significant improvements in performance for any of the parameters measured, indicating moderate evidence that cooling garments are an ineffective pre-cooling intervention.

Mixed cooling methods

Three studies evaluated the effectiveness of combined pre-cooling methods to a control condition (see Figure 5) [17,25,27]. Two studies pre-cooled athletes using cold water immersion followed by wearing a cooling jacket (torso, sleeves and hood) [17,27]. Performance measures evaluated in both studies were time taken to cycle a set distance and MPO. Although not statistically significant, Quod *et al.* [27] showed a trend towards the pre-cooling condition improving performance (d = 0.98, 0.39 for time taken and MPO respectively). Ross *et al.* [17] found no improvement. Cotter *et al.* [25] used two different, mixed methods pre-cooling procedures in their study. Subjects were cooled with an ice vest and cold air while their thighs were either kept warm or cooled using water-perfused cuffs. The performance measure evaluated was MPO. Both of these pre-cooling interventions showed a trend to performance improvement in the pre-cooled conditions (d = 0.49 and 0.55 in leg cooling and leg warming, respectively).

Comparison of pre-cooling methods

One study evaluated the effectiveness of ice slurry ingestion in enhancing endurance exercise performance compared to cold water immersion (see Figure 6) [19]. There was no statistically significant difference between the two pre-cooling methods (d = 0.54), though there was a trend to cold water immersion being more effective. There is limited evidence that ice slurry ingestion is as effective at improving endurance exercise performance as cold water immersion.

Discussion

The aim of the present systematic review was to summarize the effectiveness of different pre-cooling techniques to

Table 2 Investigation protocol for each included study.

Authors	Participant characteristics[a]	Exercise duration (min)	Cooling mode[b]	Cooling duration (min)	Environmental conditions		Performance task	Core temperature measurement	Outcome measure
					Temperature (°C)	Humidity (%)			
Arngrímsson *et al.*, 2004 [24]	9 male, 8 female; trained	15.6 to 22.8[c]	G	38	32	50	Running	Rectal	Time to complete 5 km
Booth *et al.*, 1997 [42]	5 male, 3 female; trained	30	W	60	32	62	Running	Rectal	Distance completed in a 30-minute test at self-controlled pace
Cotter *et al.*, 2001 [25]	9 male; untrained	35	G ± LC	45	35	60	Cycling	Rectal	Mean power output (W/kg) during 15 minutes at self-selected pace
Duffield *et al.*, 2010 [41]	8 male; trained	40	W	20[d]	33	50	Cycling	Rectal	Mean power output (W) during 40-minute time trial
Gonzalez-Alonso *et al.*, 1999 [40]	7 male; trained	42 to 66[c]	W	30	40	19	Cycling	Esophageal	Time to volitional fatigue at 60% VO_2max
Hasegawa *et al.*, 2006 [43]	9 male; untrained	2.5 to 8.0[e, f]	W/D/W + D	30	32	80	Cycling	Rectal	Time to volitional fatigue at 80% VO_2max
Ihsan *et al.*, 2010 [16]	7 male; trained	70 to 103[c]	I	30	30	75	Cycling	Gastrointestinal	Time to complete 40 km; mean power output (W)
Kay *et al.*, 1999 [28]	7 male; trained	30	W	58.6	31	60	Cycling	Rectal	Distance completed in a 30-minute test at self-controlled pace
Quod *et al.*, 2008 [27]	6 male; trained	40	G/W + G	40/70[g]	34	41	Cycling	Rectal	Time to complete a fixed amount of work (kJ); mean power output (W)
Ross *et al.*, 2011 [17]	11 male; trained	76 to 123[c]	W + G/I[h]	30	32 to 35	50 to 60	Cycling	Rectal	Time to complete 23 km; mean power output (W)
Siegel *et al.*, 2010 [18]	10 male; untrained	40.7 to 50.2[c]	I	30	34	55	Running	Rectal	Time to volitional fatigue at first ventilatory threshold
Siegel *et al.*, 2012 [19]	8 male; untrained	46.7 to 56.8[c]	I/W	30	34	52	Running	Rectal	Time to volitional fatigue at first ventilatory threshold
Ückert and Joch, 2007 [26]	20 male; trained	26.9 to 32.5[c]	G/WU	20	30 to 32	50	Running	Tympanic	Time to volitional fatigue during an incremental treadmill test

[a]Described as moderately trained to well trained in sports with high endurance components by the study authors.

[b]W = cold water immersion, G = cooling garment, D = cool water drink, WU = warm-up, I = ice slurry ingestion, LC = leg cooling.

[c]Mean group time.

[d]Cooling was maintained during subsequent warm-up by application of cool gel packs to hamstrings and quadriceps.

[e]Preceded by 10 minutes at 50% and 30 minutes at 70% VO_2max.

[f]Preceded by 60 minutes at 60% VO_2max.

[g]30 minutes cold water immersion, followed by 40 minutes wearing a cooling garment.

[h]While applying iced towels.

VO_2max = maximal aerobic capacity.

Table 3 Physiotherapy Evidence Database (PEDro) scale scores for each study

Factor	Authors, year and reference												
	Arngrïmsson *et al.*, 2004 [24]	Booth *et al.*, 1997 [42]	Cotter *et al.*, 2001 [25]	Duffield *et al.*, 2010 [41]	Gonzalez-Alonso *et al.*, 1999 [40]	Hasegawa *et al.*, 2006 [43]	Ihsan *et al.*, 2010 [16]	Kay *et al.*, 1999 [28]	Quod *et al.*, 2008 [27]	Ross *et al.*, 2011 [17]	Siegel *et al.*, 2010 [18]	Siegel *et al.*, 2012 [19]	Ückert and Joch, 2007 [26]
Eligibility criteria were specified (not scored)	0	0	0	0	0	0	0	0	0	0	0	0	0
Subjects were randomly allocated to groups	0	0	0	1	1	0	1	0	1	1	1	1	1
Allocation was concealed	0	0	0	0	0	0	0	0	0	0	0	0	0
Groups were similar at baseline	1	1	1	1	1	1	1	1	1	1	1	1	1
Blinding of subjects	0	0	0	0	0	0	0	0	0	0	0	0	0
Blinding of intervention administrators	0	0	0	0	0	0	0	0	0	0	0	0	0
Blinding of assessors	0	0	0	0	0	0	0	0	0	0	0	0	0
Outcome measure obtained from ≥ 85% subjects	1	1	1	1	1	1	1	1	1	1	1	1	1
All subjects received intervention/intention to treat analysis	1	1	0	1	1	1	1	1	1	1	1	1	1
Between group statistical comparisons reported	1	1	1	1	1	1	1	1	1	1	1	1	1
Between-group variability reported	1	1	1	1	1	1	1	1	1	1	1	1	1
PEDro score (out of 10)	5	5	4	6	6	5	6	5	6	6	6	6	6
Sample size calculation performed	0	0	0	0	0	0	0	0	0	0	0	0	0

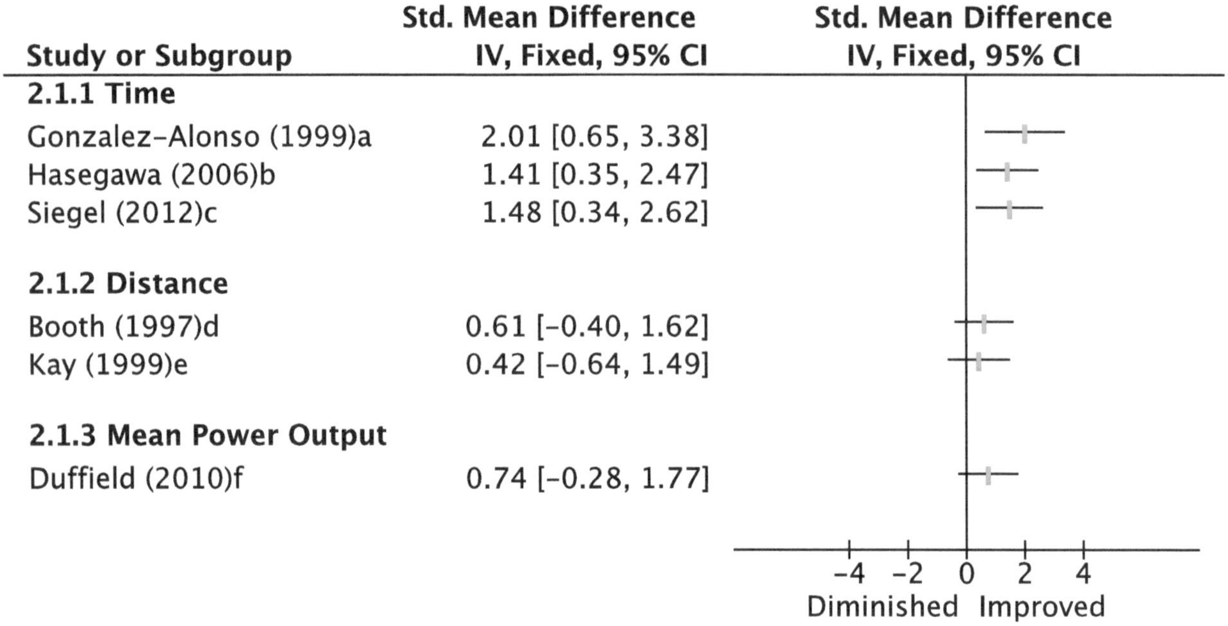

Figure 2 Effect sizes (Cohen's d) for cold water immersion versus control. Graph represents effect of intervention on exercise performance. [a]Time to volitional fatigue running at 60% VO_2max. [b]Time to volitional fatigue cycling at 80% VO_2max. [c]Time to volitional fatigue at first ventilatory threshold. [d]Distance run in 30 minutes at self-controlled pace. [e]Distance cycled in 30 minutes at self-controlled pace. [f]Mean power output during 40-minute cycling time trial.

improve endurance exercise performance in hot (≥ 28°C) environmental conditions. A total of 13 studies contained sufficient data to complete effect size calculations [16-19,24-28,40-43]. Of the three individual pre-cooling methods identified, cold water immersion was the most effective, with moderate evidence supporting its ability to improve endurance exercise performance compared to control conditions. Additionally, limited evidence indicates that ingesting ice slurry prior to competition is also effective, and potentially a more practical alternative to cold water immersion. Wearing a cooling garment prior to endurance exercise is of limited benefit to subsequent

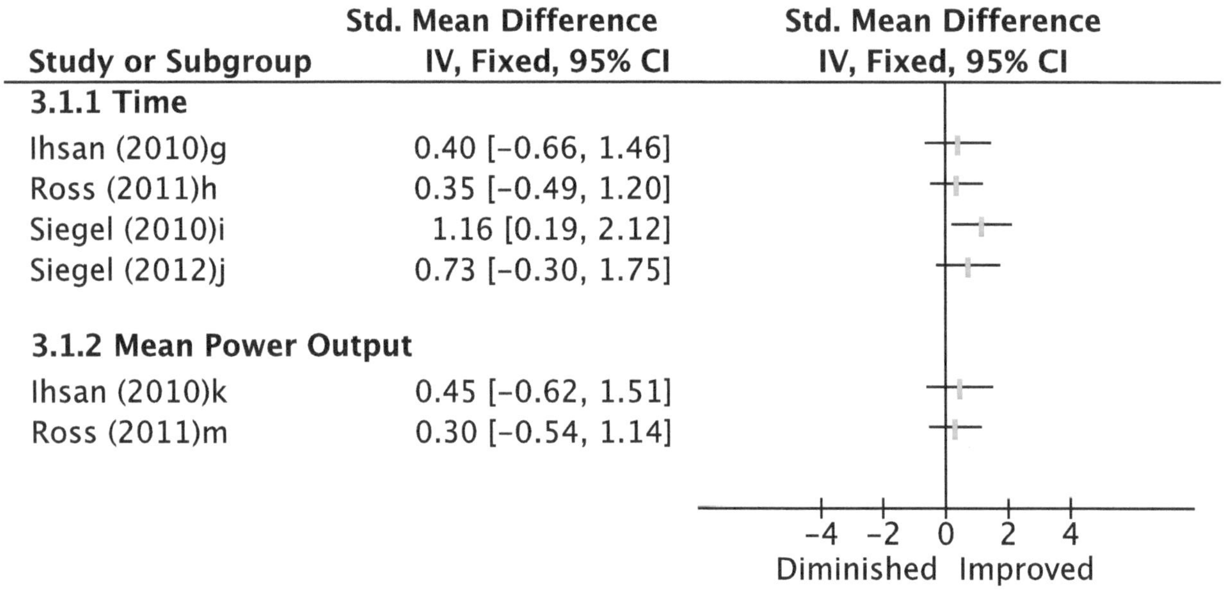

Figure 3 Effect sizes (Cohen's d) for ice slurry ingestion versus control. Graph represents effect of intervention on exercise performance. [g]Time to cycle 40 km. [h]Time to cycle 23 km. [i]Time to volitional fatigue at first ventilatory threshold. [j]Time to volitional fatigue at first ventilatory threshold. [k]Mean power output cycling 40 km. [m]Mean power output cycling 23 km.

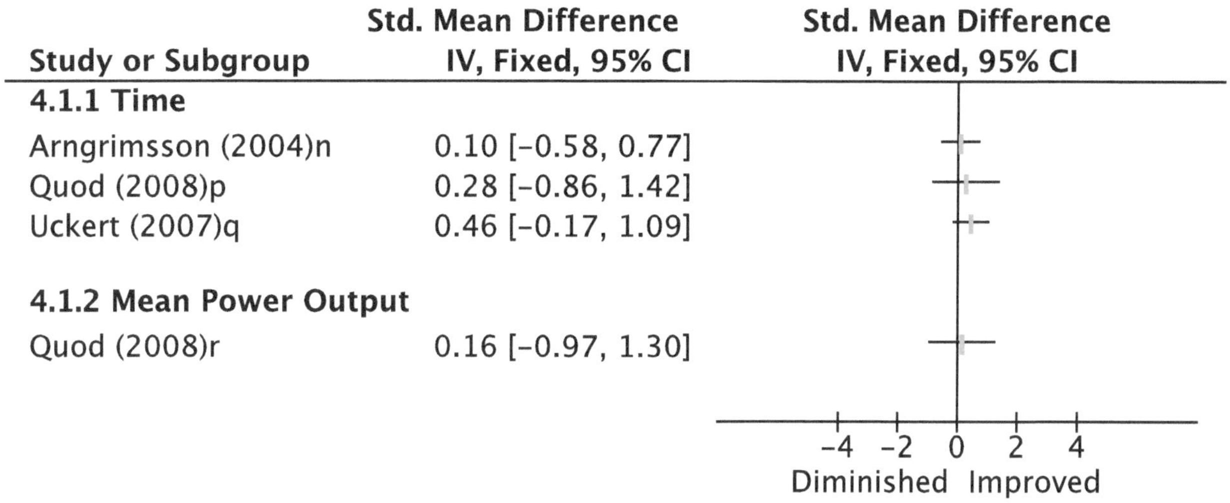

Figure 4 Effect sizes (Cohen's d) for cooling garment versus control. Graph represents effect of intervention on exercise performance. [n]Time to run 5 km. [p]Time to cycle a fixed amount of work. [q]Time to volitional fatigue during an incremental treadmill run. [r]Mean power output for duration of cycling time trial.

endurance exercise performance. Of the combined pre-cooling procedures that improved performance, the most effective protocol involved a period of cold water immersion.

Quality

Each included study used a repeated measures crossover design. However, methodological quality was varied with PEDro scores ranging from 4/10 to 6/10, indicating no high quality randomized controlled trials evaluating the effectiveness of pre-cooling to improve endurance exercise performance in the heat. Some studies did not randomize participant allocation, possibly introducing allocation bias [24,25,28,42,43]. All except four studies [18,19,25,43] used participants who were moderately to well trained (Table 4) in sports with high endurance

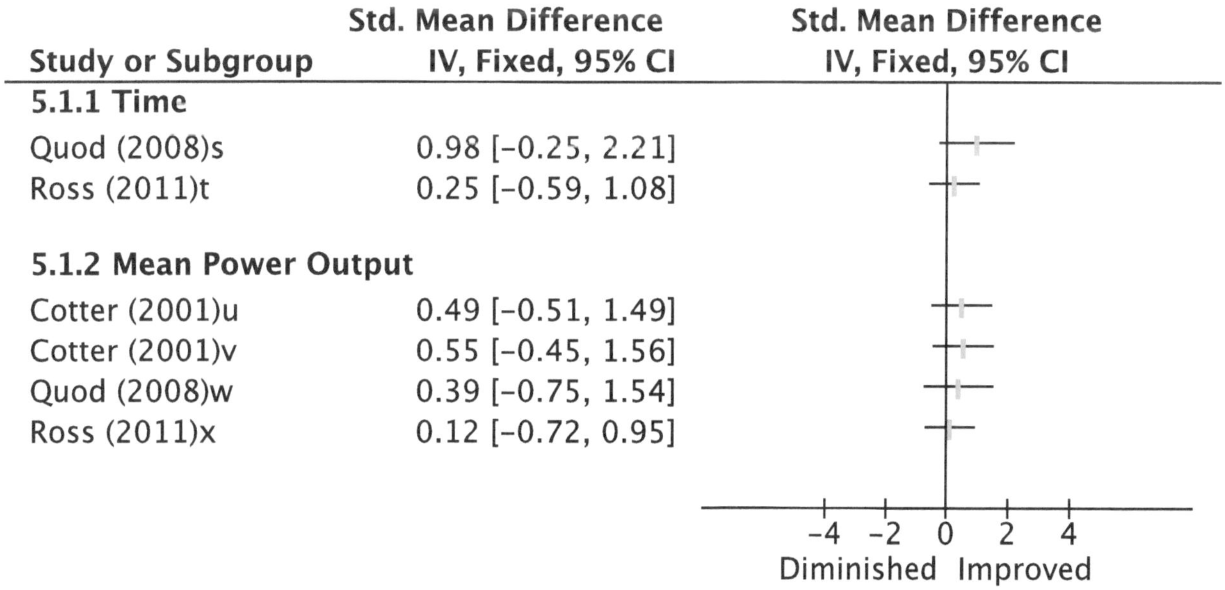

Figure 5 Effect sizes (Cohen's d) for various mixed cooling methods versus control. Graph represents effect of intervention on exercise performance. [s]Time to cycle a fixed amount of work (cold water immersion + cooling garment). [t]Time to cycle 23 km (cold water immersion + cooling garment). [u]Mean power output during 15-minute cycling time trial (cold air + cooling garment + leg cooling). [v]Mean power output during 15-minute cycling time trial (cold air + cooling garment + leg warming). [w]Mean power output for duration of cycling time trial (cold water immersion + cooling garment). [x]Mean power output cycling 23 km (cold water immersion + cooling garment).

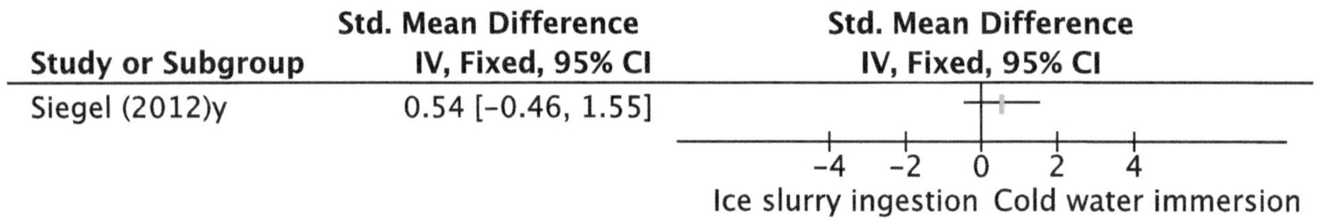

Figure 6 Effect sizes (Cohen's d) for ice slurry ingestion versus cold water immersion. Graph represents effect of intervention on exercise performance. [y]Time to volitional fatigue at first ventilatory threshold.

Table 4 Participant characteristics for each included study

Authors, year and reference	Participant characteristics
Arngrímsson *et al.*, 2004 [24]	Competitive collegiate and club middle/long distance runners
	Age men: 23.4 (4.4) years
	Age women: 22.1 (2.2) years
	Height men: 178.6 (4.4) cm
	Height women: 167.7 (5.5) cm
	Body mass men: 67.7 (4.2) kg
	Body mass women: 55.9 (4.3) kg
	Body fat men: 7.3 (2.0) %
	Body fat women: 17.8 (3.3) %
	Best 5 km run time men: 15.5 (0.8) min
	Best 5 km run time women: 17.9 (1.1) min
	VO_2max men: 4.50 (0.31) l/min
	VO_2max women: 3.24 (0.25) l/min
	Heat acclimatized
Booth *et al.*, 1997 [42][a]	Competitive runners from a local athletic club
	Age: 26.7 (1.7) years
	Height: 169.7 (4.0) cm
	Weight: 65.96 (2.87) kg
	Sum of eight skinfolds: 62.5 (9.7) mm
	Body surface area: 1.75 (0.06) m^2
	Body fat: 15.8 (1.2) %
	HR_{max}: 189.5 (2.8) beats/min
	VO_2peak: 63.1 (0.1) ml/kg/min
	Non-heat acclimatized
Cotter *et al.*, 2001 [25]	Habitually active, but were of lower average aerobic fitness than subjects used in previous studies on the effects of pre-cooling
	Age: 32.4 (3.6) years
	Height: 175.6 (6.9) cm
	Body mass: 80.9 (10.5) kg
	Body surface area: 1.96 (0.15) m^2
	VO_2peak: 51 (8) ml/min/kg
	Non-heat acclimatized
Duffield *et al.*, 2010 [41]	Moderate to well trained cyclists of club and regional standard who trained multiple times a week, competing in regional competitions
	Age: 24.8 (3.3) years
	Height: 178.3 (8.0) cm
	Body mass: 76.1 (2.7) kg
	Sum of seven skinfolds: 54.4 (10.9) mm
	Lactate threshold: 221 (42) W
	Non-heat acclimatized

Table 4 Participant characteristics for each included study *(Continued)*

Gonzalez-Alonso *et al.*, 1999 [40]*	Endurance trained
	Age: 28 (3) years
	Height: 187 (6) cm
	Body mass: 77.9 (6.4) kg
	HR_{max}: 200 (9) beats/min
	VO_2peak: 5.13 (0.30) l/min
	Non-heat acclimatized
Hasegawa *et al.*, 2006 [43]*	Untrained
	Age: 21.8 (0.8) years
	Height: 1.72 (0.02) cm
	Body mass: 61.7 (2.1) kg
	Body fat: 15.1 (1.1) %
	VO_2max: 48.5 (1.5) ml/kg/min
	Non-heat acclimatized
Ihsan *et al.*, 2010 [16]	Endurance trained regularly competing in cycling or triathlon, cycling more than four sessions and > 150 km/week
	Age: 27.7 (3.1) years
	Height: 176.7 (5.8) cm
	Body mass: 81.38 (9.09) kg
	Non-heat acclimatized
Kay *et al.*, 1999 [28]*	Moderately to well-trained and undertook bicycle riding, training and competition on a regular basis
	Age: 23.7 (2.1) years
	Height: 182 (3) cm
	Body mass: 76.1 (4.0) kg
	Sum of four skinfolds: 28.4 (2.3) mm
	Body surface area: 1.97 (0.06) m^2
	HR_{max}: 184 (3) beats/min
	VO_2peak: 4.91 (0.25) l/min
	Non-heat acclimatized
Quod *et al.*, 2008 [27]	Well trained male cyclists with 6 (5) years of experience
	Age: 28 (4) years
	Height: 182 (2) cm
	Body mass: 75.1 (3.2) kg
	Sum of seven skinfolds: 50 (11) mm
	VO_2peak: 71.4 (3.2) ml/kg/min
	Maximum aerobic power: 384 (23) W
	Non-heat acclimatized
Ross *et al.*, 2011 [17]	Well trained A-grade cyclists aged 18 to 35 years
	Age: 33 (5.1) years
	Body mass: 72.1 (5.5) kg
	Maximum aerobic power: 449 (26) W
	VO_2peak: 71.6 (6.1) ml/kg/min
	Heat acclimatized
Siegel *et al.*, 2010 [18]	Moderately active, participating in recreational sport
	Age: 28 (6) years
	Height: 178.9 (6.3) cm
	Body mass: 79.9 (11.2) kg
	Sum of nine skinfolds: 92.8 (41.4) mm
	VO_2peak: 56.4 (4.7) ml/kg/min
	Non-heat acclimatized
Siegel *et al.*, 2012 [19]	Moderately active, were partaking in recreational sport
	Age: 26 (4) years

Table 4 Participant characteristics for each included study *(Continued)*

	Height: 179.9 (6.7) cm
	Body mass: 78.1 (5.9) kg
	Sum of nine skinfolds: 87.3 (22.5) mm
	VO_2peak: 54.2 (2.5) ml/kg/min
	Non-heat acclimatized
Ückert and Joch, 2007 [26]	Regularly practiced types of sport with high endurance and strength components at a high level for example, soccer, athletics
	Age: 25.6 (3.5) years
	Height: 183.4 (7.6) cm
	Weight: 77.9 (9.5) kg
	Non-heat acclimatized

All values are mean (± SD).
[a]Values in brackets are ± (SE).
HR = heart rate; VO_2max = maximal aerobic capacity; VO_2peak = peak oxygen uptake.

components (cycling, triathlon and distance running), and within that only cycling and running exercise protocols were used, limiting the applicability of the findings to the broader, less well trained population. Lack of participant, investigator and outcome assessor blinding was consistent across all studies, likely due to practical difficulties. Consequently, some results could have been unintentionally biased, either by observer bias, such as encouraging participants in the pre-cooled group, or a placebo effect.

Participant numbers in each study were low, ranging from 6 [27] to 20 [26], limiting the validity of conclusions that can be drawn from the results. None of the reviewed studies performed sample size calculations, and therefore certain data trends could not be substantiated due to inadequate statistical power. There was a high level of methodological heterogeneity between studies, including: exercise performance protocol, pre-cooling duration, exercise duration and outcome measure, making comparison of studies and recommendations for enhancing sporting performance difficult. This was further compounded by the absence of comparisons between the three main individual pre-cooling maneuvers (cold water immersion, cooling garment and ice slurry ingestion) in all but one study [19]. Therefore, the relative efficacy and practicality of one pre-cooling method to another could not be made. In one study, subjects exercised at 60% VO_2max for 60 minutes followed by an effort at 80% VO_2max to volitional fatigue [43]. However, mean performance time ± standard error were only reported for the short effort at 80% VO_2max to fatigue. This is likely to have inflated the effect size compared to other studies.

Cold water immersion

Moderate evidence currently exists to support the use of cold water immersion as a pre-cooling intervention to improve endurance exercise performance in the heat. Three studies showed a significant performance improvement in the pre-cooled compared to control condition [19,40,43], with the remaining three studies showing a positive trend to improved performance [28,41,42]. In each of the immersion studies there was a significant reduction in core temperature compared to control at some point during the exercise protocol. Additionally, the rate of heat storage was greater in three of the four studies that reported this variable [19,28,42], conferring a greater margin for metabolic load during exercise in the pre-cooling condition. Gonzalez-Alonso *et al.* [40] reported that rate of heat storage was equal between both conditions. However, as the pre-cooled group commenced exercise with a core temperature 1.5°C lower than the control condition, their total heat storage capacity was greater. Although not conclusive evidence of a precise mechanism, it seems that pre-cooling using cold water immersion could possibly improve performance by reducing core temperature prior to exercise, or blunting the rate of rise in core temperature during exercise, increasing heat storage capacity and enabling athletes to perform at a greater relative intensity or for a greater duration [29].

Despite a more rapid reduction in core temperature with water immersion compared with traditional cold air exposure [46], the required length of pre-cooling remains significant (30 to 60 minutes) [29,30]. Marino and Booth [21], in one of the first studies investigating the potential use of pre-cooling via cold water immersion prior to endurance exercise, reduced core temperature by gradually reducing the temperature of the immersion bath over a 60-minute period. This was to avoid the potentially detrimental cold stress responses that had previously been seen with cold air exposure, such as shivering [29]. Such a regimented technique, which also precludes a concomitant warm-up, is limited in its practicality in an elite sports setting immediately prior to athletic competition, in addition to other logistical issues such as expense, transportation of equipment, and access to such a large volume of water and electricity in the field.

Ice slurry ingestion

Limited evidence currently exists to support the use of ice slurry as a pre-cooling intervention to improve endurance exercise performance in the heat. One study [18] showed a significant performance improvement in the ice slurry ingestion pre-cooled compared to the control condition and the three remaining studies showed a positive trend to improved performance [16,17,19]. Each study reported that core temperature was significantly lower in the pre-cooling condition than control after the cooling intervention and prior to the start of the exercise task, increasing heat storage capacity. Alternatively, the participants' lower core body temperatures prior to exercise may have enabled them to select a faster pacing strategy by influencing central regulation of exercise intensity [47].

Two studies [18,19] reported that the pre-cooled group exhibited a significantly higher core temperature at exhaustion. The authors suggest that this could be due to the generation of higher metabolic heat loads as a result of either a direct cooling effect on the brain, or an effect on core temperature afferent nerves [48], altering perception of effort and increasing time to exhaustion. Increased core temperature above normal tolerable limits is an important safety consideration and may be detrimental to athlete health, increasing the risk of heat-related illness, and is something that requires attention in future studies.

Ice slurry ingestion offers a number of practical benefits over cold water immersion, as it is not subject to the same logistical restrictions. The ice slurry can be produced using a commercially available machine or simply freezing and part-thawing sports drinks prior to the event, and transporting them in a cool box. This is particularly useful at events where there is no provision for electrical equipment, or where transportation is an issue. Pre-cooling athletes in this way is quick and simple. The amount of ice slurry required to achieve effective cooling is low and similar in volume to pre-exercise fluid hydration protocols, ranging from 6.8 g/kg [16] to 14 g/kg [17] of body mass. In each reviewed study, the volume of ice slurry was administered over a 30-minute period at a standardized rate that ranged from 5 [18,19] to 15 minutes [17]. Although not yet investigated, there is the potential that ice slurry ingestion could enable athletes to warm-up during cooling, making it much more time efficient than cold water immersion. In addition to providing a greater cooling effect than cold water alone [23], a much smaller volume is required to produce this response, reducing the potential for detrimental effects that the ingestion of large volumes of fluid may have. As well as cooling athletes, the ice slurry can be used to hydrate athletes too so that combined fluid and slurry ingestion is not necessary.

Cooling garments

None of the studies showed a significant improvement of wearing a cooling garment on subsequent exercise performance [24,26,27]. This likely resulted from the lack of effect on core body temperature. In two studies [26,27], despite the pre-cooling groups having significantly lower skin temperatures while wearing the cooling garment, core temperature was not significantly lower at any time point during either pre-cooling or subsequent exercise. Arngrïmsson *et al.* [24] reported significantly lower rectal temperatures in the pre-cooling group for the last 18 minutes of the warm-up and first 3.2 km of the running exercise task compared to the control group. However, this effect was not strong enough to have caused a significant improvement in performance and may have resulted from the high rectal temperatures, and therefore reduced heat storage capacity, at the start of the performance task in both the cooling garment (38.0°C) and control group (38.2°C) compared to all other studies that reported rectal temperature at the onset of the exercise task [18,19,25,27,28,41-43].

Kay *et al.* [28] suggested a reduction in core body temperature achieved through lowering skin temperature, effecting heat loss from core to skin. This is the mechanism by which cooling garments are believed to act to cool athletes prior to exercise. However, cooling in Kay *et al.'s* [28] study was achieved via whole-body cold water immersion, which likely provided a greater cooling stimulus than cooling garments, especially at peripheral areas of the body. This could explain why cooling garments were found to have little effect on core body temperature in the present study. One study reported than the application of a cooling garment reduced skin blood flow across the body by stimulating vasoconstriction, preventing efficient heat transfer between the skin and the cooling garment. Core body temperature of subjects remained unaltered, likely from the redistribution of blood to the core [44]. If the hypothesis that a critical core temperature limits exercise performance in the heat is correct, then, by failing to reduce core body temperature cooling garments were unable to improve endurance exercise performance.

Mixed methods

Some studies combined more than one pre-cooling intervention to cool participants prior to the exercise component of the trial. Two studies immersed subjects in cold water, followed by a period wearing a cooling garment [17,27]. Quod *et al.* [27] reported a significant decrease in core body temperature prior to exercise, likely as a result of an 'afterdrop' effect [49]; that is, a continued fall in core temperature after the initial hypothermic exposure, as opposed to any further cooling effect of the garment.

Indeed, the same study reported that wearing the cooling garment alone failed to reduce core temperature compared to control. Exercise performance was significantly better than control and cooling garment conditions. Conversely, Ross *et al.* [17] reported that, despite a significantly lower core body temperature after cooling and throughout warm-up compared to controls, there was no improvement in performance. The authors suggest that the larger cooling response in the combined condition may have led the athletes to select poorer pacing strategies. An alternative explanation could be that the cold water immersion protocol used may have been too abrupt compared to that used in other studies [21], and may therefore have elicited a cold stress response that was detrimental to performance, similar to that reported for cold air exposure [29].

A combination of cold air and a cooling garment, with or without thigh cooling, showed trends to improved performance in both conditions compared to control in one study [25]. Both pre-cooling groups had a lower core temperature after pre-cooling, and power output was significantly greater compared to controls during the 15-minute performance trial. There was no difference in power output between the two cooling conditions. It is difficult to determine whether the cooling garment conferred any additional benefits than have been shown to be conferred by cold air cooling alone [12,13,50]. In practice, cold air cooling has a number of logistical limitations including equipment transport and cost, the significant time required to adequately cool athletes, and a noted cold stress response that can impair exercise performance [29].

Limitations and future research

There is a high level of heterogeneity in study design examining the effectiveness of pre-cooling strategies, and optimal cooling protocols have yet to be established. Variables such as cooling duration and time between pre-cooling and commencing exercise are likely to exert considerable influence on study outcomes and require greater attention. Once repeatable pre-cooling protocols have been identified for each individual modality, then more reliable comparisons of effectiveness can be made between modalities. One study directly compared ice slurry ingestion to cold water immersion and found it to be similarly effective at improving performance (Figure 6) [19]. As potentially the cheaper, more practical strategy, this result is encouraging and warrants further investigation of ice slurry ingestion in the field. Additionally, following Quod *et al.'s* study [27], it would be instructive to determine whether the combination of a cooling garment following cold water immersion confers any additional benefit compared to immersion only.

Hydration strategies employed, and reporting of these strategies was inconsistent (Table 5). Water ingestion, especially cool water, may lower core body temperature via a similar mechanism as ice slurry ingestion. Potentially, if control participants were permitted to drink cool water either before or throughout the exercise trial this may confound the effectiveness of the pre-cooling strategy. However, this is a difficult variable to control for and depends on the comparison being made. For example, studies investigating ice slurry ingestion used water ingestion of an equal volume as the control condition to determine that any improvements in performance were a result of the pre-cooling effect of ice slurry ingestion as opposed to the ergogenic effect of adequate hydration [51]. Interestingly, Siegel *et al.* found a greater effect of ice slurry ingestion on performance when compared to controls drinking cool fluid (4°C) [18] than when compared to controls drinking warmer fluid (37°C) [19], which suggests that cool water ingestion may not blunt the effectiveness of pre-cooling as much as expected. However, more consistent hydration protocols will enable greater analysis of this relationship. Hasegawa *et al.* [43] reported that continuous cool water ingestion during exercise following cold water immersion significantly improved performance compared to cold water immersion alone and negated the rise in core body temperature towards the end of the performance protocol. The authors attributed this to increased evaporative sweat loss, sweat efficiency and decreased heat strain in the continuous water ingestion group. This finding suggests that the benefits of pre-cooling may be augmented by maintaining hydration during exercise. Ice slurry ingestion acts to pre-cool athletes and could also be used to maintain cooling and hydration during exercise. Therefore, a comparison of combined cold water immersion and water beverage with continuous ice slurry ingestion is warranted.

The level of fitness of participants varied across studies as did the consistency of reporting of fitness and experience of endurance exercise (Table 4). It is difficult, therefore, to determine whether more experienced or less experienced athletes would benefit more from pre-cooling. Furthermore, those who are less experienced are likely to be less accurate when anticipating a required pacing strategy to complete a given exercise trial [47]. By lowering core body temperature using exogenous means, participants may perceive their level of exertion to be lower than their body's thermal load should dictate, that is, a discrepancy between their perceived and actual homeostatic state, which could cause them to develop heat illness due to the masking of thermal strain. This is acknowledged in the two studies that reported participants to have an elevated core body

Table 5 Hydration practices for each included study

Authors, year and reference	Hydration practice
Arngrïmsson *et al.*, 2004 [24]	Pre-test: instructed to drink water and other non-caffeinated beverages liberally
	During the warm-up: water *ad libitum*. Tap temperature. Amount was recorded and repeated for the second condition.
	Not reported/performed during exercise
Booth *et al.*, 1997 [42]	During exercise trial: water *ad libitum*
Cotter *et al.*, 2001 [25]	Pre-test: instructed to drink at least 15 ml/kg BM 2 to 3 h before arrival at laboratory
	During the warm-up: water *ad libitum* after warm-up and before exercise trial
	Not reported/performed during exercise
Duffield *et al.*, 2010 [41]	Pre-test: 500 ml water 60 min before arrival at the laboratory
	Not reported/performed during exercise
Gonzalez-Alonso *et al.*, 1999 [40]	Pre-test: 200 to 300 ml with breakfast
	Not reported/performed during exercise
Hasegawa *et al.*, 2006 [43]	Pre-test: 500 ml 2 h before the trial
	Immersion: no fluid ingestion
	Immersion + water ingestion: water (14 to 16°C) every 5 min during exercise equal to volume sweat loss in sweat test performed at a prior visit to laboratory
	Water ingestion: water (14 to 16°C) every 5 min during exercise equal to volume sweat loss in sweat test performed at a prior visit to laboratory
	Control: no fluid ingestion
Ihsan *et al.*, 2010 [16]	Pre-test: adequate hydration was strongly encouraged before testing
	Pre-cooling: 6.8 g/kg BM ice slurry in 150 to 200 g aliquots in intervals of 8 to 10 minutes over a period of 30 minutes (1.4 ± 1.1°C)
	Control: 6.8 g/kg BM tap water slurry in 150 to 200 g aliquots in intervals of 8 to 10 minutes over a period of 30 minutes (26.8 ± 1.3°C)
	During exercise trial: 100 ml water (26.8 ± 1.3°C) at four intervals
Kay *et al.*, 1999 [28]	During exercise trial: water *ad libitum*
Quod *et al.*, 2008 [27]	Pre-test: 250 ml sport drink diluted to half the manufacturer's recommended strength
	During exercise trial: 250 ml sport drink diluted to half the manufacturer's recommended strength
Ross *et al.*, 2011 [17]	Pre-test: water (4°C) *ad libitum* throughout heat stabilization and warm-up
	Pre-cooling: 14 g/kg BM ice slurry in two 7 g/kg BM boluses 15 minutes apart
	Control: water (4°C) *ad libitum*
	During exercise trial: subjects were provided with 350 ml of a 6% carbohydrate-electrolyte drink at 12.5 and 37.5 km to consume *ad libitum* for the next km (drinks left out in heat temperature to simulate race conditions)
Siegel *et al.*, 2010 [18]	Pre-test: instructed to drink at least 2 l fluid the day before the trial, and 400 ml during the meal consumed before the trial
	Pre-cooling: 7.5 g/kg BM ice slurry (1°C) with 5% carbohydrate in 1.25 g/kg BM aliquots every 5 minutes over a period of 30 minutes
	Control: 7.5 g/kg BM water (4°C) with 5% carbohydrate in 1.25 g/kg BM aliquots every 5 minutes over a period of 30 minutes
	Not reported/performed during exercise
Siegel *et al.*, 2012 [19]	Pre-test: instructed to drink at least 2 l fluid the day before the trial, and 400 ml during the meal consumed before the trial
	Pre-cooling: 7.5 g/kg BM ice slurry (-1°C) with 5% carbohydrate in 1.25 g/kg BM aliquots every 5 minutes over a period of 30 minutes
	Immersion: 7.5 g/kg BM water (37°C) with 5% carbohydrate in 1.25 g/kg BM aliquots every 5 minutes over a period of 30 minutes
	Control: 7.5 g/kg BM water (37°C) with 5% carbohydrate in 1.25 g/kg BM aliquots every 5 minutes over a period of 30 minutes
	Not reported/performed during exercise
Ückert and Joch, 2007 [26]	Pre-test: avoid fluid for 3 h before start of test
	Not reported/performed during exercise

BM = body mass.

temperature at volitional fatigue [18,19]. Notably, these studies used untrained participants so it is possible that more experienced athletes may be better attuned to their physiological limits and hence less at risk of heat illness, but this is speculative and warrants further investigation before ice slurry ingestion can be recommended.

Given the lack of blinding of participants and researchers in the reviewed studies, a placebo effect cannot be excluded from having influenced results. Future studies should consider introducing a separate, placebo-controlled group, and participant and assessor blinding to improve methodological validity. The placebo-control could, for example, use menthol to provide a cooling sensation for participants without causing an actual change in temperature [52].

Each study included in this review was limited by low participant numbers. It was therefore difficult to determine whether certain reported trends or lack thereof were the result of the studies being underpowered. *A priori* power calculations should be performed to increase the statistical significance of any trends reported in the results. Study participants were predominantly male, therefore the findings of this review may not be applicable to females, especially because certain anthropometric and hormonal differences, including stage of the menstrual cycle [53] and body composition [54], can affect thermoregulation under heat stress. It should be acknowledged that the majority were performed with the intention of applying the findings to highly trained athletes, and that recruiting large numbers of such compliant volunteers is difficult. However, the inclusion of larger sample sizes and inclusion of similar proportions of female and male participants in future research will allow both improved external validity for broader populations and between sex comparisons to be made.

Laboratory studies grant assessors strict control of certain variables, such as the environmental conditions under which exercise is performed, which is necessary with preliminary studies to establish intervention efficacy and optimal protocols. However, future studies of pre-cooling should focus on real-world testing to determine whether the promising laboratory findings translate to tangible performance gains in the field. This is also important to evaluate the practicality of each method of pre-cooling during competition.

There was also a lack of safety or adverse event reporting. It remains unknown what effect increased heat storage capacity may have on other bodily systems other than those directly involved in thermoregulation. Therefore, until these can be elucidated, it would be prudent for future research to include consideration of athlete safety, as this will be of primary concern to coaches and athletes alike, given the physiologically stressful environment in which they will be competing.

Practicality and recommendations

Although consistently the most effective method of pre-cooling and enhancing endurance exercise performance in the heat, cold water immersion has limited practicality in sporting settings due to expense, transportation issues, difficulty accessing large volumes of water and time required to achieve a reduction in core body temperature. Ice slurry ingestion is a relatively cheap and much more practical alternative to whole body immersion and effectively lowers core body temperature, approaching the improvements in performance seen with immersion. Additionally, there is currently limited evidence from one study that indicates the effectiveness of ice slurry ingestion and cold water immersion are comparable [19]. However, safety concerns raised by two studies that reported a raised core body temperature at volitional fatigue need to be addressed before its use can be recommended for competing athletes. Cooling garments failed to improve endurance exercise performance and therefore are of limited use in this regard.

Conclusions

This systematic review suggests that pre-cooling procedures can improve endurance exercise performance in the heat, with the likely mechanism being reduced core body temperature prior to exercise, and subsequently increased heat storage capacity. Cold water immersion is the most effective method of pre-cooling, with moderate evidence to support its effectiveness. However, its limited practicality in many sporting settings must be considered. Ice slurry ingestion has shown good initial results, with limited evidence supporting its effectiveness, and may provide a more practical pre-performance option. However, larger studies with consistent protocols and further investigation of potential safety issues associated with altered levels of perceived exertion are required before its use can be recommended. Cooling garments appear of limited efficacy, but this finding may be the result of sub-optimal cooling protocols or inadequate study power. To date, most studies have focused on whether pre-cooling improves performance compared to no intervention, with only one study directly comparing individual modalities. Therefore, recommending one method over another to coaches and athletes is difficult. Further comparative research is required before best practice recommendations can be made.

Authors' contributions

PRJ conceived the review topic. All authors assisted with the review design. PRJ and CB completed searching, quality assessment and data analysis. All authors contributed to interpretation of results, editing of the manuscript and approved the final manuscript

Competing interests

The authors declare that they have no competing interests.

Author details

[1]Centre for Sports and Exercise Medicine, William Harvey Research Institute, Bart's and the London School of Medicine and Dentistry, Queen Mary University of London, Mile End Hospital, Bancroft Road, London E1 4DG, UK. [2]King's College London School of Medicine and Dentistry, King's College London, Guy's Campus, London SE1 9UL, UK.

References

1. Galloway SD, Maughan RJ: **Effects of ambient temperature on the capacity to perform prolonged cycle exercise in man.** *Med Sci Sports Exerc* 1997, **29**:1240-1249.
2. MacDougall JD, Reddan WG, Layton CR, Dempsey JA: **Effects of metabolic hyperthermia on performance during heavy prolonged exercise.** *J Appl Physiol* 1974, **36**:538-544.
3. Peiffer JJ, Abbiss CR: **Influence of environmental temperature on 40 km cycling time-trial performance.** *Int J Sports Physiol Perform* 2011, **6**:208-220.
4. El Helou N, Tafflet M, Berthelot G, Tolaini J, Marc A, Guillaume M, Hausswirth C, Toussaint JF: **Impact of environmental parameters on marathon running performance.** *PLoS One* 2012, **7**:e37407.
5. McCann DJ, Adams WC: **Wet bulb globe temperature index and performance in competitive distance runners.** *Med Sci Sports Exerc* 1997, **29**:955-961.
6. Brück K, Olschewski H: **Body temperature related factors diminishing the drive to exercise.** *Can J Physiol Pharmacol* 1987, **65**:1274-1280.
7. Nielsen B, Hales JR, Strange S, Christensen NJ, Warberg J, Saltin B: **Human circulatory and thermoregulatory adaptations with heat acclimation and exercise in a hot, dry environment.** *J Physiol* 1993, **460**:467-485.
8. Febbraio MA, Murton P, Selig SE, Clark SA, Lambert DL, Angus DJ, Carey MF: **Effect of CHO ingestion on exercise metabolism and performance in different ambient temperatures.** *Med Sci Sports Exerc* 1996, **28**:1380-1387.
9. Maughan RJ: **Distance running in hot environments: a thermal challenge to the elite runner.** *Scand J Med Sci Sports* 2010, **20**:95-102.
10. Sawka MN, Young AJ, Latzka WA, Neufer PD, Quigley MD, Pandolf KB: **Human tolerance to heat strain during exercise: influence of hydration.** *J Appl Physiol* 1992, **73**:368-375.
11. Abbiss CR, Burnett K, Nosaka AK, Green JP, Foster JK, Laursen PB: **Effect of hot versus cold climates on power output, muscle activation, and perceived fatigue during a dynamic 100-km cycling trial.** *J Sports Sci* 2010, **28**:117-125.
12. Lee DT, Haymes EM: **Exercise duration and thermoregulatory responses after whole body precooling.** *J Appl Physiol* 1995, **79**:1971-1976.
13. Hessemer V, Langusch D, Brück LK, Bödeker RH, Breidenbach T: **Effect of slightly lowered body temperatures on endurance performance in humans.** *J Appl Physiol* 1984, **57**:1731-1737.
14. Olschewski H, Brück K: **Thermoregulatory, cardiovascular, and muscular factors related to exercise after precooling.** *J Appl Physiol* 1988, **64**:803-811.
15. Martin DT, Hahn AG, Ryan-Tanner R, Yates K, Lee H, Smith JA: **Ice jackets are cool.** *Sportscience* 1998, **2**: [http://sportsci.org/jour/9804/dtm.html].
16. Ihsan M, Landers G, Brearley M, Peeling P: **Beneficial effects of ice ingestion as a precooling strategy on 40-km cycling time-trial performance.** *Int J Sports Physiol Perform* 2010, **5**:140-151.
17. Ross ML, Garvican LA, Jeacocke NA, Laursen PB, Abbiss CR, Martin DT, Burke LM: **Novel precooling strategy enhances time trial cycling in the heat.** *Med Sci Sports Exerc* 2011, **43**:123-133.
18. Siegel R, Maté J, Brearley MB, Watson G, Nosaka K, Laursen PB: **Ice slurry ingestion increases core temperature capacity and running time in the heat.** *Med Sci Sports Exerc* 2010, **42**:717-725.
19. Siegel R, Maté J, Watson G, Nosaka K, Laursen PB: **Pre-cooling with ice slurry ingestion leads to similar run times to exhaustion in the heat as cold water immersion.** *J Sports Sci* 2012, **30**:155-165.
20. Burton AC, Bazett HC: **A study of the average temperature of the tissues, of the exchanges of heat and vasomotor responses in man by means of a bath calorimeter.** *Am J Physiol* 1936, **117**:36-54.
21. Marino F, Booth J: **Whole body cooling by immersion in water at moderate temperatures.** *J Sci Med Sport* 1998, **1**:73-82.
22. Merrick MA, Jutte LS, Smith ME: **Cold modalities with different thermodynamic properties produce different surface and intramuscular temperatures.** *J Athl Train* 2003, **38**:28-33.
23. Vanden Hoek TL, Kasza KE, Beiser DG, Abella BS, Franklin JE, Oras JJ, Alvarado JP, Anderson T, Son H, Wardrip CL, Zhao D, Wang H, Becker LB: **Induced hypothermia by central venous infusion: saline ice slurry versus chilled saline.** *Crit Care Med* 2004, **32**:S425-431.
24. Arngrïmsson SA, Petitt DS, Stueck MG, Jorgensen DK, Cureton KJ: **Cooling vest worn during active warm-up improves 5-km run performance in the heat.** *J Appl Physiol* 2004, **96**:1867-1874.
25. Cotter JD, Sleivert GG, Roberts WS, Febbraio MA: **Effect of pre-cooling, with and without thigh cooling, on strain and endurance exercise performance in the heat.** *Comp Biochem Physiol A Mol Integr Physiol* 2001, **128**:667-677.
26. Uckert S, Joch W: **Effects of warm-up and precooling on endurance performance in the heat.** *Br J Sports Med* 2007, **41**:380-384.
27. Quod MJ, Martin DT, Laursen PB, Gardner AS, Halson SL, Marino FE, Tate MP, Mainwaring DE, Gore CJ, Hahn AG: **Practical precooling: effect on cycling time trial performance in warm conditions.** *J Sports Sci* 2008, **26**:1477-1487.
28. Kay D, Taaffe DR, Marino FE: **Whole-body pre-cooling and heat storage during self-paced cycling performance in warm humid conditions.** *J Sports Sci* 1999, **17**:937-944.
29. Marino FE: **Methods, advantages, and limitations of body cooling for exercise performance.** *Br J Sports Med* 2002, **36**:89-94.
30. Quod MJ, Martin DT, Laursen PB: **Cooling athletes before competition in the heat: comparison of techniques and practical considerations.** *Sports Med* 2006, **36**:671-682.
31. Ranalli GF, Demartini JK, Casa DJ, McDermott BP, Armstrong LE, Maresh CM: **Effect of body cooling on subsequent aerobic and anaerobic exercise performance: a systematic review.** *J Strength Cond Res* 2010, **24**:3488-3496.
32. Cabanac M, Massonnet B: **Thermoregulatory responses as a function of core temperature in humans.** *J Physiol* 1977, **265**:587-596.
33. Tyler C, Sunderland C: **The effect of ambient temperature on the reliability of a preloaded treadmill time-trial.** *Int J Sports Med* 2008, **29**:812-816.
34. Price MJ: **Thermoregulation during exercise in individuals with spinal cord injuries.** *Sports Med* 2006, **36**:863-879.
35. Maher CG, Sherrington C, Elkins M, Herbert RD, Moseley AM: **Challenges for evidence-based physical therapy: accessing and interpreting high-quality evidence on therapy.** *Phys Ther* 2004, **84**:644-654.
36. de Morton NA: **The PEDro scale is a valid measure of the methodological quality of clinical trials: a demographic study.** *Aust J Physiother* 2009, **55**:129-133.
37. Sedgwick P: **Meta-analysis: funnel plots.** *BMJ* 2011, **343**:d5372.
38. Sterne JA, Egger M, Smith GD: **Systematic reviews in health care: investigating and dealing with publication and other biases in meta-analysis.** *BMJ* 2001, **323**:101-105.
39. van Tulder M, Furlan A, Bombardier C, Bouter L, Editorial Board of the Cochrane Collaboration Back Review Group: **Updated method guidelines for systematic reviews in the cochrane collaboration back review group.** *Spine (Phila Pa 1976)* 2003, **28**:1290-1299.
40. González-Alonso J, Teller C, Andersen SL, Jensen FB, Hyldig T, Nielsen B: **Influence of body temperature on the development of fatigue during prolonged exercise in the heat.** *J Appl Physiol* 1999, **86**:1032-1039.
41. Duffield R, Green R, Castle P, Maxwell N: **Precooling can prevent the reduction of self-paced exercise intensity in the heat.** *Med Sci Sports Exerc* 2010, **42**:577-584.
42. Booth J, Marino F, Ward JJ: **Improved running performance in hot humid conditions following whole body precooling.** *Med Sci Sports Exerc* 1997, **29**:943-949.
43. Hasegawa H, Takatori T, Komura T, Yamasaki M: **Combined effects of pre-cooling and water ingestion on thermoregulation and physical capacity during exercise in a hot environment.** *J Sports Sci* 2006, **24**:3-9.

44. Bogerd N, Perret C, Bogerd CP, Rossi RM, Daanen HA: **The effect of pre-cooling intensity on cooling efficiency and exercise performance.** *J Sports Sci* 2010, **28**:771-779.
45. Webster J, Holland EJ, Sleivert G, Laing RM, Niven BE: **A light-weight cooling vest enhances performance of athletes in the heat.** *Ergonomics* 2005, **48**:821-837.
46. Smith RM, Hanna JM: **Skinfolds and resting heat loss in cold air and water: temperature equivalence.** *J Appl Physiol* 1975, **39**:93-102.
47. Noakes TD: **The central governor model of exercise regulation applied to the marathon.** *Sports Med* 2007, **37**:374-377.
48. Gleeson M: **Temperature regulation during exercise.** *Int J Sports Med* 1998, **19**:S96-99.
49. Romet TT: **Mechanism of afterdrop after cold water immersion.** *J Appl Physiol* 1988, **65**:1535-1538.
50. Schmidt V, Brück K: **Effect of a precooling maneuver on body temperature and exercise performance.** *J Appl Physiol* 1981, **50**:772-778.
51. Sawka MN, Montain SJ, Latzka WA: **Hydration effects on thermoregulation and performance in the heat.** *Comp Biochem Physiol A Mol Integr Physiol* 2001, **128**:679-690.
52. Eccles R: **Menthol and related cooling compounds.** *J Pharm Pharmacol* 1994, **46**:618-630.
53. Tenaglia SA, McLellan TM, Klentrou PP: **Influence of menstrual cycle and oral contraceptives on tolerance to uncompensable heat stress.** *Eur J Appl Physiol Occup Physiol* 1999, **80**:76-83.
54. Selkirk GA, McLellan TM: **Influence of aerobic fitness and body fatness on tolerance to uncompensable heat stress.** *J Appl Physiol* 2001, **91**:2055-2063.

8

The Transeurope Footrace Project: longitudinal data acquisition in a cluster randomized mobile MRI observational cohort study on 44 endurance runners at a 64-stage 4,486km transcontinental ultramarathon

Uwe HW Schütz[1,2*†], Arno Schmidt-Trucksäss[3†], Beat Knechtle[4], Jürgen Machann[5], Heike Wiedelbach[1], Martin Ehrhardt[1], Wolfgang Freund[1], Stefan Gröninger[6], Horst Brunner[1], Ingo Schulze[7], Hans-Jürgen Brambs[1] and Christian Billich[1]

Abstract

Background: The TransEurope FootRace 2009 (TEFR09) was one of the longest transcontinental ultramarathons with an extreme endurance physical load of running nearly 4,500 km in 64 days. The aim of this study was to assess the wide spectrum of adaptive responses in humans regarding the different tissues, organs and functional systems being exposed to such chronic physical endurance load with limited time for regeneration and resulting negative energy balance. A detailed description of the TEFR project and its implemented measuring methods in relation to the hypotheses are presented.

Methods: The most important research tool was a 1.5 Tesla magnetic resonance imaging (MRI) scanner mounted on a mobile unit following the ultra runners from stage to stage each day. Forty-four study volunteers (67% of the participants) were cluster randomized into two groups for MRI measurements (22 subjects each) according to the project protocol with its different research modules: musculoskeletal system, brain and pain perception, cardiovascular system, body composition, and oxidative stress and inflammation. Complementary to the diverse daily mobile MR-measurements on different topics (muscle and joint MRI, T2*-mapping of cartilage, MR-spectroscopy of muscles, functional MRI of the brain, cardiac and vascular cine MRI, whole body MRI) other methods were also used: ice-water pain test, psychometric questionnaires, bioelectrical impedance analysis (BIA), skinfold thickness and limb circumference measurements, daily urine samples, periodic blood samples and electrocardiograms (ECG).

Results: Thirty volunteers (68%) reached the finish line at North Cape. The mean total race speed was 8.35 km/hour. Finishers invested 552 hours in total. The completion rate for planned MRI investigations was more than 95%: 741 MR-examinations with 2,637 MRI sequences (more than 200,000 picture data), 5,720 urine samples, 244 blood samples, 205 ECG, 1,018 BIA, 539 anthropological measurements and 150 psychological questionnaires.

Conclusions: This study demonstrates the feasibility of conducting a trial based centrally on mobile MR-measurements which were performed during ten weeks while crossing an entire continent. This article is the reference for contemporary result reports on the different scientific topics of the TEFR project, which may reveal

* Correspondence: uwe.schuetz@rocketmail.com
† Contributed equally
[1]Department of Diagnostic and Interventional Radiology, University Hospital of Ulm, Germany
Full list of author information is available at the end of the article

additional new knowledge on the physiological and pathological processes of the functional systems on the organ, cellular and sub-cellular level at the limits of stress and strain of the human body.
Please see related articles: http://www.biomedcentral.com/1741-7015/10/76 and http://www.biomedcentral.com/1741-7015/10/77

Background

Ultramarathon

Various aspects of the physical characteristics of recreational and elite level runners up to marathon distance events have been reported [1-9]. Much less has been written about the anthropometric characteristics of ultra endurance runners [10-14]. The case and field studies of Knechtle *et al.* developed a growing knowledge about the physical characteristics of multistage ultra endurance runners in the past years [15-22]. The German Ultramarathon Association (DUV) defines foot-races of 50 km or longer as ultramarathons (UM). Multistage ultramarathons (MSUM) are races in which each stage has a distance of a UM. Besides a few case reports very little has been reported about the medical aspects of runners doing a transcontinental extended MSUM over several weeks [23]. Until now, there have been no reports published regarding UM running over more than 1,500 km. However, prolonged MSUM races offer the best opportunity to study physical adaptation and the associations of the physiological parameters of athletes in a longitudinal setting day by day.

The race

Among some very heroic solo runs, the TransEurope FootRace 2009 [24] (TEFR09) was the 11th official transcontinental competition multistage footrace within living memory (Table 1) [25-33]. This second European transcontinental MSUM took place from 19 April to 21 June 2009 from Bari, South Italy (41° 8' N, 16° 52' E) to the North Cape, Norway (71°10'N, 25°47'E) (Figure 1). Sixty-seven ultra endurance runners (mean age 50.7 years, range 26 to 74 years, male 56 (83.6%)) from 12 nations (Germany, Japan, Netherlands, France, Switzerland, Norway, Sweden, Finland, Turkey, South Korea, Taiwan, USA) met the challenge and tried to cross six countries (Italy, Austria, Germany, Sweden, Finland, Norway). This comprised running 4,487 km (2,788 miles) in 64 stages without any day of rest. Thus, they expected to complete an average stage distance of 70.1 km, representing 1.7 marathon distances (minimum: 44 km, maximum: 95.1 km) [32].

All participants organized their arrival at Bari on their own. Following breakfast at 5:00 a.m., the daily stage started at 6:00 a.m. The race director, together with his staff, planned the stages with their corresponding distances and ascent or descent and organized the accommodations for the runners in halls as well as the food for each stage. In addition, most of the runners carried individual nutrition on their own. Depending on the stage length, five to ten stop points for nutrition were placed on the daily routes. After each stage the runners had time on their own (nutrition, sleeping, regeneration). Depending on the stage length and local situation, dinner was served between 5:00 and 9:00 p.m. The runners slept in camping grounds (mainly in Italy), local sport halls or local community halls at the stage destinations (9:00 p.m. to 4:00 a.m.). Sometimes the quarters were crowded resulting in difficult sleeping conditions. In total, the runners had about 7 to 13 hours of rest per day for recuperation. The local sanitary conditions also changed daily and from country to country.

The project

The TEFR09 project is the first observational cohort study intended to produce unique and comprehensive data from longitudinal measurements of a large sample of ultra endurance runners taking part in one of the most extreme multistage endurance competitions in the world, which takes the participants to a different level, where the race becomes a way of life, and where nutrition, sleep, energy and psychological states have to be carefully managed [34,35]. It is also the first study using a mobile MRI scanner for continuous examination of the athletes while performing a transcontinental MSUM. The aim was to explain the wide spectrum of adaptive responses in humans being exposed to such a chronic physical endurance load with negative energy balancing but without enough time for regeneration and to identify factors associated with inter-individual variation in these responses. Due to the unique possibility to observe morphological and physiological changes and the reactions of different tissues and functional systems on the systemic, organ and (sub)cellular level with modern MRI techniques, a wide range of multiple questions, hypotheses and unproven assumptions regarding injury, adaptation, regeneration, reparation and overuse processes arose. Therefore, four different project modules of investigations were created, focusing on multiple open questions and unproven hypotheses regarding long distance running:

Project module I: musculoskeletal system

Pre-race injuries and deformation

It is inevitable that pre-race injuries or biomechanical deviations from the norm (for example, mal-alignment)

Table 1 History of transcontinental footraces

No	race: date	route	total distance	days, stages	mean stage distance	star -ter[a]	fin-isher[a]
C.C. Pyle's International Trans-continental Foot Races (Bunion Derbies 1928, 1929) [25-27]							
1.	1928: 4 March - 24 May	Los Angeles - New York	5,509 km 3,423 miles	84	65.6 km/d 40.8 miles/d	199	55 28%
2.	1929: 21 March - 8 June	New York - Los Angeles	5,509 km 3,423 miles	84	65.6 km/d 40.8 miles/d	80	31 39%
Trans America Foot Races 1992-95 [28,29]							
3.	1992: 20 June - 22 August	Huntington Beach - New York	4,722 km 2,935 miles	64	73.8 km/d 45.9 miles/d	28	13 46%
4.	1993: 19 June - Aug.21	Huntington Beach - New York	4,686 km 2,912 miles	64	73.8 km/d 45.9 miles/d	13	6 46%
5.	1994: June 18 - 20 August	Huntington Beach - New York	4,708 km 2,926 miles	64	73.6 km/d 45.7 miles/d	14	5 36%
6.	1995: 17 June 17 - 19 August	Huntington Beach - New York	4,676 km 2,906 miles	64	73.1 km/d 45.4 miles/d	14	10 71%
Trans Australia Foot Race 2001							
7.	2001: 6 January - 11 March	Perth - Canberra	4,109 km 2,553 miles	63	67.8 km/d 42.1 miles/d	24	14 58%
Run Across America 2002							
8.	2002: 15 June - 24 August	New York - Huntington Beach	4,961 km 3,084 miles	71	68.9 km/d 42.8 miles/d	11	8 73%
10.	2004: 15 June - 24 August	Huntington Beach - New York	4,961 km 3,084 miles	71	68.9 km/d 42.8 miles/d	10	6 60%
Trans Europe Foot Races 2003, 2009 [30-33]							
9.	2003: 19 April - 21 June	Lisbon, Portugal - Moscow	5,020 km 3,119 miles	64	79.5 km/d 49.4 miles/d	44	22 50%
11.	2009: 19 April - 21 June	Bari, Italy - North Cape	4,486 km 2,787 miles	64	70.1 km/d 43.6 miles/d	67	46 69%
Run Across America 2011: LANY (Los Angeles to New York)							
12.	2011: 19 June - 27 August	Huntington Beach - New York	5,157 km 3,205 miles	70	73.7 km/d 45.8 miles/d	14	8 57%

[a]total: 528 starters, 224 finishers. 42.4% (some of these have made more than one crossing)

will lead to progressing focal damage of the lower extremities when performing a transcontinental MSUM. If any participant who suffers from unhealed pre-race injuries or deformation of the lower extremities reaches the finish line at North Cape without deterioration, this hypothesis can be rejected. Furthermore, the TEFR project tries to detect reasons for not finishing the race in detail.

Joints

Recent investigations indicate that running a marathon does not increase pathologies of structures of the knee joint [36-39]. Some authors postulate a risk factor of repeated marathon running for osteoarthritis of the knee [40]. However, a protective effect of running for knee joint cartilage is also discussed [41,42]. Nothing is known about the effect of ultra long distance running over weeks as in MSUM on knee structures. For the knee cartilage, experimental studies on animals using quantitative microspectrophotometry and polarized light microscopy showed a decrease of the glycosaminoglycan content of the superficial femorotibial joint cartilage layer and degradation and reorganization of the superficial collagen network [43-45]. With this study, there are two hypotheses to be proven: first, in a MSUM over nine weeks, the well-trained participants show no increase in pathologies of the structures of the knee joint; and second, the cartilage of the femorotibial joint shows a degradation of the glycosaminoglycan content with quick regeneration after the end of the race. The hypothesis that MSUM running does not indicate a higher risk of osteoarthritis of the knee in well-trained endurance runners has to be proven with the TEFR project. Contrary to the femorotibial joint the following hypothesis for the femoropatellar joint has to be proven: retropatellar cartilage degeneration is not caused by MSUM running. The femoropatellar joint is not a limiting factor for ultra endurance running, although degeneration arthrosis is already present in some MSUM participating athletes, respectively. This hypothesis is based on the fact that retropatellar arthrosis has a high prevalence in older people [46] and long

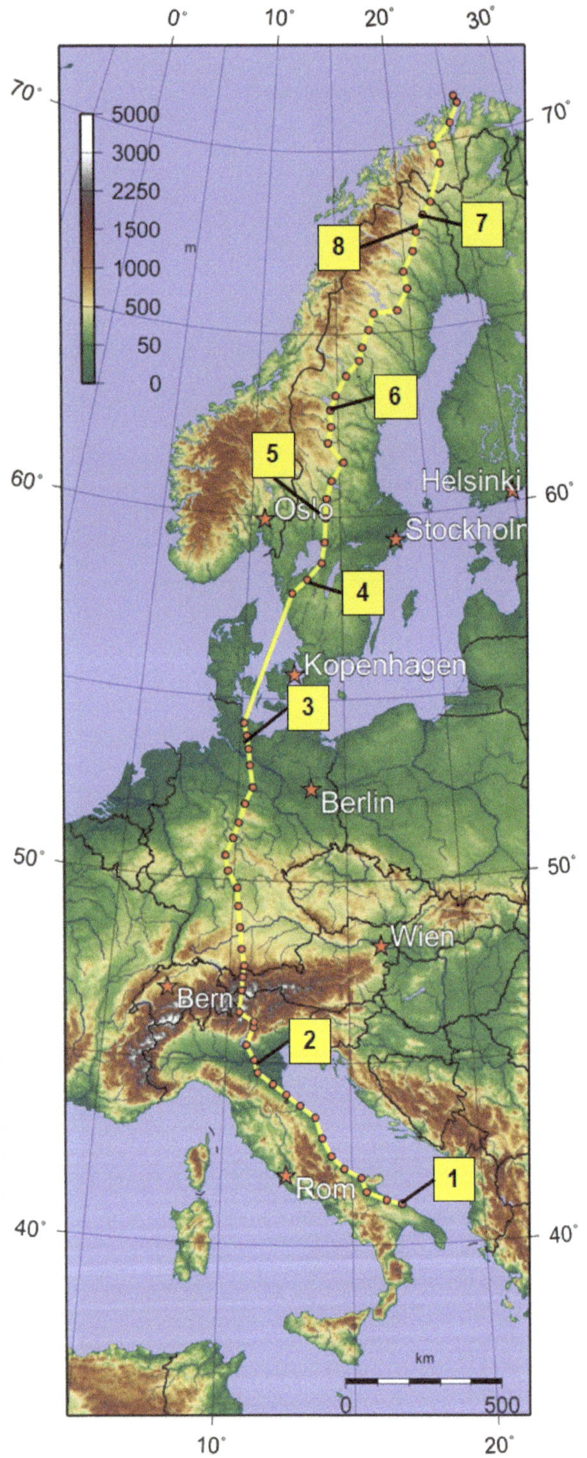

Figure 1 **Route of Trans Europe Foot Race 2009 (4,486 km from south to north of Europe).**

distance running participation rises with age [47]. This TEFR project will also prove the same hypothesis for the joints of the ankle and hindfoot. For the latter no specific studies have been published until now.

Soft tissues of the leg

The literature on long distance running demonstrates that injuries mostly occur in the active and passive soft tissues of the lower extremities [48-54]. Injuries of the muscles, tendons and fascia of the lower legs are the most obvious limiting factors for performance and the most common reasons for not finishing a transcontinental footrace. This postulation leads to the following hypothesis which has to be proven by the TEFR project: During a MSUM every participant will suffer from different injuries and overload of active and passive soft tissues of the lower musculoskeletal system, resulting in long lasting damage due to lack of recreation time.

A special problem for endurance runners is a pain syndrome of the lower leg, so-called 'shin splint'. Investigations over the past years, especially with MRI, showed that several entities caused by overuse of the lower leg due to long distance running can be differentiated. Some authors indicated that bone or periosteal reactions of the ventral tibia are a typical part of this syndrome [55,56], while others do not consider this as being mandatory [57]. Depending on the involved tissues and the lack of exact knowledge of the pathogenesis, the terminology regarding chronic lower leg pain in runners is broad and has not been differentiated and defined in detail until now: medial tibial stress syndrome, shin splint, anterior muscle syndrome, (peri-)myositis, periostitis, fasciitis, and so on [58,59]. With our study design we try to prove the hypothesis that running-associated chronic lower leg pain includes different entities, such as overuse pathologies of muscles, fascias, tendons and bone tissues of the lower leg. The problem begins in the friction areas of the fascia of the muscles and the tendons (peritendineum) and then extends to other tissues such as the muscles, periosteum and bone if the running burden continues and the pain is ignored by the athlete. As many ultra athletes reported, it seems to be possible to overrun 'shin splint' without further damage. Whether medial tibial stress syndrome can end up in a stress fracture or a chronic exertional compartment syndrome when running is continued without any further rest is not clear [56,60,61]. Perhaps further understanding and differentiation of soft tissue overuse of the leg is possible due to this observational cohort study with a mobile MRI.

Bones

Stress fractures of the lower body often occur in people doing extensive walking or running without proper training or adaption to the repeated and persistent mechanical burden their bones have to deal with. As seen in young soldiers doing their first long march with full body equipment [62] or amateur runners or beginners in (half-) marathons [63] our hypothesis is that even well trained ultra runners, such as the TEFR participants, can suffer stress fractures, because their skeletal system is not adapted to this tremendous mechanical burden that occurs while crossing a continent by foot with a speed of more than 6 km/hour without any day of rest. The TEFR project with mobile MRI tries to detect early signs of bone reaction (for example, subperiosteal new bone formation, adaptive cortical hypertrophy with little true inflammation, local bone edema or bruising) indicating overload as precursors of stress fractures [59].

For asymptomatic healthy marathon runners significantly higher red bone marrow hyperplasia has been observed compared to healthy volunteers [64]. This is postulated to be a response to 'sports anemia', which is commonly found in highly conditioned trained athletes. The TEFR project wanted to prove the hypothesis that during a MSUM lasting more than nine weeks an increase of red bone marrow occurs in the participants, even though they are adapted and well trained in ultra running.

Project module II: brain, mind and pain perception

Brain volume

Aerobic exercise protects from insular atrophy in the brain of healthy volunteers [65,66]. The normal annual volume loss due to age-related brain atrophy is about 0.11% [66,67]. Increased atrophy is shown for several diseases, such as Alzheimers (2% per year) [68,69] anorexia nervosa [70,71] or malnutrition based on other reasons [72]. Some hypotheses explain this based on the influence of the stress hormone cortisol [70] but further pathophysiological principles leading to this decrease in brain volume are not understood [73-76]. Marathon-induced changes in endocrine levels [77,78], in fluid balance [79] and amino acid blood level [80] are known to alter brain metabolism. The hypothesis that ultra endurance running leads to volume reduction of the brain cortex could be investigated by the TEFR project using high resolution cerebral MRI. Combined with specific laboratory analyses of different markers (for example S100B [81,82]) in blood and urine, reasons explaining the mechanism may be identified. On the other hand, when we postulate that an ultra long MSUM, such as the TEFR09, modifies the plastic brain (state marker) the hypothesis that the sensomotoric cortex volume - which is responsible for the lower extremities - will increase has also to be proven [83].

Brain lesions

Additionally we hypothesize that the well-known exercise-induced hyponatremia due to inappropriate arginine vasopressin secretion which can lead to encephalopathy [84-87] is not seen in the highly endurance-trained participants of the TEFR09. If an MSUM leads to brain lesions, water sensitive cerebral MRI sequences of the TEFR project will show it.

Pain perception, mind and mental stress

All participants in the TEFR09 had previously finished an ultra marathon. This unique collective of endurance athletes is eminently suitable for examining the hypothesis that ultra runners have different mental prerequisites (higher auto suggestibility) compared to the normal population (trait marker). Experienced ultra endurance runners often mentioned that finishing an ultra race is more a matter of mind than a matter of the body. The hypothesis that finishers of MSUM differ from non-finishers with regard to pain suppression and willpower can be proven by pain tests combined with functional MRI of the brain and mental stress markers in serum samples.

Project module III: cardiovascular system

Heart

The MSUM TEFR09 results in an extreme prolonged stress for the whole organism. Its effects on the heart can be discussed controversially. Cardiac dysfunction after marathon running is verified with biochemical markers and cardiac ultrasound [88,89]. Investigations with cardiac MRI are inconsistent; cardiac damage such as myocardial necrosis is seen in middle-aged marathon runners (57.2 +/- 5.7 years) [90], but not in younger marathon participants (30 to 50 years) [91,92]. Myocardial function disorders are reported with cardiac MRI tagging [93]. Until now, diagnostic analyses of long-lasting running effects on the heart using cardiac biomarkers are difficult to interpret, for example, the increase in brain natriuretic peptide (BNP) after 100 km trials [94,95] could show cytoprotective or growth regulatory effects [89,96] but also myocardial insufficiency. The TEFR project intends to prove the following hypotheses: Even in well trained ultra endurance runners, the running burden of a trans-continental MSUM of more than nine weeks induces a progressive cardiac distress and signs of cardiovascular mal-adaption. Cardiac MRI, stress laboratory tests and ECG might show signs of cardiac structural and functional restrictions, dysfunctions, damages and insufficiency. Non-finishers of the TEFR09 will show more restrictive parameters than finishers. Another hypothesis contradicting the Morganroth hypothesis [97,98] is proven: Although an aerobic endurance burden is performed, the TEFR09 finisher will show an increase in cardiac output and left ventricular mass index and in ventricular wall thickness, which might be caused by incomplete or critical left ventricular hypertrophy in some cases. Using a MR tagging technique, we will try to prove the hypothesis that the anatomical position of the heart is going to change (steep position) with a prolonged aerobic running burden [99].

Arteries

Arteries of the muscular-type, such as the common femoral artery (CFA) adapt structure and function to endurance exercise training and elastic-type arteries, such as the common carotid artery, show functional adaptations to increased endurance exercise training. Schmid-Trucksäss *et al.* [100] found an increase of diameter and compliance and a constant shear rate for CFA using noninvasive vascular ultrasound in highly endurance-trained athletes compared to sedentary controls. Other authors postulate that endurance exercise does change arterial wall stiffness and vascular (endothelial) function [101-103]. The TEFR project tries to prove the hypotheses that the MSUM burden results in cardiovascular adaptations in the form of an increase of arterial wall compliance in the lower extremities associated with an increase in the vessel lumen diameter of the femoral artery and of the central aortal pulse wave velocity even in well-trained ultra-endurance runners. This will result in a decrease of the peripheral arterial resistance leading to an increase in basic perfusion of the lower extremities.

Project module IV: body composition

Endurance exercise leads to a reduction of subcutaneous fatty tissue as demonstrated in several field studies [104-107]. It is well known that fat is the main energy-rich substrate for ultra endurance performance [105,107,108]. In contrast, muscle tissue provides lower energy, when being catabolized. A decrease in skeletal muscle mass due to ultra endurance performance has only been demonstrated in case reports [15,23,109] or small series [108].

Different effects for long-lasting or ultra endurance performances on body composition are described in the literature and seem to depend on the type of endurance burden. In ultra endurance performance with defined breaks (for example, during the night), body mass may remain stable [110-112] or even increase [105] while body fat is reduced [104,105,113], whereas skeletal muscle mass seems to be spared [111,113,114] or may even increase [104]. Ultra endurance performance over hours, days or weeks without a break, results in a decrease in body mass [23,107,109,115] in which body fat as well as skeletal muscle seems to decrease as a few case reports indicate [15,23,109]. With this cohort study we can prove the hypothesis that due to the immense negative energy balance during a transcontinental MSUM, not only fat but also lean tissue is involved in catabolism, even in the leg muscles. With its mobile whole body MRI protocol, the TEFR project will be able to measure the different amount of mass loss in the different functional muscle units of the leg. We also intend to detect the microstructural and intracellular adaption processes of leg muscle tissue with modern MRI methods (MR-spectroscopy, diffusion and perfusion MR imaging).

Purpose

This report describes the design and conduct of the TEFR project. We report the pattern of chronic endurance running exposure, characteristics of the subject groups and reasons for not finishing. Detailed descriptions of measuring methods in relation to the hypotheses and technical challenges encountered in the realization of the interdisciplinary TEFR project are presented. We discuss the strengths and limitations of the study setting.

Methods

After commitment to funding by the German Research Society (DFG) the 67 TEFR09 participants were asked to join the TEFR project, which was approved by the local ethics committee of the University Hospital of Ulm (UHU, No.: 270/08-UBB/se), Germany (in accordance with the Declaration of Helsinki) regarding the study design, risk management plan and individual protocols. Verbal and written informed consent was obtained from all concurring subjects.

Mobile MRI

The most important research tool was a 1.5 Tesla whole-body MR imager (Magnetom Avanto™ mobile MRI 02.05, software version: Syngo™ MR B15, Siemens Ltd., Erlangen, Germany) mounted on a mobile unit (MRI-Trailer Model Mob.MRI 02.05, SMIT Mobile Equipment B.V., Division AK Specialty Vehicles, Farnham, UK) pulled by a specially hired truck tractor. The semi-trailer had an internal diesel generator to power the helium cooling circuit for the MRI over the ten-week period. However, it did not generate enough electricity for continuous MRI measurements and was therefore supplemented by a more powerful custom made external diesel generator (150 KVA, Strom Rent™ e.k., Dortmund, Germany) which was pulled by an additional material van. The mobile hardware had a total weight of more than 45 tonnes and was nearly 30 meters long. All of the equipment was installed daily at each stopover and required daily checks and support of all technical systems (Figure 2).

Study participants

Forty-four (67%) of the race participants (mean age 49.7 years, range 26 to 68 years, male 40 (90.9%), f 4) were recruited for the TEFR project. The inclusion criterion obviously was an official acceptance as a participant at the TEFR09 by the organizers and the race director. The conditions of participation were: minimum age 18 years, the presence of a medical certificate not older than 30 days which indicated physical health and clear proof of appropriate running performance in the field of UM. The specific running history and performance of the individual subjects can be described by different traits, which were requested before the start of the TEFR09: years of regular endurance running training, finished (ultra-) marathons, personal best times in different defined ultra

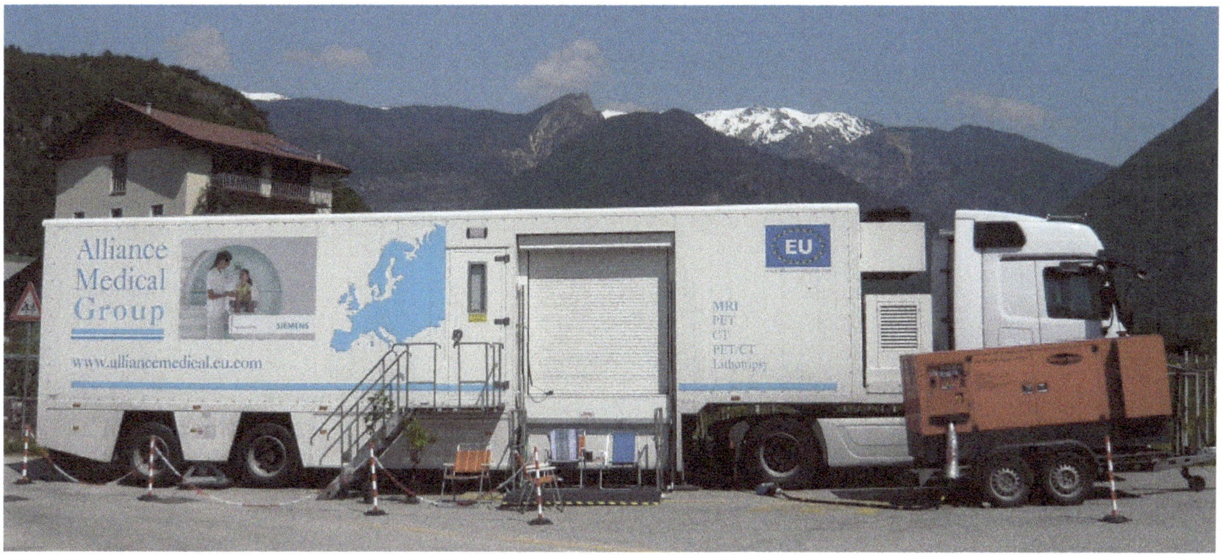

Figure 2 Truck trailer with mobile MRI and external generator in working position.

races and extent of training (volume, duration, intensity) before TEFR09.

The investigators additionally performed a resting cardiovascular check using a 12-channel PC-ECG system (Custo cardio 100™, Custo Med Ltd., Ottobrunn, Germany) and blood pressure (RR) measurement using a manual sphygmomanometer (BOSO Clinicus, JungingenGermany: to the nearest 3 mmHg). Cardiovascular exclusion criteria were resting blood pressure > 200 mmHg systolic and/or > 110 mmHg diastolic, acute systemic infection, acute chest pain and new arrhythmias or ECG changes. An orthopedic physical examination was done focusing on contraindications for endurance running such as relevant malalignment and painful joint diseases of the lower extremities. Additional specific exclusion criteria were contraindications against MRI scanning (for example, metallic foreign bodies in dangerous locations, specific cochlear or ocular implants, ferromagnetic vascular clips and relevant claustrophobia). None of the volunteers had to be excluded from study participation due to these criteria.

Investigators

Four members of the TEFR project comprised the investigator core team that accompanied the TEFR09 for direct data acquisition before and during the race: two physicians, one medical student and one radiological assistant. The latter (HW) was responsible for subject positioning in the scanner and performance of the MR examinations. One of the investigators, the initiator and main organizer of the TEFR project (US), drove the MR-trailer truck, adapted the daily research program to the actual circumstances, controlled and checked the quality of the MR examinations and was responsible for the technical readiness of the whole mobile MRI and its functional circuits and equipment with external and internal diesel generator. Being specialized in radiology and orthopedic surgery, he also did the initial and follow-up physical musculoskeletal examinations of the subjects. The second investigator (CB) was responsible for acquisition of daily anthropometric, laboratory and ECG data. The medical student (ME) made the daily anthropological measurements.

The two physicians were solely responsible for the study and gave neither training advice nor provided medical help.

Study design

The study design of the TEFR project is shown in Figure 3.

Pre-race

Baseline studies were performed within the last four days before the start of the TEFR09 in Bari on every subject. They included group specific MRI examinations and anthropometric and cardiovascular physical measurements with urine and venous blood samples.

Additionally, body height measuring using a wall-mounted stadiometer (to the nearest 5 mm, standing barefoot) and active range of motion measurement (AROM) of hip and knee joints using a manual double-armed universal goniometer (to the nearest 5°) were done before the start. One experienced orthopedic surgeon, trained in a standardized procedure for positioning both the subject and the goniometer, collected these data.

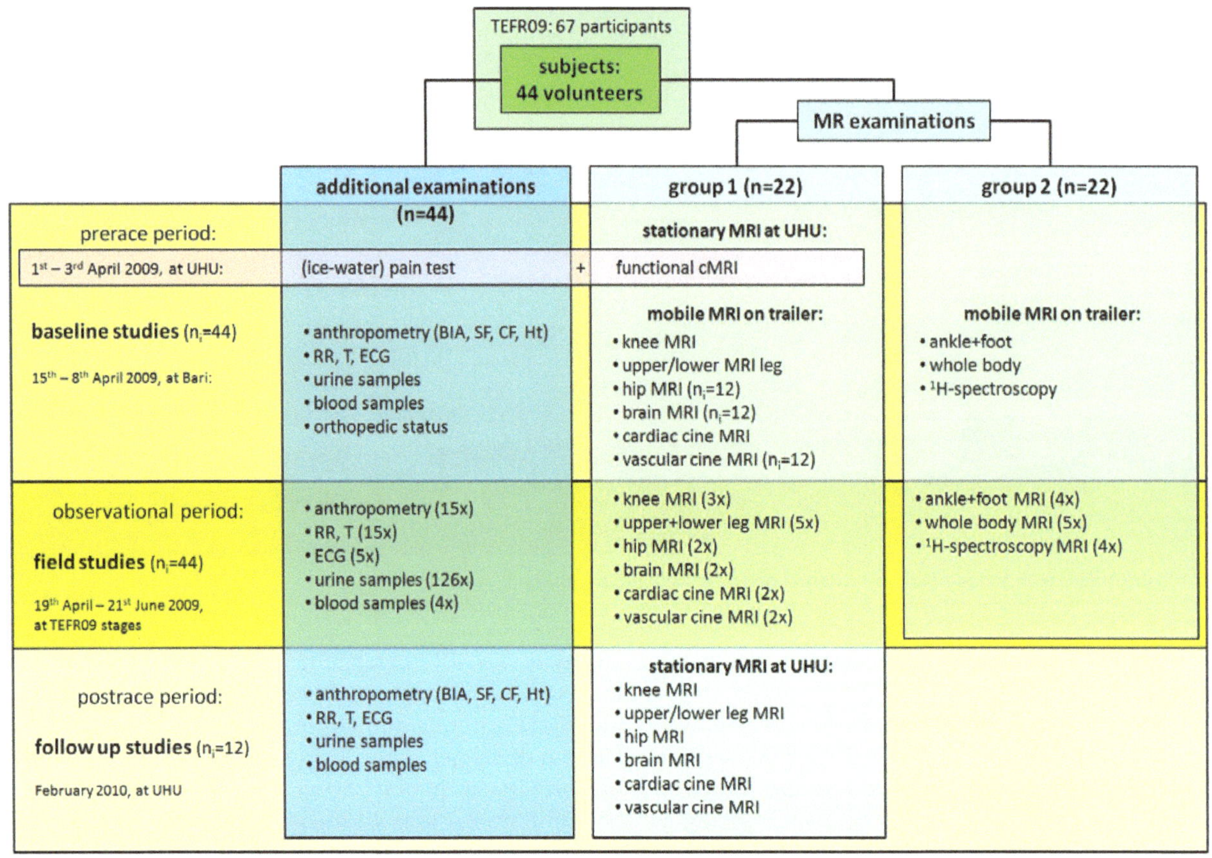

Figure 3 Study design of TEFR-project.

Adapted from the methods of Paley *et al.* [116] and Weidelich *et al.* [117], analysis of lower limb alignment was done on coronal lower body scout views of pre-race MRI with subjects in the supine position and with extended legs. Measured parameters were: leg length (LL), as the straight line from the middle of the femoral head to the midpoint of the upper talus rim; femorotibial angle (FTA), as the angle between anatomical femoral and tibial axis; the mechanical axis deviation (MAD) as the distance from the point of intersection between the perpendicular and mechanical axis of the limb (straight line from the middle of the femoral head to the midpoint of the upper talus rim) to the midpoint of the knee (medial tibial eminence) and the femoral to tibial length ratio (F/T) [116-122].

A 240-item, 31-dimensional personality temperament and character inventory (TCI) [123,124] in addition to a 10-item, 4-scaled questionnaire on self expectancy (General Self-Efficacy Scale, GSE) [125,126] were also integrated into the project before its start.

Additionally, 15 of the 44 subjects had an initial separate pre-race test on pain perception (ice-water test) combined with functional cerebral MRI two weeks before the start of the TEFR09 at UHU on 1 to 3 April 2009, because these examinations could not be implemented on the mobile MRI due to technical limitations. Due to the exorbitant physical and mental burden placed on the subjects, there was no opportunity for field experiments, invasive tests or application of psychometric instruments during the transcontinental footrace.

Field studies

The observant field studies during the TEFR09 were completed between 15 April and 21 June 2009. Every morning from 3:45 to 4:30 a.m. urine samples and anthropometric measurements were taken. The core team broke down their examination units and drove to the next stage destination. Before stage length dependent arrival of the first runner they had set their systems ready and had refuelled the generators and vehicles. MRI examination time was between 2:30 p.m. +/- 90 minutes and 9:00 p.m.). At the same time anthropometric and cardiovascular physical measurements, blood and urine samples were collected and ECG was done. The daily data acquisition also included measurement and documentation of daily weather conditions (temperature outside and inside, humidity outside) using a calibrated electronic thermometer, the stage length and the individual stage performances of the runners (stage running time).

MR measurements

For MR measurements two groups (22 subjects each) were cluster randomized according to the different research modules. The MR protocols were created in an interdisciplinary content ensuring multifold specific and diverse but precise analyses and measurements for detailed testing of the mentioned hypotheses concerning long distance running (Table 2).

MRI of feet

For high resolution investigation of the whole foot a special table fixed boot-like designed 8-channel foot-ankle coil was chosen and a sagittal orientated water sensitive T2w MR sequence (TIRM) configured a wide field of view. If on this sequence any pathology was detected, a transversal oriented focused water sensitive sequence with a more structured T2 sequence (fat saturated proton density weighted (PDw)) was added. For investigation of the joint cartilage a specific T2* mapping MR sequence (syngo™ MapIt FLASH T2*w GRE) in sagittal orientation was used [127-129], allowing quantitative measurement of hydrophilic changes in the cartilage layers of tibiotalar, talocalcaneal, calcaneocuboid, and calcaneonavicular joints. The specification of these MR sequences (Table 2) was done for detection of typical running associated overuse injuries of the feet [52]: subcutaneous edema, Achilles tendonitis [49,50], extensor digitorum tendonitis [48,49]), plantar fasciitis [50], calcaneal apophysitis, arthritis/arthrosis, stress fractures, bone edema, metatarsalgia, Morton's neuroma, and ankle inversion injuries (Figure 4).

MRI of knees

With a table-fixed 8-channel knee coil all subjects of group 1 had both knees examined with a sagittal TIRM sequence for water detection in knee-related tissues and evaluation of femorotibial joint. A transversal fat saturated PDw sequence was used to assess the femoropatellar joint. As for the hindfoot joints, specific T2* mapping MR sequences in sagittal and transversal orientations were done for quantification of cartilage layers of the femoropatellar and femorotibial joints regarding intrachondral water proportioning [127-129]. The specification of these MR sequences (Table 2) was done to evaluate running-associated overuse injuries in the knees [52]: patella tendonitis ('runner's knee'), arthritis/arthrosis [130], stress fracture, bone edema [64], retropatellar pain syndrome [48-50], chondromalacia patellae, meniscal lesions [50] and patellar tendinitis [50] (Figure 5).

MRI of hips/pelvis

One flexible 6-channel body matrix coil was used to obtain an MR overview of the pelvis with one coronal water sensitive sequence (TIRM: Table 2) to detect injuries in this part of the body: hip arthritis/arthrosis [131], sacroiliac injuries [52], stress fractures of the pelvic ring [132-134], muscle overuse injuries and so on. Additional case specific sequences were added as necessary (Figure 6).

MRI of upper/lower legs

With three to four flexible 6-channel body matrix coils total MR examination of upper and lower legs was possible. To get detailed information about soft tissue edema, muscle perfusion and injuries of the legs different sequences were adapted in transversal orientation (T1w for adipose tissue separation and acute bleeding detection, TIRM for high sensitivity in water detection, fat saturated PDw for structural detailed water sensitive imaging, DWI for perfusion analysis of muscles and separation between intra- and extra-cellular water in the muscles: Table 2). With these sequences all of the typical running-associated syndromes could be detected and differential diagnosis done [49,52]: anterior compartment pain/syndrome [48], (medial) tibial stress syndrome [50,135,136], gastrocnemius injuries, peroneal tendonitis, tibialis posterior injury, calcaneal apophysitis, iliotibial band friction syndrome [50], greater trochanteric bursitis, gluteus medius - hamstring - adductor - abductor - quadriceps injuries, such as tendonitis, strains or tears. Muscle volumetry of different compartments of the upper and lower leg muscles is possible for evaluation of changes in muscle volume: Figure 7.

Cerebral MRI, functional MRI

As for the muscles in the legs, a MRI guided volumetric analysis of the brain was one focus of the cerebral MRI measurements. Therefore, a T1 weighted high resolution (1 mm) turbo FLASH three-dimensional-sequence was used, making an isovoxel based volumetry (VBM) possible (Figure 8A). For detection of brain lesions and global edema a typical T2-sensitive sequence (FLAIR) in coronal orientation was chosen (Figure 8B). With diffusion weighted imaging (DWI), ischemia detection was possible. For all these MR sequences (Table 2) a table integrated 12-channel head matrix coil with a head restraint system was used. The same coil was used on the stationary scanner for functional MRI (fMRI) using echo-planar imaging (epi) with blood oxygenation level dependent (BOLD) contrast to analyze pain perception

Table 2 MRI protocols of the TEFR project

MRI in module I: Musculoskeletal System
ankle/foot (PP: FFS, supine):
• **TIRM** 2D sag; **PM**: FA 140, TE 60; TR 11320, IR 120, ST 2, SBS 2.4, FOV 900, MS 512*512, PS 0.586 iso, PB 130; **IAT**: 5:37
• **PDw TSE fs** 2D tra; **PM**: FA 150, TE 32, TR 5830, ST 4, SBS 4.4, FOV 256, MS 384*384, PS 0.4167 iso, PB: 150; **IAT**: 3:46
• **syngo™ MapIt FLASH** 2D sag: T2*w GRE; **PM**: FA 60, TE 4.5, TR 1010, ST 2.5, SBS 2.75, FOV 182.25, MS 320*320; PS 0.421875 iso, PB: 250, IN: 12; **IAT**: 4:15
knee (PP: FFS, supine):
• **TIRM** 2D sag; **PM**: FA 140, TE 50, TR: 4010, TI 150, ST 3, SBS 3.3, FOV 289, MS 256*256, PS 0.664 iso, PB 180; **IAT**: 3:31
• **PDw TSE fs** 2D cor; **PM**: FA 150, TE 31, TR 4400, ST 3, SBS 3.3, FOV 289, MS 512*512, PS 0.332 iso, PB 100; **IAT**: 4:11
• **syngo™ MapIt FLASH** 2D tra/sag: T2*w GRE; **PM**: FA 60, TE 4.18, TR 889/1120, ST 3, SBS 3.3, FOV 289, MS 512*512; PS 0.332 iso, PB: 250, IN: 12; **IAT**: 4:21/3:58
Hip (PP: FFS):
• **TIRM** 2D cor; PM: FA 150, TE 61, TR 6230, TI 145, ST 3.5, SBS 3.85, FOV 1444, MS 384*384, PS 0.9896 iso, PB 130; **IAT**: 03:38
upper/lower leg (PP: FFS, supine):
• **T1w SE** 2D tra, **PM**: FA 90, TE 13, TR 626, ST 5, SBS 5, FOV 1050/722, MS 512*336/256, PS 0.78125/0.7422 iso, PB 115; **IAT**: 1:54/1:30
• **TIRM** 2D tra; **PM**: FA 140, TE 62; TR 12530, TI 130, ST 3, SBS 3.9, FOV 512, MS 384*192, PS 0.833 iso, PB 180; **IAT**: 2:08
• **PDw TSE fs** 2D tra; **PM**: FA 150, TE 39, TR 6730, ST 3, SBS 3.9, FOV 512, MS 320*160, PS 1.0 iso, PB: 150; **IAT**: 2:14
• **DWI** (with **ADC**): **SPAIR** epi b-value 0-800, 2D tra; **PM**: FA 90, TE 75, TR 5100, ST 10, SBS 10, FOV 1300/1173.25, MS 128*104, PS 3.125/2.96875 iso, PB 1030; **IAT**: 2:32/3:01
MRI in module II: Brain and Pain
Brain (PP: HFS, supine):
• **(turbo) FLASH 3D** sag: T1 mpr; **PM**: FA 15, TE 4.75, TR 2100, ST 1, FOV 614.4, MS 240*256, PS 1.0 iso, PB130; **IAT**: 8:37
• **T2w fs FLAIR** 2D cor: TIRM; **PM**: FA 150, TE 120, TR 9000, TI 2500, ST 5, SBS 5.5, FOV, MS 288*384, PS 0.599 iso, PB 150; **IAT**: 4:43
• **DWI** (with **ADC**): **SPAIR** epi b-value 0-1000, 2D tra; **PM**: FA 90, TE 98, TR 3700, ST 5, SBS 6, FOV 529, MS 256*256, PS 0, 89844 iso, PB 1000; **IAT**: 0:49
functional MRI (fMRI) for pain perception: Epi 2d: epi2d_bold; **PM**: Fa 90, TE 60, TR 2600, ST 5, SBS 6, FOV, MS 384*384 (Start fMRI: 16*16), PS 3.59375, PB 2440; **IAT**: ~15:20 in total
MRI in module III: Cardiovascular System
Cardiac cine-MRI (PP: HFS, supine), **IAT**: ~25:00 in total
• **Cine SSFP**, 2D: GRE cine with retrospective 2d cardiac triggering; **PM**: FA 80, TE var, TR var, ST 6, SBS 6, FOV 1156/1089, MS 192*192/156, PS 1.771/ 1.71875 iso, PB 930, IN: 30
• **Phase contrast acquisition 2D; PM**: venc 150, FA 30, TE 2.33var, TR 41.1var, ST 6, FOV, MS 180*192, PS 1.875 iso, PB 555, IN:25
• **Cine-tagging SSFP**, 2D: GRE cine with retrospective 2d cardiac triggering; **PM**: FA 20, TE var, TR var, ST 6, SBS 18, FOV 1073.25, MS 212*256, PS 1.40625 iso, PB 500, IN: 21
Vascular cine-MRI (PP: HFS, supine), **IAT**: ~25:00 var in total
• **Carotid artery: FLASH** 2D tra: T2*w gradient-spoiled GRE cine with prospective 2d cardiac triggering; **PM**: FA 15, TE ~5.45 var, TR ~34.75 var, ST 6, FOV 289, MS 320 × 320, PS 0.53125 iso, PB 250, IN: 50/RR-cycle; **IAT**: ~5:30 var
• **Femoral artery: FLASH** 2D tra: see carotid artery; **PM**: FA 15, TE 5.00 var, TR 26.80 var, ST 6, FOV 768, MS 512 × 384, PS 0.625 iso, PB 250, IN: 50/ RR-cycle; **IAT**: ~4:20 var
• **Aortic flow** prox./dist.**: FLASH** 2D tra: **PM**: FA 20, TE 2.75 var, TR 11.55 var, ST 5, FOV 768, MS 256*192, PS 1.25 iso, PB 590, IN: 100; **IAT**: ~4:10
MRI in module IV: Morphometry, Body Composition
whole body MRI (PP: HFP/FFP, prone): **T1w TSE** 2D tra; **PM**: FA 180, TE 12, TR 490, ST 10, SBS 20, FOV 1991, MS 256*196, PS 1.9922 iso, PB 120, IN: 90-120 var; **IAT**: appr. 20:00
MR spectroscopy (PP: FFS, supine) for **evaluation** of intramyocellular lipids (IMCL): **Single-voxel STEAM**, TE 20, TR 2000, voxel of interest 11 × 11 × 20 mm^3, 40 acq., **IAT:** appr. 10:00

Tra, transversal (axial); sag, sagittal; cor, coronal; Seq., sequence; ADC, apparent diffusion coefficient; bold, blood oxygenation level dependent contrast; DWI, diffusion weighted imaging; epi, echo planar imaging; FLAIR, fluid-attenuated inversion recovery; FLASH, fast low angle shot; fs, fat saturated; GRE, gradient echo seq.; IR, inversion recovery; mpr, MPRAGE (magnetization prepared rapid gradient echo); PDw, proton density weighting; SPAIR, spectral adiabatic inversion recovery; SSFP, steady state free precision; STEAM, stimulated-echo acquisition mode; T1w, T1 contrast; T2w, T2 contrast; TIRM, turbo inversion recovery magnitude; (T)SE, (turbo) spin echo; PM, parameters; parameter abbreviations: FA, flip angle (°); TE, time to echo (ms); TR, repetition time (ms); TI, inversion time (ms); ST, slice thickness (mm), SBS, spacing between slices (mm); FOV, field of view (cm^2); MS, matrix size (pixel); PS, pixel size (mm); PB, pixel bandwith; IN, image number (n); var, variable dependency; venc, velocity encoded gradient echo imaging (cm/second); IAT, image acquisition time (min:second); PP, patient positioning; HFS, head forward supine; FFS, feet forward supine; HFP, head forward prone; FFP, feet forward prone; cardiac triggering, ECG- gating.

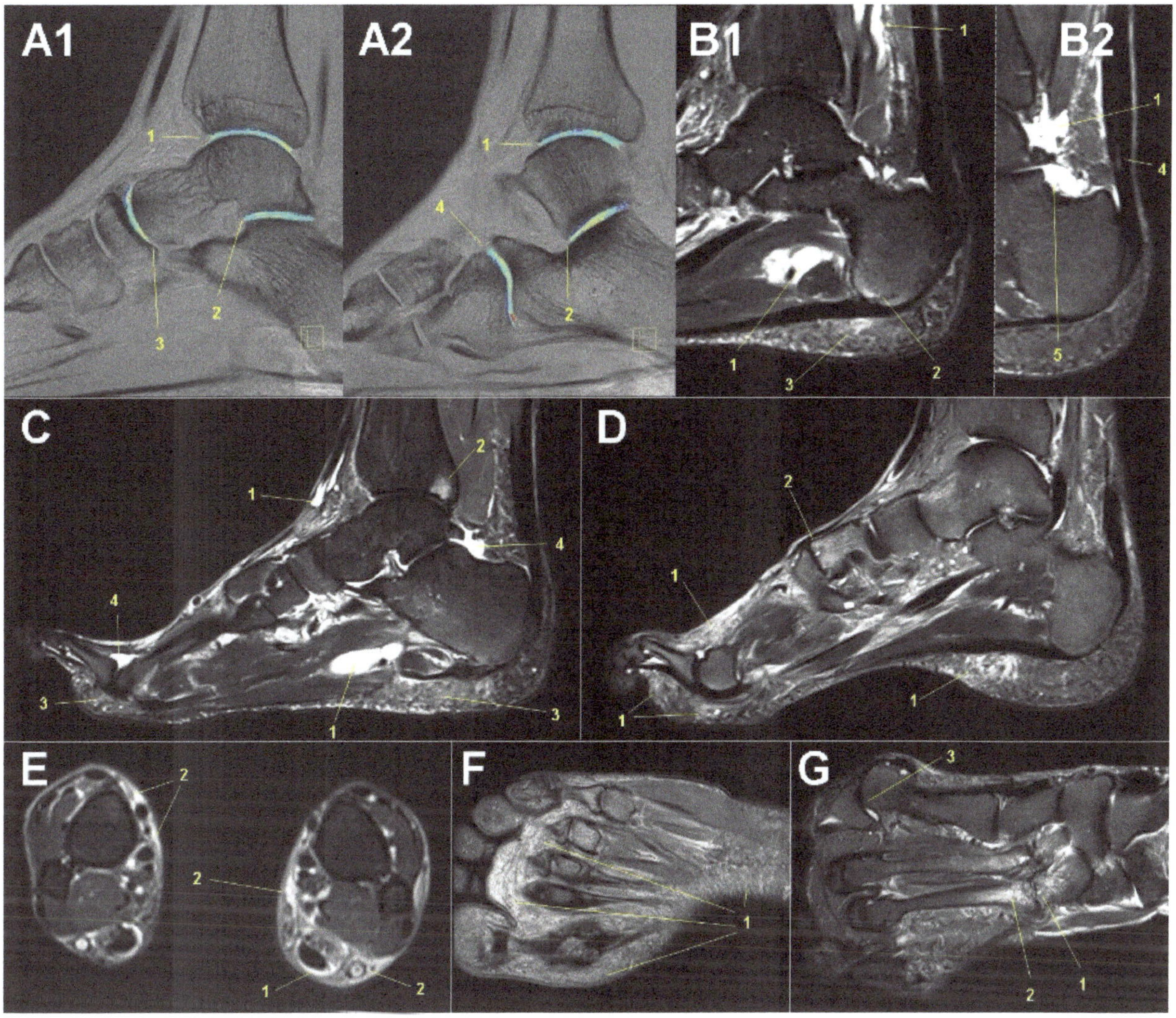

Figure 4 Mobile MRI of the feet. A: male, 39-years-old, stage 53, 3,669 km (fused colored T2* GRE map sagittal: syngo™ MapIt fusion technique, Siemens Medical solutions, Erlangen, Germany): Colored visualization of focal water concentration in cartilage layers of the ankle joint (1), subtalar joint (2), talonavicular joint (3) and calcneocuboid joint (4). **B:** male, 61-years-old, stage 23, 2,176 km (T2 TIRM sagittal): Multiple running related signs of tissue alteration. Peritendinous fluid accumulation in tendon sheaths (1). Focal bone edema at insertion of plantar fascia (2) with corresponding subcutaneous edema (3), but without plantar fasciitis. Edema in the Achilles tendon (4). Articular effusion in the ankle joint (5). **C:** male, 59-years-old, stage 45, 3,082 km (T2 TIRM sagittal): Peritendinous fluid accumulation in tendon sheaths of foot dorsiflexors (1), focal arthrosis of the ankle joint with subchondral bone edema (2), plantar subcutaneous edema (3), articular effusion in subtalar and metatarsophalangeal joint (4). **D:** male, 54-years-old, stage 32, 2,176 km (T2 TIRM sagittal): Subcutaneous edema (1), arthrosis of midfoot joints (2). **E:** male, 30-years-old, stage 12, 789 km (PDw TSE fs transversal): Peritendinous fluid accumulation in Achilles tendon sheath (1) with wide local subcutaneous edema (2). **F:** female, 68-years old, stage 15, 1,003 km (PDw TSE fs transversal): Extensive plantar subcutaneous edema (1). **G:** male, 47-years-old, stage 52, 3,609 km (PDw TSE fs transversal): Severe arthrosis of midfoot joints (1) with perifocal bone edema (2), hallux valgus (3).

in 12 participants of the TEFR09 compared to age-related normal volunteers (Figure 8C).

Cardiac cine MRI

For mobile cardiac cine MRI, a flexible six-channel body matrix coil was used. Cine SSFP gradient echo sequences with retrospective cardiac triggering were generated to obtain plane short axis four-, three- and two-chamber (Figure 9B) views of the heart. The mitral and aortic flow (Figure 9D) was measured using phase contrast sequences with 150 cm/second velocity encoded gradient echo imaging (venc). This protocol ensured measurement or secondary evaluation of parameters, such as ejection fraction (%), end diastolic and systolic volume and, therefore, stroke volume (ml), cardiac output (L/minute), myocardial mass (g) (Figure 9E), muscle volume of ventricles (ml) (Figure 9A), and so on. MR tagging using a Cine SSFP gradient echo sequence with retrospective

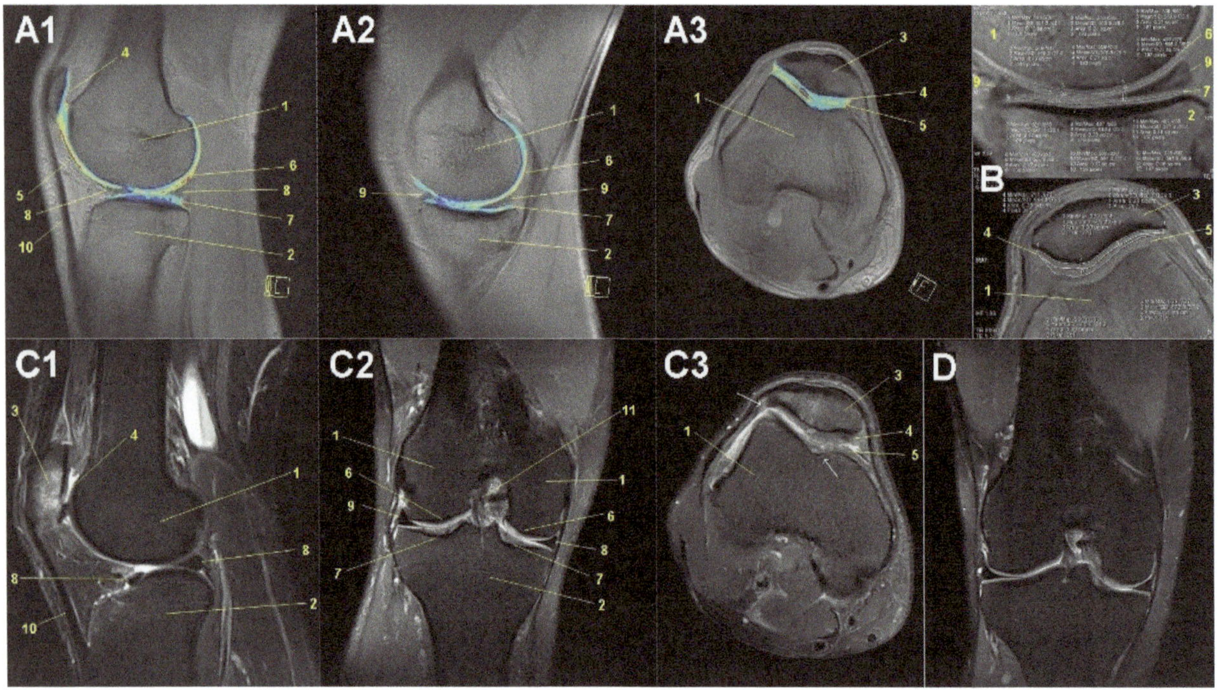

Figure 5 Mobile MRI of the knees. Femoral condyle (1), tibial head (2), patella (3), retropetallar cartilage layer (4), ventral femoral cartilage layer (5), dorsal femoral cartilage layer (6), tibial cartilage layer (7), medial meniscus (8), lateral meniscus (9), patellar tendon (10). **A:** female, 45-years-old, stage 44, 3,021 km (fused colored T2* GRE map: syngo™ Maplt fusion technique, A1: medial femorotibial joint sagittal, A2: lateral femorotibila joint sagittal, A3: femoropatellar joint transversal). **B:** male, 25-years-old, before start of TEFR09 Cartilage layer segmentation (T2* GRE map: syngo™ Maplt). **C:** male, 43-years-old, stage 40, 2,738 km (PDw TSE fs, C1: sagittal, C2: coronal, C3: transversal): Severe arthrosis of the patellofemoral joint with retropatellar cartilage defects (4, 5) and wide subchondral bone edema of the patella (3), intrachondral signal alterations of the femoral (6) and tibial (7) cartilage layers. **D:** male, 26-years-old, stage 40, 2,738 km (PDw TSE fs coronal): Nondescript cartilage layers of femorotibial joint.

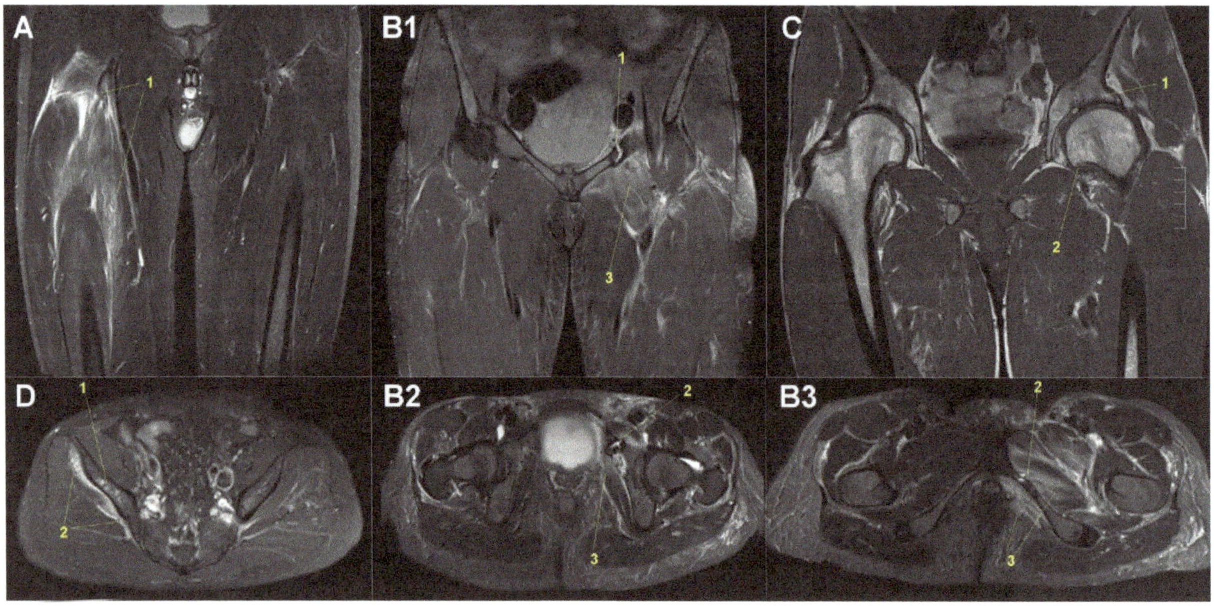

Figure 6 Mobile MRI of pelvis region and hip joints. **A:** male, 45-years-old, stage 8, 511 km (PDw TSE fs coronal): Massive edema and (peri-) myositis of right proximal quadriceps muscle (1). **B:** female, 46-years-old, stage 48, 3,290 km (PDw TSE fs, B1: coronal, B2,3: transversal): Stress fracture of left ventral pelvic ring (1: Ramus superior ossis pubis; 2: Ramus inferior ossis pubis) with perifocal soft tissue edema/inflammation (3). **C:** male, 41-years old, stage 11, 739 km (T1 TSE coronal): Arthrosis of the left hip (1: acetabular sclerosis, 2: deformation and osteophyte of the femoral head). **D:** male, 61-years-old, stage 38, 2601 km (PDw TSE fs transversal): Intraosseus edema in the right Ala ossis ileum (1) with massive peri-osseal inflammation of the gluteal muscle origin (2).

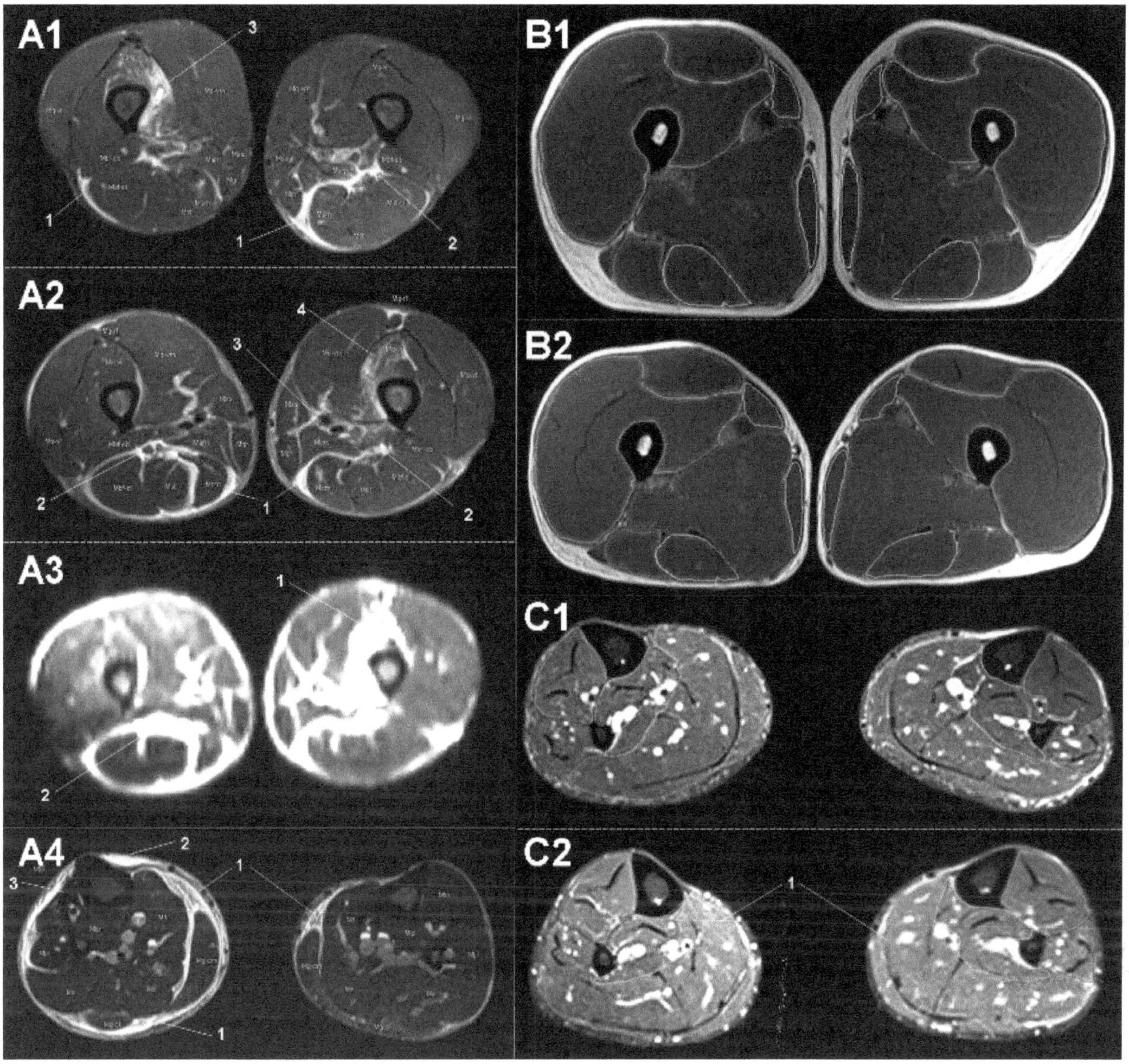

Figure 7 Mobile MRI of upper and lower legs. A: male, 49-years-old (coronal slices): A1: stage 12, 789 km, upper legs (PDw TSE fs): Subfascial intermuscular fluid, superficial (1), deep peri-neural (2). Partial quadriceps tear (M. vastus intermedius: 3). A2: stage 19, 1,260 km, upper legs (PDw TSE fs): Subfascial intermuscular fluid, superficial (1), deep peri-neural (2) and peri-vascular (3). Partial muscle edema of M. vastus intermedius (4). Specific diffusion weight imaging (A3, same slice as A2) is a sensitive method for free water detection. A4: stage 19, 1,260 km, lower legs (T2 TIRM): Subfascial intermuscular (1) and epifascial subcutaneous edema (2) indicating soft tissue inflammation such as perimyositis and panniculitis (shin splints), respectively. **B:** male, 31-years-old, B1: start, B2: stage 62, 6,358 km (PDw TSE fs transversal): Segmentation of muscle compartments of upper leg for functional muscle volumetry. **C:** male, 53-years-old: C1: start, C2: stage 46, 3,161 km (T2 TIRM transversal): Segmentation of muscle compartments of lower leg for functional muscle volumetry. Muscle edema in calf muscle (1).

cardiac triggering in plane short axis four- and two-chamber view (Table 2) made quantification of the myocardial motion with its spatial orientation (Figure 9C) possible.

Vascular cine MRI

For analysis of changes in the arterial aortic stiffness, measurement of the central pulse wave velocity using MRI is the gold standard [137]. With detection and measurement of the proximal and distal aortic flow and diameter using phase contrast acquisition with venc and prospective two-dimensional cardiac triggering on mobile MRI (Figure 10B, C), this and the central hemodynamic changes (peak and mean shear rate differences) and their influence on the vascular (aortic) diameter [100] during the TEFR09 can be calculated. Additionally, T2 weighted cine FLASH gradient echo sequences with prospective two-dimensional cardiac triggering were generated

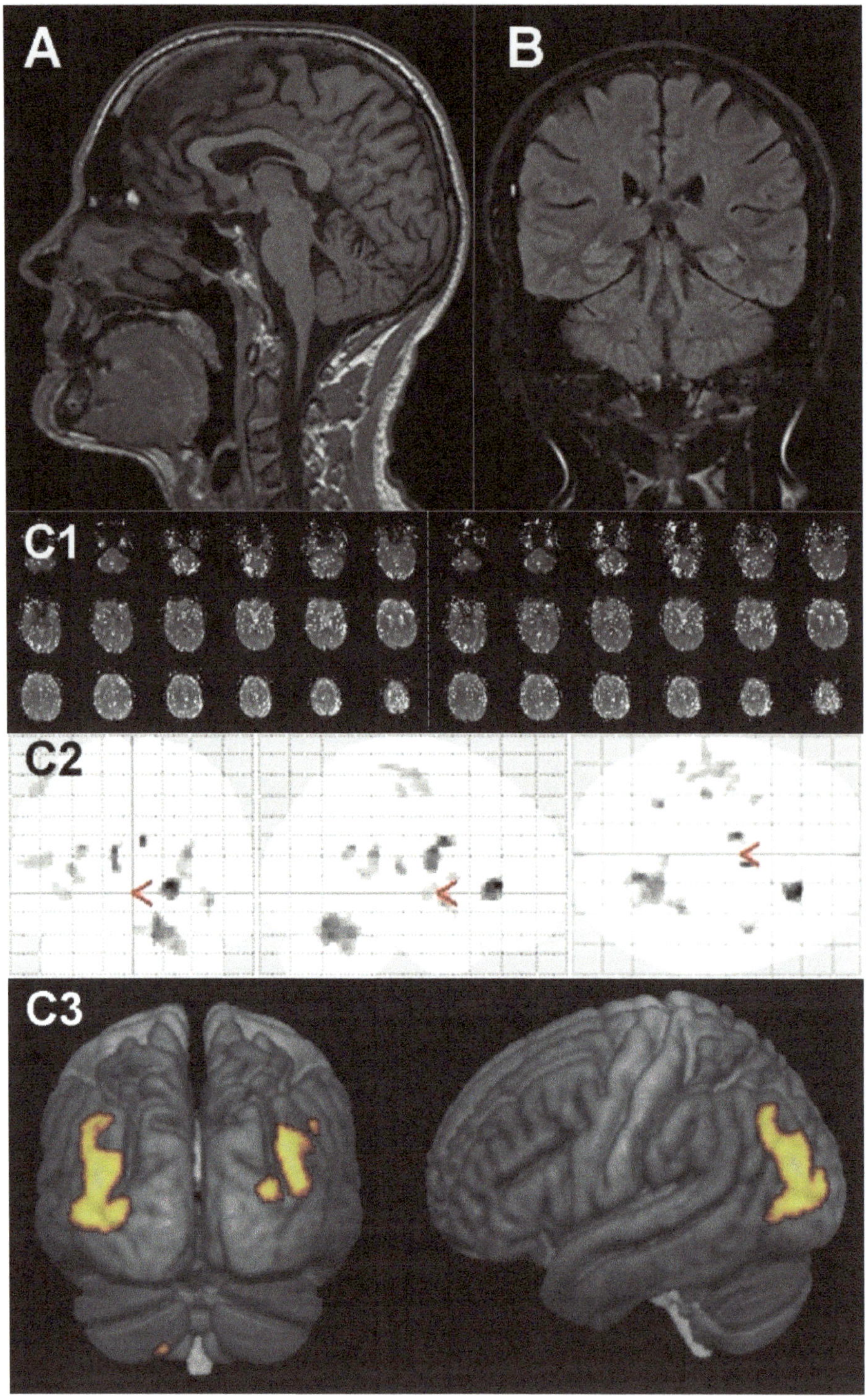

Figure 8 MRI of the brain. Male, 52-years-old. **A1:** stage 57, 3,971 km (T1w turbo FLASH 3D sagittal): High resolution isometric three-dimensional sequence (1 mm) allows isovoxel based volumetry (VBM) of the whole brain. **A2**: Three-dimensional view shows dominant areas of volume loss (colored) of grey brain matter occurring during the TEFR09. **B:** stage 36, 2,448 km (T2w FLAIR): Sensitive sequence for detection of brain lesions. In this case, no lesions visible. **C:** 20 days before the start. Functional MRI (fMRI) using blood oxygenation level dependent (BOLD) contrast for evaluation of pain perception in ultra runners (C1: without pain stimulus, C2: with pain stimulus). C3: Post-processing analysis using statistical parametric mapping (SPM) shows areas of activation.

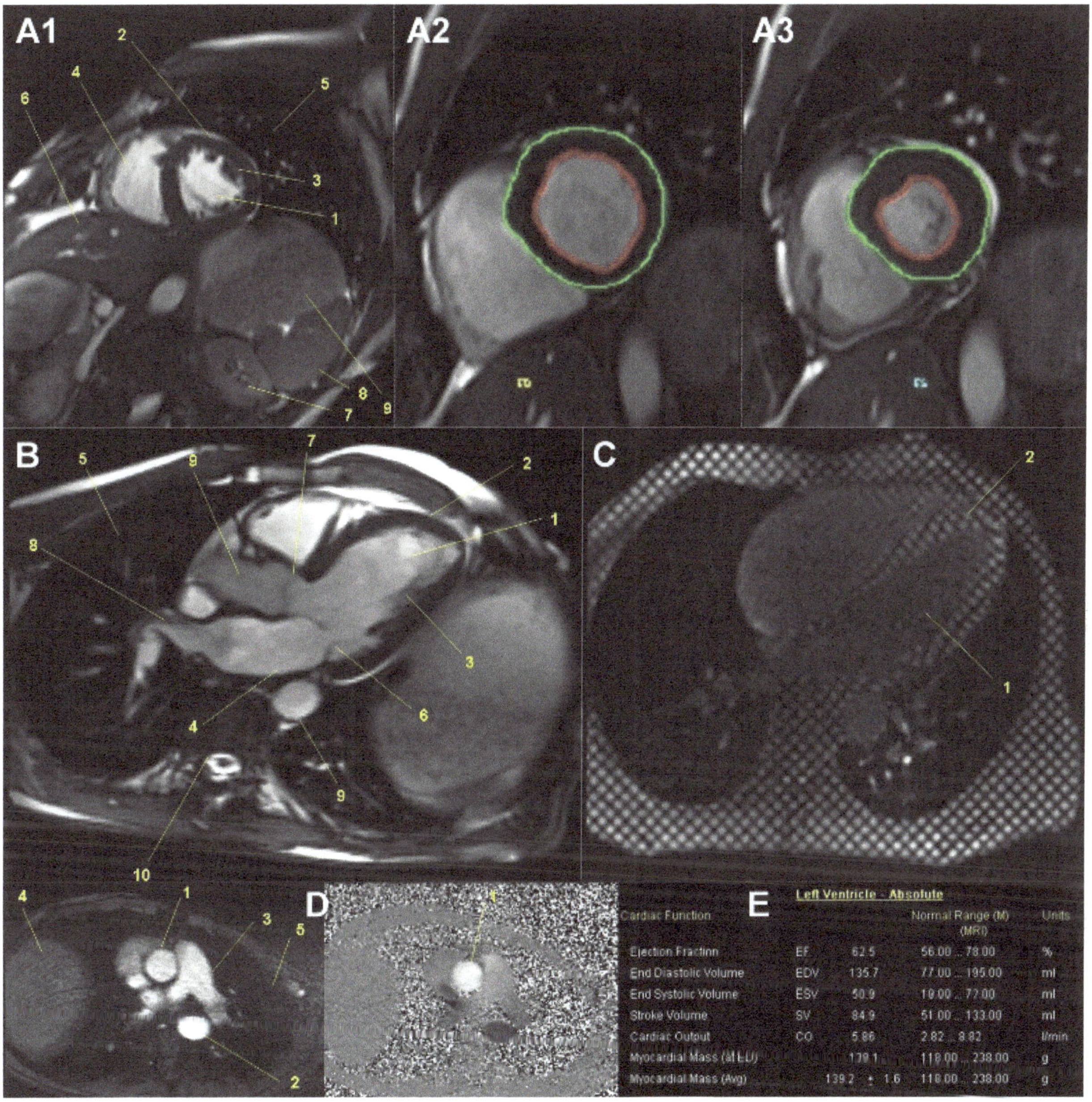

Figure 9 Mobile cardiac cine-MRI. **A:** male, 52-years-old, stage 23, 1,569 km (cine SSFP GRE, 2-chamber view): Focus is the left ventricle (1), myocardium (2). papillary muscles (3), right ventricle (4), lung (5), liver (6), left kidney (7), spleen (8), stomach (9). A2, A3: Specific post-processing makes functional volumetry of left ventricle and myocardium possible (green line: epicardium, red line: endocardium). **B:** male, 52-years-old, stage 25, 1,706 km (cine SSFP GRE, 3-chamber view): left ventricle (1), myocardium (2), papillary muscles (3), left atrium (4), lung (5), mitral valve (6), aortic valve (7), pulmonary vein (8), aorta (9), thoracic spine (10). **C:** male, 49-years-old, stage 26, 1,770 km (cine tagging SSFP GRE, four-chamber view): MR tagging of the left ventricle (1) makes quantification of the myocardial (2) motion with its spatial orientation possible. **D:** female, 45-years-old, stage 38, 2,601 km (phase contrast transversal): Ascending aortic (1) flow is measured by specific velocity-encoded (venc) MR imaging. Descending aorta (2), pulmonary artery (3), liver (4), lung (5). **E:** Selection of possible cardiac parameters measurable by cardiac cine-MRI.

(Table 2) to measure compliance changes of the vessel wall of the distal common carotid (Figure 10A) and proximal superficial femoral artery (Figure 10D). In total, for vascular MRI three flexible six-channel body matrix coils for aortic and femoral artery measurements, one four-channel phased dual mode neck matrix coil and ECG triggering makes positioning and preparation of the subjects very time consuming.

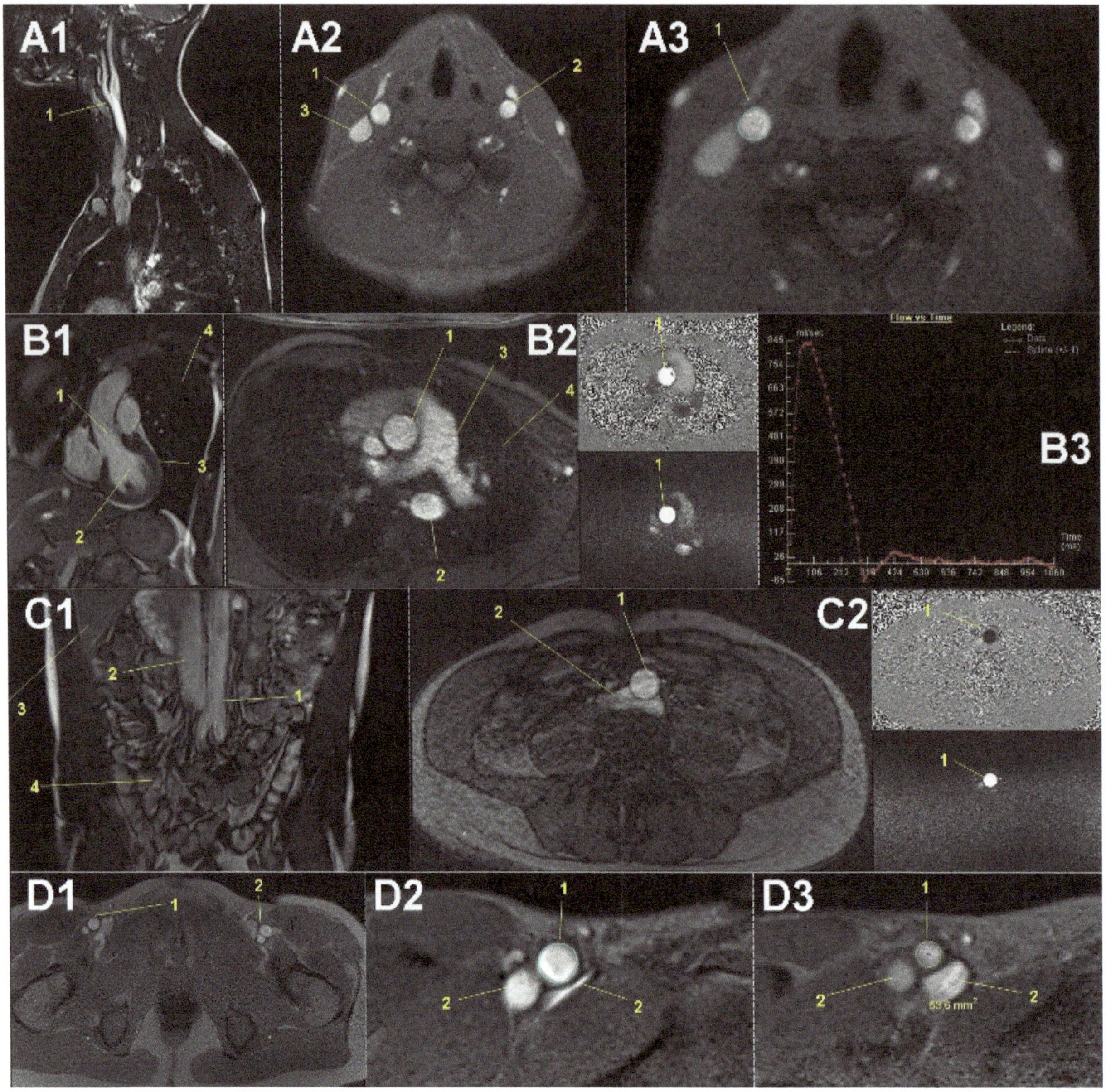

Figure 10 Mobile vascular cine-MRI: male, 52-years-old, stage 27, 1,838 km. A1: MR localizer sagittal, A2,3: FLASH transversal: Automatic functional measurement of common right carotid artery diameter just below carotid bifurcation (1). Left carotid artery (2), right deep jugular vein (3). **B1:** MR localizer, **B2:** phase contrast transversal: Ascending aortic (1) diameter and flow is measured by specific velocity-encoded (venc) MR imaging. Descending aorta (2), pulmonary artery (3), lung (4). **B3:** graphic depiction of aortic pulsatile flow (ml/second). **C1:** MR localizer coronal, **C2**: phase contrast transversal: Distal descending aortic (1) diameter and flow is measured by specific velocity-encoded (venc) MR imaging just above the aortic bifurcation. Inferior vena cava (2), liver (3), intestines (4). **D1:** FLASH transversal: Functional measurement of superficial right femoral artery diameter just below bifurcation (1), left femoral artery (2). **D2:** Manual diameter measurement (1), **D3:** Automatic diameter measurement (1). Femoral veins (2).

Whole body MRI

For total body MRI, change of subject positioning from prone head forward to prone feet forward was necessary during a T1 weighted turbo spin echo sequencing using an adapted protocol developed on adipose and diabetic volunteers [138] (Table 2). With topographic tissue segmentation and mapping of the athlete's body using a fuzzy c-means algorithm according to Würslin *et al.* [139] a simple and time-saving strategy for assessment and standardization of the tissue distribution in the entire body was possible. With additional manual adaption due to the non-fasting condition of the subjects changes in different lean and adipose body compartments could be measured during the TEFR09 (Figure 11).

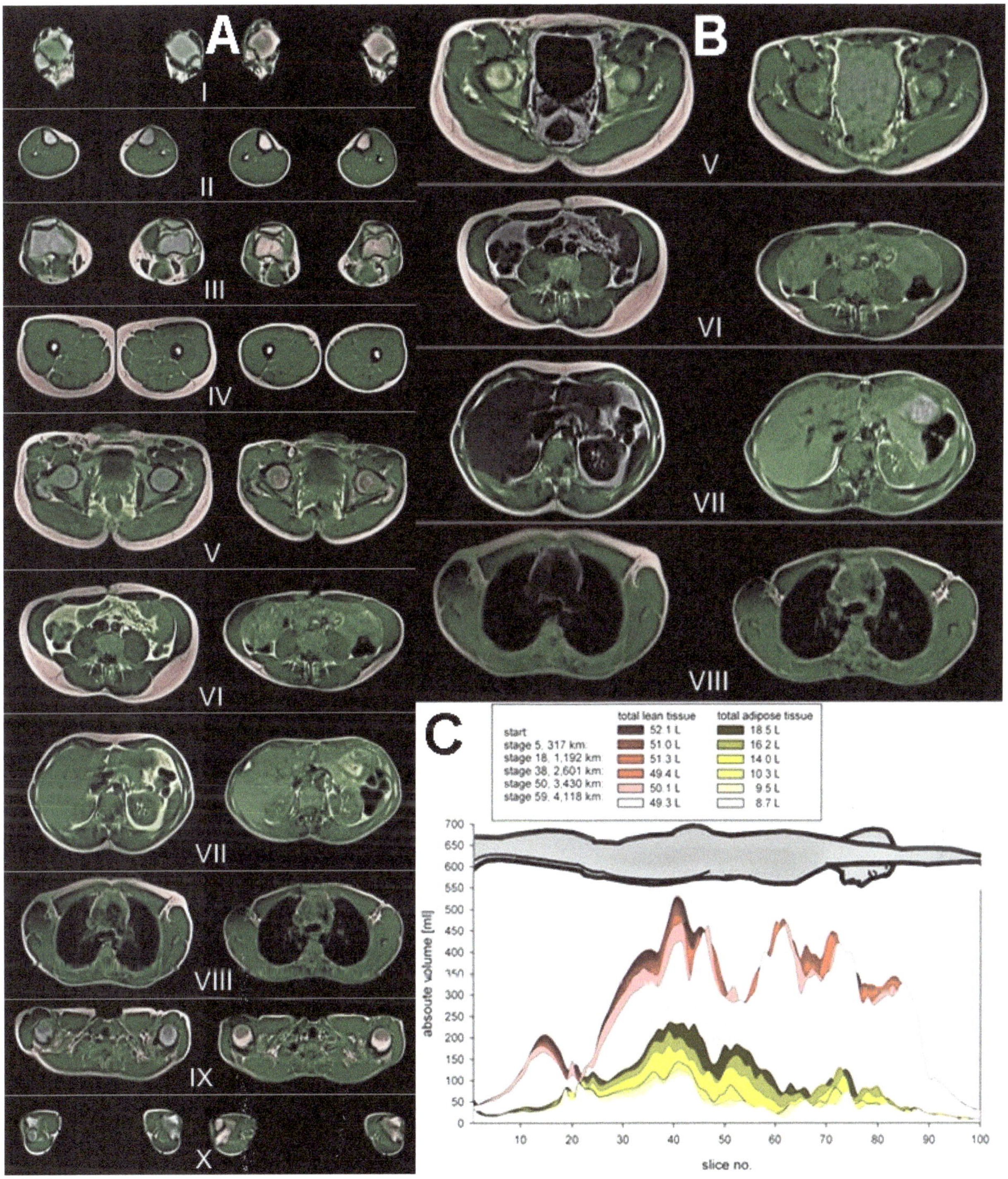

Figure 11 Semiautomatic tissue separation with mobile whole body MRI of a 32-year-old male finisher of the TEFR09. A: Right row (before start): green: total lean tissue, red: somatic adipose soft tissue, yellow: visceral adipose tissue, blue: adipose bone marrow. Left row (after 4,120 km): green: total lean tissue, red: somatic adipose tissue (= somatic adipose soft tissue + adipose bone marrow), yellow: visceral adipose tissue. (selected slices: I: ankles, II: middle of lower legs, III: knees, IV: middle of upper legs, V: hip/pelvis, VI: umbilical level, VII: upper abdomen, VIII: heart/mediastinum, IX: shoulder girth, X: elbows). **B:** Right row (before start): green: somatic lean tissue, red: somatic adipose tissue, grey: total visceral volume. Left row (after 4,120 km): green: total lean tissue, red: somatic adipose tissue (= somatic adipose soft tissue + adipose bone marrow), yellow: visceral adipose tissue, blue: intraluminal nutrition fat in intestinal tract. (selected slices: V: hip/pelvis, VI: umbilical level, VII: upper abdomen, VIII: heart/mediastinum). **C:** Loss of total lean and total adipose tissue during the TEFR09.

MR-spectroscopy

Proton MR-spectroscopy with a flexible six-channel body matrix coil for measurement of the intramyocellular lipid (IMCL) content of the tibialis anterior and soleus muscle required the stimulated-echo acquisition mode (STEAM) technique (Table 2) and manual shimming of the magnetic field [140], which makes generation of valuable results on a mobile MRI difficult and unpredictable (Figure 12).

Focused supplementary sequences

In addition to the mentioned study protocol, additional MR examinations were done on subjects and TEFR participants, if acute injuries (for example, stress fractures [52]) and pain syndromes (for example, low back pain [49,52]) occurred and a specific diagnostic finding was necessary to prevent further injuries or complications on the endurance runners (Figure 13).

Anthropometric and cardiovascular physical measurements

Anthropometric and cardiovascular physical measurements were done on all subjects (Figure 3) every fourth day. Therefore, the 44 subjects were randomly assigned to one of four groups. Body mass was measured with BIA using a Tanita BC-545™ BIA scale (Arlington Heights, IL, USA: to the nearest 0.1 kg). This balance gave additional results about percentage of body fat and lean body mass based on MR validated calculation procedures [141]. The measurements took place in the morning (between 4 a.m. and 5 a.m.) and after the stage (between 3 p.m. and 9 p.m.) together with measurement of blood pressure and body temperature (T) using an infrared ear thermometer (ThermoScan IRT 4020 ™, Braun, Germany: to the nearest 0.2°C. After the stage between 3 p.m. and 9 p.m., the skinfold (SF) thickness of the same subjects was measured using a skinfold caliper (GPM ™, Silber and Hegner, Zurich, Switzerland: to the nearest 2 mm) and their segmental body circumference (CF) was measured using a retractable measuring tape (to the nearest 1 mm). For SF, the mean value was calculated from three consecutive intra-individual measurements at eight regions on the right side of the body according to Ball *et al.* [142]: chest, midaxillary (vertical), triceps, subscapular, abdominal (vertical), suprailiac (at anterior axillary), thigh, and calf. For CF, mean value was calculated from three consecutive intra-individual measurements at six regions on the right side of the body according to Lee *et al.* [143]: upper arm (largest part of the limb), waist, hip, thigh (10 cm/20 cm above upper patella pole), and calf (largest part of the limb).

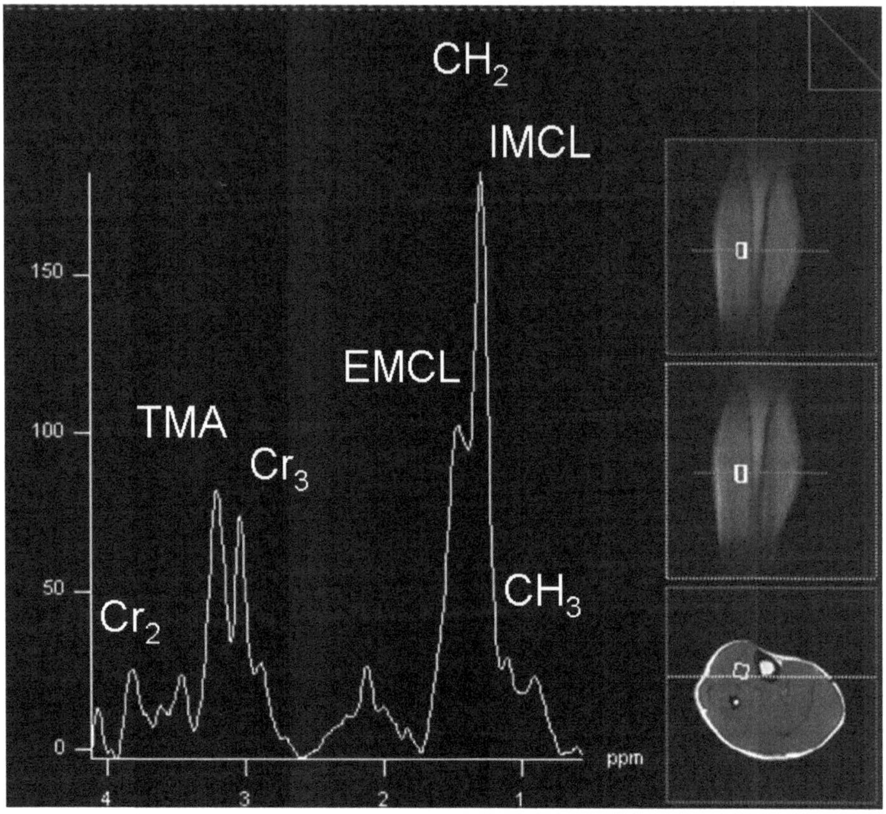

Figure 12 Mobile MRI H^1-spectroscopy.

To avoid inter-observer error all the anthropometric measurements were done by the same, specifically trained investigator. Every 800 km a short term ECG was planned on every subject.

Lab samples

Midstream urine samples were taken from all subjects twice each day. Before breakfast in the morning between 4:00 a.m. and 5:00 a.m. and after each stage in the evening after dinner between 7:00 p.m. and 9:00 p.m. Blood samples were taken every 1,000 km from the cubital vein after stage. The samples were immediately centrifuged and frozen (below -20°C) and put on -80°C after the race.

Post-race/follow-up

On the day they dropped out, non-finishers (NF) had a last complete measurement of all specific MRI protocols and physical examinations (BIA, SF, CF) and provided blood- and urine-samples. Nearly eight months after the TEFR09, 15 of the 44 subjects (all of them finishers of the TEFR09) had a follow up examination at UHU on the same topics involved during the field studies: specific MRI examinations, anthropometric measurements, ECG and blood and urine samples.

Statistical analysis

For statistical analysis the software 'SPSS 12.OG for Windows, Version 12.0.1' was used. Data are presented as mean (SD, range) and median (IQR) as appropriate. The coefficient of variation (CV (%) = 100*SD/mean) was calculated only for measured absolute data on performance. The stage severity index (SSI) is an indirect parameter calculated from the mean stage velocity of all runners without a severe handicap $\bar{v}_{STAGE^*}$ in relation to the total mean velocity of the whole race $\bar{v}_{TEFR^*}$. Therefore, the SSI represents the relative burden of each stage, which is dependent on the mentioned multiple external factors that changed daily. It reflects the sum of daily weather and route conditions:

$$SSI = v_{STAGE} \frac{\bar{v}_{STAGE^*}}{\bar{v}_{TEFR^*}}$$

*: values are only integrated in calculation, if the stage performance of the specific runner is more than 87% of his mean race performance

Results

Race conditions

The mean stage length was 70.1 km (SD 11.8 km, range 44 to 95.1 km) and influenced the SSI positively (Figure 14). Temperature and humidity were also factors influencing the SSI and showed a mean (mean of three daily measures at 6:00 a.m., 10:00 a.m. and 2:00 p.m.) of 15.2° C (SD 4.7°C, range 3.7 to 25.1°C) and 55.6% (SD 14.3, range 26.5% to 82.7%), respectively. Altitude differences were not measured. The longest stages occurred in the last third of the race and the coldest, wettest and most humid and, therefore, most severe stages, were at end of the TEFR09 which pushed the runners to their limits (Figure 14).

Changes of study plan due to hazards in TEFR

For every research topic, distance intervals of measurement (MI) throughout the TEFR09 were defined. The discrepancies between these planned and the realized MI can be shown as mean absolute deviations (Figure 15). For MRI, data showed mean deviations between 100 and 300 km. For MR spectroscopy it raised up to 400 km, because this special MR technique was highly dependent on the locations with their local magnetic field disturbances (such as, traffic and so on). However, reasons for the deviations were multifold.

Study staff had to deal with many influencing factors, which made daily adaptation of the research plan necessary: acute or chronic illness of study staff, bad weather conditions (Figure 14) which sometimes influenced operability of the mobile MRI, accidents and technical problems (Table 3) and local situations at stage destination which sometimes made a nearby commissioning of the mobile MRI difficult. However, the strongest influence forcing the staff to change and adapt the daily research work program was the athlete with more or less daily changes in mental and physical conditions and necessities: pain, fatigue, fears, doubts, illness, nutrition time schedules and specific behavior and rituals regarding regeneration from this immense physical and psychological stress. Therefore, it was not always possible to ensure the exact time of pre- and post-race measurements. Despite these uncertainties, 95% of the measurement protocol could be followed.

Figure 16 shows all performed examinations and measurements done before, during and six months after the TEFR09. The overall work load includes: 741 MRI protocols with 2,637 MRI sequences (more than 200,000 picture data), 5,600 urine samples, 1,018 BIA-, 539 SF- and CF-measurements, 250 blood samples and 205 ECGs.

Baseline characteristics and performances of subjects

The baseline characteristics of the study groups are summarized in Table 3. Age and gender did not differ between the two MR groups. None of the 44 subjects showed different AROM of the hip and knee or any functional or anatomical mal-alignment of the legs compared to normal values or between the MR groups. Only active hip extension shows a tendency to be better in endurance runners (Table 4).

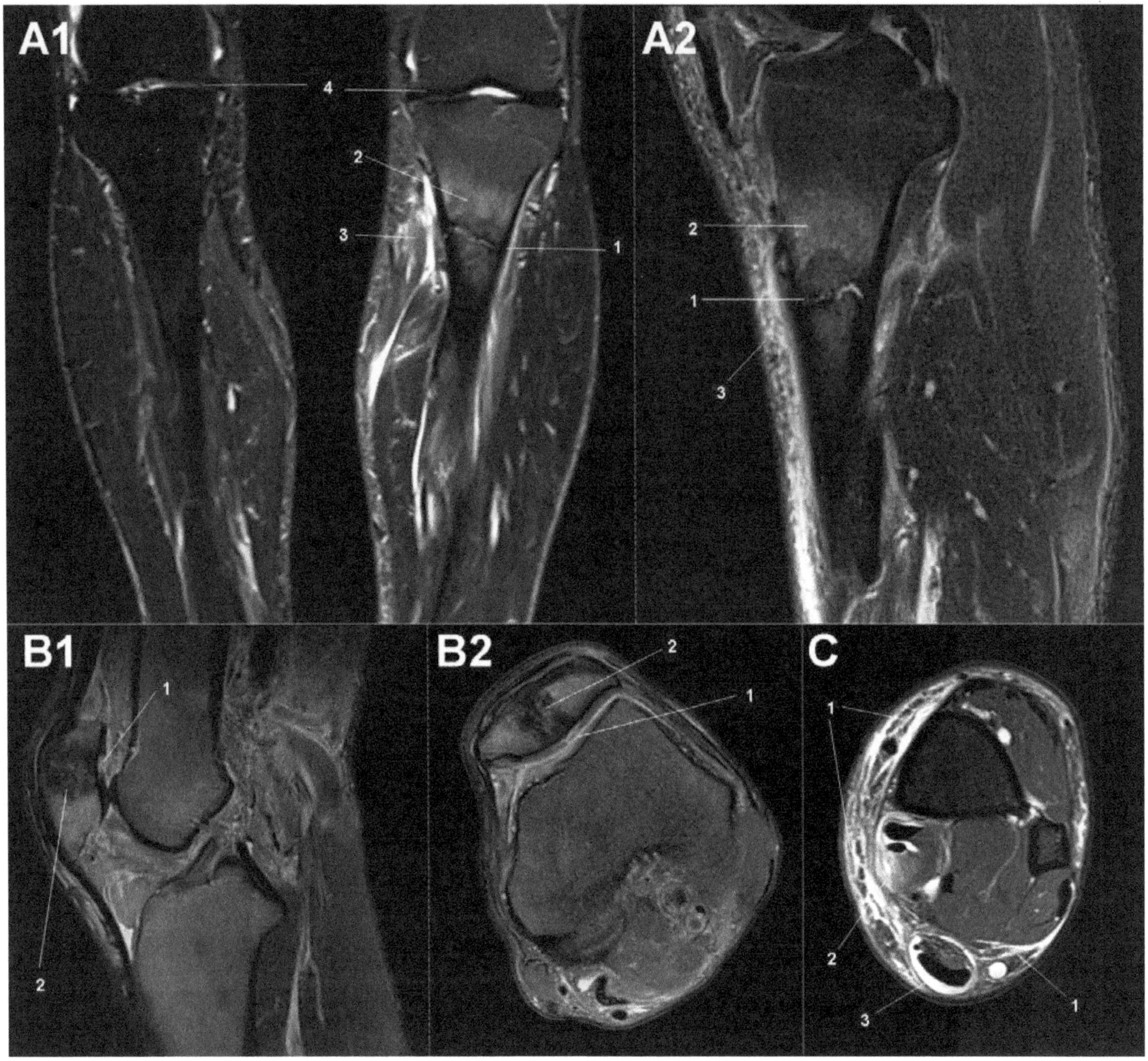

Figure 13 Supplementary mobile MRI examinations during the TEFR09. A: male, 61-years-old, stage 38, 2,601 km (PDw TSE fs, A1: coronal, A2: sagittal): Stress fracture of the proximal tibia (1) with perifocal bone edema (2) and focal subcutaneous edema (3). **B:** male, 49-years old, stage 52, 3,609 km (PDw TSE fs, B1: sagittal, B2: transversal): Retropatellar chondral ulcer (1) leading to bleeding/hematoma of the patellar bone (2). **C:** male, 41-years-old, stage 13, 857 km (PDw TSE fs transversal): Massive subcutaneous edema (panniculitis: 1) with focal myositis of deep flectors (2) and tenosynovitis of Achilles tendon (3).

Regarding the ratio of F and NF there is no relevant difference between subject group and the whole starter group (Table 5, Figure 17), but randomly between the MR groups (Table 4). Reasons for dropping out of the race were multifold (Table 5, Figure 17). The main reasons for premature exiting the race were overuse syndromes of the soft tissues of the leg, resulting in (peri-) myotendinous inflammations in the lower and upper legs (71.4%). Two subjects suffered a stress fracture in the third part of the race, one high tibia fracture (male, 60 years old) and one ventral pelvic fracture (female, 46 years old). Due to the unspecific pain and the high pain level, they ran with these fractures for about 200 km to 240 km before they gave up. There was one case of a rapidly ascending soft tissue abscess of the upper extremity due to an initially minor finger lesion (male, 39 years old) indicating the immense burden of the ultra-endurance performance to the runners and their immunological system.

Performances

Regarding all participants, the mean speed per stage was 8.35 km/hour (SD = 0.32; CV = 3.8%) and the mean total race speed of all finishers was 8.25 km/hour (SD = 1.4,

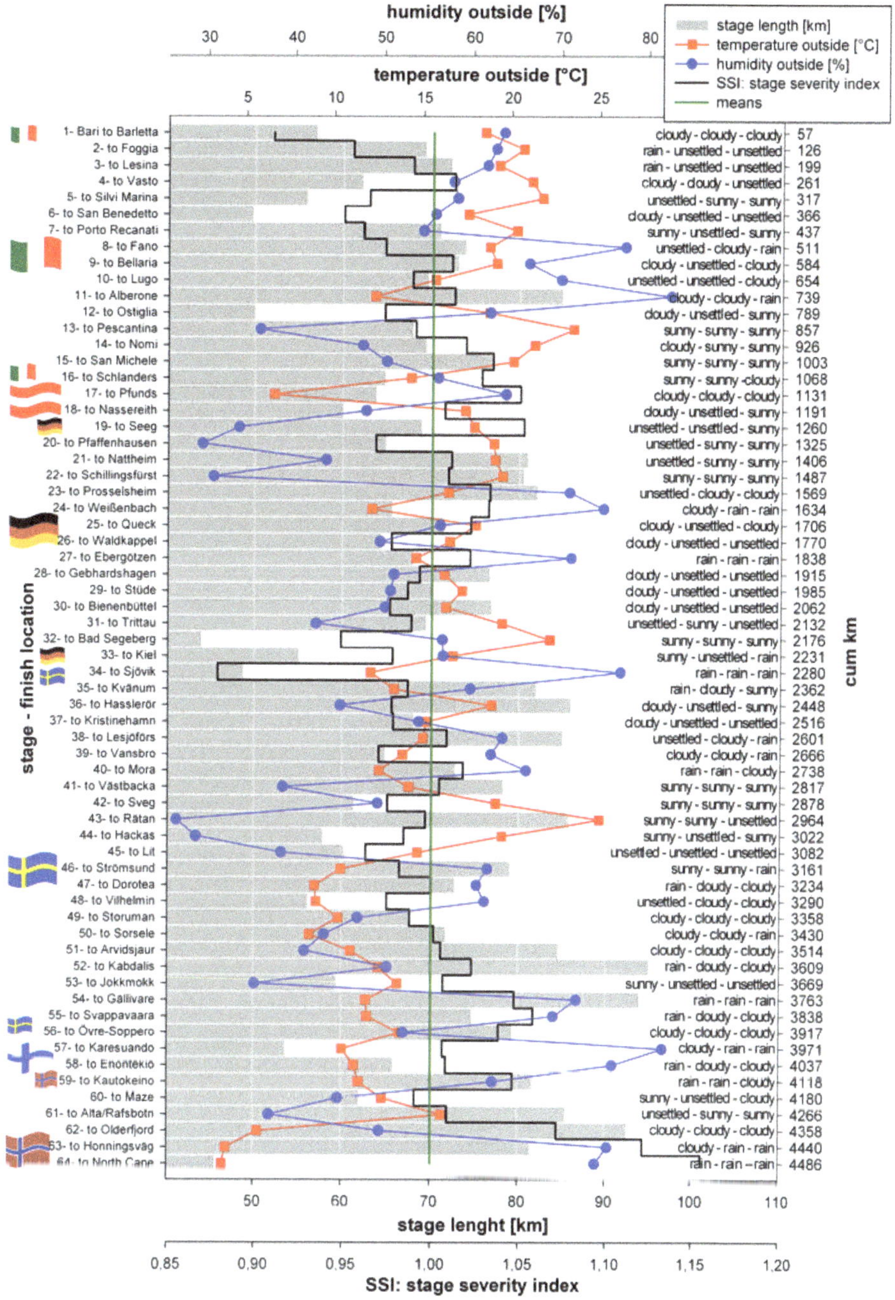

Figure 14 Daily profile of weather and stage conditions during the entire TEFR09.

CV = 17.1%). Finishers invested 552 hours (SD = 91, CV = 16.5%) for the 4,486 km in total. There was a wide range of performance difference between the best and slowest runner throughout the whole race, independent of the stage severity (Figure 18). The best runner (male, 28 years old) performed the race with a mean speed of 11.9 km/hour (total running time: 378 hours), nearly twice as fast as the slowest runner (female, 58 years old), with a mean speed of 6.2 km/hour (total running time: 723 hours. In the subject group, mean speed per stage was 8.28 km/hour (SD = 0.33; CV = 3.9%) and the mean total race speed of the subject finishers was 8.25 km/hour (SD = 1.3, CV = 15.3%), ranging from 11.1 km/hour (male, 26 years old, total running time: 407 hours, second rank) to 6.5 km/hour (male, 63 years old, total running time: 696.4 hours, 45th rank). Subjects mean stage speed was on average 8.32 km/hour (SD = 0.33, CV = 3.9%). Figure 18 shows mean performances in total and per stage.

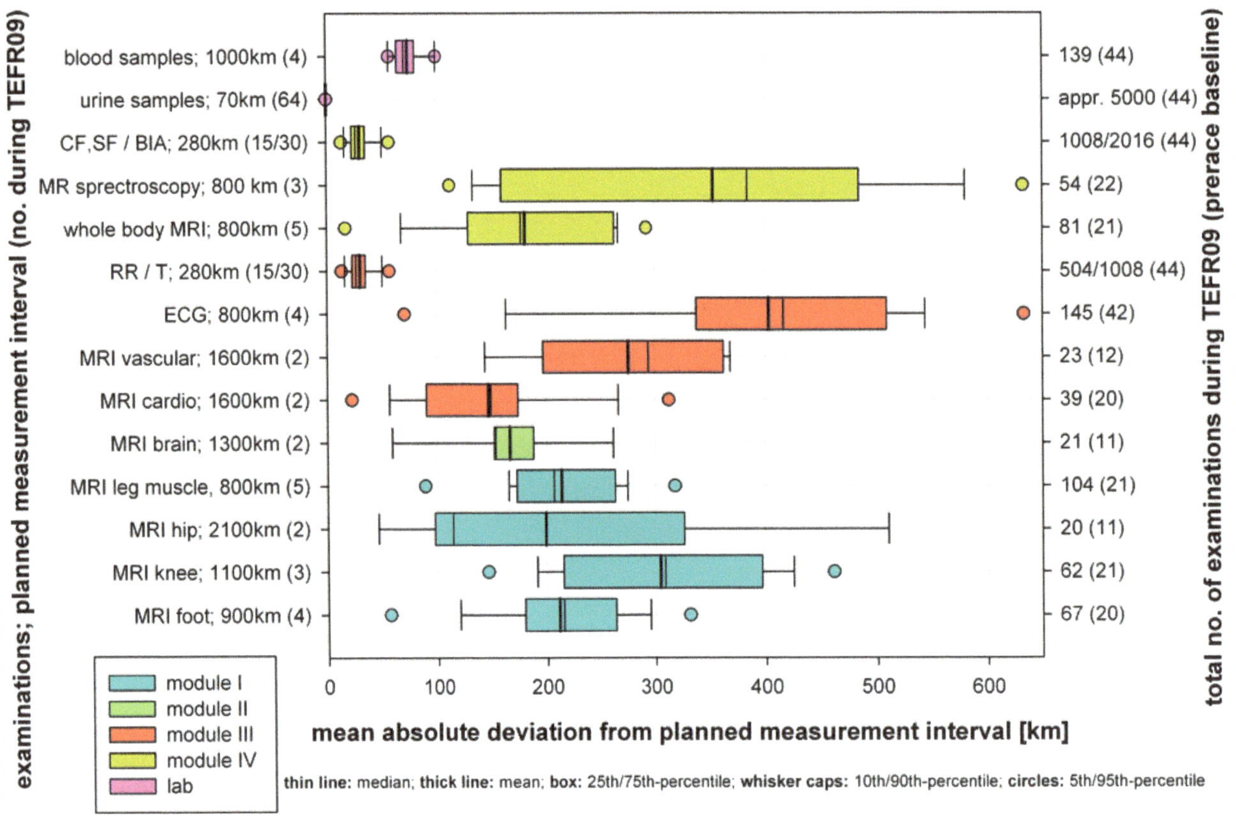

Figure 15 Deviation of measurements from projected intervals [km] during TEFR09.

Discussion

History

Looking at transcontinental footrace history, the finisher rate ranges from 28% to 73% (Table 1). The Bunion Derbies of the early twentieth century showed the lowest rate due to lower standards regarding sports equipment, nutrition features, endurance-associated behavioral knowledge and the level of organization. These two Derbies had 150 starters in mean, much more than nowadays, indicating a high rate of rookies with little or no experience in ultra running. In the TEFR09, 31% of the participants (32% of the subjects) did not reach the finish line (Table 5, Figure 17). This is 18% more finishers than at the TEFR03. This could be attributed to the longer distance in 2003 (+540 km) from Lisbon to Moscow, implying a mean difference of 8.3 km per stage between the TEFR09 and the TEFR03. Apart from the TEFR03, running distances of modern transcontinental footraces (1992 to 2009) were approximately equally long and the finishing rate of 68% in the TEFR09 lies in the upper range of the published data (Table 1). Looking at the rate of participation, being more than 200% higher

Table 3 Relevant accidents and damage to MRI and vehicles during the TEFR project

No.	stage	location (Figure 1)	event (Figure 3)	MR down time
1	0	Bari, Southern Italy	Defect of MRI table.	24 hours
2	12	Lugo to Alberone, Northern Italy	Truck collision on bridge over the river Po.	-
3	33	Bad Segeberg, Nothern Germany	Roof damage on MRI trailer.	-
4	36	Göteborg to Sjövik, Southern Sweden	Total system breakdown, damage of one compressor.	16 hours
5	38	Kristinehamn, Central Sweden	Truck sunken in football sand-field.	5 hours
6	45	Hackas, Central Sweden	Severe ankle fracture of MRI assistant.	16 hours
7	56	Svapparaava, Northern Sweden	Total rupture of tractor to trailer cables.	2 hours
8	after race	nearby Gällivare, Northern Sweden	Reindeer collision on the way back from North Cape: total damage of material van.	-

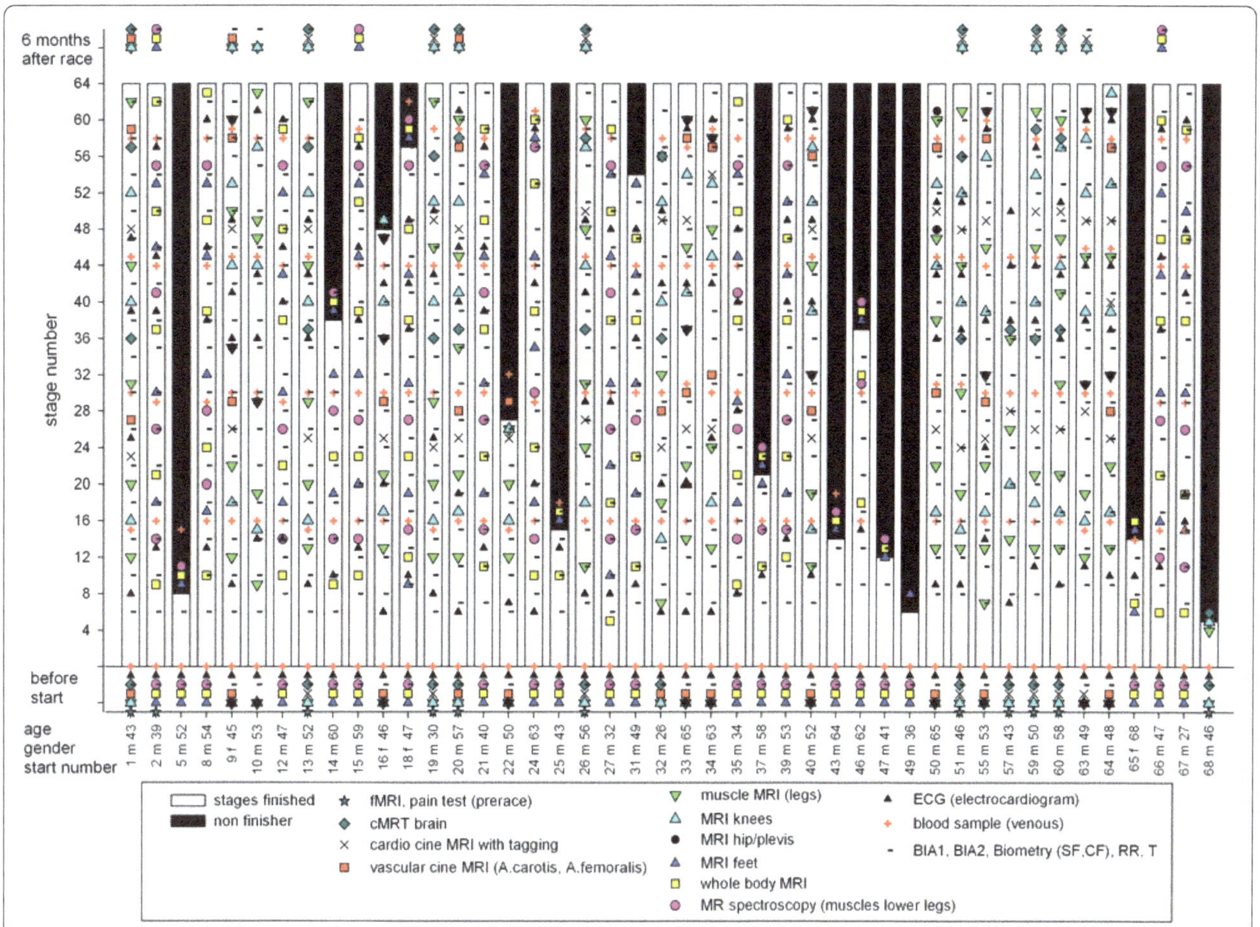

Figure 16 Realized clinical and MRI-measurements on all subjects during TEFR09.

than the mean starter rate of all modern transcontinental footraces, the comparably high finishing rate indicates a professional organization and preparation of both the runners and organizers of the TEFR09.

Performance

Due to the diverse ways and possibilities to exercise long distance running (that is, area, length, altitude, distance, weather, indoor/outdoor, on/off-road, looped course, combinations with other disciplines and so on), it is extremely difficult to compare the performances of ultra athletes in the literature [107,108,145]. Regarding the present literature, an abundant variety of physiological, anthropometrical, pre-race and training variables seem to influence running performance and associated injuries, depending upon the length and duration of the races [146-150]. In MSUM, such as the TEFR09, the daily changing environmental conditions have a direct influence on stage performances. In the last days of the TEFR09 weather conditions became more and more difficult towards the destination, North Cape, leading to a marked decrease of mean running speed (Figure 18). Only their indomitable will not to drop out at the end of race after more than 4,000 km of running, kept many emaciated participants in the race.

Drop out and injuries

Due to the likely multifactorial nature of running injuries, very few firm conclusions can be made based on the existing studies. In general, there are intrinsic factors such as individual biomechanical abnormalities (that is, mal-alignments, muscle imbalance, stiffness, weakness, instability) or extrinsic (mostly avoidable) factors such as poor running technique, improper equipment and improper changes in training extent and mode or duration and frequency of the race burden contributing to overuse injuries [151]. The one year prevalence of running injuries is 55% in male marathon runners; limb overuse injuries are the most common [152]. In UM these entities become much more important. The most common injuries for runners are multiply cited in the literature: anterior knee pain (for example, patella-femoral syndrome), iliotibial band friction syndrome, tibial stress syndrome (shin splint/injuries), plantar

Table 4 Baseline characteristics of the TEFR study population

	all subjects number (%)	MR group 1 number (%)	MR group 2 number (%)
total	44	22 (50.0)	22 (50)
men	40 (90.9)	20 (90.9)	20 (90.9)
women	4 (9.1)	2 (9.1)	2 (9.1)
Finisher (F)	30 (68.2)	19 (86.4)	11 (50.0)
Non-finisher (NF)	14 (31.8)	3 (13.6)	11 (50.0)
	mean/median (SD)	mean/median (SD)	mean/median (SD)
age (years)	49.7 (10.5)	50.3 (9.6)	49.1 (11.5)
prerace history:			
years of regular endurance running	17.9 (7.5)	19.1 (7.5)	17.1 (7.4)
finished marathons	91.7 (168.6)	62.0 (93.4)	121.47 (218.8)
finished ultra-marathons	85.4 (63.6)	81.1 (59.0)	89.8 (69.0)
finished multistage ultra-marathons	5.7 (3.6)	5.1 (4.1)	6.3 (2.9)
anthropometry:			
height (cm)	175 (8)	175 (6)	174 (9)
BMI (kg/m^2)	23.1 (2.2)	22.8 (1.8)	23.4 (2.6)
body fat percentage, BIA (%)	11.2 (4.3)	11.0 (4.1)	11.4 (4.5)
body fat percentage, calculated[a] (%)	16.6 (4.2)	15.5 (3.2)	16.6 (5.0)
body fat percentage, MRI (%)	-	-	22.7 (6.0)
muscle percentage, calculated[b] (%)	49.8 (5.1)	49.7 (4.7)	50.0 (5.7)
somatic lean tissue, MRI (%)	-	-	65.0 (5.3)
active range of hip motion (°)			
flexion, 121 (26)[c]	123 (27)	122 (26)	124 (27)
extension, 19 (16)[c]	24 (17)	25 (17)	21 (16)
abduction, 42 (22)[c]	43 (23)	43 (22)	42 (24)
internal rotation, 31 (16)[c]	31 (16)	30 (16)	32 (16)
external rotation, 32 (18)[c]	34 (19)	33 (18)	34 (19)
active range of knee motion (°):			
flexion, 132 (20)[c]	134 (19)	135 (20)	133 (19)
lower limb alignment:	-		-
LL difference [mm], 6 (95th: 11)[d]		2 (3.3), 95th: 9)	
FTR, 1.26 (0.05)[d]		1.17 (0.04)	
FTA [°], m: 178 (174-182)[e]		178 (175-182)	
w: 181 (177-185)[e]			
FTA difference		1 (0.8)	
MAD (mm), 10 (4-16)[e]		10 (4-17)	

[a]calculated by the updated DC (DEXA criterion)-equation according to Ball *et al.* [142], inputs: age, 7SF (chest, midaxillary, triceps, subscapular, abdomen, suprailiac, thigh); [b]calculated estimation of skeletal muscle mass according to Lee *et al.* [143], inputs: gender, age, race, height, 3 SF and CF (upper arm, thigh, calf); [c]normal AROM-values of hip and knee joints (goniometric data) according to the 1st National Health and Nutrition Examination Survey (NHANES I) [144]; [d]normal values of side differences in the lower limb [119], generated with computed tomography gold standard method [117]. FTR: femoro-tibial length-ratio. Leg length (LL) differences of > 14 mm (3SD) are seen as pathological [122,119,118]; [e]normal values of femorotibial angle (FTA) and mean axis distance (MAD) [116,120,121]

fasciitis, Achilles tendonitis and meniscal injuries of the knee [152-156].

Approximately two thirds of NF dropped out of the race in the first half of the TEFR09 (Figure 17). As our results show, the reasons for premature resignation of subjects were different. Conforming to the literature [20,22], in more than two thirds of the cases, overuse injuries of the lower and upper limb were the most common reasons (Table 5). However, these soft tissue overuse injuries occurred not only in less experienced ultra runners, but also in runners who had already successfully finished transcontinental races such as the TEFR03 or the 'Run Across America'. There were only a few subjects and runners without any overuse problems of the limbs in these 64 days. However, not every soft tissue overuse inflammation leads to the cessation of running. Most runners were able to 'overrun' these specific problems. They reduced running speed in adaptation to their problems, used topical application of anti-inflammatory medication and some of them took non-steroidal anti-inflammatory drugs for a

Table 5 Reason for not-finishing the TEFR09

affected region	pathology	subjects (number = 14, 31.8%)	all (number = 21, 31.3%)
Soft tissues of legs:		10 (71.4%)	14 (66.7%)
lower legs:	shin splint: myofasciitis, tenditis	5 (35.7%)	7 (33.3%)
	Achillodynia	-	1 (4.8%)
upper legs:	myo-tendino-fasciitis, perineuritis	5 (35.7%)	6 (28.6%)
Bone/joint of lower body:	stress fractures: tibia, pelvis	2 (14.3%)	2 (9.5%)
	bunion (arthritis)	1 (7.1%)	1 (4.8%)
Upper extremities:	Phlegmon of the hand	1 (7.1%)	1 (4.8%)
Gastrointestinal (GIT):	upper GIT-bleeding (NSAID)	-	1 (4.8%)
	GIT infection	-	1 (4.8%)
Mental problems:	Intolerance of crowded small halls at night	-	1 (4.8%)

GIT, gastrointestinal tract; NSAID, non-steroidal anti-inflammatory drug.

few days. With adequate behavior many, but not all, athletes recovered and were able to continue the race. Presumably some athletes could handle more pain than others [20]. An example is one extreme runner, an experienced 49-year-old male subject, who had multiple severe overuse-induced soft tissue inflammations with local muscle fiber rupture forcing him to frequently slow down his speed (Figure 7A). He also showed signs of exertional compartment syndrome, but did finish the TEFR09. His ordeal at the TEFR09 is reflected by the red line in Figure 18. Contrary to other reports, Achilles tendonitis or lower limb joint problems were not a reason for subjects to stop the TEFR09. Further results of module II research topics such as specific personality, temperament, character and pain perception will be presented soon.

Statement of principal findings

The relevance of results in field studies is determined by the appropriateness of the research questions and hypotheses, by the practicability of methods and measurements and the consistency of their specific implementation and by the correct interpretation of results. Due to the manifold open questions and unproven hypotheses in endurance running, the unique opportunity of doing real time observations of changes in the body of athletes while running at the upper limit in a MSUM was demanding.

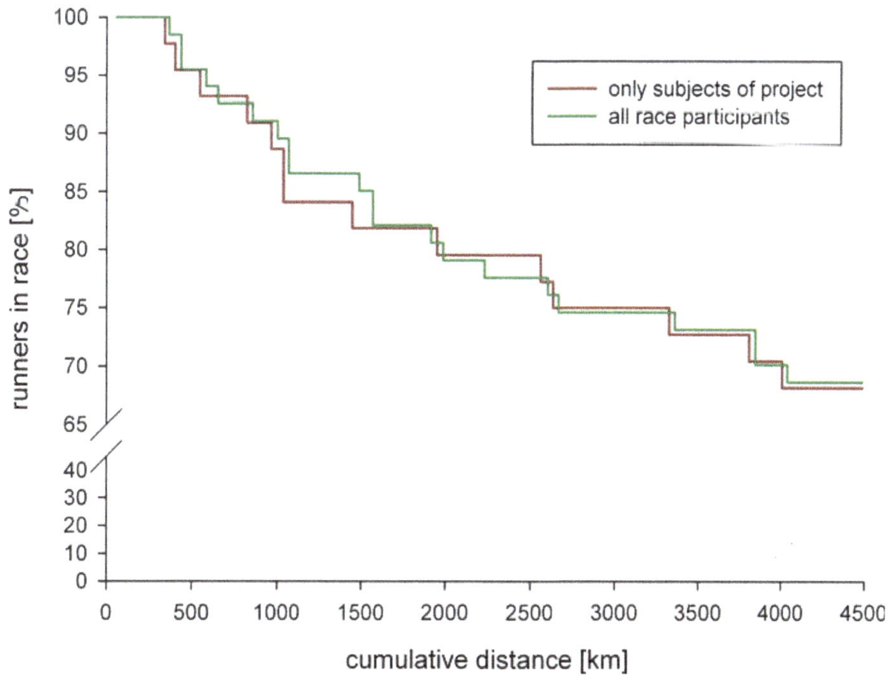

Figure 17 Drop-out rate of TEFR09.

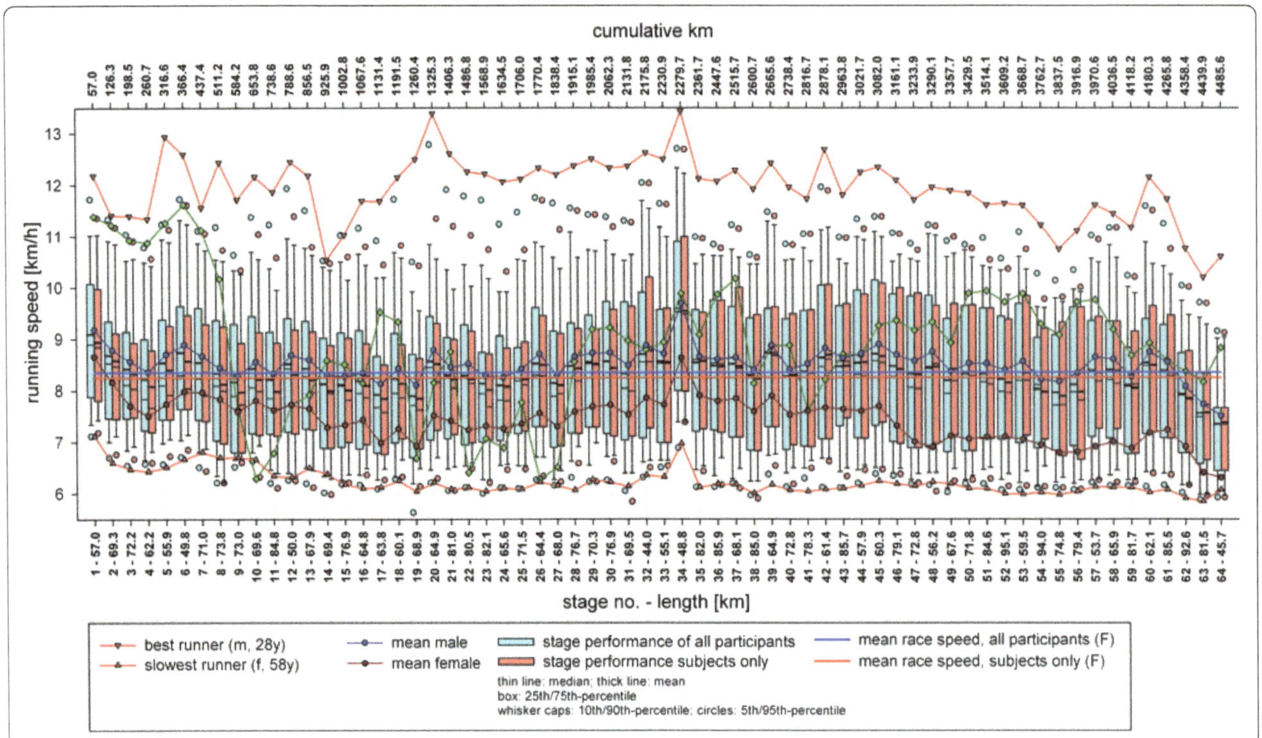

Figure 18 TEFR09 performances.

The TEFR project was designed to explore inter-individual variability in adaption to the tremendous persisting physical endurance running load on the different organic and functional systems of the body with regard to the lack of breaks and time for regeneration.

All technical equipment was tested by the specific manufacturers on reliability and validity under normal clinical conditions and usage. But daily dismantling, transport and setting up of the mobile MRI hardware sets extraordinary demands which were initially not totally verifiable and calculable. Despite some technical problems and temporal defects (Table 3), our arrival at the North Cape demonstrated the feasibility of accompanying a large group of endurance runners (67) with a mobile MRI and all its necessary equipment ensuring permanent operability during the 64 stage ultra marathon.

Throughout the whole TEFR09 our time schedules for examinations adapted to the daily changing local circumstances and the athletes mental state and problems. To avoid additional stress for the subjects, they could not and were not forced to follow the study protocol strictly. However, the efficiency of this strategy was reflected in the high rate of compliance (98%) until the end of the TEFR09. Only one subject who finished the race left the study at stage 36 (km 2,448) due to personal and, explicitly, not study related problems. Consequently, the completion rate of planned examinations over the whole running distance of 4,486 km was only limited by the drop-out rate of the subjects from the TEFR09 (Table 4, Figure 16). In particular, specific implementation of stationary validated MRI protocols on the mobile MRI on the truck trailer by a team of MRI experts and training of the research staff on the mobile MRI before the start ensures practical experience with the experimental protocols under field conditions and makes modification of them possible where necessary.

Strengths of the study

The strengths of the TEFR project are the unique chance to do a field study with the large number of 44 subjects, the realization of tests and measurements with the modern technical gold-standard equipment MRI in a daily changing and increasingly harsh and inhospitable environment (Figure 14), the complete baseline control data and the high rate of test completion. Large subject numbers provide the statistical power to discriminate between and, identify associations with, different patterns of adaptation as well as to detect differences in response between subgroups. Matched subject race profiles and baseline measurements before the start of the TEFR09 control for variability of exposure to ascending running distance and, thereby, permit valid inter-individual comparison of responses to this burden (with subjects as their own controls), maximizing the signal (true physiological differences) to noise (variations in exposure) ratio.

The avoidance of invasive or interventional tests on the subjects' mechanisms during the TEFR09 and the descriptive nature of the data may be considered a weakness of this study. However, the variety of outputs from different measurement techniques (for example, functional and cine MRI, physical anthropometrical measurements and laboratory data including proteomics, plasma and urine biomarkers) allows observation of consistent patterns of response that may be strongly suggestive of particular mechanisms.

In module I, for example, measured data of T2*-mapping of joint cartilage (Figure 4 A and 4.2A/B) will allow conclusions on the influence of long distance running on the proteoglycans in the cartilage matrix based on the current experimental experiences [43-45,157]. As in most other mobile MR associated examinations of other modules, additional laboratory analyses using specific parameters on collected blood and urine samples (for example, cartilage oligomeric matrix protein (COMP) [158-165] for joint cartilage research) will give further information for interpretation and verification of image related results.

Another example is the vascular cine MRI studies of module III. In humans, the relationships of blood flow changes to structure, function, and shear rate of conducting arteries have not been thoroughly examined. Therefore, the purpose of the vascular cine MRI study in module III (Figure 10) was to investigate these parameters of the elastic-type, common carotid artery (CCA) and the muscular-type, common femoral artery (CFA) in long-term running, assuming that the impact of activity-induced blood flow changes on conduit arteries, if any, should be seen in these highly endurance-trained athletes. These investigations using the gold standard method, MRI [137], enable further analyses on the current status of insights on the question of structural and functional vascular adaption and associated exercise-induced blood flow changes on endurance training based on sonographic B-mode measurements [100].

The manifold investigations of Knechtle *et al.* on ultra endurance athletes [15-22,113,145] focused on the question which anthropometric parameters of ultra athletes are predictors of ultra endurance performance. These authors postulated some direct connections between specific physical anthropometric markers and ultra endurance performance [16,19,166]. Examinations of module I and module IV (morphometry, body composition) of the TEFR project with its possibility of precise and differentiated morphometric analysis (for example, segmental and functional muscle volumetry) may be able to verify common experiences and to detect relationships between anthropometry and morphometry of endurance athletes and performance in MSUM.

All tissue systems - subcutaneous and visceral adipose tissues, muscles, ligaments, fascia, tendons, bones and cartilage - were studied with special quantitative and qualitative MR techniques. This should help explain how the different tissues react to the severe stress that continued for days and weeks without any pauses for regeneration or even resting phases as two marathon distances had to be completed every day.

Individual performance and ability to deal with injuries and overuse symptoms with regard to decision making for stopping MSUM is a complex psychosomatic process and more or less modulated by character traits. Strong changes of endocrine and metabolic status during marathon runs are described [78,79]. Hormonal changes can influence pain sensation and show an influence on specific brain functions [167]. Knowing this, investigations detecting reasons for dropping out of the race (14 subjects) can focus not only on MR image analysis, but must also include specific laboratory analysis and psychometric tests as done or planned in the TEFR project. Serotonin, tryptophan and endorphin are described for use as stress markers in UM [3]. The relation of branched-chain to aromatic amino acids as a model (amino acid dysbalance hypothesis) to explain running-associated fatigue is described [80]. The reduction of the pain sensation is known for cortisol [167]. Considering all these particular mechanisms influencing performance and decision making in ultra athletes, the important dimension of laboratory analysis possibilities, in addition to MR data analysis, becomes obvious for the different parts of the TEFR project.

Overall, the possibility of cross-validations between physical, MR-graphic, -functional and laboratory follow-up data on multiple organic systems during a nearly ten-week ultra run is a unique strength of this study.

Weakness of the study

The main weakness of this study is the lack of a control group of non endurance experienced subjects. However, this is not a feasible option in field studies under race conditions including such an immense amount of physical and mental load. In order to explore the influence of pre-race running experience, we will undertake subgroup analyses investigating the influence of individual pre-race performances on our findings. In the pre-race pain study (project module II, MR group 2), we recruited a parallel age-related control group that was tested over the same pain scale and functional MRI protocol as the MSUM exposed subjects. This sub-group is, therefore, not confounded by self-selection due to prior endurance tolerance.

As the first attempt in MR research, we tried to perform H^1-MR-spectroscopy for measurement of IMCL [140,168,169] with a mobile MRI on a truck trailer. MR spectroscopy needs a stable magnetic field and, therefore, a still and static environment around the scanner.

Due to the daily changing position of the mobile MRI, the possibility and feasibility of manual shimming was not predictable. This is the only measurement with uncertain validity due to changing environmental conditions in the TEFR project.

Environmental factors, such as ambient weather conditions (Figure 14), subject de- or hyperhydration and concurrent illnesses may also have confounded results. However, indoor temperature (18.7°C, SD 3.0°C, range 11.7 to 28.5°C) and temperature in the MR trailer (20.5°C, SD 0.8°C, range 18.5 to 21.8°C) was much less variable than outdoor temperature (15.2°C, SD 4.7°C, range 3.7 to 25.1°C). All subjects were encouraged to maintain adequate

hydration (guided by the production of good quantities of pale urine). There was only one Japanese subject identified with a severe illness during the race, suffering from a severe cough which persisted from stage 12 till stage 32 (day of drop out).

Another weakness of the study was that there was only rough documentation of nutrition. Nutrition depended on food availability at the TEFR stages and was provided by the TEFR organization. The use of doping substances was forbidden by the terms of participation but not controlled. Runners did not agree to close measurement and documentation of food and caloric intake, because this would have meant too much disturbance of their daily running routine and compromised compliance due to additional stress conducted by the research work. Despite initial concerns, mobile MRI examinations did not result in additional stress for the athletes. On the contrary, most of them enjoyed relaxing in the MR scanner, having no other noises and people around them while listening to their favorite music via headphones.

Strengths and weakness in relation to other studies

In comparison to previous field, laboratory and radiological, especially stationary MR studies focusing on long distance running and its effects on the human body, our study is unique in several aspects: ultra-long distance running without any day of rest, cohort size of subjects and use of a mobile MRI throughout the whole race. This is the first MR-based follow-up ultra marathon field study that ensures unique data based on repeated measurements on ascending distance burden.

We explored the possibility of conducting this study with a stationary MRI in a fixed local setting. However, this is not realizable with a large cohort size, because not many ultra endurance athletes took the challenge to run ultra long distances in circles in local regions or stadiums day by day. For example, at the Sri Chinmoy Self-Transcendence 3,100 Mile Race over 5,649 laps of one extended city block in Jamaica, Queens, New York (http://www.3100.srichinmoyraces.org) only 10 to 14 participants started regularly. If a study like this is planned, it has to be adapted to the race circumstances and not the race conditions to the study. Only exceptional runners would be willing to take such a burden under laboratory conditions. It is the experience of the distance and the environment that motivates these athletes to run thousands of kilometers. In addition, such an approach might have incurred significant additional costs; our subjects were entirely self-funded, whereas volunteers in chamber studies often expect remuneration.

Unanswered questions and future research

Further research arising from this study will follow two themes. First, studies in patients to explore the validity of our model by applying the findings of this study to pathophysiological problems in a clinical setting. Second, collecting additional healthy volunteer data from subjects exposed to an ultra endurance burden (ultra marathon, ultra triathlon, ultra cycling and) in further field studies and chamber studies.

Whether it is possible to initiate future projects using this model of a mobile MRI field study is critical. First, this was a unique cohort size in transcontinental ultra running and it would be difficult to find a size like this again: the latest Run Across America (Table 1) had only 14 participants. Second, in addition to sufficient funding a bit of luck is necessary to finish a field study successfully when using a sensitive and high-maintenance technical piece of equipment such as a mobile MRI. Future studies might answer additional questions by using alternative or additional measurement techniques or undertaking novel intervention trials.

Conclusions

The TEFR project was both a challenge and risk together. It demonstrates the feasibility and safety of conducting a large ultra endurance cohort study with a mobile MRI under 'natural' conditions over 64 stages and daily changing environment on the way across all of Europe. Thanks to the possibility offered by a modern mobile MR-imager diverse research topics from different fields of medicine could be implemented in the measurement protocol to study human adaption to an ultra endurance burden. Systematic measurements of a large set of variables were achieved with high-fidelity in 44 subjects and up to 4,500 kilometers distance running. The resulting dataset is a unique resource for the study of regeneration and adaption in relation to a high impact ultra endurance running burden which may improve specific or general scientific understanding of responses to critical illness at the limits of stress and strain of the human body.

Acknowledgements

Contributions to the study

The TransEurope FootRace 2009 Project is a research project coordinated by the Department of Diagnostic and Interventional Radiology, University Hospital of Ulm, Germany. The aim of the project is to conduct research into ultra endurance running in order to improve understanding of regeneration and adaption processes in different kind of tissues, organs and functional body systems. The TEFR project research groups members all contributed to the collection and analysis of data described in this paper.
Study funding sources
This project was mainly supported in part by the German Research Association (DFG: 'Deutsche Forschungsgemeinschaft'), under Grants SCHU 2514/1-1 and SCHU 2514/1-2. Other non-public funds were received from Siemens Healthcare Ltd. and the Medical Faculty of the University of Ulm. All funding was unrestricted. None of the funding bodies had any role in the study design, data collection, data analysis, data interpretation, manuscript preparation or decision to publish.
We cordially thank all endurance athletes who took part at this project. Considering their immense physical and mental stress they showed an extraordinary compliance every day of the TransEurope FootRace 2009.

Author details

[1]Department of Diagnostic and Interventional Radiology, University Hospital of Ulm, Germany. [2]Outpatient Rehabilitation Centre at University Hospital of Ulm, Germany. [3]Institute of Exercise and Health Sciences, Sports Medicine, University of Basel, Switzerland. [4]Health Center St. Gallen and Department of General Practice, University Hospital of Zürich, Switzerland. [5]Section on Experimental Radiology, Department of Diagnostic and Interventional Radiology, University Hospital of Tübingen, Germany. [6]Siemens Healthcare, Magnetic Resonance, Stuttgart, Germany. [7]Main organizer and race director TransEurope FootRace 2009, Horb, Germany.

Authors' contributions

US contributed to the conception and design of the study, to the funding, to the acquisition of data, the analysis of data, the interpretation of data and drafted the manuscript. AST contributed to the conception and design of the study, to the acquisition of data, and the analysis and interpretation of data. BK contributed to the design of the study and the interpretation of data. JM contributed to the design of the study, to specific MR sequence protocols and to the analysis and interpretation of data. HW contributed to the acquisition of data. ME contributed to the acquisition and analysis of data. WF contributed to the conception of the study, to the acquisition of data, the analysis of data and the interpretation of data. IS contributed to the conception and to the acquisition of data. SG contributed to the creation of specific MR sequence protocols. HB contributed to specific MR sequence protocols. IS contributed to the conception of the study. HJB contributed to the acquisition of data. CB contributed to the conception and design of the study, to the acquisition of data and the analysis and interpretation of data. All authors read and approved the final draft. Cooperators and coworkers in data post processing and analysis are permanently rising. At time of manuscript writing they are as follows: F. Birklein, M. Breimhorst, DC Cheng, J. Ellermann, S. Faust, S. Göd, L. Heisterkamp, E. Kitzenmaier, K. König, S. König, TC. Mamisch, A. Reiner, D. Schoss, C. Tassler, C. Trattnig, F. Weber, S. Wuchenauer, A. Wunderlich and C. Würslin.

Authors' information

Dr Uwe Schütz may also be contacted using his alternative email address: uwe.schuetz@uniklinik-ulm.de

Competing interests

The authors declare that they have no competing interests.

References

1. Costill DL, Bowers R, Kammer WF: **Skinfold estimates of body fat among marathon runners.** *Med Sci Sports* 1970, **2**:93-95.
2. Davies CTM, Thompson MW: **Aerobic performance of female marathon and male ultramarathon athletes.** *Eur J Appl Physiol* 1979, **41**:233-245.
3. Tittel K, Wutscherk H: **Anatomical and anthropometric fundamentals of endurance.** In *Endurance in Sport.* Edited by: Shephard RJ, Ästrand PO. Oxford: Blackwell Scientific Publications; 1992:35-45.
4. Svedenhag J, Sjödin B: **Body-mass-modified running economy and step length in elite male middle- and long-distance runners.** *Int J Sports Med* 1994, **15**:305-310.
5. Speechly DP, Taylor SR, Rogers GG: **Differences in ultra-endurance exercise in performance-matched male and female runners.** *Med Sci Sports Exerc* 1996, **28**:59-365.
6. Hetland ML, Haarbo J, Christiansen C: **Regional body composition determined by dual-energy X-ray absorptiometry. Relation to training, sex hormones, and serum lipids in male long-distance runners.** *Scand J Med Sci Sports* 1998, **8**:102-108.
7. Abe T, Kumagai K, Brechue WF: **Fascicle length of leg muscles is greater in sprinters than distance runners.** *Med Sci Sports Exerc* 2000, **32**:1125-1129.
8. Hoffman MD: **Anthropometric characteristics of ultramarathoners.** *Int J Sports Med* 2008, **29(19)**:808-811.
9. Freund W, Billich C, Brambs HJ, Weber F, Schütz UHW: **MRI changes of Achilles tendon in experienced runners and beginners during training and after (half-) marathon competition.** *Z Orthop Unfall* 2011, **149**:407-417.
10. Davies CTM, Thompson MW: **Physiological responses to prolonged exercise in ultramarathon athletes.** *J Appl Physiol* 1986, **61**:611-617.
11. Sharwood K, Collins M, Goedecke J, Wilson G, Noakes T: **Weight changes, sodium levels, and performance in the South African Ironman Triathlon.** *Clin J Sport Med* 2002, **12**:391-399.
12. Tomaszewski M, Charchar FJ, Przybycin M, Crawford L, Wallace AM, Gosek K, Lowe GD, Zukowska-Szczechowska E, Grzeszczak W, Sattar N, Dominiczak AF: **Strikingly low circulating CRP concentrations in ultramarathon runners independent of markers of adiposity: how low can you go?** *Arterioscler Thromb Vasc Biol* 2003, **23**:1640-1644.
13. Knechtle B, Wirth A, Knechtle P, Zimmermann K, Kohler G: **Personal best marathon performance is associated with performance in a 24-h run and not anthropometry or training volume.** *Br J Sports Med* 2009, **43(11)**:836-839.
14. Knechtle B, Knechtle P, Rosemann T, Senn O: **What is associated with race performance in male 100-km ultra-marathoners - anthropometry, training or marathon best time?** *J Sports Sci* 2011, **23**:1-7.
15. Knechtle B, Bircher S: **Changes in body composition during an extreme endurance run.** *Praxis* 2005, **94**:371-377.
16. Knechtle B, Knechtle P, Schulze I, Kohler G: **Upper arm circumference is associated with race performance in ultra-endurance runners.** *Br J Sports Med* 2008, **42**:295-299.
17. Knechtle B, Kohler G: **Running 338 km within 5 days has no effect on body mass and body fat but reduces skeletal muscle mass - the Isarrun 2006.** *J Sports Sci Med* 2007, **6**:401-407.
18. Knechtle B, Duff B, Schulze I, Kohler G: **The effects of running 1,200 km within 17 days on body composition in a female ultrarunner-Deutschlandlauf 2007.** *Res Sports Med* 2008, **16**:167-188.
19. Knechtle B, Duff B, Welzel U, Kohler G: **Body mass and circumference of upper arm are associated with race performance in ultraendurance runners in a multistage race–the Isarrun 2006.** *Res Q Exerc Sport* 2009, **80**:262-268.
20. Knechtle B, Duff B, Schulze I, Rosemann T, Senn O: **Anthropometry and pre-race experience of finishers and nonfinishers in a multistage ultra-endurance run–Deutschlandlauf 2007.** *Percept Mot Skills* 2009, **109**:105-118.
21. Knechtle B, Wirth A, Knechtle P, Rosemann T: **Training volume and personal best time in marathon, not anthropometric parameters, are associated with performance in male 100-km ultrarunners.** *J Strength Cond Res* 2010, **24**:604-609.
22. Knechtle B, Knechtle P, Rosemann T: **Race performance in male mountain ultra-marathoners: anthropometry or training?** *Percept Mot Skills* 2010, **110**:721-735.
23. Knechtle B, Enggist A, Jehle T: **Energy turnover at the Race across America (RAAM): a case report.** *Int J Sports Med* 2005, **26**:499-503.
24. **Transeurope Footrace.** [http://www.transeurope-footrace.org].
25. Kastner CB: *Bunion Derby: The 1928 Footrace Across America.* 1 edition. University of New Mexico Press; 2007.
26. Williams G: *C.C. Pyle's Amazing Foot Race: The True Story of the 1928 Coast-to-Coast Run Across America.* Illustrated edition. Rodale Books; 2007.
27. Griffis ML: **Great American Bunion Derby.** Eakin Press;, 1 2003.
28. Lewis B: *Running the Trans America Footrace: Trials and Triumphs of Life on the Road.* 1 edition. Stackpole Books; 1994.

29. Shapiro JE: *Meditations from the Breakdown Lane: Running Across America* Houghton Mifflin Press; 1983.
30. Schulze I: *Transeuropalauf 2003. Lissabon - Moskau 5036 km in 64 Tagesetappen.* 1 edition. Engelsdorfer Verlagsgesellschaft; 2004.
31. Biermanski B: *Der härteste Lauf der Welt: In 64 Tagen von Lissabon nach Moskau (Trans Europa Lauf).* 1 edition. Books on Demand GmbH; 2005.
32. Schulze I: *TransEurope-FootRace 2009: Bari - Nordkap - 4.487,7 km in 64 Tagesetappen. Engelsdorfer Verlag* , 1 2010.
33. Secker R: *Running across countries* Create Space; 2009.
34. Knechtle B, Knechtle P, Schulze I, Kohler G: **Vitamins, minerals and race performance in ultra-endurance runners-Deutschlandlauf 2006.** *Asia Pac J Clin Nutr* 2008, **17**:194-198.
35. Knechtle B, Schulze I: **Nutritional behaviours in ultra-endurance runners-Deutschlandlauf 2006.** *Praxis (Bern 1994)* 2008, **97**:243-251.
36. Shellock FG, Deutsch AL, Mink JH, Kerr R: **Do asymptomatic marathon runners have an increased prevalence of meniscal abnormalities? An MR study of the knee in 23 volunteers.** *AJR Am J Roentgenol* 1991, **157**:1239-1241.
37. Shellock FG, Mink JH: **Knees of trained long-distance runners: MR imaging before and after competition.** *Radiology* 1991, **179**:63.
38. Hohmann E, Wörtler K, Imhoff A: **MR imaging of the hip and knee before and after marathon running.** *Am J Sports Med* 2004, **32**:55-9.
39. Schueller-Weidekamm C, Schueller G, Uffmann M, Bader TR: **Does marathon running cause acute lesions of the knee? Evaluation with magnetic resonance imaging.** *Eur Radiol* 2006, **16**:2179-2185.
40. Krampla W, Mayrhofer R, Malcher J, Kristen KH, Urban M, Hruby W: **MR imaging of the knee in marathon runners before and after competition.** *Skeletal Radiol* 2001, **30**:72-76.
41. Cymet TC, Sinkov V: **Does long-distance running cause osteoarthritis?** *J Am Osteopath Assoc* 2006, **106**:342-345.
42. Krampla WW, Newrkla SP, Kroener AH, Hruby WF: **Changes on magnetic resonance tomography in the knee joints of marathon runners: a 10-year longitudinal study.** *Skeletal Radiol* 2008, **37**:619-626.
43. Arokoski J, Kiviranta I, Jurvelin J, Tammi M, Helminen HJ: **Long-distance running causes site-dependent decrease of cartilage glycosaminoglycan content in the knee joints of beagle dogs.** *Arthritis Rheum* 1993, **36**:1451-1459.
44. Arokoski J, Jurvelin J, Kiviranta I, Tammi M, Helminen HJ: **Softening of the lateral condyle articular cartilage in the canine knee joint after long distance (up to 40 km/day) running training lasting one year.** *Int J Sports Med* 1994, **15**:254-260.
45. Arokoski JP, Hyttinen MM, Lapveteläinen T, Takács P, Kosztáczky B, Módis L, Kovanen V, Helminen H: **Decreased birefringence of the superficial zone collagen network in the canine knee (stifle) articular cartilage after long distance running training, detected by quantitative polarised light microscopy.** *Ann Rheum Dis* 1996, **55**:253-264.
46. Lacey RJ, Thomas E, Duncan RC, Peat G: **Gender difference in symptomatic radiographic knee osteoarthritis in the Knee Clinical Assessment–CAS(K): a prospective study in the general population.** *BMC Musculoskelet Disord* 2008, **9**:82.
47. Leyk D, Erley O, Gorges W, Ridder D, Rüther T, Wunderlich M, Sievert A, Essfeld D, Piekarski C, Erren T: **Performance, training and lifestyle parameters of marathon runners aged 20-80 years: results of the PACE-study.** *Int J Sports Med* 2009, **30**:360-365.
48. Bishop GW, Fallon KE: **Musculoskeletal injuries in a six-day track race: ultramarathoner's ankle.** *Clin J Sport Med* 1999, **9**:216-220.
49. Fallon KE: **Musculoskeletal injuries in the ultramarathon: the 1990 Westfield Sydney to Melbourne run.** *Br J Sports Med* 1996, **30**:319-323.
50. Fredericson M, Misra AK: **Epidemiology and aetiology of marathon running injuries.** *Sports Med* 2007, **37**:437-439.
51. Schueller-Weidekamm C: **Long-term success and risk for marathon runners.** *Radiologe* 2010, **50**:444-452.
52. Taunton JE, Ryan MB, Clement DB, McKenzie DC, Lloyd-Smith DR, Zumbo BD: **A retrospective case-control analysis of 2002 running injuries.** *Br J Sports Med* 2002, **36**:95-101.
53. Taunton JE, Ryan MB, Clement DB, McKenzie DC, Lloyd-Smith DR, Zumbo BD: **A prospective study of running injuries: the Vancouver Sun Run "In Training" clinics.** *Br J Sports Med* 2003, **37**:239-244.
54. Van Middelkoop M, Kolkman J, van Ochten J, Bierma-Zeinstra SM, Koes BW: **Course and predicting factors of lower-extremity injuries after running a marathon.** *Clin J Sport Med* 2007, **17**:25-30.
55. Johnell O, Rausing A, Wendeberg B, Westlin N: **Morphological bone changes in shin splints.** *Clin Orthop Relat Res* 1982, **167**:180-184.
56. Aoki Y, Yasuda K, Tohyama H, Ito H, Minami A: **Magnetic resonance imaging in stress fractures and shin splints.** *Clin Orthop Relat Res* 2004, **421**:260-267.
57. Wilder RP, Sethi S: **Overuse injuries: tendinopathies, stress fractures, compartment syndrome, and shin splints.** *Clin Sports Med* 2004, **23**:55-81.
58. Detmer DE: **Chronic shin splints: classification and management of medial tibial stress syndrome.** *Sports Med* 1986, **3**:436-446.
59. Batt ME: **Shin splints–a review of terminology.** *Clin J Sport Med* 1995, **5**:53-57.
60. Verleisdonk EJ, van Gils A, van der Werken C: **The diagnostic value of MRI scans for the diagnosis of chronic exertional compartment syndrome of the lower leg.** *Skeletal Radiol* 2001, **30**:321-325.
61. Bong MR, Polatsch DB, Jazrawi LM, Rokito AS: **Chronic exertional compartment syndrome: diagnosis and management.** *Bull Hosp Jt Dis* 2005, **62**:77-84.
62. Lee D, Armed Forces Health Surveillance Center (AFHSC): **Stress fractures, active component, U.S. Armed Forces, 2004-2010.** *MSMR* 2011, **18**:8-11.
63. Harrast MA, Colonno D: **Stress fractures in runners.** *Clin Sports Med* 2010, **29**:399-416.
64. Shellock FG, Morris E, Deutsch AL, Mink JH, Kerr R, Boden SD: **Hematopoietic bone marrow hyperplasia: high prevalence on MR images of the knee in asymptomatic marathon runners.** *AJR Am J Roentgenol* 1992, **158**:335-338.
65. Gondoh Y, Sensui H, Kinomura S, Fukuda H, Fujimoto T, Masud M, Nagamatsu T, Tamaki H, Takekura H: **Effects of aerobic exercise training on brain structure and psychological well-being in young adults.** *J Sports Med Phys Fitness* 2009, **49**:129-135.
66. Peters J, Dauvermann M, Mette C, Platen P, Franke J, Hinrichs T, Daum I: **Voxel-based morphometry reveals an association between aerobic capacity and grey matter density in the right anterior insula.** *Neuroscience* 2009, **163**:1102-1108.
67. Good CD, Johnsrude IS, Ashburner J, Henson RN, Friston KJ, Frackowiak RS: **A voxel-based morphometric study of ageing in 465 normal adult human brains.** *Neuroimage* 2001, **14**:21-36.
68. O'Brien JT, Paling S, Barber R, Williams ED, Ballard C, McKeith IG, Gholkar A, Crum WR, Rossor MN, Fox NC: **Progressive brain atrophy on serial MRI in dementia with Lewy bodies, AD, and vascular dementia.** *Neurology* 2001, **56**:1386-1388.
69. Fox NC, Crum WR, Scahill RI, Stevens JM, Janssen JC, Rossor MN: **Imaging of onset and progression of Alzheimer's disease with voxel-compression mapping of serial magnetic resonance images.** *Lancet* 2001, **358**:201-205.
70. Katzman DK, Lambe EK, Mikulis DJ, Ridgley JN, Goldbloom DS, Zipursky RB: **Cerebral gray matter and white matter volume deficits in adolescent girls with anorexia nervosa.** *J Pediatr* 1996, **129**:794-803.
71. Castro-Fornieles J, Bargalló N, Lázaro L, Andrés S, Falcon C, Plana MT, Junqué C: **A cross-sectional and follow-up voxel-based morphometric MRI study in adolescent anorexia nervosa.** *J Psychiatr Res* 2009, **43**:331-340.
72. Geibprasert S, Gallucci M, Krings T: **Alcohol-induced changes in the brain as assessed by MRI and CT.** *Eur Radiol* 2010, **20**:1492-1501.
73. Gunston GD, Burkimsher D, Malan H, Sive AA: **Reversible cerebral shrinkage in kwashiorkor: an MRI study.** *Arch Dis Child* 1992, **67**:1030-1032.
74. Golden NH, Ashtari M, Kohn MR, Patel M, Jacobson MS, Fletcher A, Shenker IR: **Reversibility of cerebral ventricular enlargement in anorexia nervosa, demonstrated by quantitative magnetic resonance imaging.** *J Pediatr* 1996, **128**:296-301.
75. Knudsen L, Drummond PD: **Cold-induced limb pain decreases sensitivity to pressure-pain sensations in the ipsilateral forehead.** *Eur J Pain* 2009, **13**:1023-1029.
76. Van den Eynde F, Treasure J: **Neuroimaging in eating disorders and obesity: implications for research.** *Child Adolesc Psychiatr Clin N Am* 2009, **18**:95-115.
77. Kraemer WJ, Fragala MS, Watson G, Volek JS, Rubin MR, French DN, Maresh CM, Vingren JL, Hatfield DL, Spiering BA, Yu-Ho J, Hughes SL, Case HS, Stuempfle KJ, Lehmann DR, Bailey S, Evans DS: **Hormonal responses to a 160-km race across frozen Alaska.** *Br J Sports Med* 2008, **42**:116-120.
78. Agawa H, Yamada N, Enomoto Y, Suzuki H, Hosono A, Arakawa K, Ghadimi R, Miyata M, Maeda K, Shibata K, Tokudome M, Goto C,

Tokudome Y, Hoshino H, Imaeda N, Marumoto M, Suzuki S, Kobayashi M, Tokudome S: **Changes of mental stress biomarkers in ultramarathon.** *Int J Sports Med* 2008, **29**:867-871.
79. Hew-Butler T, Noakes TD, Soldin SJ, Verbalis JG: **Acute changes in endocrine and fluid balance markers during high-intensity, steady-state, and prolonged endurance running: unexpected increases in oxytocin and brain natriuretic peptide during exercise.** *Eur J Endocrinol* 2008, **159**:729-737.
80. Lehmann M, Huonker M, Dimeo F, Heinz N, Gastmann U, Treis N, Steinacker JM, Keul J, Kajewski R, Häussinger D: **Serum amino acid concentrations in nine athletes before and after the 1993 Colmar ultra triathlon.** *Int J Sports Med* 1995, **16**:155-159.
81. Pickering A, Carter J, Hanning I, Townend W: **Emergency department measurement of urinary S100B in children following head injury: can extracranial injury confound findings?** *Emerg Med J* 2008, **25**:88-89.
82. Gazzolo D, Frigiola A, Bashir M, Iskander I, Mufeed H, Aboulgar H, Venturini P, Marras M, Serra G, Frulio R, Michetti F, Petraglia F, Abella R, Florio P: **Diagnostic accuracy of S100B urinary testing at birth in full-term asphyxiated newborns to predict neonatal death.** *PLoS One* 2009, **4**: e4298.
83. Jäncke L, Koeneke S, Hoppe A, Rominger C, Hänggi J: **The architecture of the golfer's brain.** *PLoS One* 2009, **4**:e4785.
84. Stuempfle KJ, Lehmann DR, Case HS, Bailey S, Hughes SL, McKenzie J, Evans D: **Hyponatremia in a cold weather ultraendurance race.** *Alaska Med* 2002, **44**:51-55.
85. Hew TD, Chorley JN, Cianca JC, Divine JG: **The incidence, risk factors, and clinical manifestations of hyponatremia in marathon runners.** *Clin J Sport Med* 2003, **13**:41-47.
86. Almond CS, Shin AY, Fortescue EB, Mannix RC, Wypij D, Binstadt BA, Duncan CN, Olson DP, Salerno AE, Newburger JW, Greenes DS: **Hyponatremia among runners in the Boston Marathon.** *N Engl J Med* 2005, **352**:1550-1556.
87. Noakes TD, Sharwood K, Speedy D, Hew T, Reid S, Dugas J, Almond C, Wharam P, Weschler L: **Three independent biological mechanisms cause exercise-associated hyponatremia: evidence from 2,135 weighed competitive athletic performances.** *Proc Natl Acad Sci USA* 2005, **102**:18550-18555.
88. Urhausen A, Scharhag J, Herrmann M, Kindermann W: **Clinical significance of increased cardiac troponins T and I in participants of ultra-endurance events.** *Am J Cardiol* 2004, **94**:696-698.
89. Neilan TG, Januzzi JL, Lee-Lewandrowski E, Ton-Nu TT, Yoerger DM, Jassal DS, Lewandrowski KB, Siegel AJ, Marshall JE, Douglas PS, Lawlor D, Picard MH, Wood MJ: **Myocardial injury and ventricular dysfunction related to training levels among nonelite participants in the Boston marathon.** *Circulation* 2006, **114**:2325-2333.
90. O'Connor DT, Frigon RP: **Chromogranin A, the major catecholamine storage vesicle soluble protein. Multiple size forms, subcellular storage, and regional distribution in chromaffin and nervous tissue elucidated by radioimmunoassay.** *J Biol Chem* 1984, **259**:3237-3247.
91. Mousavi N, Czarnecki A, Kumar K, Fallah-Rad N, Lytwyn M, Han SY, Francis A, Walker JR, Kirkpatrick ID, Neilan TG, Sharma S, Jassal DS: **Relation of biomarkers and cardiac magnetic resonance imaging after marathon running.** *Am J Cardiol* 2009, **103**:1467-1472.
92. Trivax JE, Franklin BA, Goldstein JA, Chinnaiyan KM, Gallagher MJ, deJong AT, Colar JM, Haines DE, McCullough PA: **Acute cardiac effects of marathon running.** *J Appl Physiol* 2010, **108**:1148-1153.
93. Hanssen H, Keithahn A, Hertel G, Drexel V, Stern H, Schuster T, Lorang D, Beer AJ, Schmidt-Trucksäss A, Nickel T, Weis M, Botnar R, Schwaiger M, Halle M: **Magnetic resonance imaging of myocardial injury and ventricular torsion after marathon running.** *Clin Sci (Lond)* 2011, **120**:143-152.
94. Scharhag J, Herrmann M, Urhausen A, Haschke M, Herrmann W, Kindermann W: **Independent elevations of N-terminal pro-brain natriuretic peptide and cardiac troponins in endurance athletes after prolonged strenuous exercise.** *Am Heart J* 2005, **150**:1128-1134.
95. Scharhag J, George K, Shave R, Urhausen A, Kindermann W: **Exercise-associated increases in cardiac biomarkers.** *Med Sci Sports Exerc* 2008, **40**:1408-1415.
96. Montgomery HE, Clarkson P, Dollery CM, Prasad K, Losi MA, Hemingway H, Statters D, Jubb M, Girvain M, Varnava A, World M, Deanfield J, Talmud P, McEwan JR, McKenna WJ, Humphries S: **Association of angiotensin-converting enzyme gene I/D polymorphism with change in left ventricular mass in response to physical training.** *Circulation* 1997, **96**:741-747.
97. Morganroth J, Henry WL, Maron RJ, Clark CE, Epstein SE: **Idiopathic left ventricular hypertrophy.** *N Engl J Med* 1974, **290**:1047-1050.
98. Morganroth J, Maron BJ, Henry WL, Epstein SE: **Comparative left ventricular dimensions in trained athletes.** *Ann Intern Med* 1975, **82**:521-524.
99. Naylor LH, George K, O'Driscoll G, Green DJ: **The athlete's heart: a contemporary appraisal of the 'Morganroth hypothesis'.** *Sports Med* 2008, **38**:69-90.
100. Schmidt-Trucksäss A, Schmid A, Brunner C, Scherer N, Zäch G, Keul J, Huonker M: **Arterial properties of the carotid and femoral artery in endurance-trained and paraplegic subjects.** *J Appl Physiol* 2000, **89**:1956-1963.
101. Kasikcioglu E, Oflaz H, Kasikcioglu HA, Kayserilioglu A, Umman S, Meric M: **Endothelial flow-mediated dilatation and exercise capacity in highly trained endurance athletes.** *Tohoku J Exp Med* 2005, **205**:45-51.
102. Petersen SE, Wiesmann F, Hudsmith LE, Robson MD, Francis JM, Selvanayagam JB, Neubauer S, Channon KM: **Functional and structural vascular remodeling in elite rowers assessed by cardiovascular magnetic resonance.** *J Am Coll Cardiol* 2006, **48**:790-797.
103. Naylor LH, O'Driscoll G, Fitzsimons M, Arnolda LF, Green DJ: **Effects of training resumption on conduit arterial diameter in elite rowers.** *Med Sci Sports Exerc* 2006, **38**:86-92.
104. Raschka C, Plath M, Cerull R, Bernhard W, Jung K, Leitzmann C: **The body muscle compartment and its relationship to food absorption and blood chemistry during an extreme endurance performance.** *Z Ernährungswiss* 1991, **30**:276-288.
105. Raschka C, Plath M: **Body fat compartment and its relationship to food intake and clinical chemical parameters during extreme endurance performance.** *Schweiz Z Sportmed* 1992, **40**:13-25.
106. Höchli D, Schneiter T, Ferretti G, Howald H, Claassen H, Moia C, Atchou G, Belleri M, Veicsteinas A, Hoppeler H: **Loss of muscle oxidative capacity after an extreme endurance run: the Paris-Dakar Foot-Race.** *Int J Sports Med* 1995, **16**:343-346.
107. Helge JW, Lundby C, Christensen DL, Langfort J, Messonnier L, Zacho M, Andersen JL, Saltin B: **Skiing across the Greenland icecap: divergent effects on limb muscle adaptations and substrate oxidation.** *J Exp Biol* 2003, **206**:1075-1083.
108. Frykman PN, Harman EA, Opstad PK, Hoyt RW, DeLany JP, Friedl KE: **Effects of a 3-month endurance event on physical performance and body composition: the G2 trans-Greenland expedition.** *Wilderness Environ Med* 2003, **14**:240-248.
109. Bircher S, Enggist A, Jehle T: **Effects of an extreme endurance race on energy balance and body composition: a case study.** *J Sports Sci Med* 2006, **5**:154-162.
110. Nagel D, Seiler D, Franz H, Leitzmann C, Jung K: **Effects of an ultra-long-distance (1000 km) race on lipid metabolism.** *Eur J Appl Physiol* 1989, **59**:16-20.
111. Dressendorfer RH, Wade CE: **Effects of a 15-d race on plasma steroid levels and leg muscle fitness in runners.** *Med Sci Sports Exerc* 1991, **23**:954-958.
112. Väänänen II, Vihko V: **Physiological and psychological responses to 100 km crosscountry skiing during 2 days.** *J Sports Med Phys Fitness* 2005, **45**:301-305.
113. Knechtle B, Salas OF, Andonie JL, Kohler G: **Effect of a multistage ultra-endurance triathlon on body composition: World Challenge Deca Iron Triathlon 2006.** *Br J Sports Med* 2008, **42**:121-125.
114. Reynolds RD, Lickteig JA, Deuster PA, Howard MP, Conway JM, Pietersma A, deStoppelaar J, Deurenberg P: **Energy metabolism increases and regional body fat decreases while regional muscle mass is spared in humans climbing Mt. Everest.** *J Nutr* 1999, **129**:1307-1314.
115. Lehmann M, Huonker M, Dimeo F: **Serum amino acid concentrations in nine athletes before and after the 1993 Colmar Ultra Triathlon.** *Int J Sports Med* 1995, **16**:155-159.
116. Paley D, Herzenberg JE, Tetsworth K, McKie J, Bhave A: **Deformity planning for frontal and sagittal plane corrective osteotomies.** *Orthop Clin North Am* 1994, **25**:425-465.
117. Waidelich HA, Strecker W, Schneider E: **Computed tomographic torsion-angle and length measurement of the lower extremity. The methods, normal values and radiation load.** *Rofo* 1992, **157**:245-251.

118. Blustein SM, D'Amico JC: **Limb length discrepancy. Identification, clinical significance, and management.** *J Am Podiatr Med Assoc* 1985, **75**:200-206.
119. Strecker W, Keppler P, Gebhard F, Kinzl L: **Length and torsion of the lower limb.** *J Bone Joint Surg Br* 1997, **79**:1019-1023.
120. Keppler P, Strecker W, Kinzl L: **Analysis of leg geometry–standard techniques and normal values.** *Chirurg* 1998, **69**:1141-1152.
121. Keppler P: **Normwerte des Beines. 8. Kurs zur Analyse und Korrektur von Beindeformitäten.** *Schloss Reisensburg, Günzburg, Germany* 2005, **03**:16-19.
122. Keppler P, Kinzl L: **Diagnostik der posttraumatischen Beindeformitäten.** *Trauma Berufskrankh* 2006, **8(Suppl 3)**:303-316.
123. Nagoshi CT, Waler D, Muntaner C, Haertzen CA: **Validation of the Tridimensional Personality Questionnaire in a sample of male drug users.** *Personality and Individual Differences* 1992, **13**:401-409.
124. Hansenne M, Delhez M, Cloninger CR: **Psychometric properties of the temperament and character inventory-revised (TCI-R) in a Belgian sample.** *J Pers Assess* 2005, **85**:40-49.
125. Schwarzer R, Jerusalem M: **Generalized Self-Efficacy scale.** In *Measures in Health Psychology: A User's Portfolio. Causal and Control Beliefs.* Edited by: Weinman J, Wright S, Johnston M. Windsor; 1995:35-37.
126. Luszczynska A, Scholz U, Schwarzer R: **The general self-efficacy scale: multicultural validation studies.** *J Psychol* 2005, **139**:439-457.
127. Mamisch TC, Trattnig S, Quirbach S, Marlovits S, White LM, Welsch GH: **Quantitative T2 mapping of knee cartilage: differentiation of healthy control cartilage and cartilage repair tissue in the knee with unloading–initial results.** *Radiology* 2010, **254**:818-826.
128. Welsch GH, Trattnig S, Hughes T, Quirbach S, Olk A, Blanke M, Marlovits S, Mamisch TC: **T2 and T2* mapping in patients after matrix-associated autologous chondrocyte transplantation: initial results on clinical use with 3.0-Tesla MRI.** *Eur Radiol* 2010, **20**:1515-1523.
129. Apprich S, Welsch GH, Mamisch TC, Szomolanyi P, Mayerhoefer M, Pinker K, Trattnig S: **Detection of degenerative cartilage disease: comparison of high-resolution morphological MR and quantitative T2 mapping at 3.0 Tesla.** *Osteoarthritis Cartilage* 2010, **18**:1211-1217.
130. Schueller-Weidekamm C, Schueller G, Uffmann M, Bader T: **Incidence of chronic knee lesions in long-distance runners based on training level: findings at MRI.** *Eur J Radiol* 2006, **58**:286-293.
131. Schmitt H, Rohs C, Schneider S, Clarius M: **Is competitive running associated with osteoarthritis of the hip or the knee?** *Orthopade* 2006, **35**:1087-1092.
132. Major NM, Helms CA: **Sacral stress fractures in long-distance runners.** *AJR Am J Roentgenol* 2000, **174**:727-729.
133. Shah MK, Stewart GW: **Sacral stress fractures: an unusual cause of low back pain in an athlete.** *Spine* 2002, **27**:E104-108.
134. Alsobrook J, Simons SM: **Sacral stress fracture in a marathon runner.** *Curr Sports Med Rep* 2007, **6**:39-42.
135. Fredenicson M, Bergman AG, Hoffman KL, Dillingham MS: **Tibial stress reaction in runners: correlation of clinical symptoms and scintigraphy with a new magnetic resonance imaging grading system.** *Am Sports Med* 1995, **23**:472-481.
136. Bergman AG, Fredericson M: **MR imaging of stress reactions, muscle injuries, and other overuse injuries in runners.** *Magn Reson Imaging Clin N Am* 1999, **7**:151-174, ix.
137. Bolster BD Jr, Atalar E, Hardy CJ, McVeigh ER: **Accuracy of arterial pulse-wave velocity measurement using MR.** *J Magn Reson Imaging* 1998, **8**:878-888.
138. Machann J, Thamer C, Schnoedt B, Haap M, Haring HU, Claussen CD, Stumvoll M, Fritsche A, Schick F: **Standardized assessment of whole body adipose tissue topography by MRI.** *J Magn Reson Imaging* 2005, **21**:455-462.
139. Würslin C, Machann J, Rempp H, Claussen C, Yang B, Schick F: **Topography mapping of whole body adipose tissue using a fully automated and standardized procedure.** *J Magn Reson Imaging* 2010, **31**:430-439.
140. Brechtel K, Niess AM, Machann J, Rett K, Schick F, Claussen CD, Dickhuth HH, Haering HU, Jacob S: **Utilisation of intramyocellular lipids (IMCLs) during exercise as assessed by proton magnetic resonance spectroscopy (1H-MRS).** *Horm Metab Res* 2001, **33**:63 66.
141. Jebb SA, Cole TJ, Doman D, Murgatroyd PR, Prentice AM: **Evaluation of the novel Tanita body-fat analyser to measure body composition by comparison with a four-compartment model.** *Br J Nutr* 2000, **83**:115-122.
142. Ball SD, Altena TS, Swan PD: **Comparison of anthropometry to DXA: a new prediction equation for men.** *Eur J Clin Nutr* 2004, **58**:1525-1531.
143. Lee RC, Wang Z, Heo M, Ross R, Janssen I, Heymsfield SB: **Total-body skeletal muscle mass: development and cross-validation of anthropometric prediction models.** *Am J Clin Nutr* 2000, **72**:796-803.
144. Roach KE, Miles TP: **Normal hip and knee active range of motion: the relationship to age.** *Phys Ther* 1991, **71**:656-665.
145. Knechtle B, Knechtle P, Andonie JL, Kohler G: **Influence of anthropometry on race performance in extreme endurance triathletes: World Challenge Deca Iron Triathlon 2006.** *Br J Sports Med* 2007, **41**:644-648.
146. Marti B, Abelin T, Minder CE: **Relationship of training and life-style to 16-km running time of 4000 joggers. The '84 Berne "Grand-Prix" Study.** *Int J Sports Med* 1988, **9**:85-91.
147. Marti B, Vader JP, Minder CE, Abelin T: **On the epidemiology of running injuries. The 1984 Bern Grand-Prix study.** *Am J Sports Med* 1988, **16**:285-294.
148. Macera CA, Pate RR, Woods J, Davis DR, Jackson KL: **Postrace morbidity among runners.** *Am J Prev Med* 1991, **7**:194-198.
149. Pate RR, Macera CA, Bailey SP, Bartoli WP, Powell KE: **Physiological, anthropometric, and training correlates of running economy.** *Med Sci Sports Exerc* 1992, **24**:1128-1133.
150. Saunders PU, Pyne DB, Telford RD, Hawley JA: **Factors affecting running economy in trained distance runners.** *Sports Med* 2004, **34**:465-485.
151. Wilder RP, Sethi S: **Overuse injuries: tendinopathies, stress fractures, compartment syndrome, and shin splints.** *Clin Sports Med* 2004, **23**:55-81.
152. Van Middelkoop M, Kolkman J, Van Ochten J, Bierma-Zeinstra SM, Koes BW: **Risk factors for lower extremity injuries among male marathon runners.** *Scand J Med Sci Sports* 2008, **18**:691-697.
153. Wen DY, Puffer JC, Schmalzried TP: **Injuries in runners: a prospective study of alignment.** *Clin J Sport Med* 1998, **8**:187-194.
154. Satterthwaite P, Norton R, Larmer P, Robinson E: **Risk factors for injuries and other health problems sustained in a marathon.** *Br J Sports Med* 1999, **33**:22-26.
155. Taunton JE, Ryan MB, Clement DB, McKenzie DC, Lloyd-Smith DR, Zumbo BD: **A retrospective case-control analysis of 2002 running injuries.** *Br J Sports Med* 2002, **36**:95-101.
156. Fredericson M, Misra AK: **Epidemiology and aetiology of marathon running injuries.** *Sports Med* 2007, **37**:437-439.
157. Mosher TJ, Liu Y, Torok CM: **Functional cartilage MRI T2 mapping: evaluating the effect of age and training on knee cartilage response to running.** *Osteoarthritis Cartilage* 2010, **18**:358-364.
158. Neidhart M, Müller-Ladner U, Frey W, Bosserhoff AK, Colombani PC, Frey-Rindova P, Hummel KM, Gay RE, Häuselmann H, Gay S: **Increased serum levels of non-collagenous matrix proteins (cartilage oligomeric matrix protein and melanoma inhibitory activity) in marathon runners.** *Osteoarthritis Cartilage* 2000, **8**:222-229.
159. Kim HJ, Lee YH, Kim CK: **Biomarkers of muscle and cartilage damage and inflammation during a 200 km run.** *Eur J Appl Physiol* 2007, **99**:443-447.
160. Kim HJ, Lee YH, Kim CK: **Changes in serum cartilage oligomeric matrix protein (COMP), plasma CPK and plasma hs-CRP in relation to running distance in a marathon (42.195 km) and an ultra-marathon (200 km) race.** *Eur J Appl Physiol* 2009, **105**:765-770.
161. Addison S, Coleman RE, Feng S, McDaniel G, Kraus VB: **Whole-body bone scintigraphy provides a measure of the total-body burden of osteoarthritis for the purpose of systemic biomarker validation.** *Arthritis Rheum* 2009, **60**:3366-3373.
162. Liphardt AM, Mündermann A, Koo S, Bäcker N, Andriacchi TP, Zange J, Mester J, Heer M: **Vibration training intervention to maintain cartilage thickness and serum concentrations of cartilage oligometric matrix protein (COMP) during immobilization.** *Osteoarthritis Cartilage* 2009, **17**:1598-1603.
163. Berry PA, Maciewicz RA, Wluka AE, Downey-Jones MD, Forbes A, Hellawell CJ, Cicuttini FM: **Relationship of serum markers of cartilage metabolism to imaging and clinical outcome measures of knee joint structure.** *Ann Rheum Dis* 2010, **69**:1816-1822.
164. Niehoff A, Kersting UG, Helling S, Dargel J, Maurer J, Thevis M, Brüggemann GP: **Different mechanical loading protocols influence serum cartilage oligomeric matrix protein levels in young healthy humans.** *Eur J Appl Physiol* 2010, **110**:651-657.
165. Pelletier JP, Raynauld JP, Caron J, Mineau F, Abram F, Dorais M, Haraoui B, Choquette D, Martel-Pelletier J: **Decrease in serum level of matrix metalloproteinases is predictive of the disease-modifying effect of**

osteoarthritis drugs assessed by quantitative MRI in patients with knee osteoarthritis. *Ann Rheum Dis* 2010, **69**:2118-2124.

166. Knechtle B, Knechtle P, Rosemann T: Upper body skinfold thickness is related to race performance in male Ironman triathletes. *Int J Sports Med* 201, **32**:20-27.
167. al'Absi M, Petersen KL, Wittmers LE: Adrenocortical and hemodynamic predictors of pain perception in men and women. *Pain* 2002, **96**:197-204.
168. Thamer C, Machann J, Bachmann O, Haap M, Dahl D, Wietek B, Tschritter O, Niess A, Brechtel K, Fritsche A, Claussen C, Jacob S, Schick F, Häring HU, Stumvoll M: Intramyocellular lipids: anthropometric determinants and relationships with maximal aerobic capacity and insulin sensitivity. *J Clin Endocrinol Metab* 2003, **88**:1785-1791.
169. Machann J, Etzel M, Thamer C, Haring HU, Claussen CD, Fritsche A, Schick F: Morning to evening changes of intramyocellular lipid content in dependence on nutrition and physical activity during one single day: a volume selective 1H-MRS study. *MAGMA* 2011, **24**:29-33.

9

Characteristics, changes and influence of body composition during a 4486 km transcontinental ultramarathon: results from the Transeurope Footrace mobile whole body MRI-project

Uwe HW Schütz[1,2*], Christian Billich[1], Kathrin König[3], Christian Würslin[3], Heike Wiedelbach[1], Hans-Jürgen Brambs[1] and Jürgen Machann[3,4]

Abstract

Background: Almost nothing is known about the medical aspects of runners doing a transcontinental ultramarathon over several weeks. The results of differentiated measurements of changes in body composition during the Transeurope Footrace 2009 using a mobile whole body magnetic resonance (MR) imager are presented and the proposed influence of visceral and somatic adipose and lean tissue distribution on performance tested.

Methods: 22 participants were randomly selected for the repeated MR measurements (intervals: 800 km) with a 1.5 Tesla MR scanner mounted on a mobile unit during the 64-stage 4,486 km ultramarathon. A standardized and validated MRI protocol was used: T1 weighted turbo spin echo sequence, echo time 12 ms, repetition time 490 ms, slice thickness 10 mm, slice distance 10 mm (breath holding examinations). For topographic tissue segmentation and mapping a modified fuzzy c-means algorithm was used. A semi-automatic post-processing of whole body MRI data sets allows reliable analysis of the following body tissue compartments: Total body volume (TV), total somatic (TSV) and total visceral volume (TVV), total adipose (TAT) and total lean tissue (TLT), somatic (SLT) and visceral lean tissue (VLT), somatic (SAT) and visceral adipose tissue (VAT) and somatic adipose soft tissue (SAST). Specific volume changes were tested on significance. Tests on difference and relationship regarding prerace and race performance and non-finishing were done using statistical software SPSS.

(Continued on next page)

* Correspondence: uwe.schuetz@rocketmail.com
[1]Department of Diagnostic and Interventional Radiology, University Hospital of Ulm, Albert-Einstein-Allee 23, 89081, Ulm, Germany
[2]Outpatient Rehabilitation Centre at University Hospital of Ulm, Pfarrer-Weiß-Weg 10, 89073, Ulm, Germany
Full list of author information is available at the end of the article

(Continued from previous page)

Results: Total, somatic and visceral volumes showed a significant decrease throughout the race. Adipose tissue showed a significant decrease compared to the start at all measurement times for TAT, SAST and VAT. Lean adipose tissues decreased until the end of the race, but not significantly. The mean relative volume changes of the different tissue compartments at the last measurement compared to the start were: TV −9.5% (SE 1.5%), TSV −9.4% (SE 1.5%), TVV −10.0% (SE 1.4%), TAT −41.3% (SE 2.3%), SAST −48.7% (SE 2.8%), VAT −64.5% (SE 4.6%), intraabdominal adipose tissue (IAAT) −67.3% (SE 4.3%), mediastinal adopose tissue (MAT) −41.5% (SE 7.1%), TLT −1.2% (SE 1.0%), SLT −1.4% (SE 1.1%). Before the start and during the early phase of the Transeurope Footrace 2009, the non-finisher group had a significantly higher percentage volume of TVV, TAT, SAST and VAT compared to the finisher group. VAT correlates significantly with prerace training volume and intensity one year before the race and with 50 km- and 24 hour-race records. Neither prerace body composition nor specific tissue compartment volume changes showed a significant relationship to performance in the last two thirds of the Transeurope Footrace 2009.

Conclusions: With this mobile MRI field study the complex changes in body composition during a multistage ultramarathon could be demonstrated in detail in a new and differentiated way. Participants lost more than half of their adipose tissue. Even lean tissue volume (mainly skeletal muscle tissue) decreased due to the unpreventable chronic negative energy balance during the race. VAT has the fastest and highest decrease compared to SAST and lean tissue compartments during the race. It seems to be the most sensitive morphometric parameter regarding the risk of non-finishing a transcontinental footrace and shows a direct relationship to prerace-performance. However, body volume or body mass and, therefore, fat volume has no correlation with total race performances of ultra-athletes finishing a 4,500 km multistage race.

Keywords: Magnetic resonance imaging, MRI, Body mass, Body volume, Body composition, Running, Marathon, Ultramarathon, Performance, Adipose tissue, Body fat, Lean tissue, Visceral, Somatic, Topography, Segmentation, Mapping

Background

With the worldwide growing number of people running, endurance sports have experienced differentiation into multiple (sub-) disciplines in the last decades. Concerning distance running, the ultramarathon (UM) seems to be the greatest challenge in endurance running. The German Ultramarathon Association (DUV) defines footraces of 50 km or longer as UM. However, as in every field of human physical activities, some people try to push themselves to the limits and beyond. For these ultra-athletes a multistage ultramarathon (MSUM) is the ultimate test of endurance performance. Sometimes, the worldwide small group of ultra-endurance runners meet with each other trying to achieve the impossible: finishing a multistage transcontinental footrace over thousands of kilometers. These most extreme multistage endurance competitions in the world take the runner to a different level, where nutrition, sleep, energy and psychological states have to be carefully managed. Besides a few case reports, almost nothing has been reported about the medical aspects of runners doing a transcontinental extended MSUM over several weeks [1]. Until now, there have been no series published regarding UM running over more than 1,500 km. However, prolonged ultra-endurance footraces offer the best opportunity to study physical adaptations and the relationships of the physiological parameters in endurance athletes.

The Transeurope Footrace Project (TEFR-project) [2] is the first observational cohort field study of a transcontinental MSUM, the Transeurope Footrace 2009 (TEFR09) [3]. A unique group of 67 endurance runners (mean age 50.7 years, standard deviation (SD) 10.5 years, range 26 to 74 years, m 56 (83.6%)) met the challenge and tried to cross six countries while running 4,486 km in 64 stages (mean 70.1 km, min 44 km, max 95.1 km) without any day of rest [4]. The central aspect of the TEFR-project was the use of a mobile magnetic resonance imaging (MRI) scanner accompanying the TEFR09 participants on a truck trailer over 64 days under their 'natural' conditions [2].

One focus of this presentation is on the descriptive presentation of characteristics and changes in body composition during TEFR09 in a new way, differentiating between somatic and visceral and segmental volumes of defined fat and lean tissue compartments measured by continuous mobile whole body MRI. In addition, possible associations of body volume composition and prerace and race performance were analyzed to test the following hypotheses: it is hypothesized, that prerace endurance running performance is related to specific body fat and lean tissue composition in ultra-athletes. Secondarily, it is supposed, that although the running distance of a transcontinental UM cannot be trained for concerning the running volume (km), participants need specific prerace performance skills and fat and lean tissue volume distribution, if they want to finish such a race. Due to the expected huge energy burden a transcontinental footrace without any day of rest implies, another assumption is that it is mandatory for every participant to lose body mass and total body volume (TV) due to massive adipose tissue decrease and more or less lean tissue catabolism. At least, with the continuous differentiated measurement of body tissue compartments throughout the entire TEFR09, it should be shown indirectly, that although the participants are preselected in regard to their ultra endurance running expertise, they will develop further economical adaptations as the 4,500 km race progresses.

Methods

Subjects

Every TEFR09 participant was asked to join the TEFR-project, which was approved by the local ethics committee of the University Hospital of Ulm (UHU, No.: 270/08-UBB/se) in accordance with the Declaration of Helsinki, regarding the study design, risk management plan and individual protocols [2]. Forty-four participants (67%) were recruited for the study and gave their informed written consent. Every second subject (n = 22, 20 men, mean age 49.1 years, SD 11.5 yrs., range 27 to 69 years) was randomly selected for whole body MRI measurements regarding body composition. According to project protocol these subjects underwent a whole body MRI before the start at Bari (South Italy) and during the race in measurement intervals of approximately 800 km. Due to various reasons, deviations from planned measurement intervals (MI: t0 to t6) occurred. The mean deviation of actual from planned measurement intervals was 187.8 km (SD = 141.3 km) [2].

Prerace performance

Before the start of TEFR09 all subjects filled out specific questionnaires concerning their prerace experience in endurance running. This history includes the years of regular endurance running (PRY), the number of finished (n_F) marathons (M), UM and MSUM, and the prerace records (PRR) for marathon and specific UM (50 km, 100 km, 6 hours, 12 hours, 24 hours) races within the last decade before TEFR. It also includes the extent of prerace training (PRT) 16 months before TEFR09: training volume (Vol: km/week), training duration (Time: hours/week) and the training intensity (Int: km/hour). The self-disclosures about n_F and PRR were cross checked with the archive of the DUV and discrepancies were clarified. However, for PRT and PRY we had to rely solely on the self-disclosures; these could not be compared with any official lists.

Body composition analysis

Different techniques for quantification of body fat are described and more or less commonly used in the literature:. *In vivo*, two-compartment model methods are the hydrodensitometry [5] and the body fat percentage and muscle mass calculation from anthropometric data such as skinfold thickness (SF) calipometry and/or segmental body circumferences (CF) [6-8]. Three-compartment methods are the bioelectrical impedance analysis (BIA) [9] and dual-energy X-ray absorptiometry (DEXA) [10]. Using these methods, indirect measurement, approximated calculation or simple estimation of total, regional or local adipose or lean tissue [11-14] is possible. In contrast, a whole body MRI assessment of adipose tissue as a multi-compartment method is the only method enabling exact topographic tissue mapping and tissue segmentation. Therefore, it is the gold standard imaging tool for differentiated assessment of adipose or lean tissue distribution in the body [15-18].

Subjects who finished TEFR09 had whole body MRI six times during TEFR09 (seven measurements in total). Measurement of body mass (BM) was done at the same time as MRI and every fourth day: BIA balance Tanita BC-545 to the nearest 0.1 kg (Tanita, Arlington Heights, IL, U.S.A.). Body height was measured with a wall-mounted stadiometer (to the nearest 5 mm, standing barefoot) and body mass index (BMI) was calculated.

Mobile whole body MRI

For whole body magnetic resonance (MR) measurements a 1.5 Tesla MRI scanner (Magnetom Avantot™, Siemens Ltd., Erlangen, Germany) mounted on a mobile unit (MRI-Trailer, SMIT Mobile Equipment B.V., Great Britain) was used. The total 45 tonnes of equipment (MRI-trailer, truck tractor, external 105KVA diesel-generator, and material van) was built up and taken down daily at each stopover of TEFR09, requiring daily checks and support of all technical systems [2].

Several MRI techniques have been described for the measurement and quantification of body fat composition: T1-weighted imaging by spin-echo or gradient-echo techniques [14,16,19], chemical shift selective (CHESS) imaging [20-22], or DIXON techniques [23,24]. All of them have specific advantages and disadvantages, the details of which are beyond the scope of this article. For analysis of body composition a standardized assessment of whole body adipose tissue measurement based on a MRI protocol according to Machann *et al.* [25] was used. A two-dimensional T1-weighted turbo spin echo sequence with an echo train length of seven was applied (Siemens Ltd.). Measurement parameters were set to be: flip angle 180°, echo time 12 ms, repetition time 490 ms, slice thickness 10 mm, slice distance 10 mm, 5 slices per sequence, field of view 1,991 cm^2, matrix size 256 × 196 was recorded in a measuring time of 12 seconds (allowing breath holding examinations in the trunk area), bandwidth 120 Hz/pixel. A total of 90 to 120 images were generated, depending on the size of the subject. Total examination time was between 20 and 25 minutes including one rearrangement of prone positioned subject (head forward and arms extended for upper body, feet forward for lower body), as total table feed of the MR-imager is limited to 110 cm. In order to guarantee identical slice positions after repositioning, the subjects were marked at the iliac crest. A body coil was used.

Image post-processing

For topographic tissue segmentation and mapping of the athletes body a fuzzy c-means algorithm according to Würslin *et al.* [26] was used. This approach provides a simple and time-saving strategy for assessment and standardization of individual adipose tissue distribution in the entire body. Due to standardization using defined internal markers, it enables a completely automatic, reliable analysis and creation of adipose tissue distribution profiles of the whole body from the multislice MR datasets and makes a reliable comparison of subjects with different body structure possible [25,26].

The signal of intestinal content with a short T1can be interpreted as visceral adipose tissue (VAT) in the absence of intraluminal gastroenteric nutrition fat (INF). If the scanned subject is in a non-fasting condition, the visceral T1 signal occurs from both, VAT and INF. Reliability (mean absolute deviation of three repeated measurements) is noted with 3.08% for total volume (TV), 1.48% for total adipose tissue (TAT) and 1.13% for visceral adipose tissue (VAT) [26].

Due to their immense mental and physical stress caused by the daily ultra-endurance burden, the runners' biggest fear was losing too much energy over the course of TEFR09. Their primary effort after stage finishing was to get as much nutrition and calories as possible before falling asleep. Therefore, it was not always possible to ensure fasting conditions of the subjects for mobile MRI measurements. Some subjects were motivated enough to do the MR examination directly after the daily stage before eating in a fasting but exhausted condition, so they sometimes were not able to lie absolutely still on the MR table and follow the breath commands exactly. These specific circumstances resulted in the image post-processing analysis being less automated than that mentioned by Machann and Würslin [25,26]: Movement artifacts had to be cleared manually more often before automatic post-processing. Compared to normal or overweight patients, in thin and lean bodies the amount of adipose bone marrow (ABM) and INF is more relevant in relation to whole body adipose and lean tissue. At the start of TEFR09, ABM and INF together accounted for 13.2% of total adipose tissue. Due to the continuous loss of adipose body tissue, this ratio rises up to 28.2% until the end of the race. For visceral adipose tissue, INF rose from 3% at the start up to 65.4% at the end of TEFR09. Therefore, a manual separation of ABM (Figure 1) and INF (Figure 2) was done on all MR slices of the subjects. Looking at the mean differences, Würslin *et al.* [26] calculated between manual tissue segmentation and their automatic procedure (2.07% for TV, 8.13% for TAT, 3.21% for VAT), the described additional manual corrections regarding the small volumes of ABM and INF are appropriate.

After these procedures a specific and extensive topographic mapping and segmentation of body tissue was possible (Table 1). Total volume (TV) can be subdivided into total somatic volume (TSV) and total visceral volume (TVV, Figure 2) or can be subdivided into total adipose tissue (TAT; without INF) and total lean tissue (TLT). TLT can be separated into somatic (SLT) and visceral lean tissue (VLT). Subtraction of ABM from TAT leads to total adipose soft tissue (TAST). TAST can be subdivided into VAT and somatic adipose soft tissue (SAST). Therefore, somatic adipose tissue (SAT, Figure 1) is the same as SAST plus ABM or TAT minus VAT, respectively. VAT can be subdivided into intraabdominal (retro- and intraperitoneal) adipose tissue (IAAT) and intrathoracic, mainly mediastinal adipose tissue (MAT). Body segmentation was done into upper extremities (UE), trunk (TR) and lower extremities (LE). TV, lean tissue (LT) and SAST volume was calculated for the upper and lower extremities (UE and LE) and for the trunk (TR). For nomenclature of specific segmented tissues see Table 1.

Statistical analysis

For data elaboration specific software was used: Microsoft™ Office Excel™ (Release 12.0.6665.5003, Microsoft Home and Student Suite, 2007, Microsoft Inc.) for data documentation, SPSS (IBM™ SPSS™ Statistics, Release 19.0.0, 2010, SPSS Inc.) for statistical analysis and SigmaPlot for Windows Version 11.0 (Release 11.2.0.5, 2008, Systat Software Inc.) for graphical data presentation.

The measured volumes of tissue compartments are presented as percentage volumes (vol%) and as absolute [1] and relative differences (%) to start. For every measurement interval (t0 to t5) the dispersion measures are presented graphically in box plot figures (median, 25th/75th percentile, 10th/90th percentile and all outliers) for all subjects (finishers and non-finishers) and location measures (mean and standard error, SE) are presented graphically in line figures for finishers only. Calculated total changes (t5 versus t0) of volumes and volume percentages are presented in text as means and standard deviation (SD) with minimum (min) and maximum (max) as appropriate.

Analyses on volume changes during TEFR09

For analysis of the significance regarding volume changes of the specific tissue compartments during TEFR09, a

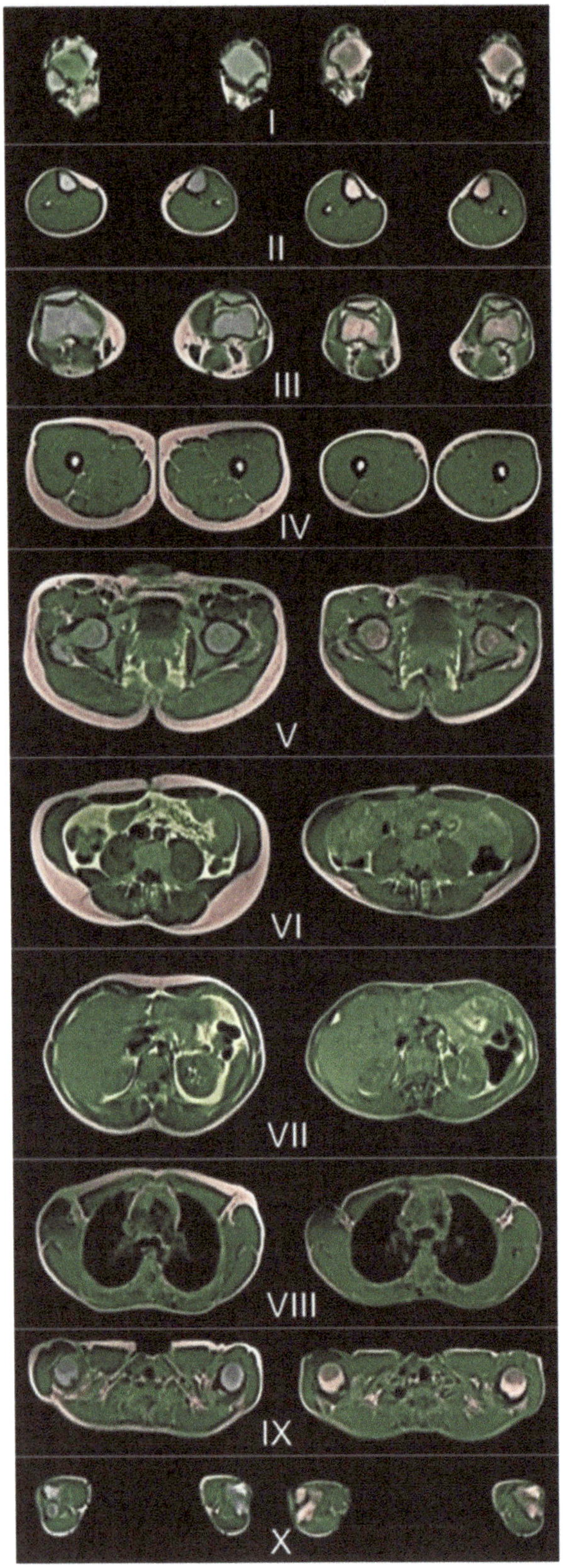

Figure 1 Semiautomatic separation of adipose bone marrow: selected slices from whole body MRI of a 32-year-old male finisher of TEFR09. I: ankles, II: middle of lower legs, III: knees, IV: middle of upper legs, V: hip/pelvis, VI: umbilical level, VII: upper abdomen, VIII: heart/mediastinum, IX: shoulder girth, X: elbows. Left row: before start (t0), green: TLT, red: SAST, yellow: VAT+INF, blue: ABM. Right row: after 4,120 km of running (t5), green: TLT, red: SAT (=SAST + ABM), yellow: VAT + INF. ABM, adipose bone marrow; INF, intraluminal nutrition fat; MRI, magnetic resonance imaging; SAST, somatic adipose soft tissue; SAT, somatic adipose tissue; TEFR09, Transeurope Footrace 2009; TLT, total lean tissue; VAT, visceral adipose tissue.

univariate variance analysis (ANOVA) for repeated measurements was preferred (only subjects who had the whole body MRI at every measurement interval (t0 to t5): n = 12). Therefore, a common linear model for repeated measurements (with *post hoc* analysis on the significance between the different times of measurement) was chosen. For correction of accumulation of the alpha level due to multiple testing (of hypothesis: 'The means at stage intervals are significantly different to means at start'), the Bonferroni-

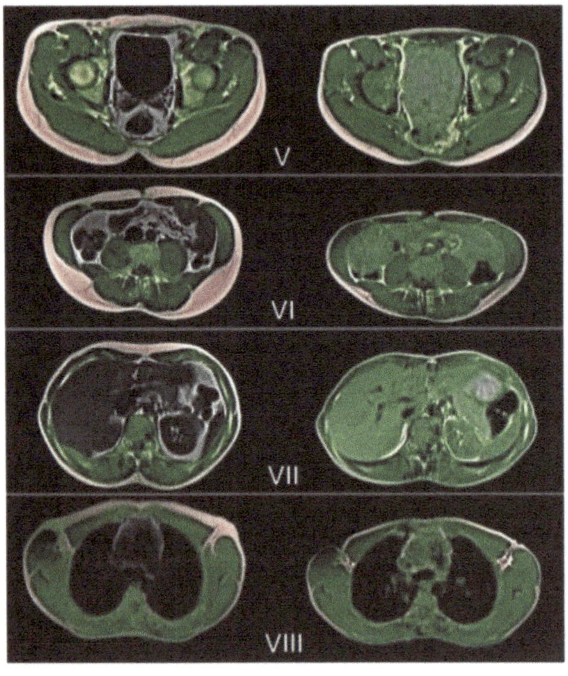

Figure 2 Semiautomatic separation of somatic and visceral volume (right row) and intraluminal nutrition fat (left row): selected slices from whole body MRI of a 32-year-old male finisher of TEFR09. V: hip/pelvis, VI: umbilical level, VII: upper abdomen, VIII: heart/mediastinum. Left row: before start (t0), green: SLT, red: TSAT, grey: TVV. Right row: after 4,120 km of running (t5), green: TLT, red: SAT (=SAST+ABM), yellow: VAT, blue: INF. ABM, adipose bone marrow; INF, intraluminal nutrition fat; MRI, magnetic resonance imaging; SAT, somatic adipose tissue; SLT, somatic lean tissue; TEFR09, Transeurope Footrace 2009; TLT, total lean tissue; TSAT, total somatic adipose tissue; TVV, total visceral volume; VAT, visceral adipose tissue.

Table 1 Abbreviations of compartments after tissue mapping and segmentation with mobile whole body MRI data sets (T2*)

Abbreviation	Description, Definition
	Tissue mapping in specific compartments
ABM	Adipose bone marrow
TV	Total volume of the body (from ankle to wrist), without INF
TVV	Total visceral volume: includes intrathoracic and intraabdominal volume.
TSV	Total somatic volume (TV without TVV).
TLT	Total lean tissue
VLT	Visceral lean tissue: includes lean tissue of intrathoracic and intraabdominal organs.
SLT	Somatic lean tissue: mostly muscles
TAT	Total adipose tissue (without INF)
SAT	Somatic adipose tissue (TAT without VAT)
TAST	Total adipose soft tissue (TAT without ABM)
SAST	Somatic adipose soft tissue (TAT without ABM and VAT)
SCAT	Subcutaneous adipose tissue (SAST without IMAT)
IMAT	Intermuscular adipose tissue (SAST without SCAT)
VAT	Visceral adipose tissue (IAAT + MAT without INF)
IAAT	Intraabdominal adipose tissue: retroperitoneal and intraperitoneal (mesenteric, omental) fat depots (without INF)
MAT	Intrathoracic, mainly mediastinal adipose tissue
INF	(Undigested) intraluminal nutrition fat in the gastrointestinal tract
	Tissue mapping of body segments
TV-LE	Total volume of lower extremities (apex trochanter major to ankle joint)
TV-TR	Total volume of trunk (acromion to apex of trochanter major)
TV-UE	Total volume of upper extremities (wrist to acromion level)
LT LE	Lean tissue volume of lower extremities (apex trochanter major to ankle joint)
LT-TR	Lean soft tissue volume of trunk (acromion to apex of trochanter major)
LT-UE	Lean soft tissue volume of upper extremities (wrist to acromion level)
SAST-LE	Adipose soft tissue volume of lower extremities (apex trochanter major to ankle joint)
SAST-TR	Adipose soft tissue volume of trunk (acromion to apex of trochanter major)
SAST-UE	Adipose soft tissue volume of upper extremities (wrist to acromion level)

procedure for confidence-interval (CI) adaption was applied. For the univariate ANOVA model, one precondition, the sphericity of data (homogenity between the variance of differences of two measurements) is necessary and was proven by the Mauchly-Test. Because of the small number of subjects, the power of the Mauchly-Test regarding sphericity is low. Therefore, the 'Greenhouse-Geisser' (SPSS) correction procedure was used. Looking at result reliability and test power, in cases of severe injury of the sphericity assumption, a multivariate ANOVA test was used. In cases of missing values, the specific dependent variable (specific tissue compartment) was excluded from ANOVA analysis.

Analyses of difference

For dependence analysis including all stages of and total TEFR09, analyses of difference between the dichotomous nominally scaled dependent variables of the sample finishing status (finisher/non-finisher: F/NF) regarding prerace running performance history and regarding total, lean and adipose tissue volumes were carried out. Depending on normal or free distribution of the independent interval scaled variables, the parametric independent t-test (variance homogeneity was calculated with Levene`s test) or nonparametric Mann–Whitney-U-test was used. Due to the higher power in small cohorts, the Shapiro-Wilk [27,28] test (and not the Kolmogorov-Smirnov statistic [29]) was used to check for normal distribution of the independent prerace variables of performance (PRY, PRT, PRR).

Analysis of relationships

For analyses of relationships, the Pearson correlation coefficient (CC_P) and Spearman-rho correlation coefficient (CC_S) were calculated for parametric and non-parametric parameters, respectively, using bivariate (two-sided) or univariate (one-sided) testing as appropriate:

- BM versus TV and its distribution throughout the race: bivariate CC_S
- Prerace performance versus percentage total, lean and adipose volumes: univariate CC_S / CC_P
- Race performance versus percentage total, lean and adipose volumes: univariate CC_P

For interpretation of CC-values the effect size according to Cohen (r = 1: low, r = 3: medium, r = 5: high) was used [30]. For all tests, an alpha level (*P*-value) of 0.05 was used to indicate significance.

Results

Case presentation

Figure 3 shows the topographical mapping of changes of lean and adipose tissue of a subject (male, 32 years, finisher) with one of the largest decreases of SAST and VAT during TEFR09. Runners often had discomfort or pain after stage finishing, so the investigators tried to adapt body positioning in the MR scanner to the athletes' current problems to make it as comfortable as possible for them. Therefore, a reliable and strictly standardized lying

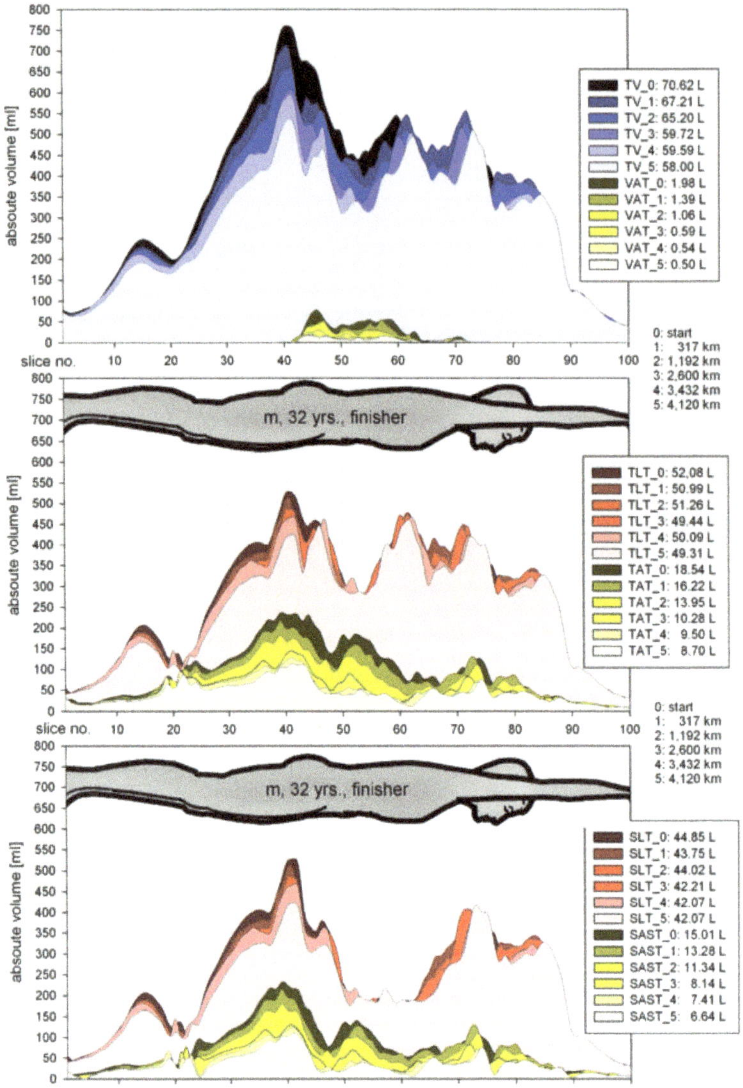

Figure 3 Topography of lean and adipose tissue changes in a 32-year-old male finisher.

position on the MRI table was not possible at each time of measurement. Sometimes, knees or elbows were positioned more or less straightened. This explains the sometimes visible but small topographical phase shifting between different times of measurement in Figure 3.

Total body volume versus body mass/body mass index

The absolute volumes of all investigated body tissue compartments and segments are shown in Table 2. Over all subjects, mean loss of BM and BMI at the end of the race was 5.23 kg (SD 3.72 kg) and 1.49 kg/m^2 (SD 1.18 kg/m^2), respectively (Tables 3 and 4). There was a high correlation (CC_S: 0.978, P <0.001) between BM (kg) and TV [1] regarding mean absolute value changes throughout the race (Figure 4).

Percentage body composition

At the start of the TEFR09, the mean percentage volume of TSV was 84.8 (SD 1.36 vol.%). TSV could be differentiated into mean SLT 65.0 vol% (SD 5.33 vol%), mean ABM 3.2 vol% (SD 0.89 vol%) and mean SAST 16.6 vol% (SD 5.58 vol%). The mean TVV of 15.2 vol% (SD 1.36 vol%) is consistent and divides into mean VLT 12.3 vol% (SD 1.23 vol%) and mean VAT 2.9 vol% (SD 1.37 vol%). From these data the changes in mean vol% of tissue compartments regarding the overall population of ultrarunners could be calculated for transcontinental MSUM races (Figure 5).

Total volumes

Percentage volume changes of TSV and TVV were not significant (Table 3, Figure 6). For absolute volumes (TV,

Table 2 Mean volumes (l) of body compartments and segments (all subjects)

Abbreviation	t0: start	t1: 317 to 789 km	t2: 1,003 to 1,635 km	t3: 2,516 to 2,738 km	t4: 3,234 to 3,669 km	t5: 4,037 to 4,440 km
			Tissue mapping in specific compartments			
TV	57.70	56.63	54.75	53.39	54.16	52.65
TVV	8.74	8.34	7.93	7.64	7.65	7.58
TSV	48.97	48.29	46.82	45.74	46.51	45.08
TLT	44.34	44.61	45.07	45.38	46.20	45.52
VLT	7.02	7.04	7.01	7.10	7.14	7.12
SLT	37.32	37.56	38.06	38.28	39.06	38.40
TAT	13.36	12.02	9.68	8.00	7.96	7.14
SAT	11.65	10.73	8.76	7.46	7.45	6.68
TAST	11.52	10.19	7.76	6.05	6.01	5.19
SAST	9.81	8.89	6.84	5.51	5.50	4.73
VAT	1.71	1.30	0.92	0.54	0.51	0.45
IAAT	1.55	1.15	0.77	0.39	0.36	0.33
MAT	0.17	0.15	0.15	0.15	0.14	0.13
INF	0.05	0.21	0.36	0.57	0.70	0.86
ABM	1.98	1.93	1.92	1.95	1.95	1.95
			Tissue mapping of body segments			
TV-LE	23.51	22.49	21.46	21.65	22.02	20.60
TV-TR	28.83	28.63	27.86	26.57	27.03	27.00
TV-UE	5.79	5.89	5.75	5.73	5.64	5.60
TLT-LE	17.51	16.97	16.82	17.45	17.83	16.97
TLT-TR	23.22	23.12	23.46	23.02	23.39	23.39
TLT-UE	4.79	4.62	4.70	4.81	4.74	4.77
SAST-LE	4.84	4.36	3.43	2.96	2.96	2.40
SAST-TR	4.31	3.47	2.12	1.02	0.99	0.81
SAST-UE	0.98	0.95	0.72	0.57	0.54	0.48

ABM, adipose bone marrow; IAAT, intraabdominal adipose tissue; INF, intraluminal nutrition fat; LE, lower extremities; MAT, mediastinal adipose tissue; SAST, somatic adipose soft tissue; SAT, somatic adipose tissue; SLT, somatic lean tissue; TAT, total adipose tissue; TLT, total lean tissue; TR, trunk; TSV, total somatic volume; TV, total volume; TVV, total visceral volume; UE, upper extremities; VAT, visceral adipose tissue; VLT, visceral lean tissue.

TSV, TVV), however, a significant change could be evaluated with a very high test power (Table 5). Except for TSV at the first measurement interval, significant decreases for TV, TSV and TVV could be shown at all MIs throughout TEFR09 (Figure 7). Paired comparison of MI after the start showed no significant difference for TVV but partial differences for TV and TSV (Figure 7).

Total volume

After more than 4,000 km of running the mean TV showed a mean decrease of 9.5% (SD 5.1%, min –2.7%, max –17.9%) compared to the start. Depending on the total sample the mean TV decrease for the overall population of ultrarunners ranges between 8% to 11% (SE 1.5%), (Figure 8). Looking only at the group of finishers, the absolute amount of mean TV loss at the last MI was 6.1 L (SD 3.4 L, min–2.5 L, max –12.6 L (Figure 9). Mean loss of TV per km was 3.5 ml (SD 2.9 ml/km) in the beginning and became smaller, like a reversed parabolic function, during TEFR09 down to 1.5 ml/km (SD 0.8 ml/km) at the end of the race (Figure 10).

Total somatic volume

The relative decrease of TSV during TEFR09 showed a nearly similar curve as TV (Figure 8), but was less pronounced (mean –9.4% after more than 4,000 km, SD 5.3%, min –2.1%, max –18.1%) with the same SE of 1.5%. For the finisher group the absolute loss of TSV increased to 5.2 L in the mean (SD 3.0 L, min –1.7 L, max –11.1 L) at the end of the race (Figure 9). This is consistent with a mean TSV loss of 1.3 ml/km (SD –0.7 ml/km) at the end of TEFR09, starting with 2.7 ml/km (SD 2.7 ml/km) in the first eight stages of TEFR09 (Figure 10).

Total visceral volume

Compared to TV and TSV, the relative decrease of TVV occurred much faster but ended in a nearly similar

Table 3 BM and BMI loss during TEFR09

Number			Distance run (km)	BM (kg)						BMI (kg/m²)					
all	F	NF		all		F		NF		all		F		NF	
			mean	mean	SD	mean	SD	mean	SD	mean	SD	mean	SD	mean	SD
22	12	10	0.00	71.75	11.13	72.07	11.23	71.38	11.60	23.58	2.55	23.36	2.58	23.84	2.62
15	10	5	116.1	72.43	10.82	71.38	12.48	74.54	7.14	23.33	2.47	22.98	2.75	24.02	1.87
20	11	9	354.2	70.53	11.67	72.20	11.63	68.49	12.07	23.18	2.68	23.26	2.58	23.08	2.95
21	12	9	618.5	70.20	11.20	70.51	11.04	68.08	12.22	22.98	2.59	22.84	2.35	22.95	3.07
20	12	8	893.8	68.73	10.96	70.04	10.60	66.76	11.92	22.68	2.51	22.70	2.23	22.67	3.05
17	12	5	1,168.2	69.52	10.65	69.83	10.78	68.76	11.56	22.72	2.31	22.62	2.23	22.96	2.77
16	12	4	1,456.9	68.18	10.72	68.93	10.70	65.93	12.09	22.20	2.21	22.33	2.25	21.80	2.35
15	12	3	1,754.0	68.39	10.61	68.65	10.45	67.37	13.59	22.26	2.08	22.24	2.12	22.38	2.34
15	12	3	2,026.1	67.64	10.93	67.94	10.57	66.43	14.78	22.01	2.18	22.01	2.19	22.02	2.65
14	11	3	2,294.2	68.01	10.81	68.19	10.75	67.37	13.47	22.11	2.13	22.03	2.18	22.39	2.35
14	12	2	2,594.5	67.05	10.83	67.44	10.30	64.70	18.53	21.73	2.05	21.85	2.18	20.98	0.81
14	12	2	2,852.0	68.88	9.85	67.66	10.14	76.20	2.12	22.17	2.19	21.92	2.09	23.69	3.06
13	12	1	3,134.2	68.45	9.95	67.73	10.04	77.00		21.90	1.95	21.95	2.03	21.33	
13	12	1	3,401.7	68.58	10.07	67.78	10.06	78.30		21.93	1.91	21.95	1.99	21.69	
12	12		3,724.8	67.35	10.16	67.35	10.16			21.82	2.15	21.82	2.15		
12	12		4,010.8	67.48	9.91	67.48	9.91			21.87	2.06	21.87	2.06		
12	12		4,307.3	66.83	10.50	66.83	10.50			21.64	2.12	21.64	2.12		

BM,body mass; BMI, body mass index; F, finisher; NF, non-finisher; TEFR09, Transeurope Footrace 2009.

amount with a mean of 10.0% (SD 4.9%, min −3.8%, max −19.3%) in a negative parabolic graph shape (see Figure 8). The mean loss of absolute TVV was 0.9 L (SD 0.5 L, min −0.3 L, max −1.7 L) for finishers (Figure 9). Mean absolute TVV loss per km during TEFR09 had a maximum of 0.75 ml/km (SD 0.5 ml/km) at the beginning and 0.2 ml/km (SD 0.1 ml/km) at the end (Figure 10).

Adipose tissue

In total (TAT), somatic (SAST) and visceral (VAT) adipose tissue, a significant change of absolute volumes (Table 5) and percentage volumes (Table 3) could be evaluated with a very high test power at the different MIs during TEFR09. A significant decrease for TAT, SAST and VAT could be shown at all MIs throughout TEFR09 compared to the start and for TAT and SAST compared to the first MI after the start (stage 5 to 12) (Figure 11). For other MIs the paired comparison showed no significant change.

Total adipose tissue

There was a continuous decrease of TAT that ended in a relative mean loss of 41.3% (SD 8.0%, min −25.4%,

Table 4 Significance of topographic tissue volume changes regarding percentage volume (vol. %)

	Mauchly-Test	Univariate ANOVA[b]			Multivariate ANOVA[c]		
(vol.%)	*P*-value	F value	*P* value	test power	F value	*P* value	test power
TSV	0.322	2.565	**0.058**	0.640	-	-	-
TVV	0.322	2.565	**0.058**	0.640	-	-	-
TLT[a]	0.000	44.605	0.000	1.000	51.592	**0.000**	1.000
SLT[a]	0.000	43.573	0.000	1.000	19.556	**0.001**	1.000
VLT[a]	0.005	22.980	0.000	1.000	6.699	**0.013**	0.884
TAT[a]	0.000	44.655	0.000	1.000	52.762	**0.000**	1.000
SAST[a]	0.000	44.721	0.000	1.000	57.109	**0.000**	1.000
VAT[a]	0.000	23.718	0.000	1.000	8.598	**0.007**	0.950

[a]mean differences are significant; [b]'Greenhouse-Geisser' correction procedure was used; [c]Pillai-Spur, Wilks-Lambda, Hotelling-Spur and 'biggest characteristical root of Roy'. ANOVA, analysis of variance; SAST, somatic adipose soft tissue; SLT, somatic lean tissue; TAT, total adipose tissue; TLT, total lean tissue; TSV, total somatic volume; TVV, total visceral volume; VAT, visceral adipose tissue; VLT, visceral lean tissue.
Bold numbers mark the prefered *P*-value of the prevered ANOVA regarding sphericity assumption proven by Mauchly-Test.

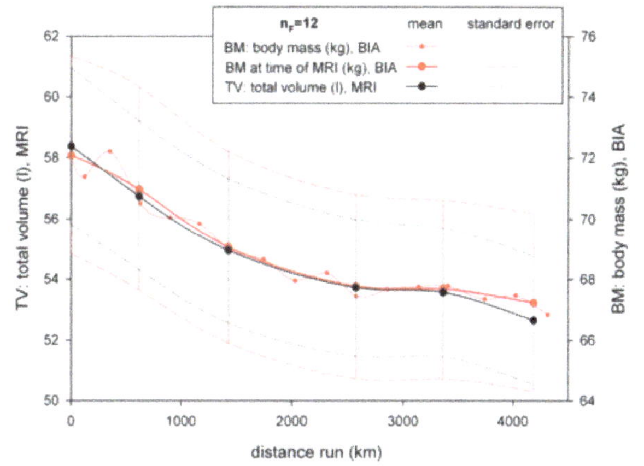

Figure 4 Comparison of total body volume versus body mass during TEFR09 (finisher, n_F = 12). TEFR09, Transeurope Footrace 2009.

max −53.2%) with a small SE of 2.3% (Figure 8) at the last MI. Looking at the absolute loss of TAT, a finisher lost 5.3 L in the mean (SD 2.6 L min −2.7 L, max −9.8 L) until the end of the race (Figure 9). The mean TAT loss per km in finishers was 3.2 ml (SD −1.7 ml/km) at the beginning and 1.2 ml (SD 0.6 ml/km) at the end of TEFR09 (Figure 10).

Somatic adipose soft tissue

The relative SAST decrease compared to the start showed a steeper graph than TAT and ended in a mean loss of 48.7% (SD 9.9%, min −25.9%, max −65.5%) after more than 4,000 km (Figure 8). The absolute SAST decrease in finishers showed a mean of 4.4 L (SD 2.2 L, min −2.2 L, max −8.4 L) at the end of TEFR09 (Figure 9). This corresponds to a mean loss of SAST of 1.1 ml/km (SD 0.5 ml/km) at the end of TEFR09 compared to 2.4 ml/km (SD 1.4 ml/km) at the start (Figure 10).

Visceral adipose tissue

The relative decrease of VAT occurred much more rapidly in the mean and ended in a relative VAT volume

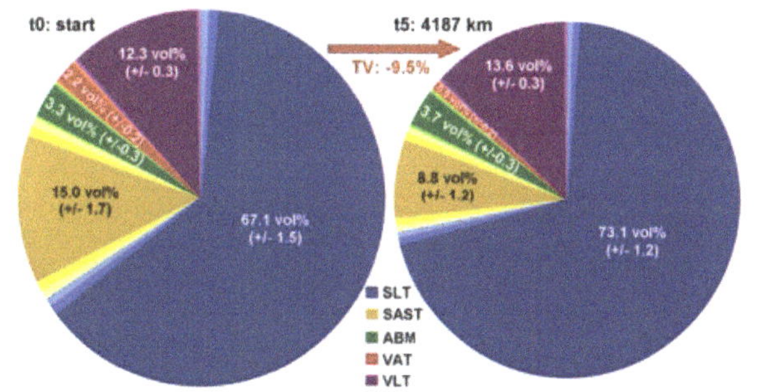

Figure 5 Adipose and lean volume percentage distribution in finishers at the start and end of TEFR09 (finisher, n_F = 12). TEFR09, Transeurope Footrace 2009, SE is indicated in brackets.

loss of 64.5% (SD 15.9%, min −27.7%, max −88.8%) at the end of the race (Figure 8) compared to the start and a SE up to 4.6%. The percentage volume of VAT decreased more quickly and severely compared to absolute VAT volume (Figure 12). In absolute values, this rapid and continuous loss of VAT ended in a mean of −0.9 L (SD 0.5 L, min −0.3 L, max −1.7 L) in the finisher group (Figure 9), which was nearly the same as the absolute TVV loss. Therefore, the mean VAT volume loss per km was the same as for TVV in the finishers (Figure 10).

The subdivision of VAT into IAAT and MAT shows that IAAT decreased a bit faster than VAT in total and ended in a relative volume loss of 67.3% (SD 14.8%, min −31.7%, max −88.8%) at the end (Figure 13). MAT initially decreased as rapidly as IAAT with respect to VAT but reached a plateau of 30% volume loss after nearly 1,000 km of running before it decreased again in the last third of the race up to 41.5% with a larger variance (SD 24.7%, min −0.1%, max −89.0%).

Lean tissue

Due to significant and continuous loss of different adipose tissue volumes the percentage volume of TLT, SLT and VLT increased during TEFR09 significantly without relevant changes in absolute volumes, respectively (Table 3, Figure 12); analysis of the means of absolute volume showed no significant changes for total, somatic and visceral lean tissue at the different MIs during TEFR09 (Table 5).

Total lean tissue, somatic lean tissue, visceral lean tissue

TLT volume showed undulating relative changes duringTEFR09 in the mean compared to the start. Just at the end, after more than 4,000 km running, the mean relative changes were −1.2% TLT (SD 3.3%, min 6.3%, max −5.5%) with an SE of 1.0% (Figure 8). Due to nearly stable volume regarding VLT during TEFR09, the SLT data during TEFR09 was similar to that of TLT relative to the start: mean −1.4% (SD 3.9%, min 7.5%, max −6.6%). Not every finisher showed a decrease of absolute TLT and SLT; some of them showed increases, some decreases: mean −0.9 l (SD 1.2 L, min 1.1 L, max −2.8 L); see Figure 9. Mean loss of TLT and SLT per km changed between 0.3 and 0.2 ml with a wide range (SD at beginning 1.9 ml/km, at the end 0.3 ml/km), see Figure 10.

Segmental volume analysis

The significance of the volume changes in the different body segments is shown in Table 6. For the lower extremities the change of volumes was only significant for SAST_LE but not for TV_LE or LT_LE; for the trunk and upper extremities decreases were significant for adipose soft tissue volume (SAST_TR, SAST_UE) and total volume (TV_TR, TV_UE) but not for lean tissue volume

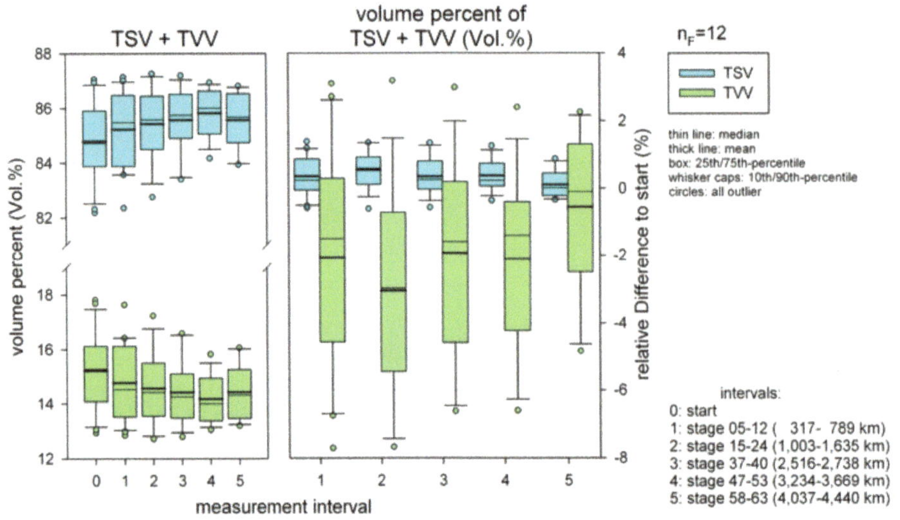

Figure 6 Changes of somatic and visceral percentage volumes during TEFR09 (finisher, n_F = 12). TEFR09, Transeurope Footrace 2009.

(LT_TR, LT_UE). Most decrease of somatic adipose tissue occurred in the trunk (t5: mean −50.3%, SD 12.0%), followed by the arms (t5:mean −39.1%, SD 8.3%); in the legs the adipose tissue lose was the smallest, but significant (t5: mean −29.2%, SD 13.4%), Figure 14. Although changes of lean tissue were not significant in any segment, mean values demonstrate a mean increase in the legs in the first half of TEFR09, and in the trunk in the first third of the race, while in the arms lean tissue loss was already detectable at the first MI t1 (Figure 14).

Finisher/non-finisher

A total of 45.5% of the subjects did not finish the race. The dropout rate of subjects compared to all race participants is shown in Figure 15. The main reason (70%, n_i = 7) for premature dropping out of the race was intolerable pain in the legs due to an overload of muscle and tendons (soft tissues) leading to intermuscular and peritendinous inflammation (fasciitis): lower legs (40%), upper legs (30%). Other reasons were a high tibial stress fracture, a painful bunion and one rapidly progressing phlegmonia from the thumb up to the forearm needing immediate surgical intervention.

Figure 16 shows the distribution of percentage volumes for all tissue compartments at the start time (t0) and MI t1 (317 to 789 km) for finishers (n_F = 12) and non-finishers (n_{NF} = 10) of TEFR09. At both times the finisher group had significantly more percentage volume regarding total somatic tissue (mean TSV) than non-finishers of TEFR09 (at t0 +1.8%: 85.5 vol% versus 84.0 vol%, at t1 +1.6%: 85.8% versus 84.4%) and, therefore, significantly less percentage volume of mean TVV (at t0 -10.5%: 14.5 vol% versus 16.0 vol%, at t1 -9.5%: 14.2 vol% versus 15.6 vol%), Table 7. The finisher group showed significantly less adipose tissue volume percentage

Table 5 Significance of topographic tissue volume changes regarding absolute volume measurements (l) (n_F = 12)

	Mauchly-Test	Univariate ANOVA[b]			Multivariate ANOVA[c]		
(l)	*P* value	F value	*P* value	test power	F value	*P* value	test power
TV[a]	0.000	20.162	0.000	0.999	5.758	**0.020**	0.828
TSV[a]	0.001	18.607	0.000	0.999	4.937	**0.030**	0.762
TVV[a]	0.000	21.516	0.000	0.999	8.678	**0.007**	0.952
TLT	0.516	1.209	**0.322**	0.307	-	-	-
SLT	0.516	1.209	**0.322**	0.307	-	-	-
TAT[a]	0.000	32.274	0.000	1.000	18.577	**0.001**	1.000
SAST[a]	0.000	32.692	0.000	1.000	15.624	**0.001**	0.998
VAT[a]	0.000	21.607	0.000	0.999	8.594	**0.007**	0.950

[a]mean differences are significant; [b]'Greenhouse-Geisser' correction procedure was used; [c]'Pillai-Spur, Wilks-Lambda, Hotelling-Spur and 'biggest characteristical root of Roy.' ANOVA, analysis of variance; SAST, somatic adipose soft tissue; SLT, somatic lean tissue; TAT, total adipose tissue; TLT, total lean tissue; TSV, total somatic volume; TVV, total visceral volume; VAT, visceral adipose tissue.
Bold numbers mark the prefered *P*-value of the prevered ANOVA regarding sphericity assumption proven by Mauchly-Test.

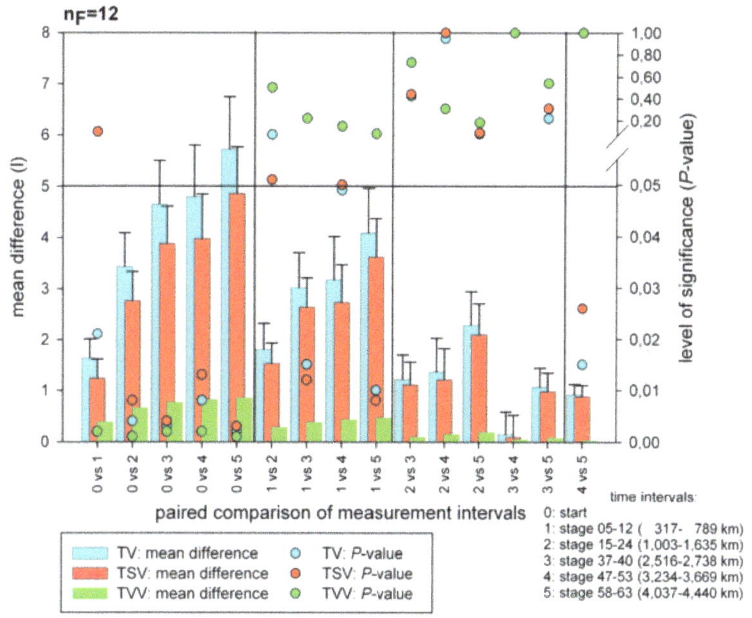

Figure 7 Post hoc analysis of significance of paired comparison of total volume measurements at different time intervals (finisher, $n_F = 12$).

than the non-finishers for TAT and VAT at t0 and t1, and also for SAST at t1 (Table 7). At the start, non-finishers had 71.5% more VAT volume percent (mean VAT at t0: 2.2 vol% versus 3.8 vol%), 28.0% more SAST volume percent (mean SAST at t0: 15.0 vol% versus 19.2 vol%) and in total 26.6% more TAT volume percent (mean TAT at t0: 20.6 vol% versus 26.1 vol%) than the finishers (Table 7). At the first MI, t1, the difference between finisher and non-finisher was significantly further on; non-finishers had 96.8% more VAT volume percent (mean VAT at t0: 1.6 vol% versus 3.2 vol%), 39.7% more SAST volume percent (mean SAST at t0: 13.3 vol% versus 18.5 vol%) and in total, 34.9% more TAT volume percent (mean TAT at t0: 18.3 vol% versus 24.7 vol%) than finishers (Table 7). These differences for adipose tissue compartments were no longer detectable as the race proceeded (t2 to t5); either there are not enough numbers to treat in the group of non-finishers for further analysis on the difference with finishers or no difference could be shown. Conversely, the lean tissue difference of percentage volume was significantly smaller in non-finishers compared to finishers for TLT (at t0: -6.9%, at t1: -7.8%) and SLT (at t0: -8,1%, at t1: -8.9%) (Table 7). VLT showed no significant difference between finishers and non-finishers at any MI (t0 to t5). Table 8 and Figure 17 demonstrate a significant relative volume loss at MI t1 and t2 compared to the start only for SAST and no other tissue compartment.

Prerace performance

Although there is a wide range of finished long distance foot races in the subject group (Table 9), every participant of TEFR09 had already finished nearly one UM and MSUM, but not every subject had finished a single marathon. The endurance training extent of one year and three months before TEFR09 also varied for training volume (km), time (hours) and intensity (km/hour) in the subject group (Table 9). For the number of finished marathons, UM and MSUM no difference between finisher and non-finisher could be evaluated (Table 10). However, regarding prerace training volume and intensity one year before TEFR09 and their 50 km- and 24 hour-race record, finishers had a significantly higher prerace-performance compared to non-finishers (Table 10). Only these five prerace-performance parameters (PRT_{Vol08}, PRT_{Vol09}, PRT_{Int08}, PRR_{50km}, PRR_{24hr}) also showed a mainly high and medium correlation with the volume percentage of adipose tissue compartments (VAT, SAST, TAT), TLT and SLT (Figure 18).

Race-performance

No relevant correlation between percentage fat and lean volumes of different compartments at the start and the race performances of the subjects at TEFR09 could be detected (Figure 19). For SAST at the beginning of TEFR09 (stage 1 to 8) a significant correlation between percentage volume at the start and cumulative performance is given, but only at a medium to low effect size. For TAT, TLT and SLT the significance for such a correlation is shown at the first 12 to 15 stages and during the last third of TEFR09 at a medium effect size (Figure 19). A correlation of percentage fat and lean volumes to performance at the individual stages can only be shown for

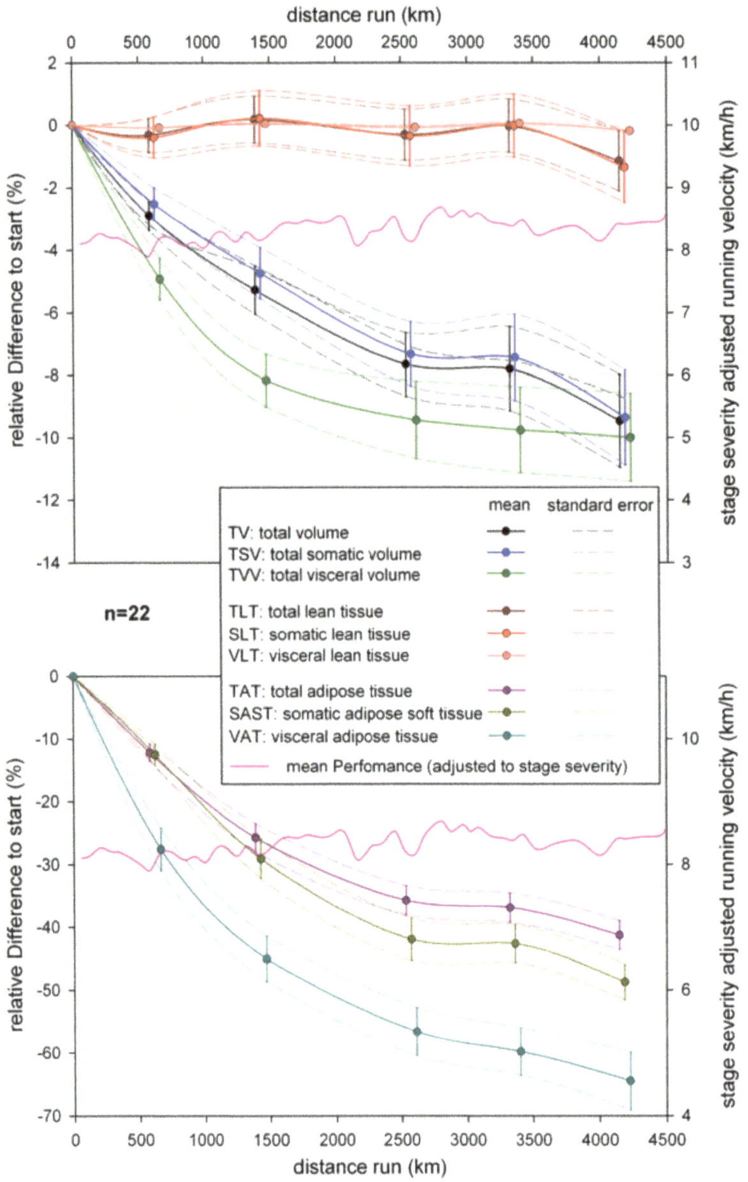

Figure 8 Mean and standard error of relative changes of specific tissue volume during TEFR09 compared to the start (total sample, n = 22). TEFR09, Transeurope Footrace 2009.

a few stages at a middle to low effect size. None of the relative changes in the investigated volumes duringTEFR09 were significantly correlated with performance.

Discussion

Almost nothing is known about the influence of the endurance burden on the specific changes in body composition regarding distribution of adipose and lean tissues in somatic and visceral compartments and in the body segments. Field studies on this topic mostly use methods which only allow indirect measurements and approximated calculations or simple estimations of total or local adipose or lean tissue proportions [11-14]. For TAT and subcutaneous adipose tissue (SCAT = SAST without intermuscular adipose tissue (IMAT) [31]), some of these indirect methods show more or less correlation to MRI findings [17]. These methods are not able to predict the amount of visceral (VAT) or somatic adipose tissue (SAT) in the body [16,32]. Being the first investigation in endurance field studies using the gold standard method [18] whole body MRI for such analyses, our results provide new data on the volume changes of fat and lean tissue in these different parts of the athlete's body.

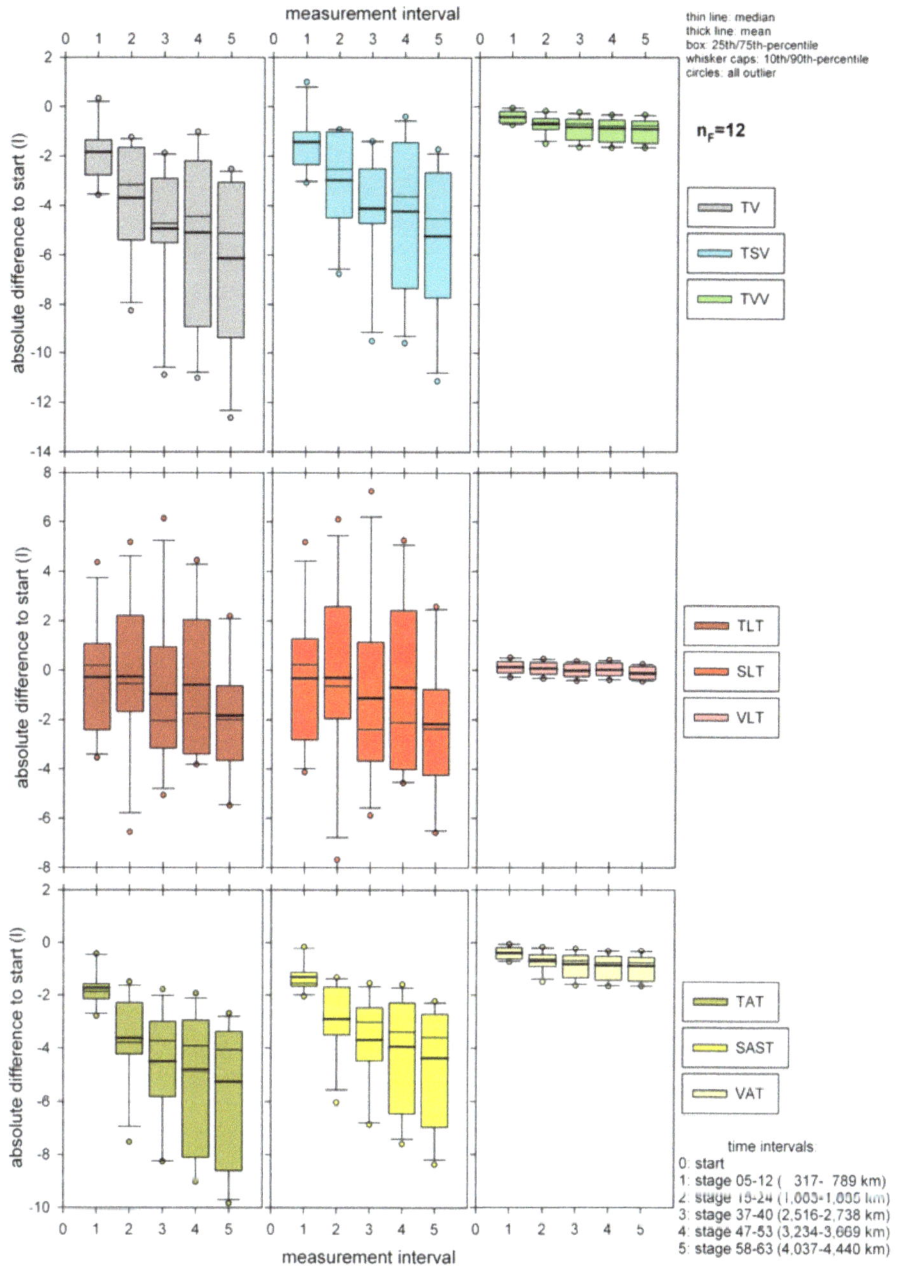

Figure 9 Absolute changes of specific tissue volume during TEFR09 compared to the start (finisher, n_F = 12). TEFR09, Transeurope Footrace 2009.

Age and gender related differences

Bale *et al.* [33] found a lower percentage of body fat in female elite marathon runners. In obese patients (BMI >27 kg/m^2) Machann *et al.* [25] found that the amount and distribution of adipose tissue correlated with age (VAT increasing with age) and with gender (%SAT female > male, % VAT male > female). They found no consistent differences in TAT profiles between the selected age groups for both females (n = 40, mean age 45 years, SD 12 yrs., range 23 to 64 yrs.) and males (n = 40, mean age 45years SD 12 yrs., range 24 to 65 yrs.) in their group. Naturally, our group of ultra-runners with a comparable age distribution (n = 22, mean age 49 years, SD 12 years, range 27 to 69 years) showed a very low absolute mean volume of VAT at the start of TEFR09 (females: 0.5 L, males 1.8 L) compared to obese patients (females 1.5 to 4 L, males 4 to 6.8 L) [25]. Statistical analysis of gender-related differences was not possible (only two females) in our group, but even these data indicate that a difference in VAT between men and women is not only visible in obese people, but is also visible

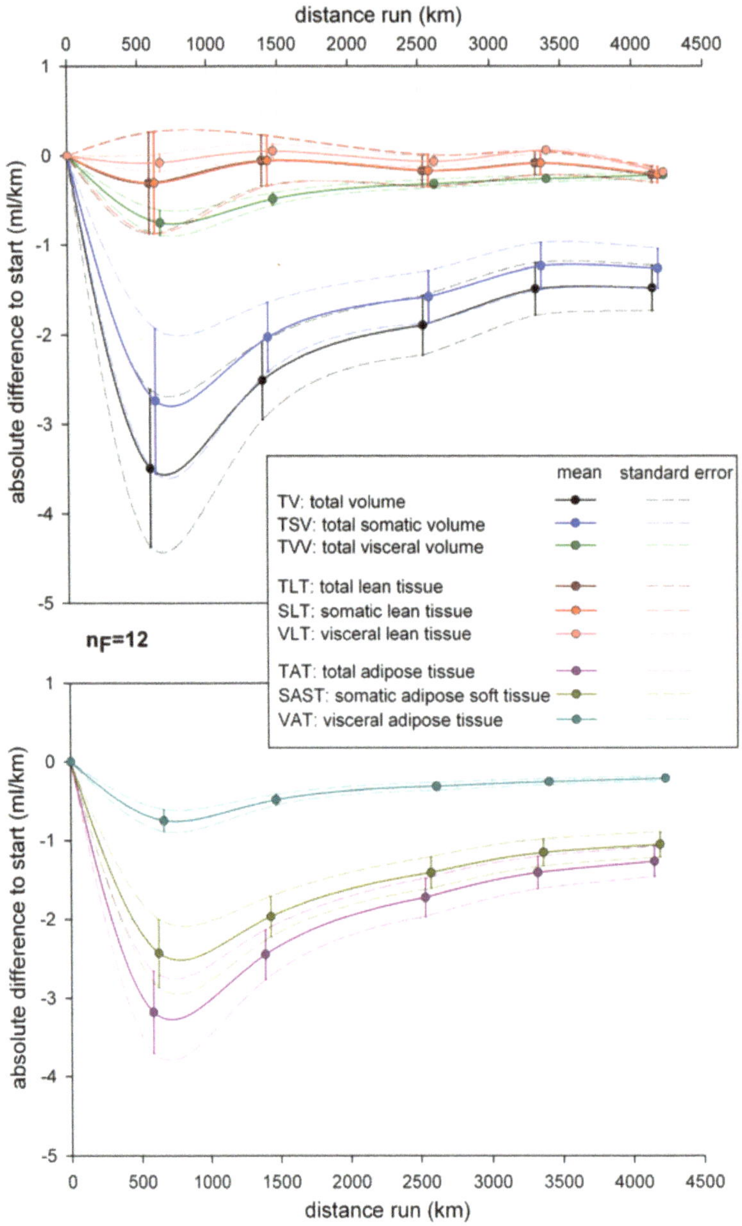

Figure 10 Absolute volume changes per km compared to the start in the finisher group (finisher, n_F = 12). TEFR09, Transeurope Footrace 2009.

in thin ultra-endurance athletes. Analysis based on age showed no correlation to fat distribution at the start (TAT, SAST, VAT) or to volume changes of lean and adipose tissue during TEFR09.

Changes in body composition

Different effects of endurance performance on body composition are described in the literature. Beyond dispute is the fact that endurance performance leads to a decrease in body mass, mainly body fat. Body fat is the main energy-rich substrate for endurance performance [34-37]. Therefore, endurance exercise leads to a reduction of subcutaneous tissue as demonstrated in several field studies [34,36,38].

The specific influence on energy turnover seems to depend on the type of endurance burden [1,39]. In general, non-stop ultra-endurance races over hours, days or weeks without a break result in a decrease in body mass [1,36,40,41] in which body fat as well as skeletal muscle seems to decrease [1,36,40-42]. In ultra-endurance performances with defined breaks, body mass may remain stable [43-45] or even increase [34] and body fat is reduced [34,46,47], whereas skeletal muscle mass seems to be spared [35,43,47] or may even increase [46]. Our

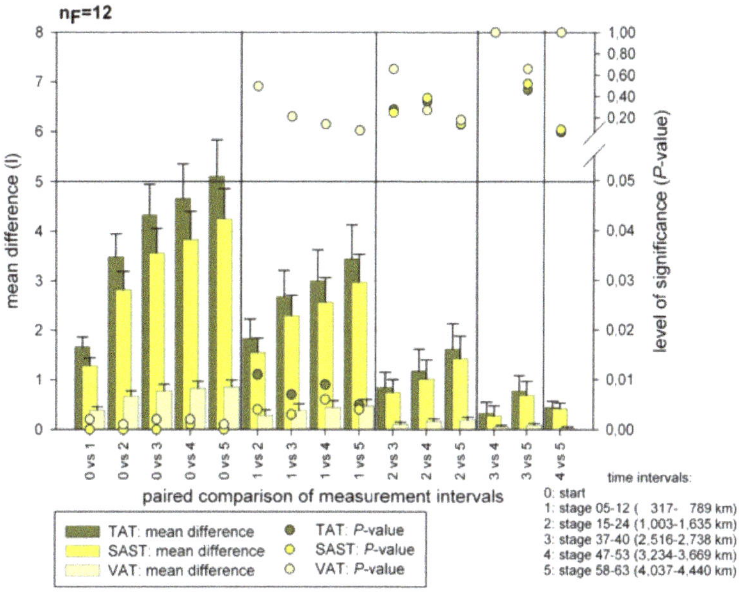

Figure 11 Post hoc analysis of the significance of the paired comparison of total fat tissue measurements at different time intervals (finisher, n_F = 12).

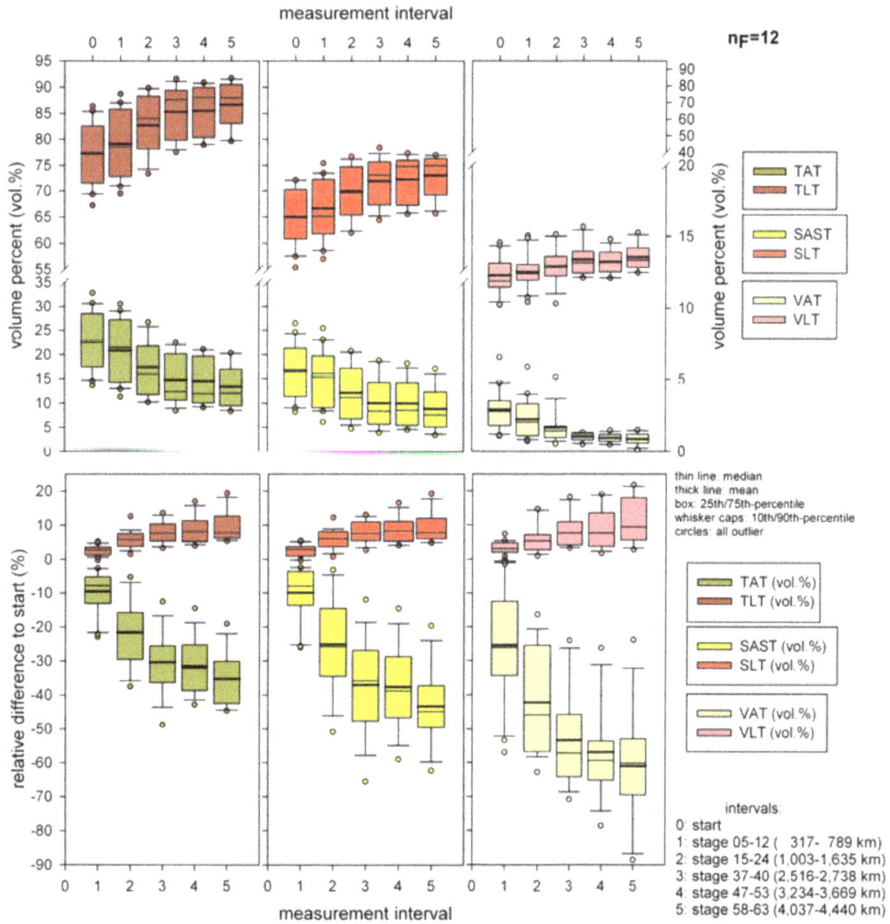

Figure 12 Changes of adipose and lean tissue percentage volumes during TEFR09 (finisher, n_F = 12). TEFR09, Transeurope Footrace 2009.

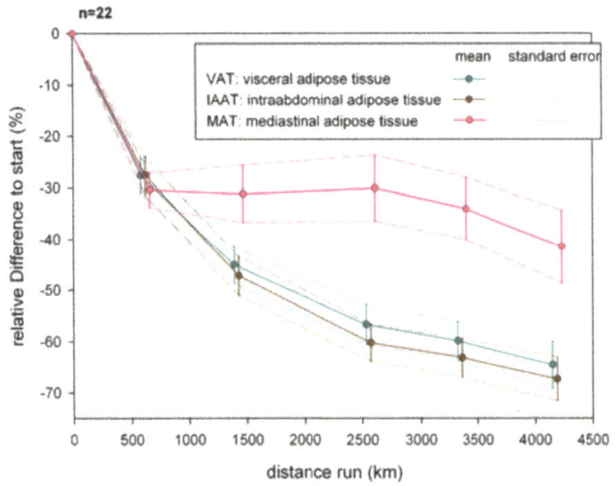

Figure 13 Relative changes of visceral adipose volume during TEFR09 compared to the start (total sample, n = 22). TEFR09, Transeurope Footrace 2009.

whole body MRI results show comparable results for an ultra-long MSUM over 64 days without any day rest; every subject decreased in BM(I), TV, TSV and TVV due to massive loss of TAT, SAT and VAT, respectively. Not every runner lost TLT and SLT during the TEFR09. Some of them showed increases, some decreases. Knechtle *at al.* found the same individual differences for lean tissue in ultra runners during a 1,200 km MSUM across Germany [48]. If there are not sufficiently long breaks in ultra-endurance races, some participants might not find enough time for regeneration and restoration of their energy depots before the next stage. As the race progresses this leads to the utilization of muscle tissue for energy provision.

Mass loss

Raschka and Plat observed a mean loss of 1.75 kg body mass in an ultra-endurance run over 1,000 km within 20 days [34]. In their investigation, there was a statistically significant decrease in body mass after day 8 until day 11, which then remained stable until the finish. In another investigation of 10 ultra runners (BIA), the mean loss of BM after a 1,200 km footrace was also not significant, but the loss of 3.9 kg fat mass was [48]. Unfortunately, the authors gave no information about the relative changes of fat and lean body mass. Our results determined that a transcontinental ultra-long MSUM of 64 stages leads to a significant three times higher loss of body volume (9.5%) than published for body mass loss in deca-triathlons or 20 stage MSUMs [34,47].

The relation of water and lipid to the density of human adipose tissue ranges from 0.925 to 0.97 kg/L [49]. Assuming the middle value (0.948 g/L), in our investigation the ultra-athletes lost a total fat mass (TAT) of 4.8 kg in the mean (SAST 4.0 kg, VAT 0.8 kg), resembling the main part (91.8%) of body mass loss of 5.2 kg. The lean tissue of the human body has a higher density than adipose tissue and muscle tissue (range 1.05 to 1.06 g/L) and varies with age [49,50], ranging between 1.10 and 1.11 g/L [51,52]. With these data and knowing the mean relative reduction of TLT (1.2%), the mean loss of lean body mass can be calculated as about −0.67 kg at the end of TEFR09 in our subject group.

Visceral adipose tissue

Mediastino-abdominal lipomatosis is described as being associated with exertional dyspnea [53], non−insulin-dependent diabetes, type IV hyperlipidemia, and

Table 6 Significance of segmental volume changes regarding repeated absolute volume (l) measurements (n_F = 12)

	Mauchly-Test	Univariate ANOVA[b]			Multivariate ANOVA[c]		
(l)	*P* value	F-value	*P* value	test power	F-value	*P* value	test power
TV_LE	0.003	7.763	0.002	0.946	2.341	**0.149**	0.423
TV_TR[a]	0.133	6.349	**0.003**	0.918	-	-	-
TV_UE[a]	0.001	27.504	0.000	1.000	13.942	**0.002**	0.996
SLT_LE	0.003	6.411	0.20	0.733	14.587	**0.095**	0.597
SLT_TR	0.252	3.534	**0.21**	0.769	-	-	-
SLT_UE	0.700	3.128	**0.29**	0.734	-	-	-
SAST_LE[a]	0.000	63.294	0.000	1.000	20.644	**0.000**	1.000
SAST_TR[a]	0.000	17.388	0.000	0.996	13.387	**0.002**	0.995
SAST_UE[a]	0.000	16.151	0.000	0.987	3.389	**0.041**	0.584
TV_LE[a]	0.001	27.504	0.000	1.000	13.942	**0.002**	0.996
TV_TR[a]	0.133	6.349	**0.003**	0.918	-	-	-
TV_UE	0.003	7.763	0.002	0.946	2.341	**0.149**	0.423

[a]mean differences are significant; [b]'Greenhouse-Geisser' correction procedure was used; [c]Pillai-Spur, Wilks-Lambda, Hotelling-Spur and 'biggest characteristical root of Roy'. ANOVA, analysis of variance; LE, lower extremities; SAST, somatic adipose soft tissue; SLT, somatic lean tissue; TR, trunk; TV, total volume; UE, upper extremities.
Bold numbers mark the prefered *P*-value of the prevered ANOVA regarding sphericity assumption proven by Mauchly-Test.

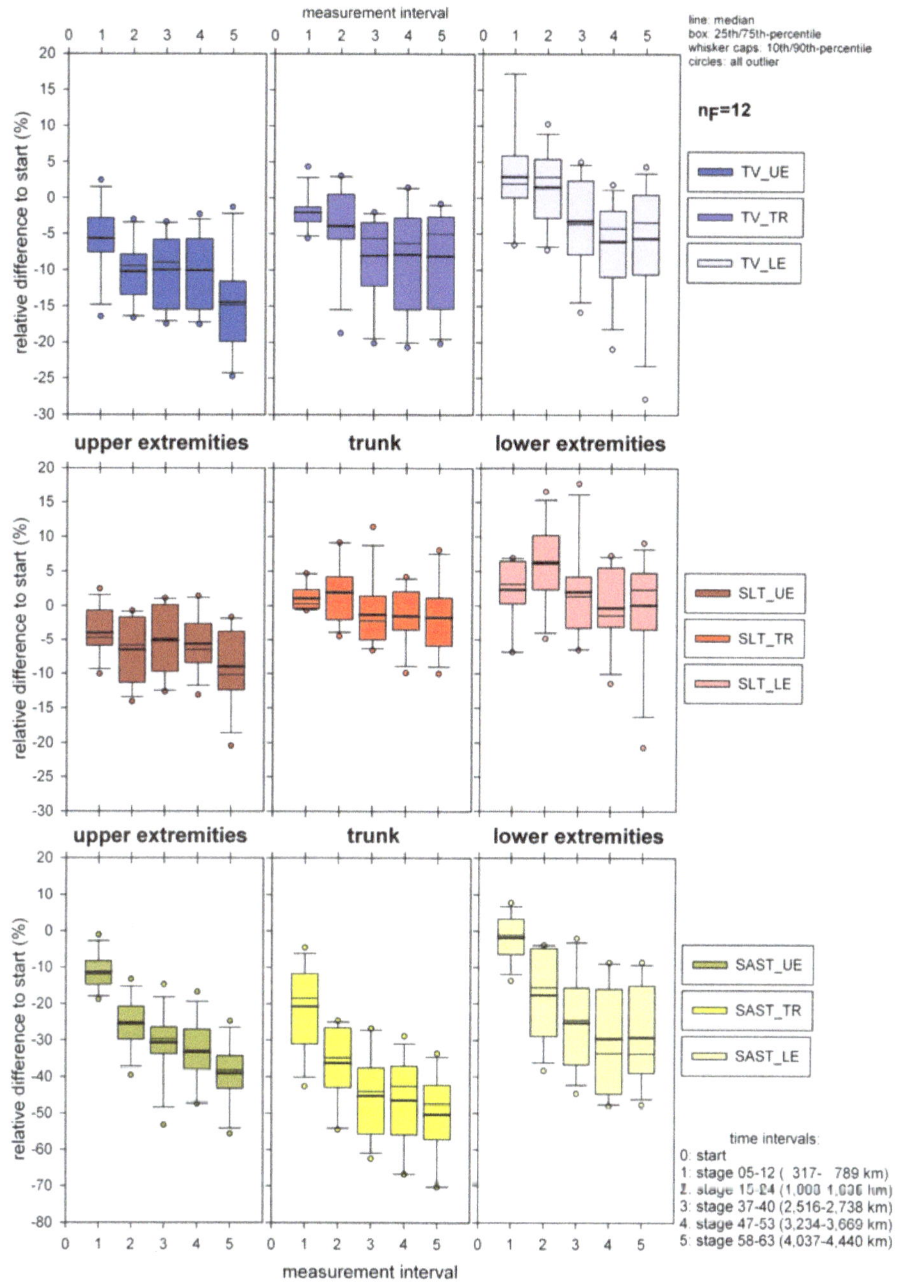

Figure 14 Relative changes of segmented tissue volume (UE, TR, LE) during TEFR09 compared to the start (finisher, n_F = 12). LE, lower extremities; TEFR09, Transeurope Footrace 2009, TR, trunk; UE, upper extremities.

hyperuricemia. The abdominal VAT is an important independent risk factor for metabolic diseases in the older patient [54] and there is evidence that mainly abdominal VAT, which is morphologically and functionally different from abdominal SAST, is associated with the metabolic syndrome (insulin resistance, dyslipidemia, hypertension, obesity) and hyperinsulinemia [55-60], as well as linked inflammatory diseases [61]. The real mean loss of relative IAAT while running a MSUM of nearly 4,500 km, was more than two thirds compared to the start in our group (Figure 13). We showed that endurance running also has an direct influence on intrathoracic fat, especially MAT, which decreased up to more than 40% in the mean (Figure 13). MAT is associated with hypertension, obesity, and iatrogenic Cushing syndrome [57,62-65].

Until now, a specific treatment for the selective reduction of VAT is not known [66] and as our MR analyses showed that VAT decreased much more rapidly and

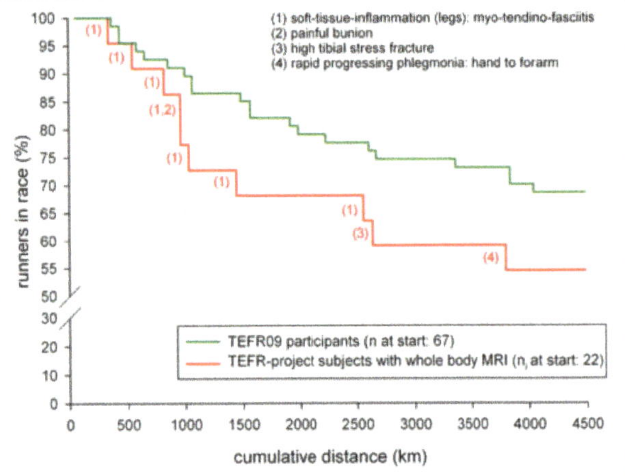

Figure 15 Dropout rate.

vigorously than SAST (Figure 8), a very good and effective way to reduce the risk of metabolic disease is endurance running. As VAT decreases much faster and more than SAST, our investigation indicates that three-compartment measurement methods, such as SF-analyses and BIA, cannot give accurate assumptions or calculations for IAAT and MAT. Even the results of the four-compartment method cadaver study are false, when post mortem findings are transferred to physiological effects which occur from the impact of long lasting running on fat and lean tissue in vivo [67].

Finishers versus non-finishers

55% (n = 12) of the 22 ultra-runners treated with mobile whole body MRI for this study reached the last measurement interval; 10 dropped out earlier. In contrast, the dropout rate for all starters at TEFR09 and all subjects taking part in the TEFR project was 31% [2]. Reasons for dropping out of this transcontinental MSUM race were overuse reactions of the musculoskeletal system of the lower extremities (80%, Figure 15), mainly concerning the myotendinous fascial system.

In a 17-day MSUM (1,200 km) Knechtle et al. found no differences between finishers and non-finishers regarding the anthropometric parameters, BMI, SF, CF, estimated skeletal muscle mass (estimated from SF and CF) and percent body fat (BIA) [68]. With whole body MRI for differentiated body composition analysis, however, we found significant differences between finishers and non-finishers between both somatic and visceral volumes and between adipose and lean tissue volumes at the start and early beginning of the 4,500 km MSUM TEFR09 (Figure 16). Out results indicate that the risk of dropping out of such an ultra-long transcontinental footrace is significantly higher when the total body fat percentage is more than 21% to 25% at the start, in which the visceral fat percentage (VAT) shows a higher difference between finishers and non-finishers (71.5% in the mean) than the somatic fat compartment (SAST, 28.0%). Because VAT is affected by the endurance running burden most quickly and most deeply compared to somatic fat and other lean tissue (Figure 9) and is highly correlated with prerace performance regarding training volume and intensity and specific ultramarathon race-performance (50 km-race), our results indicate,that VAT is the most sensible predictor for the risk of non-finishing a transcontinental MSUM, such as the TEFR09. In ultra-runners there is not a high SAST or TAT, if the VAT is low.

Although training a distance of 4,500 to 5,000 km is not possible, participants of such MSUMs should

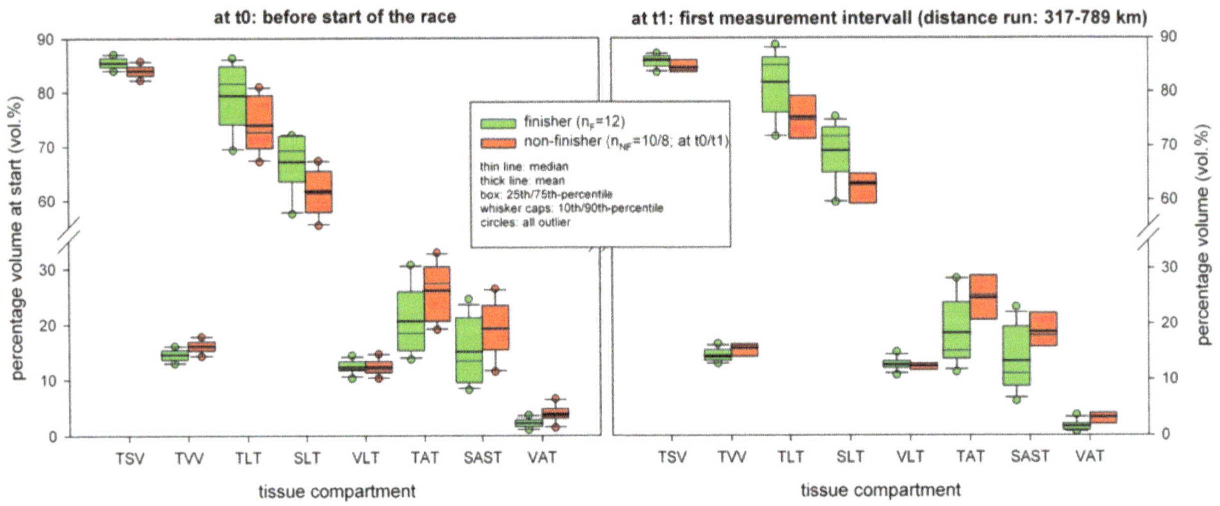

Figure 16 Difference between F and NF regarding percentage tissue volumes before the start of TEFR09 and at MI t1. F, finisher; measurement interval; NF, non-finisher; TEFR09, Transeurope Footrace 2009.

Table 7 Analysis of the difference of percentage volume (vol%) between F/NF at the start (t0) and MI (t1, t2) for total, lean and adipose tissue compartments

	t0: $n_F = 12$, $n_{NF} = 10$		t1: $n_F = 12$, $n_{NF} = 8$		t2: $n_F = 12$, $n_{NF} = 6$	
	Mean difference of percentage volume (vol.%)	*P* value (ITT)	Mean difference of percentage volume (vol.%)	*P* value (ITT)	Mean difference of percentage volume (vol.%)	*P* value (ITT)
TSV	1.52	**0.005**[a]	1.35	**0.036**[a]	1.07	0.182
TVV	−1.52	**0.005**[a]	1.35	**0.036**[a]	1.07	0.182
TLT	4.04	**0.031**[a]	6.39	**0.015**[a]	5.05	0.088
SLT	4.16	**0.014**[a]	6.18	**0.010**[a]	4.65	0.058
VLT	0.032	0.953	0.21	0.707	0.39	0.604
TAT	−5.47	**0.031**[a]	−6.39	**0.015**[a]	−5.04	0.088
SAST	−4.21	0.080	−5.27	**0.032**[a]	−3.64	0.184
VAT	−1.60	**0.006**[a]	−1.56	**0.021**[a]	−1.46	0.060

[a]mean differences between finishers and non-finishers are significant. t0: at start of TEFR09, t1: stage 5 to 12 (317–789 km), t2: stage 15 to 24 (1,003 to 1,635 km). F, finishers; ITT, t-test for independent samples; MI, magnetic imaging; NF, non-finishers; SAST, somatic adipose soft tissue; SLT, somatic lean tissue; TAT, total adipose tissue; TERF09, Transeurope Footrace 2009; TLT, total lean tissue; TSV, total somatic volume; TVV, total visceral volume; VAT, visceral adipose tissue; VLT, visceral lean tissue.
Bold numbers mark significant *P*-values.

acquire specific characteristics and levels regarding body composition and performance skills even before the race if they want to have a good chance to finish: VAT near 20% to 21%, training volumes of more than 100 km/week one year before the race and the performance intensity of 7.5 km/hour at a minimum allowing specific ultra-race records of less than 5 hours in 50 km-races or more than 178 km in 24-hour races. In other words, if these levels of prerace performance are reached for at least 15 months before the transcontinental race, the VAT (and SAST, TAT) as the sensible marker for specific body composition adaptation is also in an optimal range for low risk of non-finishing, because these parameters correlate in a mostly high level.

Because the subjects mainly fall out of the race due to overuse injuries in the myotendinous fascial system of the lower extremities, we tend to assume that the mentioned interdependent parameters of body composition and prerace ultra-running performance, lead to overuse injuries in the main stressed musculoskeletal organs, if they are not highly adapted as mentioned above; too little specific ultra endurance adaption and too much of VAT (and SAST) results in a high risk of severe soft tissue overuse in the legs and mostly happens in the early phase (Figure 15) of a transcontinental foot race.

Nearly every starter of TEFR09 showed, more or less often, overuse soft tissue problems of the myotendinous

Table 8 Analysis of the difference in relative volume changes (%) at MI t1 and t2 compared to start between F/NF for total, lean and adipose tissue compartments

	t1 versus t0: $n_F = 11$, $n_{NF} = 9$		t2 versus t0: $n_F = 11$, $n_{NF} = 7$	
	Mean diff. of relative changes (%)	*P* value (ITT)	Mean diff. of relative changes (%)	*P* value (ITT)
TV	0.47	0.608	−1.49	0.306
TSV	0.41	0.690	−2.06	0.190
TVV	0.69	0.640	1.35	0.410
TLT	1.09	0332	−0.18	0.913
SLT	1.34	0.319	−0.21	0.917
VLT	0.07	0.923	−0.24	0.545
TAT	−4.86	0.086	−9.52	0.078
SAST	−6.93	**0.031**[a]	−14.27	**0.046**[a]
VAT	−8.92	0.191	−8.88	0.276

[a]mean differences between finishers and non-finishers are significant. F, finishers; ITT, t-test for independent samples; measurement interval; NF, non-finishers; SAST, somatic adipose soft tissue; SLT, somatic lean tissue; t0, at start of TEFR09; t1,stage 5 to 12 (317 to 789 km); t2, stage 15 to 24 (1,003-1,635 km); TAT, total adipose tissue; TEFR09, Transeurope Footrace 2009; TLT, total lean tissue; TSV, total somatic volume; TV, total volume; TVV, total visceral volume; VAT, visceral adipose tissue; VLT, visceral lean tissue.
Bold numbers mark significant *P*-values.

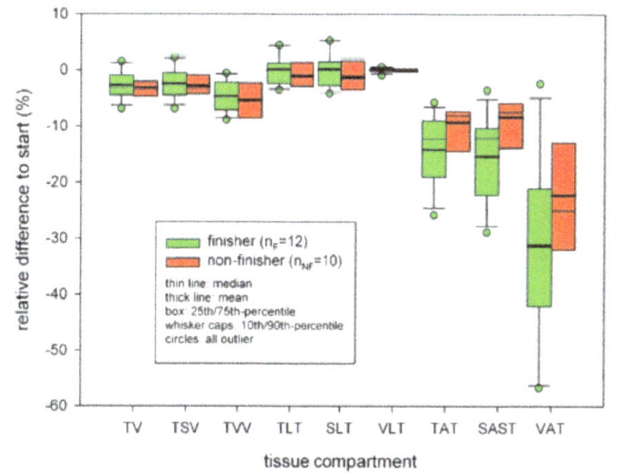

Figure 17 Difference between F and NF regarding relative volume changes of tissue compartments at first measurement interval (t1) of TEFR09. F, finishers; NF, non-finishers; TEFR09, Transeurope Footrace 2009.

Table 9 Endurance running history of subjects (n = 22)

	Mean	SD	95%-percentile	Range
Years of regular endurance running	17.4	7.6	6.3 to 31.8	6 to 32
M finished (number)	123,1	218,2	2 to 297.8	2 to 988
UM finished (number)	90,8	68	11.3 to 248.9	11 to 255
MSUM finished (number])	6,3	2,9	1.3 to 13.6	1 to 14
	Endurance training extent 2008 (one year before TEFR)			
Annual running distance (km/year)	5,468	1,720	3,000 to 9,000	2,580 to 9,152
PRT08 volume (km/week)	105.1	32.4	50.8 to 175.4	50 to 176
PRT08 time (hours/week)	12.5	3.1	7.1 to 19.6	7 to 20
PRT08 intensity (km/hour)	8.3	1.5	6.5 to 10.9	7 to 11
	Endurance training extent last two months before TEFR			
Total running distance ([km)	898	267	500 to 1260	500 to 1,500
PRT09 volume (km/week)	110.5	33.8	60.5 to 186	60 to 190
PRT09 time (hours/week)	13.2	3.5	8 to 21.6	8 to 22

M, marathon; MSUM, multistage ultramarathon; PR, prerace; TEFR, Transeurope Footrace; UM, ultramarathon.

fascial structures of the legs during the race, but the feet are not a region for problems for experienced endurance runners in a MSUM [69]. So the immense amount of mechanical stress on the musculoskeletal system when running nearly two marathons daily over a period of nine weeks can lead to these overuse syndromes without the obligatory necessity of prevalent (intrinsic) factors, such as 'overweight' (high VAT), suboptimal ultra-endurance prerace performance or mal-alignment of the legs (which was only seen in one female subject suffering from a bunion). The majority of the participants was able to 'overrun' more or less severe overuse soft tissue syndromes in the legs and reached the finish line [2]. This indicates, that, despite the mentioned somatic parameters, other mentally based factors, such as pain resistance and personality traits, are also relevant for

Table 10 Distribution type and analyses of the difference between F/NF regarding prerace performance indices

	Values			Mean (SD)		Test on normal distribution Shapiro-Wilk [29]		Test on difference F/NF	
	Valid	Missing							
	n	n	(%)	F	NF	statistic	*P*	test type[a]	*P* [b]
PRY (years)	21	1	4.5	16.5	18.7	0.936	0.185[c]	ITT	0.530
n_F M (n)	19	3	13.6	81.5	194.3	0.481	0.000	MWU	0.211
n_F UM (n)	22	0	0	94.8	86.0	0.858	0.005	MWU	0.895
n_F MSUM (n)	22	0	0	7.0	5.4	0.936	0.165[c]	ITT	0.146
PRT_{Vol08} (km/week)	21	1	4.5	**117.9** (34.3)	**88.0** (20.8)	0.959	0.505[c]	ITT	**0.032**[d]
PRT_{Time08} (hour/week)	21	1	4.5	13.0	11.9	0.971	0.761[c]	ITT	0.427
PRT_{Int08} (km/hour)	22	0	0	**9.0** (1.47)	**7.5** (0.93)	0.909	0.044	MWU	**0.040**[d]
PRT_{Vol09} (km/week)	21	1	4.5	**126.1** (35.2)	**89.7** (17.4)	0.956	0.435[c]	ITT	**0.010**[d]
PRT_{Time09} (hours/week)	21	1	4.5	14.2	12.0	0.947	0.303[c]	ITT	0.159
PRR_M (hours)	15	7	31.8	3.1	3.1	0.851	0.018	MWU	0.676
PRR_{50km} (hours)	9	13	59.1	**4.3** (0.57)	**5.1** (0.26)	0.914	0.343[c]	ITT	**0.026**[d]
PRR_{100km} (hours)	17	5	22.7	9.5	10.4	0.933	0.248[c]	ITT	0.241
PRR_{6hr} (km)	13	9	40.9	67.9	59.7	0.918	0.238[c]	ITT	0.218
PRR_{12hr} (km)	10	12	54.5	99.9	87.3	0.940	0.548[c]	ITT	0.558
PRR_{24hr} (km)	16	6	27.3	**199.8** (22.5)	**168.5** (26.0)	0.961	0.672[c]	ITT	**0.036**[d]

[a]ITT: independent t-test; [b]bilateral (asymptotic) test; [c]significance not shown (P >0.05): normal distribution accepted; [d]mean differences between finishers and non-finishers are significant. F, finishers; M, marathon; MSUM, multistage ultramarathon; MWU: Mann–Whitney-U test; n, number; NF, non-finishers; PRR, prerace records; PRT, prerace training; PRY, years of regular endurance running; IM, ultramarathon.
Bold numbers mark significant *P*-values of the test on difference between F and NF.

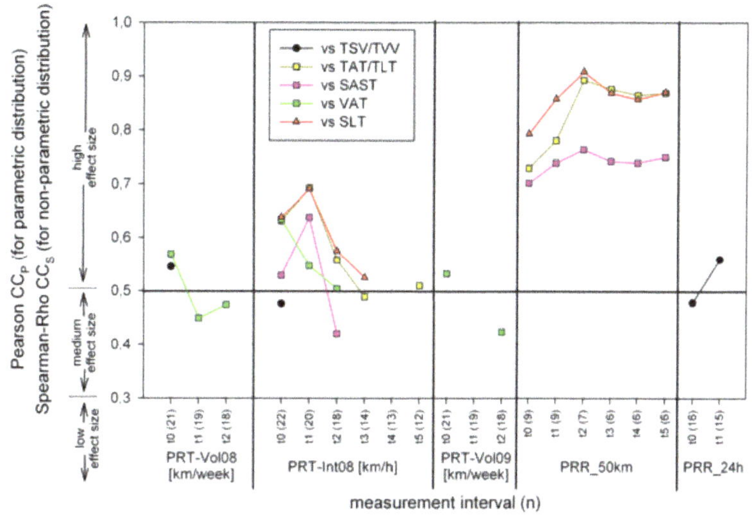

Figure 18 **Correlation (one-tailed test) of percentage volumes and prerace performance.**

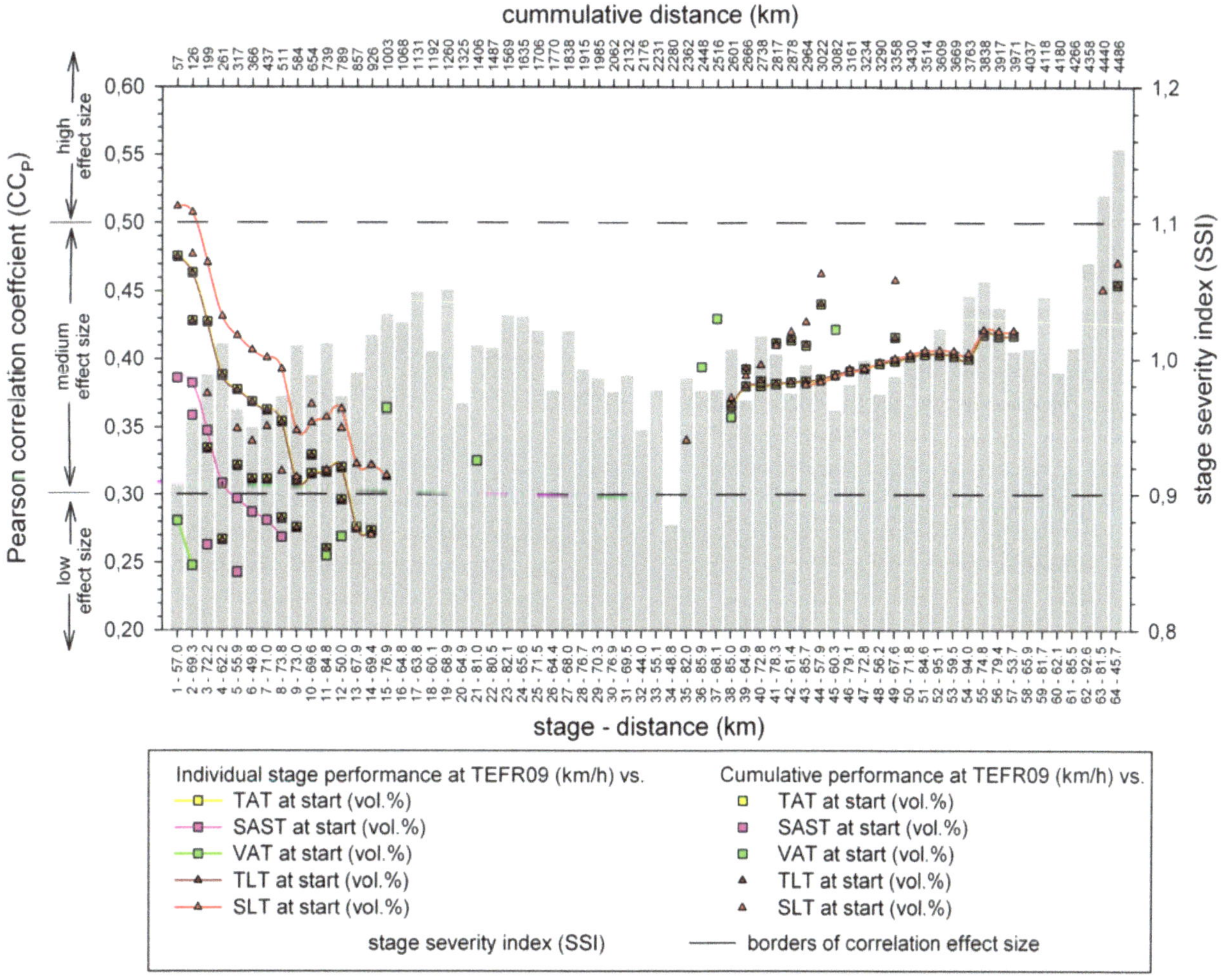

Figure 19 **Correlation of adipose and lean volumes at start with performance at TEFR09.** TEFR09, Transeurope Footrace 2009.

finishing or non-finishing a transcontinental footrace [70]. One subject (male, 61 years old) had to stop the race after stage 38 (2,601 km run) due to a high tibial stress fracture which was detected in a specific MRI on at this day (Figure 15). The astonishing thing is not the stress fracture, because this can happen to every ultra runner when starting a transcontinental race, but the fact that the major pain and massive performance (running velocity) loss had already started at stage 36. This subject ran 228 km (three stages) with a complete high tibial fracture before stopping the race, because he interpreted the pain as a soft tissue injury due to overuse and tried to 'overrun' it before he asked for MRI control. Another participant (female, 46 years old) showed the same behavior when running 208 km (stage 46 to 48) with a ventral pelvic ring stress fracture before diagnosis could be done with mobile MRI [2]. These examples and our prerace test on pain tolerance demonstrate that the resilience of the ultra athletes regarding pain is significantly higher than in a normal control group [70].

Body composition and performance

In specific treadmill investigations under laboratory settings, Millet *et al.* showed that a good single ultramarathon performance needs specific running economy depending on the ability of maximal oxygen uptake being highly correlated with citrate synthase activity and capillary network [71]. These physiological factors have not been investigated directly under race conditions in ultra-endurance events until now. Concerning this matter, only indirect parameters, such as anthropometric characteristics, are examined.

Several anthropometric factors are reported to affect performance in runners, but the presented data are inconsistent and often contradictory. Such differences are also present in the specific literature regarding anthropometrical predictors of performance outcome in ultra-marathons. Several factors are responsible for this. The numbers of volunteers are different, and in most reports they are limited and differ in gender and ethnic origin. Furthermore, the investigations are based on manifoldly different types of UM races. They can differ in the distance of running and number of stages, but also in altitude and/or external conditions.

Anthropometric parameters related to good performance are different in marathons and middle distance (half-marathon, 10 km) events [72]. Knechtle *et al.* reported that anthropometry is not associated with performance in single mono-stage UM races (24 hours [73]).

In MSUM Knechtle *et al.* found no correlation between BM or body fat (BIA) and race performance in a 17-stage MSUM ('Deutschlandlauf 2007', 1,200 km) [68]. In a cohort of 392 athletes, Hoffman found a significant relationship of BMI to finishing times in mono-stage UM running (161 km UM) [74]. In single marathon runners abdominal and front thigh SF are correlated [75]. The sum of eight SF-locations correlated significantly to 100 km race-time in a survey of three races in Knechtle *et al.* [76].

According to our results with a group of 22 subjects and using gold standard whole body MRI, in athletes taking part in a 64-day MSUM there are no relevant correlations between total volume, percentage fat and lean volumes of different compartments at the start and total race performance of subjects participating in TEFR09. For SAST, a significant correlation between percentage volume at the start and cumulative performance is seen at the beginning of TEFR09 (stages 1 to 8), but only at a medium to low effect size. Correlation of percentage fat and lean volumes to performance at the individual stages could only be shown in a few stages at a medium to low effect size. Looking at percentage volume distribution, the participants already started with a low percentage of body fat. Therefore, our results might confirm earlier findings of a negative relationship between the amount of subcutaneous fat tissue (thickness or volume), being the main fat tissue compartment of the body, and performance in single or multiday ultramarathon races. However, in a multistage ultramarathon over thousands of kilometers we found no relationship between body fat percentage or BM or BV and race performance using specific whole body MRI, as Knechtle *et al.* did with BIA [68]. The majority of transcontinental MSUM participants ran not for winning but for finishing the race; therefore, running velocity was a priority only for a few of them. For single UM races, the race time and, therefore, the performance plays a more important role for the ultra-athletes, and body composition and fat distribution have a more significant influence, respectively.

Similar interpretation has to be done, when looking at segmental (somatic) tissue changes in the arms, legs and trunk during TEFR09. As for adipose and lean total somatic and visceral volumes (Figure 19), we also did an analysis of the relationship between segmental tissue volume changes and race performance (results not demonstrated graphically) and detected only a small to low medium effect size for correlations between SAST of all segments (UE, TR, LE) with cumulative race performance in the first eight stages of TEFR09. So, in our investigation, all segments show a significant relationship to race performance that is similar to that of SAST over all (Figure 19) without any exceptional segment findings, which explains the inconstant finding in the literature. Knechtle *et al.* [77] found an association between triceps SF thickness and performance in female 100 km ultrarunners. Tanaka and Matsuura mentioned this for CF of the thigh in the early eighties [78].

Some ultra athletes show adaption to the intense running burden of TEFR09 with muscle (SLT) increase in the legs, although they are already specialized in ultra running. These findings were not significant in the mean. For the trunk, a mean increase of SLT could also be detected in the first third of the race. This is explained by the gluteal and psoas muscles, which are part of the active motor system of the lower extremities but anatomically are placed in the trunk in our segmentation. All lean tissue segments showed a decrease in their volumes towards the end of TEFR09, indicating the high negative energy burden of transcontinental running.

Metabolic changes

After the first thousand kilometers the mean loss of TV per km, mainly caused by the SAST and VAT decrease, declined constantly up to more than half until the end of race (Figure 11). Despite lack of documentation of the nutrition and caloric intake but knowing that the subjects tried to ensure an optimum of energy intake, the decrease of fat volume loss can be explained by two factors: relevant metabolic changes regarding energy balancing [79] and improvement and optimization of running style during progression of the race. Not in multistage but in single stage ultra-running conditions such economical adaptations have already been shown by Millet *et al.* [80-82]. They could show significant changes of running mechanics and spring-mass behavior towards a higher mean step frequency (+4.9%) with shorter ground-feet contact time (−4.5%) and lower ground reaction force (−4.4%) due to functional leg length decrease (−13%) and increase of leg (+9.9%) and vertical stiffness (+8.6%) during the support phase of running between the early phase and the end of a 24-hour treadmill run [80]. Millet *et al.* speculated that these changes in running mechanics contributed to the overall limitation of the potentially harmful consequences of such a long-duration run on the subjects' musculoskeletal system. Transferred to MSUM conditions, such changes in running mechanics may also contribute to the necessity of the organism to optimize the running economy to a high-end level (as low an energy consumption as possible) due to the massive negative energy burden a transcontinental race requires. The changes Millet *et al.* [80] and other researchers had measured [83,84] describe a running technique which requires only a low muscle power, because forceful eccentric load and step length are reduced. Besides the reduction of overuse risk for the musculoskeletal system this reduces the energy demand of the organism as well [85], even if the underlying mechanisms of the relation between energy cost of running and step variability remains unclear until now. If running economy could not be sacrificed in ultramarathons [86,87] and the amount of change in running mechanics depends on the duration of running and distance towards a fatigue state, respectively [81,85], it is even mandatory in transcontinental MSUM. Every subject in the TEFR-project showed a significant loss of BM and TV throughout the race, independent of the prerace overall status of body composition and performance or nutrition behavior during the race. The massive negative energy burden of a 4,500 km MSUM is also indicated by the significant loss of the grey matter in the brain [88]. The analysis of specific laboratory markers of the required blood and urine samples may give more data about the metabolic changes during TEFR09 in the near future.

Limitations

There was no general or individual nutrition plan offered or generated for the participants of TEFR09 or subjects of the TEFR-project, respectively. The athletes had a breakfast and a dinner served in different locations at the stage destinations, but these meals were organized and oriented at the local level at the last minute. The food supply points during the stages also offered products that changed every day and the athletes took additional individual food on their own throughout the race [2]. Therefore, documentation and measurement of nutrition and caloric intake was not possible and a stringent documentation of nutrition by the subjects implied the risk of compliance problems.

Whole body mobile MRI protocols did not measure ectopic fat such as intracellular fat of organs (for example liver) and muscles (intramyocellular lipids: IMCL). For IMCL measurement, specific protocols for mobile ^{1}H-MR-spectroscopy of the muscles of the lower legs were implemented in the TEFR-project [2]. However, due to the dependence of this MR-method on a stable external magnetic field around the magnetom, the analysis of mobile^{1}H-MR-spectroscopy during TEFR09 did not lead to valid data and needed further development and implementation of post-imaging proof algorithms.

Conclusions

With this mobile MRI field study a complex change in body composition during an ultra-long MSUM could be demonstrated in detail. IAAT (VAT) shows the fastest and highest decrease compared to SAST and lean tissue compartments during TEFR09. Participants lost more than half of their adipose soft tissue and even lean tissue volume decreased (mainly skeletal muscle tissue). Without exception, every subject showed a significant loss of body volume. This indicates that running an MSUM of nearly 4,500 km without any day of rest is linked with an unpreventable chronic negative energy balance due to the massive running burden. The ratio of adipose tissue contribution between the visceral and somatic compartments has a significant influence on dropping out of the race during the first third in a MUSM due to overuse injuries of the myotendinous fascial system of the legs. Body volume or body mass and, therefore, fat volume has no correlation with the performance of ultra-athletes finishing a 64-stage UM. Two- and three-compartment methods, such as bioelectrical impedance analysers and skinfold-equations, cannot give estimations about the relationship between the visceral and somatic compartments and, therefore, cannot measure the most sensitive anthropometric predictor of not finishing a MSUM: VAT. Running economy is mandatory for trans-continental MSUM races and, even in well trained ultra-athletes, such events lead to further adaptation of running mechanics and to metabolic changes as performance analysis compared to body composition changes throughout the race indicates.

Abbreviations

ABM: Adipose bone marrow; ANOVA: Analysis of variance; BIA: Bioelectrical impedance analysis; BM: Body mass; BMI: Body mass index; CF: Body circumference; CF: Body circumference; CHESS: Chemical shift selective (imaging); CCP: Pearson correlation coefficient; CCS: Spearman-rho correlation coefficient; DEXA: Dual-energy X-ray absorptiometry; F: Finisher; IAAT: Intraabdominal adipose tissue: retroperitoneal and intraperitoneal fat depots; IMAT: Intermuscular adipose tissue; IMCL: Intramyocellular lipids; INF: Intraluminal nutrition fat in the gastrointestinal tract; LT-LE: Lean tissue volume of lower extremities; LT-TR: Lean soft tissue volume of trunk; LT-UE: Lean soft tissue volume of upper extremities; MAT: Intrathoracic, mainly mediastinal adipose tissue; max: Maximum; MI: Measurement interval; min: Minimum; MR: Magnetic resonance; MRI: Magnetic resonance imaging; MSUM: Multistage ultramarathon; NF: Non-finisher; PRY: Prerace years of regular endurance running; PRR: Prerace records; PRR_M: Prerace record in marathon; PRR_{50km}: Prerace record in 50 km-races; PRR_{100km}: Prerace record in 100 km-races; PRR_{6hr}: Prerace record in 6 hours-races; PRR_{12hr}: Prerace record in 12 hours-races; PRR_{24hr}: Prerace record in 24 hours-races; PRT: Prerace training; PRT_{Int08}: Prerace training intensity (km per week) in 2008; PRT_{Vol08}: Prerace training volume (hours per week) in 2008; PRT_{Vol09}: Prerace training volume (hours per week) in 2009; PRT_{Time08}: Prerace training hours per week in 2008; PRT_{Time09}: Prerace training hours per week in 2009; SAST: Somatic adipose soft tissue; SAT: Somatic adipose tissue; SCAT: Subcutaneous adipose tissue; SD: Standard deviation; SF: Skinfold thickness; SLT: Somatic lean tissue: mostly muscles; TAST: Total adipose soft tissue; TAT: Total adipose tissue; TEFR09: Transeurope Footrace 2009; TEFR-project: Transeurope Footrace Project; TLT: Total lean tissue; TSV: Total somatic volume; TV: Total volume of the body; TV-LE: Total volume of lower extremities; TV-TR: Total volume of trunk; TV-UE: Total volume of upper extremities; TVV: Total visceral volume; UM: Ultramarathon; VAT: Visceral adipose tissue; VLT: Visceral lean tissue: includes lean tissue of intrathoracic and intraabdominal organs.

Competing interests

The authors declare they have no competing interests.

Authors' contributions

All authors of this manuscript made substantial contributions to the conception and design or acquisition, analysis and interpretation of data; all revised it critically for important intellectual content and gave final approval to the version to be published. SUHW conceived the study, implemented the project, participated in the data collection (MRI measurements), data evaluation with statistical analysis and drafted the manuscript. BC participated in the implementation of the project and in the data collection (MRI measurements). KK participated in the data evaluation. WC participated in the data evaluation. WH participated mainly in the data collection (MRI measurements) and in the implementation of the project. BHJ participated in the implementation of the project. MJ participated in the design of the study, its technical implementation and data evaluation. All authors read and approved the final manuscript.

Acknowledgements

We really want to thank all the athletes of TEFR09 who took part at this project. Considering their immense physical and mental stress they showed an extraordinary compliance on every day of the race.

Financial disclosure

This work is supported in part by the German Research Association (DFG: "Deutsche Forschungsgemeinschaft"), under Grants SCHU 2514/1-1 and SCHU 2514/1-2. The funders had no role in study design, data collection and analysis, decision to publish, or preparation of the manuscript. No additional external funding was received for this study.

Author details

[1]Department of Diagnostic and Interventional Radiology, University Hospital of Ulm, Albert-Einstein-Allee 23, 89081, Ulm, Germany. [2]Outpatient Rehabilitation Centre at University Hospital of Ulm, Pfarrer-Weiß-Weg 10, 89073, Ulm, Germany. [3]Section on Experimental Radiology, Department of Diagnostic and Interventional Radiology, University Hospital of Tübingen, Tübingen, Germany. [4]Institute for Diabetes Research and Metabolic Diseases (IDM), Metabolic Imaging – of the Helmholtz Center Munich at University of Tübingen (Paul Langerhaus Institute Tübingen), Tübingen, Germany.

References

1. Knechtle B, Enggist A, Jehle T: **Energy turnover at the Race across America (RAAM): a case report.** *Int J Sports Med* 2005, **26**:499–503.
2. Schütz UH, Schmidt-Trucksäss A, Knechtle B, Machann J, Ehrhardt M, Wiedelbach H, Freund W, Gröninger S, Brunner H, Schulze I, Brambs HJ, Billich C: **The Transeurope Footrace Project: Longitudinal data acquisition in a cluster randomized mobile MRI observational cohort study on 44 endurance runners at a 64-stage 4,486km transcontinental ultramarathon.** *BMC Med* 2012, **19**:78.
3. *Transeurope Footrace.* http://www.transeurope-footrace.org.
4. Schulze I: *TransEurope-FootRace 2009: Bari - Nordkap - 4.487,7 km in 64 Tagesetappen.* 1st edition. Leipzig, Germany: Engelsdorfer Verlag; 2010.
5. Brodie DA, Stewart AD: **Body composition measurement: a hierarchy of methods.** *J Pediatr Endocrinol Metab* 1999, **12**:801–816.
6. Lee RC, Wang Z, Heo M, Ross R, Janssen I, Heymsfield SB: **Total-body skeletal muscle mass: development and cross-validation of anthropometric prediction models.** *Am J Clin Nutr* 2000, **72**:796–803.
7. Janssen I, Heymsfield SB, Baumgartner RN, Ross R: **Estimation of skeletal muscle mass by bioelectrical impedance analysis.** *J Appl Physiol* 2000, **89**:465–471.
8. Chan DC, Watts GF, Barrett PHR, Burke V: **Waist circumference, waist-to-hip ratio and body mass index as predictors of adipose tissue compartments in men.** *QJM* 2003, **96**:441–447.
9. Gualdi-Russo E, Toselli S: **Influence of various factors on the measurement of multifrequency bioimpedance.** *Homo* 2002, **53**:1–16.
10. Lee SY, Gallagher D: **Assessment methods in human body composition.** *Curr Opin Clin Nutr Metab Care* 2008, **11**:566–572.
11. Daniel JA, Sizer PS Jr, Latman NS: **Evaluation of body composition methods for accuracy.** *Biomed Instrum Technol* 2005, **39**:397–405.
12. Vasudev S, Mohan A, Mohan D, Farooq S, Raj D, Mohan V: **Validation of body fat measurement by skin folds and two bioelectric impedance methods with DEXA – the Chennai Urban Rural Epidemiology Study (CURES-3).** *J Assoc Physicians India* 2004, **52**:877–881.
13. Broeder CE, Burrhus KA, Svanevik LS, Volpe J, Wilmore JH: **Assessing body composition before and after resistance or endurance training.** *Med Sci Sports Exerc* 1997, **29**:705–712.
14. Vogt FM, Ruehm S, Hunold P, de Greiff A, Nuefer M, Barkhausen J, Ladd SC: **Rapid total body fat measurement by magnetic resonance imaging: quantification and topography.** *Rofo* 2007, **179**:480–486.
15. Ross R, Léger L, Morris D, de Guise J, Guardo R: **Quantification of adipose tissue by MRI: relationship with anthropometric variables.** *J Appl Physiol* 1992, **72**:787–795.
16. Thomas EL, Saeed N, Hajnal JV, Brynes A, Goldstone AP, Frost G, Bell JD: **Magnetic resonance imaging of total body fat.** *J Appl Physiol* 1998, **85**:1778–1785.

17. Ludescher B, Machann J, Eschweiler GW, Vanhöfen S, Maenz C, Thamer C, Claussen CD, Schick F: **Correlation of fat distribution in whole body MRI with generally used anthropometric data.** *Invest Radiol* 2009, **44**:712–719.
18. Abate N, Burns D, Peshock RM, Garg A, Grundy SM: **Estimation of adipose tissue mass by magnetic resonance imaging: validation against dissection in human cadavers.** *J Lipid Res* 1994, **35**:1490–1496.
19. Ross R, Shaw KD, Martel Y, de Guise J, Avruch L: **Adipose tissue distribution measured by magnetic resonance imaging in obese women.** *Am J Clin Nutr* 1993, **57**:470–475.
20. Poon CS, Szumowski J, Plewes DB, Ashby P, Henkelman RM: **Fat/water quantitation and differential relaxation time measurement using chemical shift imaging technique.** *Magn Reson Imaging* 1989, **7**:369–382.
21. Lunati E, Marzola P, Nicolato E, Sbarbati A: **In-vivo quantitative hydrolipidic map of perirenal adipose tissue by chemical shift imaging at 4.7 Tesla.** *Int J Obes Relat Metab Disord* 2001, **25**:457–461.
22. Schick F, Machann J, Brechtel K, Strempfer A, Klumpp B, Stein DT, Jacob S: **MRI of muscular fat.** *Magn Reson Med* 2002, **47**:720–727.
23. Huang TY, Chung HW, Wang FN, Ko CW, Chen CY: **Fat and water separation in balanced steady-state free precession using the Dixon method.** *Magn Reson Med* 2004, **51**:243–247.
24. Donnelly LF, O'Brien KJ, Dardzinski BJ, Poe SA, Bean JA, Holland SK, Daniels SR: **Using a phantom to compare MR techniques for determining the ratio of intraabdominal to subcutaneous adipose tissue.** *AJR Am J Roentgenol* 2003, **180**:993–998.
25. Machann J, Thamer C, Schnoedt B, Haap M, Haring HU, Claussen CD, Stumvoll M, Fritsche A, Schick F: **Standardized assessment of whole body adipose tissue topography by MRI.** *J Magn Reson Imaging* 2005, **21**:455–462.
26. Würslin C, Machann J, Rempp H, Claussen C, Yang B, Schick F: **Topography mapping of whole body adipose tissue using a fully automated and standardized procedure.** *J Magn Reson Imaging* 2010, **31**:430–439.
27. Stephens MA: **Test of fit for the logistic distribution based on the empirical distribution function.** *Biometrika* 1979, **66**:591–595.
28. D'Agostino RB, Belanger A, D'Agostino RB Jr: **A suggestion for using powerful and informative test of normality.** *Am Stat* 1990, **44**:316–321.
29. Yazici B, Yolacan S: **A comparison of various tests of normality.** *J Stat Comput Simul* 2007, **77**:175–183.
30. Cohen J: **A power primer.** *Psychol Bull* 1992, **112**:155–159.
31. Boettcher M, Machann J, Stefan N, Thamer C, Häring HU, Claussen CD, Fritsche A, Schick F: **Intermuscular adipose tissue (IMAT): association with other adipose tissue compartments and insulin sensitivity.** *J Magn Reson Imaging* 2009, **29**:1340–1345.
32. Gray DS, Fujioka K, Colletti PM, Kim H, Devine W, Cuyegkeng T, Pappas T: **Magnetic-resonance imaging used for determining fat distribution in obesity and diabetes.** *Am J Clin Nutr* 1991, **54**:623–627.
33. Bale P, Rowell S, Colley E: **Anthropometric and training characteristics of female marathon runners as determinants of distance running performance.** *J Sports Sci* 1985, **3**:115–126.
34. Raschka C, Plath M: **Body fat compartment and its relationship to food intake and clinical chemical parameters during extreme endurance performance.** *Schweiz Z Sportmed* 1992, **40**:13–25.
35. Reynolds RD, Lickteig JA, Deuster PA, Howard MP, Conway JM, Pietersma A, De Stoppelaar J, Deurenberg P: **Energy metabolism increases and regional body fat decreases while regional muscle mass is spared in humans climbing Mt.** *Everest. J Nutr* 1999, **129**:1307–1314.
36. Helge JW, Lundby C, Christensen DL, Langfort J, Messonnier L, Zacho M, Andersen JL, Saltin B: **Skiing across the Greenland icecap: divergent effects on limb muscle adaptations and substrate oxidation.** *J Exp Biol* 2003, **206**:1075–1083.
37. Frykman PN, Harman EA, Opstad PK, Hoyt RW, DeLany JP, Friedl KE: **Effects of a 3-month endurance event on physical performance and body composition: the G2 trans-Greenland expedition.** *Wilderness Environ Med* 2003, **14**:240–248.
38. Höchli D, Schneiter T, Ferretti G, Howald H, Claassen H, Moia C, Atchou G, Belleri M, Veicsteinas A, Hoppeler H: **Loss of muscle oxidative capacity after an extreme endurance run: the Paris-Dakar Foot-Race.** *Int J Sports Med* 1995, **16**:343–346.
39. Knechtle B, Knechtle P, Andonie JL, Kohler G: **Influence of anthropometry on race performance in extreme endurance triathletes: World Challenge Deca Iron Triathlon 2006.** *Br J Sports Med* 2007, **41**:644–648.
40. Bircher S, Enggist A, Jehle T: **Effects of an extreme endurance race on energy balance and body composition: a case study.** *J Sports Sci Med* 2006, **5**:154–162.
41. Lehmann M, Huonker M, Dimeo F: **Serum amino acid concentrations in nine athletes before and after the 1993 Colmar Ultra Triathlon.** *Int J Sports Med* 1995, **16**:155–159.
42. Knechtle B, Bircher S: **Changes in body composition during an extreme endurance run.** *Praxis* 2005, **94**:371–377.
43. Dressendorfer RH, Wade CE: **Effects of a 15-d race on plasma steroid levels and leg muscle fitness in runners.** *Med Sci Sports Exerc* 1991, **23**:954–958.
44. Nagel D, Seiler D, Franz H, Leitzmann C, Jung K: **Effects of an ultra-long-distance (1000 km) race on lipid metabolism.** *Eur J Appl Physiol* 1989, **59**:16–20.
45. Väänänen II, Vihko V: **Physiological and psychological responses to 100 km crosscountry skiing during 2 days.** *J Sports Med Phys Fitness* 2005, **45**:301–305.
46. Raschka C, Plath M, Cerull R, Bernhard W, Jung K, Leitzmann C: **The body muscle compartment and its relationship to food absorption and blood chemistry during an extreme endurance performance.** *Z Ernährungswiss* 1991, **30**:276–288.
47. Knechtle B, Salas OF, Andonie JL, Kohler G: **Effect of a multistage ultra-endurance triathlon on body composition: World Challenge Deca Iron Triathlon 2006.** *Br J Sports Med* 2008, **42**:121–125.
48. Knechtle B, Duff B, Schule I, Kohler G: **A multi-stage ultra-endurance run over 1,200 km leads to a continuous accumulations of total body water.** *J Sports Sci Med* 2008, **7**:357–364.
49. Martin AD, Daniel MZ, Drinkwater DT, Clarys JP: **Adipose tissue density, estimated adipose lipid fraction and whole body adiposity in male cadavers.** *Int J Obes Relat Metab Disord* 1994, **18**:79–83.
50. Mernagh JR, Harrison JE, Krondl A, McNeill KG, Shepard RJ: **Composition of lean tissue in healthy volunteers for nutritional studies in health and disease.** *Nutrition Res* 1986, **6**:499–507.
51. Wells JC, Williams JE, Chomtho S, Darch T, Grijalva-Eternod C, Kennedy K, Haroun D, Wilson C, Cole TJ, Fewtrell MS: **Pediatric reference data for lean tissue properties: density and hydration from age 5 to 20 y.** *Am J Clin Nutr* 2010, **91**:610–618.
52. Schutte JE, Townsend EJ, Hugg J, Shoup RF, Malina RM, Blomqvist CG: **Density of lean body mass is greater in blacks than in whites.** *J Appl Physiol* 1984, **56**:1647–1649.
53. Enzi G, Digito M, Marin R, Carraro R, Baritussio A, Manzato E: **Mediastino-abdominal lipomatosis: deep accumulation of fat mimicking a respiratory disease and ascites. Clinical aspects and metabolic studies in vitro.** *Q J Med* 1984, **53**:453–463.
54. Brochu M, Starling RD, Tchernof A, Matthews DE, Garcia-Rubi E, Poehlman ET: **Visceral adipose tissue is an independent correlate of glucose disposal in older obese postmenopausal women.** *J Clin Endocrinol Metab* 2000, **85**:2378–2384.
55. Kahn BB, Flier JS: **Obesity and insulin resistance.** *J Clin Invest* 2000, **106**:473–481.
56. Wajchenberg BL: **Subcutaneous and visceral adipose tissue: their relation to the metabolic syndrome.** *Endocr Rev* 2000, **21**:697–738.
57. Sironi AM, Gastaldelli A, Mari A, Ciociaro D, Postano V, Buzzigoli E, Ghione S, Turchi S, Lomabardi M, Ferrannini E: **Visceral fat in hypertension: influence on insulin resistance and β-cell function.** *Hypertension* 2004, **44**:127–133.
58. Yusuf S, Hawken S, Ounpuu S, Dans T, Avezum A, Lanas F, McQueen M, Budaj A, Pais P, Varigos J, Lisheng L, INTERHEART Study Investigators: **Effect of potentially modifiable risk factors associated with myocardial infarction in 52 countries (the INTERHEART study): case–control study.** *Lancet* 2004, **364**:937–952.
59. Montague CT, O'Rahilly S: **The perils of portliness: causes and consequences of visceral adiposity.** *Diabetes* 2000, **49**:883–888.
60. Kern PA, Ranganathan S, Li C, Wood L, Ranganathan G: **Adipose tissue tumor necrosis factor and interleukin-6 expression in human obesity and insulin resistance.** *Am J Physiol Endocrinol Metab* 2001, **280**:E745–E751.
61. Marette A: **Molecular mechanisms of inflammation in obesity-linked insulin resistance.** *Int J Obes Relat Metab Disord* 2003, **27**:S46–S48.
62. Sharma AM: **Mediastinal fat, insulin resistance, and hypertension.** *Hypertension* 2004, **44**:117–118.
63. Lee WJ, Fattal G: **Mediastinal lipomatosis in simple obesity.** *Chest* 1976, **70**:308–309.

64. Price JE Jr, Rigler LG: **Widening of the mediastinum resulting from fat accumulation.** *Radiology* 1970, **96**:497–500.
65. Stummvoll HK, Wolf A, Pinggera WF, Lobenwein E, Seidl G: **Rare localizations of fat deposition in iatrogenous Cushing's syndrome.** *Munch Med Wochenschr* 1976, **118**:445–446.
66. Kopelman PG: **The effects of weight loss treatments on upper and lower body fat.** *Int J Obes Relat Metab Disord* 1997, **21**:619–625.
67. Martin AD, Janssens V, Caboor D, Clarys JP, Marfell-Jones MJ: **Relationships between visceral, trunk and whole-body adipose tissue weights by cadaver dissection.** *Ann Hum Biol* 2003, **30**:668–677.
68. Knechtle B, Duff B, Schulze I, Rosemann T, Senn O: **Anthropometry and pre-race experience of finishers and nonfinishers in a multistage ultra-endurance run–Deutschlandlauf 2007.** *Percept Mot Skills* 2009, **109**:105–118.
69. Freund W, Weber F, Billich C, Schütz UH: **The foot in multistage ultra marathon runners: Experience in a cohort study of 22 participants of the Trans Europe Footrace project with mobile MRI.** *BMJ Open* 2012, **2**. doi:10.1136/bmjopen-2012-001118.
70. Freund W, Weber F, Billich C, Birklein F, Breimhorst M, Schütz UH: **Ultra marathon runners are different. Investigations into pain tolerance and personality traits of participants of the TransEurope FootRace 2009.** *Pain Pract* 2013. doi:10.1111/papr.12039.
71. Millet GY, Banfi JC, Kerherve H, Morin JB, Vincent L, Estrade C, Geyssant A, Feasson L: **Physiological and biological factors associated with a 24 h treadmill ultra-marathon performance.** *Scand J Med Sci Sports* 2011, **21**:54–61.
72. Maldonado S, Mujika I, Padilla S: **Influence of body mass and height on the energy cost of running in highly trained middle- and long-distance runners.** *Int J Sports Med* 2002, **23**:268–272.
73. Knechtle B, Wirth A, Knechtle P, Zimmermann K, Kohler G: **Personal best marathon performance is associated with performance in a 24-h run and not anthropometry or training volume.** *Br J Sports Med* 2009, **43**:836–839.
74. Hoffman MD: **Anthropometric characteristics of ultramarathoners.** *Int J Sports Med* 2008, **29**:808–811.
75. Arrese AL, Ostáriz ES: **Skinfold thicknesses associated with distance running performance in highly trained runners.** *J Sports Sci* 2006, **24**:69–76.
76. Knechtle B, Knechtle P, Rosemann T, Senn O: **What is associated with race performance in male 100-km ultra-marathoners - anthropometry, training or marathon best time?** *J Sports Sci* 2011, **23**:1–7.
77. Knechtle B, Knechtle P, Rosemann T, Lepers R: **Predictor variables for a 100 km race time in female ultra-marathoners.** *Medicina Sportiva* 2010, **14**:214–220.
78. Tanaka K, Matsuura Y: **A multivariate analysis of the role of certain anthropometric and physiological attributes in distance running.** *Ann Hum Biol* 1982, **9**:473–482.
79. Tomaszewski M, Charchar FJ, Przybycin M, Crawford L, Wallace AM, Gosek K, Lowe GD, Zukowska-Szczechowska E, Grzeszczak W, Sattar N, Dominiczak AF: **Strikingly low circulating CRP concentrations in ultramarathon runners independent of markers of adiposity: how low can you go?** *Arterioscler Thromb Vasc Biol* 2003, **23**:1640–1644.
80. Morin JB, Samozino P, Millet GY: **Changes in running kinematics, kinetics, and spring-mass behavior over a 24-h run.** *Med Sci Sports Exerc* 2011, **43**:829–836.
81. Degache F, Guex K, Fourchet F, Morin JB, Millet GP, Tomazin K, Millet GY: **Changes in running mechanics and spring-mass behaviour induced by a 5-hour hilly running bout.** *J Sports Sci* 2013, **31**:299–304.
82. Borrani F, Candau R, Perrey S, Millet GY, Millet GP, Rouillon JD: **Does the mechanical work in running change during the VO2 slow component?** *Med Sci Sports Exerc* 2003, **35**:50–57.
83. Brisswalter J, Legros P, Durand M: **Running economy, preferred step length correlated to body dimensions in elite middle distance runners.** *J Sports Med Phys Fitness* 1996, **36**:7–15.
84. Svedenhag J, Sjödin B: **Body-mass-modified running economy and step length in elite male middle- and long-distance runners.** *Int J Sports Med* 1994, **15**:305–310.
85. Candau R, Belli A, Millet GY, Georges D, Barbier B, Rouillon JD: **Energy cost and running mechanics during a treadmill run to voluntary exhaustion in humans.** *Eur J Appl Physiol Occup Physiol* 1998, **77**:479–485.
86. Millet GP: **Economy is not sacrificed in ultramarathon runners.** *J Appl Physiol* 2012, **113**:686.
87. Millet GY, Hoffman MD, Morin JB: **Sacrificing economy to improve running performance–a reality in the ultramarathon?** *J Appl Physio* 2012, **113**:507–509.
88. Freund W, Faust S, Birklein F, Gaser C, Wunderlich AP, Mueller M, Billich C, Juchems MS, Schmitz BL, Groen G, Schütz UH: **Substantial and reversible brain gray matter reduction but no acute brain lesions in ultramarathon runners: experience from the TransEurope-FootRace Project.** *BMC Med* 2012, **21**:10–170.

Cycling and bone health: a systematic review

Hugo Olmedillas[1,2†], Alejandro González-Agüero[1,2*†], Luis A Moreno[1,3], José A Casajus[1,2] and Germán Vicente-Rodríguez[1,2]

Abstract

Background: Cycling is considered to be a highly beneficial sport for significantly enhancing cardiovascular fitness in individuals, yet studies show little or no corresponding improvements in bone mass.

Methods: A scientific literature search on studies discussing bone mass and bone metabolism in cyclists was performed to collect all relevant published material up to April 2012. Descriptive, cross-sectional, longitudinal and interventional studies were all reviewed. Inclusion criteria were met by 31 studies.

Results: Heterogeneous studies in terms of gender, age, data source, group of comparison, cycling level or modality practiced among others factors showed minor but important differences in results. Despite some controversial results, it has been observed that adult road cyclists participating in regular training have low bone mineral density in key regions (for example, lumbar spine). Conversely, other types of cycling (such as mountain biking), or combination with other sports could reduce this unsafe effect. These results cannot yet be explained by differences in dietary patterns or endocrine factors.

Conclusions: From our comprehensive survey of the current available literature it can be concluded that road cycling does not appear to confer any significant osteogenic benefit. The cause of this may be related to spending long hours in a weight-supported position on the bike in combination with the necessary enforced recovery time that involves a large amount of time sitting or lying supine, especially at the competitive level.

Keywords: cyclists, osteopenia, osteoporosis, sport, training

Background

Participation in cycling has been shown to confer several health benefits in terms of improvements in cardiovascular fitness, reductions in mortality, and reduced cardiovascular risk factors as well as a reduced risk of cancer [1]. From a public health point of view, cycling is a widely practiced non-weight-bearing sport around the world, especially in Europe [2] and the bicycle is also used as a vehicle by millions of people in many different countries, accounting for an important part of their daily physical activity. However, as a non-weight-bearing activity, cycling practice is frequently associated with lower levels of bone mass [3]; in fact, two-thirds of the professional and master adult road cyclists could be classified as osteopenic [4].

* Correspondence: alexgonz@unizar.es
† Contributed equally
[1]GENUD 'Growth, Exercise, NUtrition and Development' Research Group, Universidad de Zaragoza, Zaragoza, Spain
Full list of author information is available at the end of the article

Osteoporosis generally affects older populations and is characterized by 'low bone density and microarchitectural deterioration of bone tissue with a consequent increase in bone fragility and susceptibility to fracture' [5]. Low levels of bone mineral density (BMD) during earlier stages of life may contribute to the development of osteoporosis later on in life [6].

Many aspects of bones account for bone strength and resistance against fracture: bone mineral content (BMC), BMD, bone size, structure and microarchitecture, among others [7]. Genetic predisposition, dietary patterns, endocrine and environmental factors also play determining roles in bone health and maintenance throughout life [8,9]. Among the many environmental factors, physical activity and participation in sport promote health benefits in bone mass across all ages among different populations [10-14].

With regard to endocrine factors, the net product of bone formation and bone resorption, namely bone turnover, may be estimated by biomarkers involved with bone metabolism such as bone alkaline phosphatase (BAP), osteocalcin (OC) or C-terminal collagen crosslinks (CTX), which are among the most commonly studied in sport sciences [15].

This review aims to summarize the current available literature concerning bone mass and bone metabolism in cyclists, to observe whether the findings of the collective research are commensurate with the general idea that cycling has a deleterious effect on bone mass.

Methods

Search strategy

Journal articles were identified from MedLine (1965 to April 2012), EMBASE, Web of Science and SportDiscus. The search strategy used to identify the articles was: '((bone) or (bmc) or (bmd) or (osteoporosis)) AND ((cyclist) or (cyclists) or (cycling sport) or (triathlon) or (triathletes))' to identify the articles on the topic of this review. Additional articles were added after reviewing the references of the previous researches. This produced a total of 214 citations. MOOSE [16] and PRISMA [17] guidelines for the reporting of systematic reviews were followed for observational and interventional studies respectively.

Inclusion criteria

The inclusion criteria for this review were: (a) bone mass or bone metabolism markers, and not fractures or any other topic, had to be the main subject of each study; (b) the studies had to include cyclists or triathletes and not only athletes or sportspeople; (c) the type of studies to be included had to be original research manuscripts (cross-sectional, interventional, follow-up or retrospective studies); reviews or published abstracts were not included; (d) only papers written entirely in English were included in this review.

Exclusion criteria

The inclusion criteria were applied to the 215 citations by 2 authors independently; if disagreement occurred, all authors reviewed the data until consensus was achieved. Of the total of 215 citations, 31 references fulfilled the inclusion criteria (Figure 1). A total of 184 citations were excluded for the following reasons: 145 did not include bone mass or bone metabolism markers as their main topic, 17 were not original articles and 22 were not written in English.

Data extraction

Each study was independently evaluated. General information about the article title and type of the study, author(s), characteristics of the participants (age, sex, and exercise), comparison group(s) (if available), data source and results were also extracted.

Table 1 summarizes all the studies concerning bone mass and cycling participation included in this review. Different age stages (adolescents, adults, older adults), genders, competitive levels, years of practice and groups of comparison (that is, sedentary controls, runners, and so on) were included in this review, making the comparison between studies rather difficult; however, efforts have been made to summarize and clarify the current knowledge on this topic despite discrepancies in these variables.

Strength of evidence

The guidelines of Hadorn *et al.* [18] were used to rate the quality of evidence of every study and the qualifications were also stated in Table 1. This method includes three levels of quality, as outlined below.

Level A: well conducted randomized control trials (RCT) with 100 participants or more (including multicenter and meta-analyses); well conducted RCT with fewer than 100 participants (one or more institutions and meta-analysis; well conducted study).

Level B: well conducted case-control study, poorly controlled or uncontrolled (including RCT with one or more major or three or more minor methodological flaws), observations studies with high potential for bias (case series with comparison to historical controls), case series or case reports, conflicting evidence with more support.

Level C: expert opinion

Additional file 1 evaluates the quality and strength of evidence of each study, providing a final score based on several objective questions.

Results and discussion

Cycling and bone mass

BMC and BMD

The vast majority of the reviewed studies used dual energy X-ray absorptiometry (DXA) devices for their investigations; in fact only 2 out of 31 studies did not include any DXA measurement in their results.

Heinonen *et al.*, in 1993, first described and compared bone mass of young adult female cyclists with other different sportswomen and controls. They found that cyclists had lower BMD at all body sites than weightlifters, but no differences were observed with other sports or with controls [19]. Subsequent studies reinforced the finding that no differences in BMC or BMD were observed between cyclists and controls, in both males and females, either in adolescents [20,21] or adults [22-26], or compared with other competitive sportspeople [27]. Furthermore, Warner *et al.* found that adult cross-country cyclists had higher BMD than road cyclists and controls [28].

Despite the above-mentioned studies, the available literature largely describes lower levels of BMD and BMC for different bodily regions in cyclist participants almost at all ages and in both genders. The lumbar spine has

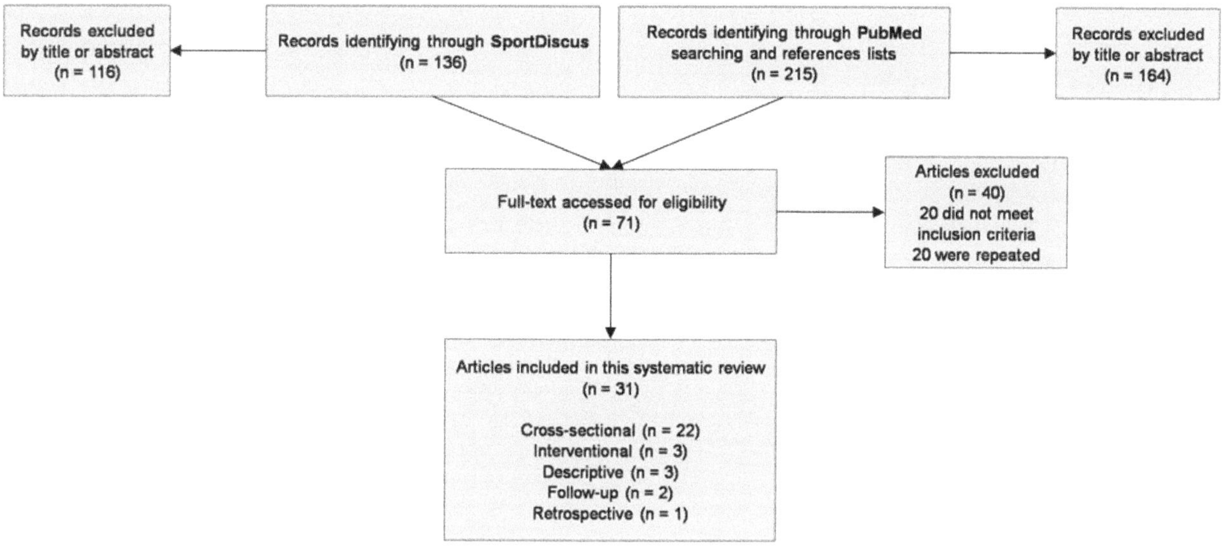

Figure 1 Flow chart diagram of the study selection process.

probably been the most studied region in this regard, with fairly conclusive results that lower BMD can be observed in cyclists compared with controls [29-35], practitioners of other sports [19,35-37] or reference values [4,38,39]. Moreover, the pelvic and hip regions, as key areas for osteoporotic fractures, and the whole body have been studied with concerning results. Lower values of pelvis, hip and femoral neck BMD in male cyclists were found compared with controls at all ages [29,32,34,40], with higher differences in the older cyclists.

Longitudinal studies may help to understand whether the observed low bone mass is acquired during a period of time and then maintained, or whether in fact, cycling training has a harmful effect on this tissue. In this regard, Beshgetoor *et al.* showed that 18 months of training in competitive female cyclist resulted in maintenance of the femur BMD, but a declination in lumbar spine BMD [41]. More recently, Nichols *et al.* showed that not only were more master cyclists classified as osteoporotic compared to age-matched and weight-matched non-athletes, but also the percentage of osteoporotic cyclists increased significantly over a 7-year period [42]. Also, Barry *et al.* studied two groups of adult cyclists supplementing them with high and low calcium intakes; they observed that the declination in hip BMD was the same in both groups [43].

Most of the studies reviewed showed that cycling does not appear to have a beneficial effect on BMD, especially at the lumbar spine, with some cases showing detrimental effects compared to other osteogenic sports. Very few studies have been conducted on child or adolescent cyclists, but the available manuscripts allow us to hypothesize that the differences in BMD become greater with age. Also, longitudinal studies point to this by showing declinations even with calcium supplementation.

Bone geometry and structure

The DXA device creates a two-dimensional image of the bone that does not provide information about volumetric BMD (vBMD) and does not differentiate cortical and trabecular bone. Osteoporosis is highly related to BMD; however, strength indexes and, therefore, the risk of fracture have a close relationship with structural aspects of bones such as cortical thickness and bone cross-sectional area, among others [44]. Peripheral quantitative computed tomography (pQCT) and magnetic resonance imaging (MRI) are alternative bone densitometry techniques that allow separate evaluation of those bone regions. These techniques are also able to assess actual vBMD at peripheral sites as well as estimating geometric properties of bone that are related to bone strength, going beyond the scope of current DXA determinations.

Two studies of this nature performed on cyclists were identified. Using MRI, Duncan *et al.* found that female adolescent cyclists had lower bone cross-sectional area, moment of inertia and mid-femur vBMD than their runner counterparts, while no differences were observed with controls [45]. Wilks *et al.* compared pQCT values of male distance-trained and sprint-trained master cyclists (aged 30 to 82 years) with age-matched sedentary controls, finding that distance-trained athletes presented higher values at the tibial sites, and sprinters at both tibial and radial sites, than controls [46].

Due to the abundance of factors contributing to bone strength, it seems that, regardless of the lower values of BMD observed in studies with DXA, cycling does not

Table 1 Studies concerning bone mass, bone metabolism and cycling participation

Study	Participants: Number	Sex	Age	Exercise	Years of cycling training	Study design	Data source	Results[a]	Strength of evidence
Barry *et al.* (2007) [47]	CYC (20)	M	22 to 45	Competitive level		2-h exercise bout at 60% to 75% VT	Hormones, calcium	Parathyroid was increased after 2 h of cycling.	B: observational
Barry *et al.* (2008) [43]	CYC (14)	M	27 to 44	>450 h/year	4.9 ± 2.4	Two groups: HIGH and LOW calcium supplementation over 1-year season	DXA	Both groups decreased BMD over 1 year in total hip and subregions, without differences for HIGH or LOW calcium.	A: RCT
Barry *et al.* (2011) [39]	CYC and TRI (20)	M	37 ± 7.6	-	6.0 ± 6.5	Different calcium supplementation groups over three 35-km trials	DXA, hormones	30% of participants had LS BMD T-score over -1.0. Calcium supplementation attenuates disruption of parathyroid hormone.	A: RCT
Beshgetoor *et al.* (2000) [41]	CYC (12); RUN (9); CON (9)	F	49.6 ± 7.9	-	-	18 months follow-up	DXA, calcium intake	Femur BMD maintained in CYC and RUN, decline CON. LS BMD maintained RUN, decline CYC and CON. No relationship between BMD and calcium intake.	B: case-control
Brown *et al.* (2000) [49]	CYC (32)	M/F	16 to 62	Competitive cycling	>2	Two groups: HIGH FAT and HIGH CARBOHYDRATE intake; 12-week intervention	DXA	No differences in fat or lean accumulation between groups. BMD increased in HIGH FAT group.	A: RCT
Campion *et al.* (2010) [34]	CYC (30) CON (30)	M	29 ± 3.4 28 ± 4.5	22 to 25 h/week <1 h/week	-	Cross-sectional	DXA	CYC lower WB, LS, pelvis, femoral neck, upper and lower limbs than CON	B: case-control
Duncan *et al.* (2002) [21]	CYC (15) RUN (15) SWI (15) TRI (15) CON (15)	F	16 to 17	≥8 h/week ≥8 h/week ≥8 h/week ≥8 h/week <2 h/week	3.1 ± 1.8	Cross-sectional	DXA	CYC lower legs BMD than RUN. No differences with CON.	B: case-control
Duncan *et al.* (2002) [45]	CYC (10) RUN (10) SWI (10) TRI (10) CON (10)	F	16 to 17	≥8 h/week ≥8 h/week ≥8 h/week ≥8 h/week <2 h/week	3.1 ± 1.8	Cross-sectional	MRI, DXA	CYC lower cortical CSA, moment of inertia and mid-femur BMD than RUN. No differences with CON.	B: case-control
Fiore *et al.* (1996) [36]	CYC (14); CAN (18); CON (28)	M	-	-	-	Cross-sectional	DXA	CYC lower WB, LS and pelvic BMD than CAN. No differences with CON.	B: case-control
Guillaume *et al.* (2012) [38]	CYC (29)	M	26.5 ± 5.3	25,000 to 30,000 km/year	4.5 ± 4	Descriptive	DXA, bone markers	CYC lower LS BMD Z-scores. Bone turnover markers were in a normal range.	B: case series
Heinonen *et al.* (1993) [19]	CYC (22); ORI (30); SKI (28); CYC (29); WL (18); CON (25)	F	18 to 32	-	-	Cross-sectional	DXA, calcium intake	CYC lower BMD at all sites than WL. No differences with CON. No relationship between BMD and calcium intake.	B: case-control
Hinrichs *et al.* (2010) [35]	CYC (16) RUN (37) TRI (22) TEAM (62) POW (45) BAL (13) STU (126) CON (61)	M/F	17 to 30	15 h/week 12.5 h/week 15 h/week 10 h/week 10 h/week 27 h/week 7.5 h/week -	>4	Cross-sectional	DXA	CYC low values of LS and femur BMD than the other groups	B: case-control

Table 1 Studies concerning bone mass, bone metabolism and cycling participation *(Continued)*

Maïmoun *et al.* (2003) [25]	CYC (11) SWI (13) TRI (14) CON (10)	M	18 to 39	10.6 h/week 10.7 h/week 15.2 h/week <2 h/week	-	Cross-sectional	DXA, hormones	CYC and TRI induce androgen deficiency compared to CON, without alteration in BMD	B: case-control
Maïmoun *et al.* (2004) [24]	CYC (11) SWI (13) TRI (14) CON (10)	M	18 to 39	10.6 h/week 10.7 h/week 15.2 h/week <2 h/week	9.3 ± 6.8	Cross-sectional	DXA, bone markers, calcium intake	CYC lower BAP than all groups. No differences in BMD. No relationship between BMD and calcium intake.	B: case-control
Medelli *et al.* (2009) [29]	CYC (73) CON (30)	M	25.8 ± 4.3 28.3 ± 4.5	≥3 to 6 h/day <1 h/week	-	Cross-sectional	DXA, calcium intake	CYC had higher calcium intake and lower LS and femoral neck BMD than CON.	B: case-control
Medelli *et al.* (2009) [4]	CYC (23)	M	28.5 ± 3.9	≥3 to 6 h/day	-	Descriptive	DXA	Two-thirds of participants had lower values of LS BMD	B: case series
Morel *et al.* (2001) [27]	CYC (47); other sports (657)	M	30	7 h/week	-	Cross-sectional. Sportsmen classed as amateur when 11 to 18 years old.	DXA	No differences between different sports	B: case-control, retrospective
Nevill *et al.* (2004) [23]	CYC (16) CON (15) Others (90)	M	28.6 ± 6 24.9 ± 5.4 -	>4 h/week - -	>3	Cross-sectional	DXA	CYC had no differences in BMD compared to CON, as other sports do	B: case-control
Nichols *et al.* (2003) [32]	Young CYC (16) Master CYC (27) CON (24)	M	31.7 ± 3.5 51.2 ± 5.3 51.2 ± 2	≥10 h/week ≥10 h/week <2 days/week	10.9 ± 3.2 20.2 ± 8.4 -	Cross-sectional	DXA	Master CYC lower WB BMD than young CYC. Master CYC lower LS and hip BMD than young CYC and CON.	B: case-control
Nichols *et al.* (2010) [42]	CYC (19) CON (18)	M	50.7 ± 4 50.7 ± 4.1	11.1 h/week 4.5 h/week	27.5 ± 6.8	Longitudinal, 7-year follow-up	DXA	Higher percentage of CYC osteopenic/osteoporotic than CON. Greater increment in this percentage in CYC.	B: case-control
Nikander *et al.* (2005) [26]	CYC (29) SWI (27) VOL (21) HUR (24) SQU (20) SOC (19) SKA (15) AER (27) WL (19) ORI (29) CRO (25) CON (30)	F	20 to 30	10.2 ± 6.8 13.5 ± 4.5 9.9 ± 2.5 9.1 ± 2.4 6.0 ± 3.1 8.6 ± 5.5 6.4 ± 3.6 6.6 ± 3.7 8.3 ± 2.6 8.6 ± 1.4 10.9 ± 12 2.9 ± 2.0	5.9 ± 3.1 10.6 ± 4.3 8.6 ± 3.3 10.4 ± 3.0 6.4 ± 4.7 10.7 ± 3.8 9.4 ± 7.2 8.3 ± 2.7 3.3 ± 1.3 13.0 ± 3.1 10.7 ± 3.5 -	Cross-sectional	DXA, calcium intake	CYC and SWI no differences with CON in BMD and CSA, as the rest of the sports. No differences in calcium intake.	B: case-control

Table 1 Studies concerning bone mass, bone metabolism and cycling participation *(Continued)*

Olmedillas *et al.* (2011) [40]	CYC (21) CON (23)	M	15 to 21	10 h/week 4 h/week	2 to 7	Cross-sectional	DXA	CYC lower BMC at WB, pelvis, FN and legs, and lower BMD at pelvis, hip and legs. Greater differences in CYC over 17 years compared to CON.	B: case-control
Penteado *et al.* (2001) [22]	CYC (31) CON (28)	M	24 26	21 h/week 0	5.2 ± 3.3	Cross-sectional	DXA	No differences with CON.	B: case-control
Rector *et al.* (2008) [37]	CYC (27) RUN (16)	M	20 to 39	≥6 h/week ≥6 h/week	>2	Cross-sectional	DXA, bone markers	CYC lower WB and LS BMD, and 7 times more likely to have osteopenia than RUN. No differences in bone turnover markers.	B: case-control
Rico *et al.* (1993) [20]	CYC (22) CON (27)	M	16	≥10 h/week -	>2	Cross-sectional	DXA, calcium intake	CYC lower legs BMC than CON, without adjustment. No differences when adjusting by weight. No relationship between BMD and calcium intake.	B: case-control
Rico *et al.* (1993) [50]	CYC (22) CON (27)	M	16	≥10 h/week -	>2	Cross-sectional	DXA	CYC lower WB BMC and BMD than CON	B: case-control
Sabo *et al.* (1996) [30]	CYC (6) WL (28) BOX (6) CON (21)	M	21 to 24	3,000 to 10,000 km in pre-competition	-	Cross-sectional	DXA	CYC lower LS BMD than CON	B: case-control
Stewart *et al.* (2000) [31]	CYC (14) RUN (12) RUN+CYC (13) CON (23)	M	18 to 43	8.7 h/week 10.7 h/week 9.4 h/week 0 h/week	>2	Cross-sectional	DXA	CYC lower LS BMD than CON. RUN higher WB BMD than CON. RUN+CYC higher WB BMD than CON.	B: case-control
Smathers *et al.* (2009) [33]	CYC (32) CON (30)	M	20 to 45	≥1 year 3 days/week	9.4 ± 1.1	Cross-sectional	DXA, calcium intake, hormones	CYC higher calcium intake. No differences for testosterone. CYC lower LS BMD than CON.	B: case-control
Warner *et al.* (2002) [28]	Cross-country CYC (16) Road CYC (14) CON (15)	M	20 to 40	≥10 h/week ≥10 h/week <2 h/week	5.9 ± 2.8 9.9 ± 4.4 -	Cross-sectional	DXA, hormones	Cross-country CYC higher BMD at all sites that road CYC and CON. No differences in testosterone levels.	B: case-control
Wilks *et al.* (2009) [46]	Sprint CYC (52) Distance CYC (19) CON (32)	M/F	30 to 82 50 ± 13	<2 h/week	26 ± 15 29 ± 16 Start age	Cross-sectional	pQCT	Sprint CYC higher index of strength in tibia and radius than CON. Distance CYC higher tibial BMC than CON.	B: case-control

[a]Unless stated, the results indicate significant differences between two or more groups.

AER = step aerobicists; BAP = bone alkaline phosphatase; BMC = bone mineral content; BMD = bone mineral density; BOX = boxers; CAN = canoeists; CIC = cyclists; CON = controls; CRO = cross-country skiers; CTX = C-terminal collagen crosslinks; DXA = dual energy X-ray absorptiometry; HUR = hurdlers; LS = lumbar spine; MRI = magnetic resonance imaging; OC = osteocalcin; ORI = orienteers; pQCT = peripheral quantitative computed tomography; RCT = randomized control trial; RUN = runners; SKA = speed skaters; SKI = skiers; SQU = squash players; SWI = swimmers; TRI = triathletes; VOL = volleyball players; WB = whole body; WL = weightlifters.

negatively affect the geometry and/or structure of the bones measured with pQCT. What appears to be clear is that more in-depth studies are required in order to corroborate these findings, and to evaluate possible changes over different periods of time and life stages in these variables.

Endocrine factors related with bone mass

Bone turnover markers

Bone turnover markers related to bone formation, such as BAP or OC and also CTX related to bone resorption, have been barely investigated in cyclist populations.

Rector *et al.* showed no differences between adult cyclists and runners in bone metabolism markers [37], and Guillaume *et al.* reinforced that by showing these markers in normal ranges in a group of young cyclists [38]. However, Maïmoun *et al.* [24] studied three groups of adult athletes (cyclists, triathletes and swimmers), compared to controls, and showed lower BAP in cyclists compared to any other group. No differences were found for OC or CTX among the three groups of athletes.

Hormonal profile

Smathers *et al.* and Warner *et al.* showed no differences in testosterone levels between adult male cyclists and controls [28,33]; however, Maïmoun *et al.* showed lower testosterone levels in adult male cyclists and triathletes compared with controls [25]. Two different interventional studies focused on the effects of cycling on parathyroid hormone concluded that it increased after 2 h of cycling [47], and that calcium supplementation attenuated its disruption [39].

Inconclusive results can be obtained from the few heterogeneous studies available on neuroendocrine factors affecting bone mass in cyclists; nevertheless, it may be stated that the hormonal status seems to be within normal ranges in this specific population and that the formation of bone appears to be somewhat reduced in a group of adult cyclists with a long history of training (over 9 years on average). For that reason, as bone metabolism does not seem to be the main factor regarding the general low mineral accumulation in cyclists' bones, other mechanical factors such as the lack of osteogenic impacts might also have an influence.

Factors affecting bone mass

Diet and calcium intake

Some authors found that cyclists take in a higher amount of calcium than controls [29,33], but as it is believed that cyclists have a higher energy intake than controls due to higher energy expenditure [48], total energy intake is a factor that must be taken into account. However, no associations were found between calcium intake and BMD for adults and young adult cyclists [19,20,24,41]. In addition, Barry *et al.* found that BMD was decreased in a group of cyclists independently of their high or low calcium intake over a 1-year season [43], and that acute calcium supplementation decreased the parathyroid hormone disruption after cycling [39]. Werner *et al.* did not find differences in calcium or vitamin D intake between road and mountain cyclists and controls [28]. Brown *et al.* showed that a fat-rich diet yielded higher increments in BMD in cyclists than other carbohydrate-rich diets without variation in fat or lean masses over a period of 12 weeks [49].

Studies appear to indicate that there are no observable effects in consuming higher amounts of calcium to reduce the supposed detrimental effect of cycling on bone mass. Furthermore, from these data it is difficult to define whether or not cyclists do in fact require any additional calcium supplements. Further studies are necessary in order to confirm previous results and to elucidate whether diet may be a more important factor for cyclists during years of growth in comparison to athletes in other disciplines.

Age

As previously stated, adult cyclists showed lower BMD at several sites of the body (mainly then lumbar spine) compared to controls or practitioners of other sports; however, few of the included studies incorporated adolescents within their samples. These studies showed similar results in that, under the age of 18, the differences in BMD between cyclists and controls were not observable [40,45,50], as observed in adolescent runners [21]. In addition, Maïmoun *et al.* [24] stated that age, among other factors, could influence BMD in people that practice sports including cycling. Though using a different measurement technique (that is, pQCT) Wilks *et al.* [46] suggested that cycling activity could prevent bone strength losses in older people.

The positive effect that general sport practice has on bone is well known [10], and that maximizing bone mineral mass during growth may help to prevent fractures during adolescence and at an older age [51]. We have observed that cycling during the early years of life does not negatively affect the bones, yet it does not exert as much of a positive influence as other sports clearly do. Consequently, the age factor for cycling must be taken into account.

Gender

It is widely known that women have lower bone mass than men throughout life and that are at higher risk of suffering from osteoporosis; therefore it is important to ascertain whether gender has any influential effect on the accumulation of bone mass in cyclists.

The studies included in this review incorporating only women within their samples showed similar results in bone mass to studies on men or both genders when they are compared with other sportswomen or controls [19,21,41,45].

Therefore, because females are more likely to become osteoporotic, pre-participation examinations (that is, DXA scans) should be conducted in adult female cyclists training at a high level.

Training level and type of cycling practice

Few studies have been performed in low-level cyclist populations; Morel *et al.* studied amateur sportsmen without finding differences in bone mass between cycling and other sports [27]. In general, studies included in this review had samples of adult cyclists with a high level of training; however, some of them were performed in amateur or adolescent cyclists, showing that in fact the level of practice and/or the years of training might increase the risk of low bone mass.

The two studies by Duncan *et al.* showed no differences in BMD between cyclists and controls, but it is worth noting the sample of adolescents that they used [21,45]. The study by Wilks *et al.*, which is discussed below, showed greater bone strength surrogates in cyclists compared to controls in a sample of adults and older adults with a high level of cycling practice during their adolescence and adulthood.

Cycling is a widespread activity that involves different disciplines (that is, mountain biking, road cyclists, BMX, and so on) and, in combination with swimming and/or running, forms part of triathlon or duathlon events.

What has been observed regarding combination of cycling with running is that this practice counteracts the effect that cycling has on bone mass by an increased total body BMD compared with controls not observed in the cycling alone group [31]. In triathletes Maïmoun *et al.* demonstrated a similar behavior to cyclists in terms of testosterone deficiency without differences in BMD [25]. Concerning different types of cycling, as expected, Wilks *et al.* demonstrated that sprint-trained cyclists had stronger bones than those training for longer distances [46], and Warner *et al.* showed that cross-country cycling practitioners acquire higher BMD than road cyclists [28].

From a review of the current available literature described herein it can be concluded that road cycling at a competitive level might be more detrimental for bone health than other forms of cycling such as mountain biking in a recreational way. However, it should be mentioned that an upper threshold of training level may exist which protects bones from fractures, perhaps by improving their geometry and/or structure. Moreover, and especially where elite cyclists are concerned, it is also possible that resistance training also provides significant positive influences on bone mass. It is noteworthy that duathlon and triathlon do not have the same harmful effect that cycling alone seems to have on bone mass.

Limitations

Different sources of bias inherent to systematic reviews should be addressed. First, we excluded non-English publications; thus a possible language bias is inherent.

Second, the studies included in our systematic review were too heterogeneous to perform a meta-analysis. The lack of this type of analysis makes difficult to reach strong conclusions. However, Table 1 contains quantitative information on each individual study.

Third, we classified articles into categories based on their assessment method, and afterwards we discussed some factors affecting bone mass. We believe that the results are more easily read and understood with this categorization. Although we systematically assessed articles before assigning them into categories, categorization is not a closed issue.

Conclusions

To date, a considerable number of studies have reported on the possible harmful effect of cycling on bone health; however there are still some pending issues that need to be addressed. In general, cycling participation seems to have a neutral effect on bone health in terms of low BMD at several sites of the body; however, some factors need to be taken into account regarding this assumption. Road endurance cycling at a professional level could be more detrimental to bone mass than performing this activity recreationally, or worse than performing other disciplines such as cross-country cycling or combinations of cycling with running [28]. In addition, there is some evidence that the practice of this sport during adolescence and adulthood could help to maintain a better bone geometry and strength later in life [46]. Few studies described bone mass in young cyclist populations, however, it can be hypothesized that the differences in BMD between cyclists and controls or other sport practitioners become greater from 17 years of age onwards [40]. It is important to note that, contrary to other sports, there have been no reports of any positive effects of cycling on bone mass during adolescence.

Factors affecting bone mass such as calcium intake and hormonal profile were found to be within the regular range in cyclists [28,29,33]; allowing us to believe that the lack of impact might be one of the main reasons for the low bone mass acquisition in this population. It is also thought that professional cyclists spend several hours daily resting after training time, and sedentary time has been associated with low bone mass [52]; this factor should be taken into account as it may also partially explain the low BMD observed in these athletes.

In general it can be concluded that individuals who practice non-weight-bearing sports such as cycling are more likely to develop osteopenia or osteoporosis [53]; and the high incidence of falls while cycling makes this fact even more relevant for this population [42,54].

In conclusion, road cycling at a competitive level is less effective at improving bone mass when compared with weight-bearing sports. Based on the available evidence, in general, cycling as a sole form of exercise is not recommended for people who are at risk of developing osteoporosis, unless it is complemented with some kind of osteogenic training.

Practical recommendations and future research

The likelihood of a cyclist to develop osteopenia or osteoporosis at clinical sites due to low levels of BMD must be taken into account by health organizations, federations, trainers and athletes. In accordance with Maïmoun *et al.* there may exist a threshold, since BMD measurements are inadequate to detect slight and acute changes in bone metabolism [55], and therefore further research on bone metabolism, bone strength and structure in cyclists at different ages, based on previous studies [46], could help to better understand the actual bone weakness in cyclists. Also, longitudinal studies aimed at identifying whether the key periods of bone mass acquisition are affected by cycling are needed.

Secondly, Beatty *et al.* [56] and Nichols *et al.* [42] proposed to incorporate impact activities in training programs for cyclists, as it has been demonstrated that plyometric jumps increase bone mass in different populations [14,57]. Generally, amateur cyclists are unwilling to include resistance and/or plyometric exercise in their routine throughout the season despite there being no scientific evidence of performance impairment. Therefore, studies on the effects of different training implementations will define whether these interventions are enough to counteract the effect of cycling.

Acknowledgements
This review was funded by Ministerio de Ciencia e Innovacion, Instituto de Salud Carlos III (DPS2008-06999) and Presidencia del Gobierno de España, Consejo Superior de Deportes (21/UPB20/10). Special thanks are given to Scott G Mitchell from the Institute of Nanoscience of Aragon (INA) for his work in reviewing the English style and grammar.

Author details
[1]GENUD 'Growth, Exercise, NUtrition and Development' Research Group, Universidad de Zaragoza, Zaragoza, Spain. [2]Faculty of Health and Sport Sciences (FCSD), Department of Physiatry and Nursing, Universidad de Zaragoza, Huesca, Spain. [3]School of Health Science (EUCS), Universidad de Zaragoza, Zaragoza, Spain.

Authors' contributions
All authors made substantive intellectual contributions to the final manuscript, and read and approved it.

Competing interests
The authors declare that they have no competing interests.

References

1. Oja P, Titze S, Bauman A, de Geus B, Krenn P, Reger-Nash B, Kohlberger T: **Health benefits of cycling: a systematic review.** *Scand J Med Sci Sports* 2011, **21**:496-509.
2. García Ferrando M: **Posmodernidad y deporte: entre la individualización y la masificación.** *Book Posmodernidad y Deporte: Entre la Individualización y la Masificación* Madrid, Spain: Consejo Superior de Deportes y Centro de Investigaciones Sociológicas; 2006.
3. Nagle KB, Brooks MA: **A systematic review of bone health in cyclists.** *Sports Health* 2011, **3**:235-243.
4. Medelli J, Lounana J, Menuet JJ, Shabani M, Cordero-MacIntyre Z: **Is osteopenia a health risk in professional cyclists?** *J Clin Densitom* 2009, **12**:28-34.
5. Consensus development conference: **Consensus development conference: diagnosis, prophylaxis, and treatment of osteoporosis.** *Am J Med* 1993, **94**:646-650.
6. Rizzoli R, Bianchi ML, Garabedian M, McKay HA, Moreno LA: **Maximizing bone mineral mass gain during growth for the prevention of fractures in the adolescents and the elderly.** *Bone* 2010, **46**:294-305.
7. Seeman E: **An exercise in geometry.** *J Bone Miner Res* 2002, **17**:373-380.
8. Ralston SH, Uitterlinden AG: **Genetics of osteoporosis.** *Endocr Rev* 2010, **31**:629-662.
9. Smith RW Jr: **Dietary and hormonal factors in bone loss.** *Fed Proc* 1967, **26**:1737-1746.
10. Vicente-Rodriguez G: **How does exercise affect bone development during growth?** *Sports Med* 2006, **36**:561-569.
11. Vicente-Rodriguez G, Ara I, Perez-Gomez J, Serrano-Sanchez JA, Dorado C, Calbet JA: **High femoral bone mineral density accretion in prepubertal soccer players.** *Med Sci Sports Exerc* 2004, **36**:1789-1795.
12. Vicente-Rodriguez G, Jimenez-Ramirez J, Ara I, Serrano-Sanchez JA, Dorado C, Calbet JA: **Enhanced bone mass and physical fitness in prepubescent footballers.** *Bone* 2003, **33**:853-859.
13. Gomez-Cabello A, Ara I, Gonzalez-Aguero A, Casajus JA, Vicente-Rodriguez G: **Effects of training on bone mass in older adults: a systematic review.** *Sports Med* 2012, **42**:301-325.
14. González-Agüero A, Vicente-Rodriguez G, Gómez-Cabello A, Ara I, Moreno LA, Casajús JA: **A 21-week bone deposition promoting exercise programme increases bone mass in youths with Down syndrome.** *Dev Med Child Neurol* 2012, **54**:552-556.
15. Banfi G, Colombini A, Lombardi G, Lubkowska A: **Metabolic markers in sports medicine.** *Adv Clin Chem* 2012, **56**:1-54.
16. Stroup DF, Berlin JA, Morton SC, Olkin I, Williamson GD, Rennie D, Moher D, Becker BJ, Sipe TA, Thacker SB: **Meta-analysis of observational studies in epidemiology: a proposal for reporting. Meta-analysis Of Observational Studies in Epidemiology (MOOSE) group.** *JAMA* 2000, **283**:2008-2012.
17. Moher D, Liberati A, Tetzlaff J, Altman DG: **Preferred reporting items for systematic reviews and meta-analyses: the PRISMA statement.** *PLoS Med* 2009, **6**:e1000097.
18. Hadorn DC, Baker D, Hodges JS, Hicks N: **Rating the quality of evidence for clinical practice guidelines.** *J Clin Epidemiol* 1996, **49**:749-754.
19. Heinonen A, Oja P, Kannus P, Sievanen H, Manttari A, Vuori I: **Bone mineral density of female athletes in different sports.** *Bone Miner* 1993, **23**:1-14.
20. Rico H, Revilla M, Hernandez ER, Gomez-Castresana F, Villa LF: **Bone mineral content and body composition in postpubertal cyclist boys.** *Bone* 1993, **14**:93-95.
21. Duncan CS, Blimkie CJ, Cowell CT, Burke ST, Briody JN, Howman-Giles R: **Bone mineral density in adolescent female athletes: relationship to exercise type and muscle strength.** *Med Sci Sports Exerc* 2002, **34**:286-294.
22. Penteado VS, Castro CH, Pinheiro Mde M, Santana M, Bertolino S, de Mello MT, Szejnfeld VL: **Diet, body composition, and bone mass in well-trained cyclists.** *J Clin Densitom* 2010, **13**:43-50.
23. Nevill A, Holder R, Stewart A: **Do sporting activities convey benefits to bone mass throughout the skeleton?** *J Sports Sci* 2004, **22**:645-650.
24. Maimoun L, Mariano-Goulart D, Couret I, Manetta J, Peruchon E, Micallef JP, Verdier R, Rossi M, Leroux JL: **Effects of physical activities that induce**

moderate external loading on bone metabolism in male athletes. *J Sports Sci* 2004, **22**:875-883.
25. Maimoun L, Lumbroso S, Manetta J, Paris F, Leroux JL, Sultan C: **Testosterone is significantly reduced in endurance athletes without impact on bone mineral density.** *Horm Res* 2003, **59**:285-292.
26. Nikander R, Sievanen H, Heinonen A, Kannus P: **Femoral neck structure in adult female athletes subjected to different loading modalities.** *J Bone Miner Res* 2005, **20**:520-528.
27. Morel J, Combe B, Francisco J, Bernard J: **Bone mineral density of 704 amateur sportsmen involved in different physical activities.** *Osteoporos Int* 2001, **12**:152-157.
28. Warner SE, Shaw JM, Dalsky GP: **Bone mineral density of competitive male mountain and road cyclists.** *Bone* 2002, **30**:281-286.
29. Medelli J, Shabani M, Lounana J, Fardellone P, Campion F: **Low bone mineral density and calcium intake in elite cyclists.** *J Sports Med Phys Fitness* 2009, **49**:44-53.
30. Sabo D, Bernd L, Pfeil J, Reiter A: **Bone quality in the lumbar spine in high-performance athletes.** *Eur Spine J* 1996, **5**:258-263.
31. Stewart AD, Hannan J: **Total and regional bone density in male runners, cyclists, and controls.** *Med Sci Sports Exerc* 2000, **32**:1373-1377.
32. Nichols JF, Palmer JE, Levy SS: **Low bone mineral density in highly trained male master cyclists.** *Osteoporos Int* 2003, **14**:644-649.
33. Smathers AM, Bemben MG, Bemben DA: **Bone density comparisons in male competitive road cyclists and untrained controls.** *Med Sci Sports Exerc* 2009, **41**:290-296.
34. Campion F, Nevill AM, Karlsson MK, Lounana J, Shabani M, Fardellone P, Medelli J: **Bone status in professional cyclists.** *Int J Sports Med* 2010, **31**:511-515.
35. Hinrichs T, Chae E, Lehmann R, Allolio B, Platen P: **Bone mineral density in athletes of different disciplines: a cross-sectional study.** *Open Sports Sci J* 2010, **3**:129-133.
36. Fiore CE, Dieli M, Vintaloro G, Gibilaro M, Giacone G, Cottini E: **Body composition and bone mineral density in competitive athletes in different sports.** *Int J Tissue React* 1996, **18**:121-124.
37. Rector RS, Rogers R, Ruebel M, Hinton PS: **Participation in road cycling vs running is associated with lower bone mineral density in men.** *Metabolism* 2008, **57**:226-232.
38. Guillaume G, Chappard D, Audran M: **Evaluation of the bone status in high-level cyclists.** *J Clin Densitom* 2012, **15**:103-107.
39. Barry DW, Hansen KC, van Pelt RE, Witten M, Wolfe P, Kohrt WM: **Acute calcium ingestion attenuates exercise-induced disruption of calcium homeostasis.** *Med Sci Sports Exerc* 2011, **43**:617-623.
40. Olmedillas H, Gonzalez-Aguero A, Moreno LA, Casajus JA, Vicente-Rodriguez G: **Bone related health status in adolescent cyclists.** *PLoS One* 2011, **6**:e24841.
41. Beshgetoor D, Nichols JF, Rego I: **Effect of training mode and calcium intake on bone mineral density in female master cyclist, runners, and non-athletes.** *Int J Sport Nutr Exerc Metab* 2000, **10**:290-301.
42. Nichols JF, Rauh MJ: **Longitudinal changes in bone mineral density in male master cyclists and nonathletes.** *J Strength Cond Res* 2012, **25**:727-734.
43. Barry DW, Kohrt WM: **BMD decreases over the course of a year in competitive male cyclists.** *J Bone Miner Res* 2008, **23**:484-491.
44. Kontulainen SA, Johnston JD, Liu D, Leung C, Oxland TR, McKay HA: **Strength indices from pQCT imaging predict up to 85% of variance in bone failure properties at tibial epiphysis and diaphysis.** *J Musculoskelet Neuronal Interact* 2008, **8**:401-409.
45. Duncan CS, Blimkie CJ, Kemp A, Higgs W, Cowell CT, Woodhead H, Briody JN, Howman-Giles R: **Mid-femur geometry and biomechanical properties in 15- to 18-yr-old female athletes.** *Med Sci Sports Exerc* 2002, **34**:673-681.
46. Wilks DC, Gilliver SF, Rittweger J: **Forearm and tibial bone measures of distance- and sprint-trained master cyclists.** *Med Sci Sports Exerc* 2009, **41**:566-573.
47. Barry DW, Kohrt WM: **Acute effects of 2 hours of moderate-intensity cycling on serum parathyroid hormone and calcium.** *Calcif Tissue Int* 2007, **80**:359-365.
48. Burke LM: **Nutritional practices of male and female endurance cyclists.** *Sports Med* 2001, **31**:521-532.
49. Brown RC, Cox CM, Goulding A: **High-carbohydrate versus high-fat diets: effect on body composition in trained cyclists.** *Med Sci Sports Exerc* 2000, **32**:690-694.
50. Rico H, Revilla M, Villa LF, Gomez-Castresana F, Alvarez del Buergo M: **Body composition in postpubertal boy cyclists.** *J Sports Med Phys Fitness* 1993, **33**:278-281.
51. Rizzoli R, Bianchi ML, Garabedian M, McKay HA, Moreno LA: **Maximizing bone mineral mass gain during growth for the prevention of fractures in the adolescents and the elderly.** *Bone* 2010, **46**:294-305.
52. Vicente-Rodriguez G, Ortega FB, Rey-Lopez JP, Espana-Romero V, Blay VA, Blay G, Martin-Matillas M, Moreno LA: **Extracurricular physical activity participation modifies the association between high TV watching and low bone mass.** *Bone* 2009, **45**:925-930.
53. Tenforde AS, Fredericson M: **Influence of sports participation on bone health in the young athlete: a review of the literature.** *Pm R* 2011, **3**:861-867.
54. Finch C, Valuri G, Ozanne-Smith J: **Sport and active recreation injuries in Australia: evidence from emergency department presentations.** *Br J Sports Med* 1998, **32**:220-225.
55. Maimoun L, Sultan C: **Effects of physical activity on bone remodeling.** *Metabolism* 2011, **60**:373-388.
56. Beatty T, Webner D, Collina SJ: **Bone density in competitive cyclists.** *Curr Sports Med Rep* 2010, **9**:352-355.
57. Witzke KA, Snow CM: **Effects of plyometric jump training on bone mass in adolescent girls.** *Med Sci Sports Exerc* 2000, **32**:1051-1057.

Changes in hydration status of elite Olympic class sailors in different climates and the effects of different fluid replacement beverages

Evan JH Lewis[1], Sarah J Fraser[2], Scott G Thomas[3] and Greg D Wells[3,4*]

Abstract

Background: Olympic class sailing poses physiological challenges similar to other endurance sports such as cycling or running, with sport specific challenges of limited access to nutrition and hydration during competition. As changes in hydration status can impair sports performance, examining fluid consumption patterns and fluid/ electrolyte requirements of Olympic class sailors is necessary to develop specific recommendations for these elite athletes. The purpose of this study was to examine if Olympic class sailors could maintain hydration status with self-regulated fluid consumption in cold conditions and the effect of fixed fluid intake on hydration status in warm conditions.

Methods: In our cold condition study (CCS), 11 elite Olympic class sailors were provided *ad libitum* access to three different drinks. Crystal Light (control, C); Gatorade (experimental control, G); and customized sailing-specific Infinit (experimental, IN) (1.0:0.22 CHO:PRO), were provided on three separate training days in cold 7.1°C [4.2 – 11.3]. Our warm condition study (WCS) examined the effect of fixed fluid intake (11.5 $mL \cdot kg^{-1} \cdot h^{-1}$) of C, G and heat-specific experimental Infinit (INW)(1.0:0.074 CHO:PRO) on the hydration status of eight elite Olympic Laser class sailors in 19.5°C [17.0 - 23.3]. Both studies used a completely random design.

Results: In CCS, participants consumed 802 ± 91, 924 ± 137 and 707 ± 152 mL of fluid in each group respectively. This did not change urine specific gravity, but did lead to a main effect for time for body mass ($p < 0.001$), blood sodium, potassium and chloride with all groups lower post-training ($p < 0.05$). In WCS, fixed fluid intake increased participant's body mass post-training in all groups ($p < 0.01$) and decreased urine specific gravity post-training ($p < 0.01$). There was a main effect for time for blood sodium, potassium and chloride concentration, with lower values observed post-training ($p < 0.05$). C blood sodium concentrations were lower than the INW group post-training ($p = 0.031$) with a trend towards significance in the G group ($p = 0.069$).

Conclusion: *Ad libitum* fluid consumption in cold conditions was insufficient in preventing a decrease in body mass and blood electrolyte concentration post-training. However, when a fixed volume of 11.5 $mL \cdot kg^{-1} \cdot h^{-1}$ was consumed during warm condition training, hydration status was maintained by preventing changes in body mass and urine specific gravity.

Keywords: Hydration, Sailing, Nutrition, Performance, Temperature

* Correspondence: greg.wells@utoronto.ca
[3]Faculty of Kinesiology and Physical Education, The University of Toronto, 55 Harbord Street, Toronto, ON M5R 2W6, Canada
[4]Physiology and Experimental Medicine, The Hospital for Sick Children, 555 University Avenue, Toronto, ON M5G 1X8, Canada
Full list of author information is available at the end of the article

Background

The maintenance of hydration status during training and competition has been repeatedly identified as a rate-limiting factor for athletic performance [1-3]. The continued intake of fluids fortified with carbohydrates and electrolytes during activities lasting longer than one hour has been found to prevent deteriorations in endurance, strength, blood volume [4-6] and cognitive function [7].

As such, the study of hydration requirements of Olympic class sailors is lacking when compared to other endurance sports such as cycling and running [8,9]. While population size and sport specific challenges may be an influencing factor, the physiologic demands of Olympic class sailing, coupled with the strategic/tactical requirements make hydration a logical variable for success that has not been adequately studied [8]. When 28 elite Olympic class sailors from New Zealand were surveyed about their sport sciences practices, 68% reported being dehydrated during racing from inadequate fluid intake that was likely related to 86% of athletes reporting a loss of concentration at the end of races and 50% reporting feelings of frustration about race results [10]. Examination of the hydration practices of novice Laser class (Men's singlehanded Olympic dinghy) sailors competing in hot climates and moderate wind velocities, revealed participants did not consume sufficient fluids to prevent a >2% loss of body mass after racing [9], a level that has previously been associated with reduced athletic performance [3]. In both studies, the authors attributed a lack of sport science knowledge to the reported change in hydration status. Since the findings of Slater and Tan [9], we are not aware of any additional findings on the impact of environmental conditions on the hydration practices or requirements of elite or novice Olympic class sailors.

Examination of the energy demands of Laser class sailors, revealed there is a direct correlation between wind velocity and the energy demand during sailing [11]. The Laser and other Olympic class dinghies require sailors to have well-developed strength endurance, especially in the quadriceps, abdominal and upper back muscles. To navigate the boat upwind, the sailor must leverage his body out of the boat to counteract the force of the wind on the sail (for a detailed figure and description see Castagna & Brisswalter [11]). Previous examination of the physiologic response to sailing in moderate winds has determined energy requirements are largely met by aerobic metabolism. Higher skilled Laser sailors sail at 45 to 68% of maximal aerobic power during 30 or more minutes of upwind sailing in moderate conditions (14–22 $km{\cdot}h^{-1}$) [11,12]. Sweating rates at similar intensities measured in America's Cup sailors can results in mean water losses of 1340 $mL{\cdot}h^{-1}$ [13]. As there are many differences between America's Cup and Olympic class sailing [8,13] it is important to determine the changes in hydration status and subsequent hydration requirements of Olympic class sailors.

Sweat rate and water loss are affected by environmental conditions [6] but it is unclear how sweat losses are compensated for by sailors in cold conditions. Furthermore, increased sweat losses in warm and hot conditions are not appropriately compensated for by increased fluid intake in elite football players [14,15] amateur Laser sailors [9] and America's Cup sailors [13]. As such, the purpose of the CCS was to examine if Olympic class sailors could self-regulate fluid requirements in cold conditions by providing them *ad libitum* access to different fluid replacement beverages during training and examining how this affected hydration status. The purpose of the WCS was to test the effect of fixed fluid intake of different fluid replacement beverages on hydration status during training in warm conditions. Examining relative fluid intakes may be a novel way of developing hydration recommendations for sailors. Previous work examining the effect relative fluid intake rates on gastric emptying during cycle exercise determined that consuming 11.5 $mL{\cdot}kg^{-1}{\cdot}h^{-1}$ of a 7.5% carbohydrate solution had a higher percentage gastric emptying compared to 17.1 and 23.0 $mL{\cdot}kg^{-1}{\cdot}h^{-1}$ [16]. While absolute gastric emptying in this study was greater in the higher fluid intake groups, these intakes equated to approximately 1200 and 1600 $mL{\cdot}h^{-1}$ and resulted in gastric discomfort [16]. Therefore, the a second purpose of this study was to determine the optimal composition of a fluid replacement drink specific to elite Olympic class sailors and test if consuming 11.5 $mL{\cdot}kg^{-1}{\cdot}h^{-1}$ was sufficient to maintain hydration status.

Methods

Research design

Two studies were performed to examine the changes in hydration status of elite Olympic class sailors during training. The first was a cold condition study (CCS) that examined *ad libitum* fluid consumption of three different fluid replacement drinks (Table 1) on hydration status and blood electrolyte concentration before and after training in cold (4.2 – 11.3°C) temperatures. WCS examined the effect of fixed volume (11.5 $mL{\cdot}kg^{-1}{\cdot}h^{-1}$) fluid consumption of three different fluid replacement drinks on hydration status and blood electrolyte concentration before and after in warm temperatures (17.0 - 23.3°C). Both studies used a single blinded, placebo-controlled, repeated-measures design. Participants were randomly assigned to each condition on three separate days using a completely randomized design. In CCS, participants completed all three conditions over five days with a maximum of one day between conditions. Training sessions were limited to 2.5 hours because of the cold temperatures. In WCS participants completed each condition on consecutive days. All training sessions were three hours in length.

Table 1 Composition of experimental drinks in CCS and WCS

Drink	CHO (g·L^{-1})	Protein (g·L^{-1})	CHO : PRO	[Na$^+$] mmol·L^{-1}	[K$^+$] mmol·L^{-1}	Energy (kcal·L^{-1})
Crystal Light (C)	0	0	-	0	0	0
Gatorade (G) Study 1	66.0 [13.0 – 43.2]	0	-	18.3	3.3	264
Gatorade (G) Study 2	66.0 [59.1- 64.2]	0	-	18.3	3.3	264
Infinit (IN) Study 1	60 [6.3 – 39.3]	13.3 [3.5 - 8.7]	1.0 : 0.22	21.8	4.3	296.7
Infinit (INW) Study 2	90.0 [80.5 – 87.6]	6.7 [6.0 – 6.5]	1.0 : 0.074	72.5	21.3	386.7

Carbohydrate (CHO) and protein (PRO) content is shown with the CHO:PRO, range of ingestion per hour based on fluid consumption (Study 1) the weight of subjects (Study 2).

In both studies, all training activities were performed in identical order for the same duration each day.

Experimental drinks

CCS and WCS had three different drink conditions, Crystal Light (C) (Kraft Foods Canada, Toronto, Ontario), Gatorade (G) (Gatorade, Barrington, Illinois) and Infinit (IN) (Infinit Nutrition Canada, Windsor, Ontario). All drinks were flavoured similarly in attempts to blind the participants. The composition of the C and G conditions were consistent between both studies; however the Infinit condition was altered to reflect the hypothesized fluid replacement and electrolyte requirements of the participants determined during sweat rate testing (INW) (Table 1).

The carbohydrate content in the G drink was entirely sucrose. In the CCS, the carbohydrate content in the IN drink was approximately 60 : 40 ratio of dextrose and maltodextrin with a carbohydrate concentration of 60 g·L^{-1}. The INW drink in WCS had a carbohydrate ratio of 2 : 1 dextrose and fructose. Protein in both drinks was whey protein isolate with 13.3 g·L^{-1} and 6.7 g·L^{-1} in the IN and INW drinks respectively.

Participants in CCS were provided *ad libitum* access to their drink condition. To measure the amount of fluid consumed during training, the content of each subject's water bottles was measured to the nearest 1.0 mL before and after training and the difference was recorded.

In WCS participants were instructed to consume one water bottle per hour containing 11.5 mL·kg^{-1}·h^{-1} of fluid based on pre-training body weight. At the beginning of each hour, participants were provided with an individually pre-measured sport bottle with their respective drink and instructed to ingest all of the fluid within the hour. Each participant had a secure bottle holder in their boat to provide convenient access to their drink throughout each hour of training. Participants in both studies were asked to refrain from consuming any other fluids or food within the hour before training, during training and until all post-training measures had been completed.

Subjects

CCS Eleven males (mean [range]) (age 23.3 y [19.5 – 31.6]; height 182.8 cm [177.5 - 187.0]; mass 81.5 kg [74.2 – 95.9]) were recruited for this study. All participants competed in Olympic class boats (Men's Laser n = 6; 49er skiff n = 3; Men's Finn n = 1 and Men's RS:X n = 1). WCS had eight male participants that competed in the Men's Laser (age 22.9 y [19.9 – 27.0]; height 183.4 cm [180.2 – 190.0]; mass 81.1 kg [78.8 - 84.5]). All participants in both studies had a minimum of four years experience competing at the international level in their respective class. The subjects were studied during training camps designed to replicate competitive conditions with the environmental condition being the variable between each study. Potential risks from participating in each study were explained to the subjects prior to obtaining written consent. The University of Toronto Research Ethics Board approved all study procedures.

Sweat rate

Prior to the each study, sweat rate and sodium loss were determined during cycle exercise in controlled laboratory conditions (CCS 21.3°C, 57.4% relative humidity; WCS 21.8°C, 59.1% relative humidity). For the day of testing, participants were instructed to drink 500 mL of water upon waking, refrain from eating breakfast and report to the laboratory at 08:30. After voiding, participants were weighed to the nearest 0.1 kg (Precision Scale UC-321PL, A&D Medical, San Jose, California, USA) wearing only dry lightweight shorts. Participants had four adhesive sweat patches (Tegaderm, 3 M, London, Ontario, Canada) affixed to their, chest, upper-back, forearm and thigh to measure whole-body sodium as previously described [17]. Participants were fitted to an electronically braked ergometer (Velotron Dynafit Pro, Seattle, WA, USA) with Computrainer Software, which allowed them to adjust their resistance to maintain desired heart rate. Subjects were instructed to warm up for five minutes before completing 30 minutes of cycling. Intensity was set at 80% of age-predicted maximum heart rate (Equation 1) as this is an average heart rate observed during racing in windy conditions [18]. Patches were removed once saturated or at the conclusion of the test and sweat concentration from all patches were analyzed (Sweat Chek 3120, Wescor Biomedical Systems, Logan, Utah, USA). This protocol produced profuse sweating in all participants and was similar to previously validated testing procedures [19].

Blood electrolytes
In CCS finger prick blood samples were collected into heparinized capillary tubes for immediate analysis in CHEM8+ cartridges inserted into an iSTAT point of care monitor (Abbott, Princeton, NJ, USA). The CHEM8+ cartridge analyses sodium, potassium, chloride, glucose, hematocrit and hemoglobin as previously described [20]. In WCS, venous blood samples were collected from the antecubital vein into heparinized tubes. Two participants were uncomfortable with venous sampling so finger prick blood samples were collected as described in CCS. Samples were pipetted into iSTAT CHEM8+ cartridges and analyzed as described in CCS.

Hydration status
Before and after training, participants provided a mid-stream urine sample in a polyurethane collection container for immediate analysis of urine specific gravity (USG) in triplicate (4410 PAL-10S, Novatech International, Houston, Texas, USA). At this time, participants voided completely and were then weighted to the nearest 0.1 kg (Precision Scale UC-321PL, A&D Medical, San Jose, California, USA), wearing only dry lightweight shorts. Differences in body mass were used to estimate hydration status and to calculate sweat rate (Equation 3). Urine excreted by each participant during training in WCS was collected in a large airtight container, carried by a support boat. There was no correction made for respiratory water loss or metabolic fluid changes. Changes in plasma volume were calculated using changes in hematocrit and hemoglobin according to the methods of Dill and Costill [21].

Environmental conditions
Environmental conditions were measured every 30 minutes during training using a portable weather station with anemometer (Kestrel 4000, Nielsen-Kellerman, Mckellar, Australia).

Calculations
Participant's target heart rate during sweat rate testing was calculated by subtracting participants' age from 220 and then multiplying by 80%.

$$\text{Heart rate} = (220 - \text{age}) * 0.80 \tag{1}$$

Mean whole body sodium output was calculated based on the equation of Patterson et al. [17].

$$\begin{aligned}\text{Whole} - \text{body}[\text{Na}] = {} & 28.2\%\ \text{chest}[\text{Na}] \\ & + 28.2\%\ \text{back}[\text{Na}] \\ & + 11.3\%\ \text{forearm}[\text{Na}] \\ & + 32.3\%\ \text{thigh}[\text{Na}]\end{aligned} \tag{2}$$

This data was pooled and used as a guide to determine the electrolyte content of the Ex drink (Table 1).

Sweat rate (millilitres per hour) was estimated as change in body mass (kilograms), with the assumption 1 kg = 1 L, during the 3 hour practice plus total fluid intake (milliliters) and minus total urine output during practice (millilitres).

$$\text{Sweat rate} = \frac{(\text{Pre body mass} - \text{Post body mass}) + \text{Fluid intake} - \text{Urine output}}{\text{Practice length}} \tag{3}$$

Total sweat sodium loss (grams) for participants was calculated by multiplying their sweat sodium concentration (millimoles per litre) with the molecular weight of sodium (22.99 grams per mol) with the total sweat volume lost (litres).

$$\text{Sodium loss} = \text{Sweat sodium concentration} * 22.99 * \text{Sweat loss} \tag{4}$$

The total sodium intake (grams) of each participant was calculated by multiplying the sodium concentration of each drink (Table 1) with the molecular weight of sodium (22.99 grams per mol) with the total volume of each drink consumed (litres).

$$\text{Sodium intake} = \text{Drink sodium concentration} * 22.99 * \text{Fluid intake} \tag{5}$$

Statistical analysis
Data is presented as the mean [range] for all descriptive statistics and mean ± SE for comparison between and within conditions with the level of confidence set at $p < 0.05$ to determine significance. Differences from pre to post training between and within conditions were examined first using a multivariate analysis of variance (MANOVA) for the blood electrolytes and hemoglobin concentrations. Analysis of variance (ANOVA) tests were then applied to each variable to determine which conditions differed and a Tukey's honestly significant difference post-hoc analysis applied when appropriate. Electrolytes with no differences detected using MANOVA, blood glucose, USG and body mass changes were analyzed using repeated measures ANOVA. There was no difference between the athletes sailing different boats in CCS so all participants were pooled into a single group. In WCS, participants' sweat rate and sodium balance variables and glucose intake were analyzed using a one-way ANOVA with Tukey's honestly significant difference. Analysis was performed using SPSS version 20.

Results

Cold condition study

Environmental conditions

During training the wet bulb temperature was 7.1°C [4.2 – 11.3] with 62.7% [32 – 87] relative humidity. Wind velocity was 23.5 km·h^{-1} [17.0 - 36.9].

Hydration status

Pre-training USG values showed that participants arrived for training in a borderline hypohydrated state. There were at least three participants in each group that had USG values greater than 1.025. Examination of USG after training showed no effect of time ($p = 0.318$) (Table 2). At least two participants per group had USG values greater than 1.025. Measurement of plasma volume supports our USG measurements, as there was no difference from pre- to post-training ($p = 0.871$). Participants consumed an average of 811.1 mL [242–1638] of fluid during training (Table 2). This resulted in an average decrease in body mass of 0.40 kg [0 – 1.0]. Body mass changes were not different between groups but there was a main effect for time ($p < 0.001$).

Hematological measurements

Blood sodium concentrations were lower post-training with a main effect for time ($p = 0.02$). The group by time interaction for sodium trended toward significance ($p = 0.084$) (Figure 1A). Participants' blood potassium concentration were lower after training C −19.4%, G −13.7% and IN −13.0%, with a main effect for time ($p < 0.001$) (Figure 1B) and blood chloride concentrations also lower after training with a main effect for time ($p = 0.007$) (Figure 1C). There was a trend towards a main effect for time for blood glucose ($p = 0.074$) (Figure 1D).

Warm condition study

Environmental conditions

Wet bulb temperature during training was 19.5°C [17.0 - 23.3] with 82.3% relative humidity [76.0 – 89.1]. Wind velocity was 24.3 $km{\cdot}h^{-1}$ [15.0 – 36.0).

Hydration status

Examination of USG and body mass revealed a main effect for time for both measures respectively ($p = 0.01$, $p = 0.003$) with no difference between drink conditions (Table 3). Before training participants' USG was higher in all groups with the C and G groups having near hypohydrated values of 1.019 and 1.020 respectively. Two participants in the C group had USG values >1.030. Body mass increased after training for all groups ($p = 0.01$). Participants gained an average of 0.31 kg or 0.44% body mass.

Blood hemoglobin concentration was significantly lower in the G group after training when compared to controls pre-training ($p > 0.05$) (Table 3). When changes in hemoglobin and hematocrit were used to calculate changes in plasma volume there was a main effect for time ($p < 0.001$), indicating a significant increase from pre to post-training; however, there were no differences between groups (Table 2).

Electrolytes

Blood sodium concentrations were reduced 2.6% in the C and 2.3% in the G condition when compared to INW ($p = 0.031$, $p = 0.069$) (Figure 2). Post-training sodium concentration was different between C and INW conditions only ($p = 0.031$) (Figure 2A). Sodium intake was different between each group; however, the amount lost through sweat was not different (Table 2). This resulted in only the INW group having a near neutral sodium balance compared to C and G groups ($p = 0.022$) There was a main effect for time for both blood potassium and chloride concentration ($p < 0.001$, $p < 0.001$) (Figure 2). One-way ANOVA of the post-training measurements of these electrolytes suggested a trend towards difference in groups for chloride ($p = 0.072$).

Blood glucose

Despite the different carbohydrate concentrations between groups, there was no difference between conditions for blood glucose levels (Figure 2D). A main effect for time was found ($p = 0.006$), suggesting an increase in blood glucose after training.

Discussion

The present studies measured changes in hydration status of elite Olympic class sailors in cold and warm conditions. CCS revealed participants consumed insufficient fluids to prevent a decrease in body mass during training, regardless of drink condition, causing a reduction in blood electrolyte concentration. WCS showed that consuming 11.5 $mL{\cdot}kg^{-1}{\cdot}h^{-1}$ of fluid from any condition prevented a decrease in body mass, lowered USG in all conditions and blood sodium concentration and sodium

Table 2 Changes hydration status measured during the CCS

	Crystal Light (C)	Gatorade (G)	Infinit (IN)
USG pre (AU)	1.021 ± 0.002	1.019 ± 0.003	1.020 ± 0.003
USG post (AU)	1.018 ± 0.003	1.019 ± 0.002	1.020 ± 0.002
Fluid Intake (mL)	802 ± 91 [242 – 1110]	924 ± 137 [493 – 1638]	707 ± 152 [186 – 1638]
Change in plasma volume (%)	3.2 ± 2.4	5.4 ± 2.7	4.8 ± 6.7
Change in body mass (kg) *	−0.5 ± 0.1 [0 – -1.0]	−0.4 ± 0.1 [−0.2 – -0.1]	−0.4 ± 0.1 [0 – -0.7]

*Main effect for time. Significantly different from pre-sailing values (p < 0.001).
Data is presented as mean ± SEM [range].

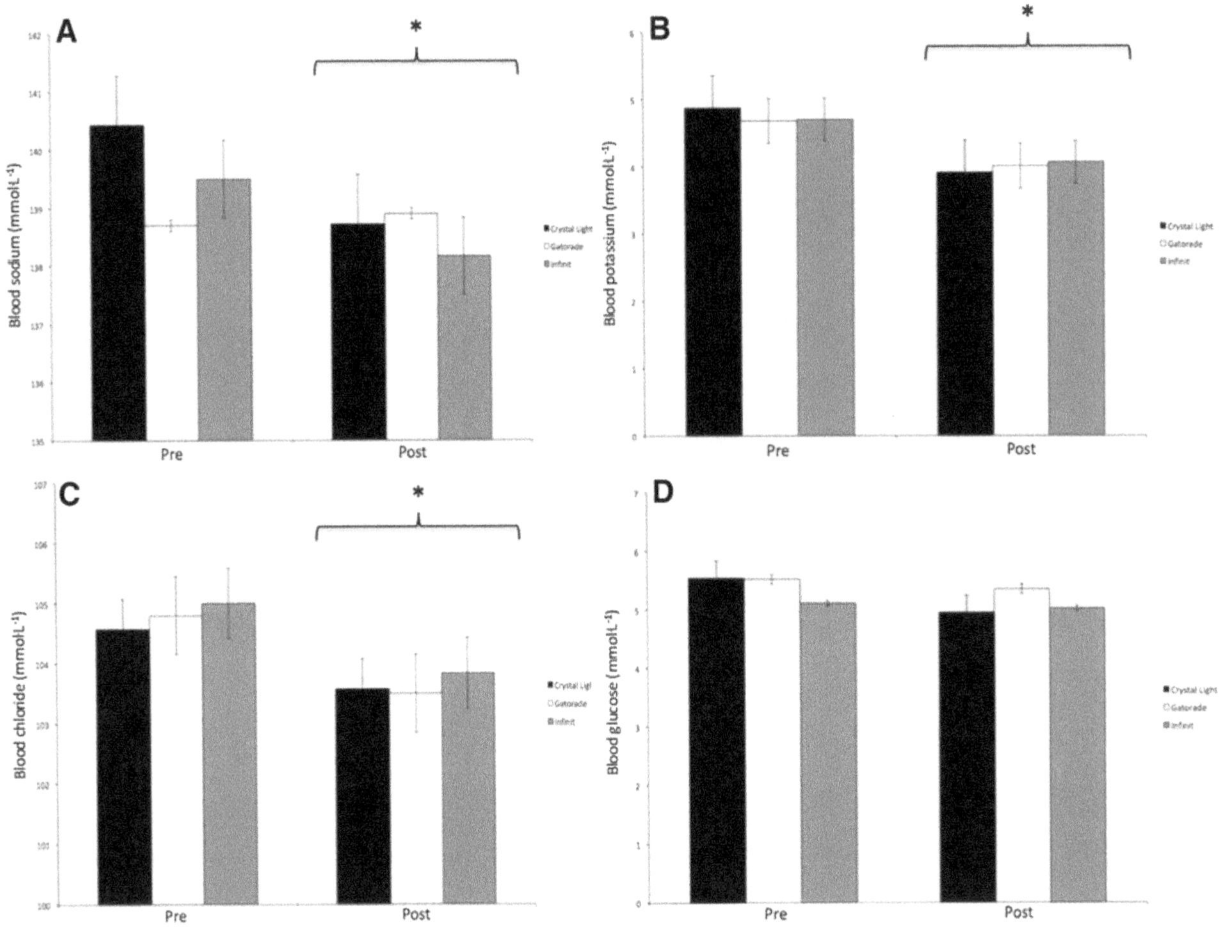

Figure 1 Changes in blood variables from the cold condition study (CCS). A – Blood sodium concentration, **B** – Blood potassium concentration, **C** - blood chloride concentration, **D** – Blood glucose concentration. * Above a bracket indicates a main effect for time ($p < 0.05$). All data are shown as mean ± SE.

Table 3 Changes of hydration variables measured in the WCS

	Crystal Light (C)	Gatorade (G)	Infinit (INW)
USG pre (AU)	1.020 ± 0.003	1.020 ± 0.002	1.018 ± 0.002
USG post (AU)[c]	1.015 ± 0.006	1.007 ± 0.002	1.014 ± 0.002
Change in body mass (kg)	0.3 ± 0.1	0.4 ± 0.2	0.3 ± 0.2
Change in hemoglobin (%)[+]	−4.1 ± 1.5	−7.5 ± 1.6	−4.5 ± 3.0[b]
Change in plasma volume (%)[+]	1.3 ± 0.28	1.7 ± 0.33	1.5 ± 0.82
Sweat rate ($mL{\cdot}h^{-1}$)	510.1 [20.9 -841.1]	597.3 [401.1 – 848.0]	727.2 [456.2-849.0]
Sodium intake (g)*	0	1.2 [1.1 – 1.2]	4.7 [4.4 – 4.7]
Sodium loss (g)	3.1 [0.94 – 5.9]	3.7 [2.0 – 5.8]	4.9 [2.0 – 7.4]
Sodium balance (g)	−3.1 [−4.4 – 0.94]	−2.5 [2.9 - -0.77]	−0.23 [−1.2 – 2.7][a]

* - All groups are significantly different from each other ($p < 0.001$). a – Significantly different from Crystal Light ($p = 0.022$). + Main effect for time indicating that there was an increase in plasma volume in all groups following training ($p < 0.001$). b – Significantly different from pre-training ($p < 0.05$). c – different from pre-training USG with a main effect for time ($p = 0.003$).
Values are shown as the mean (range) for each condition.

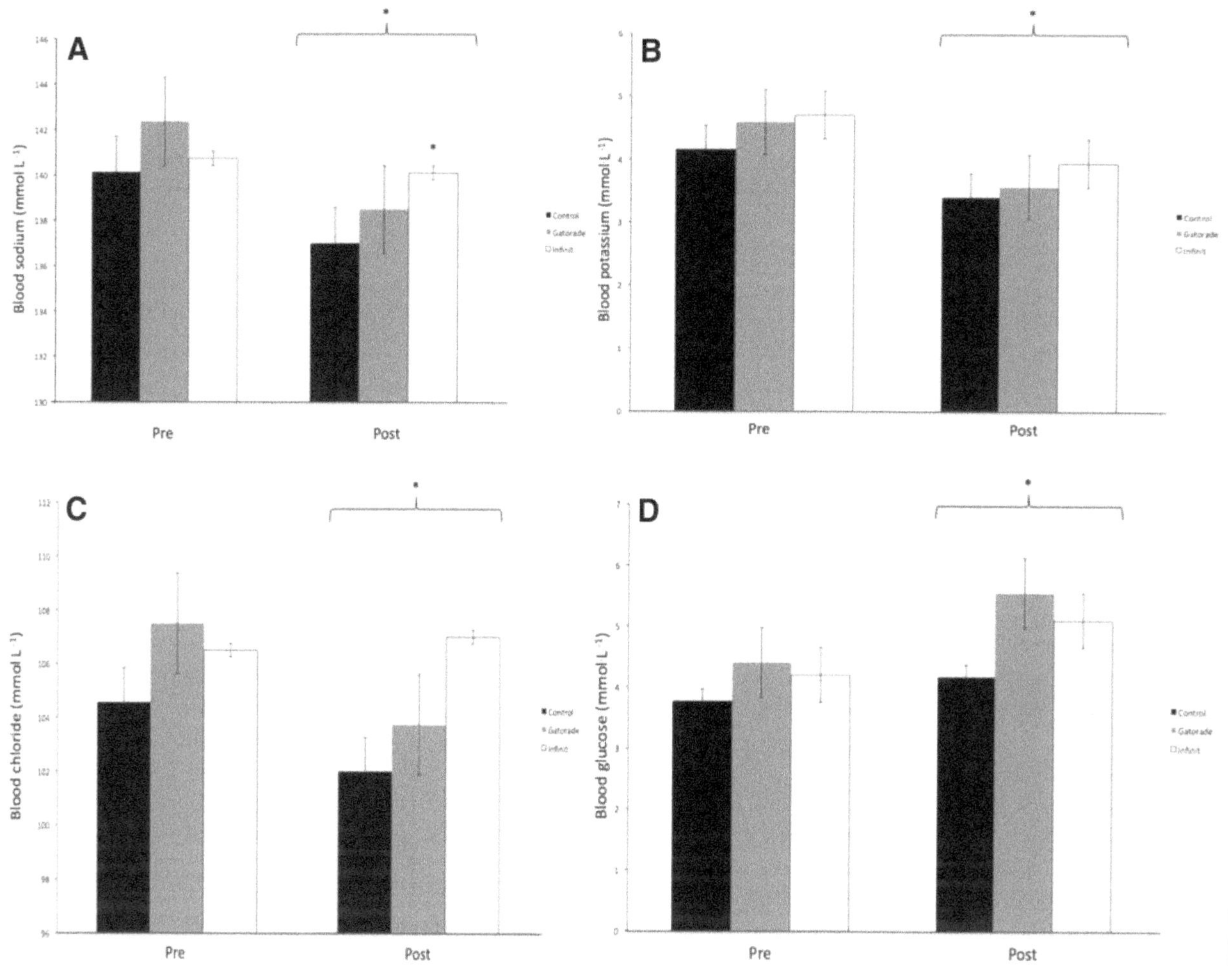

Figure 2 Change in blood variables for the warm condition study (WCS). **A** - Blood sodium concentration (* significantly different from Control p = 0.031), **B** - Blood potassium concentration, **C** - Blood chloride concentration and **D** - Blood glucose. * Above a bracket indicates a main effect for time ($p < 0.05$). All data are shown as mean ± SE.

balance were maintained with the custom drink condition (INW) only.

Hydration

The average pre-training USG value for all groups in both studies was 1.019 (Table 2 and 3), which is very close to the 1.020 threshold that has been associated with hypohydration [22]. As participants were encouraged to consume fluids ad libitum prior to training, this finding suggests individual practices are inadequate. Hamouti et al. [23] have suggested an athlete's muscle mass may influence USG values and therefore a USG measurement of 1.020 may not be an accurate cut-off for hypohydration. While developing an exact cut-off for hypohydration in athletes given their developed muscle mass compared the average population may require further study, the observed pre-practice USG values recorded during both studies were at the higher end of optimal. Since training began at 11:00 am daily, there was adequate time for athletes to consume fluids prior to arriving at the sailing centre. Furthermore, the variability between participants in pre-training USG measurements, especially in the WCS, favours inadequate fluid consumption as opposed to a higher rate of urine protein metabolites due to high muscle mass.

In the WCS, participants' fluid intake was standardized to 11.5 $mL \cdot kg^{-1} \cdot h^{-1}$ to reflect previous recommendations on relative fluid intake [16] and enable the comparison of hydration status and sodium balance between subjects and drinks. The decision to standardize participants' fluid intake was also based partially on the variability of fluid intake observed during the CCS and from inadequate fluid intake reported in previous studies [9,14]. A leading cause of insufficient fluid intake for athletes training and competing in cold temperatures is reduced thirst, which is restored in warm conditions [24]. Examination of elite football players training in cool (5°C) temperatures revealed athletes consumed far less fluid than was lost from sweating [15]. Furthermore, runners have been found to underestimate their sweat rates in cool conditions, despite accurate estimations of their fluid consumption [25]. These and our findings suggest athlete's perception of sweat rates in cool climates is impaired, which reinforces the need for specific hydration guidelines. The fluid requirements of participants in WCS (19.5°C [17.0 - 23.3]), were anticipated to reflect the average laboratory sweat rate of 1470 $mL \cdot h^{-1}$ measured at 21.8°C. The fluid intake rate of 11.5 $mL \cdot kg^{-1} \cdot h^{-1}$ was selected to deliver approximately 65% of the average laboratory sweat rate and a volume less than one litre (906.2 – 971.8 $mL \cdot h^{-1}$), with a carbohydrate content between 6-9%. This range of carbohydrate consumption in fluid replacement drinks has been identified as an optimal range for absorption and gastric emptying [6]. Furthermore, consuming volumes greater than 1000 $mL \cdot h^{-1}$ during exercise has caused gastro-intestinal discomfort in highly trained individuals [26]. None of the participants in the study commented on any bloating or gastro-intestinal issues during or after training.

Surprisingly, participants' average on-water sweat rate was only 611.8 ± 47.2 $mL \cdot h^{-1}$. This was 41.5% lower than the pre-study laboratory sweat rate of 1470 $mL \cdot h^{-1}$. As a result, participants mean fluid intake was 933.33 ± 5.13 $mL \cdot h^{-1}$ or 153.0% fluid replacement. Since on-water temperatures were similar to that of the laboratory sweat rate testing, it appears the cooling effect of splashing waves and brief pauses in activity between training drills did not elicit the same physiologic sweat response during sailing as seen during cycle exercise. This suggests laboratory based sweat rate testing over estimates sweat rates observed on-water in this study. Therefore, the on water environmental conditions experienced by Olympic class sailors may have a direct modulating influence on sweat rate and fluid requirements. Based on our observations, a lower fluid replacement rate would be more appropriate for the conditions experienced in this study. Extrapolating from the data presented, a fluid intake rate of 7.4 $mL \cdot kg^{-1} \cdot h^{-1}$ would achieve the desired hydration state.

USG and electrolytes

The greater fluid consumption compared to fluid loss during WCS may account for some of our results. Analysis of USG showed an effect for time ($p = 0.003$) with lower values after training in all groups (Table 3). This was coupled with a main effect for time for body weight, whereby all groups increased body mass during training as direct result of fluid intake. This was a clear difference from CCS during which there was no difference in USG and a decrease in body mass post-training ($p < 0.001$). In CCS it was not surprising to see no difference between groups for measures of hydration status; however, given the 3 and 4 fold higher concentrations of sodium and potassium between the INW and G drink conditions in WCS, we anticipated a difference between groups post-training. While it is clear that all groups retained fluid during training, an effect of the positive fluid balance, the higher sodium concentration in the INW condition did not have a compounding effect on fluid retention as could have been anticipated as observed in previous findings [27].

The sweat sodium loss of participants in WCS (Table 3) is similar to values reported by other groups studying elite athletes [15,28]. While there was no difference in sodium loss with the different drinks, sodium balance was almost unchanged in the INW group compared to C and G conditions. This was a result of the INW drink being designed for full sodium replacement. Sodium intake is essential for the absorption and retention of fluid during exercise [27]. Results from hydration testing in other sports have shown elite athletes have difficulty replacing sodium lost during training using fluid replacement drinks [19,29]. These finding, coupled with our results from CCS, can be explained in part by the ad libitum fluid consumption study protocol. This indicates athletes may have difficulty self-regulating their hydration requirements particularly in cold conditions, as it is easy to become caught-up in the focus and intensity of training and/or competition. This further supports the need for individual, sport specific or relative fixed volume fluid replacement recommendations.

Blood glucose carbohydrates intake

Examination of the energy demands of Laser sailing by Castagna and Brisswalter [11] revealed aerobic metabolism is the main energy source used by elite sailors to fulfill muscle energy demands. As such, blood glucose levels in CCS were trending towards a decrease over time ($p = 0.074$), despite the supply of exogenous carbohydrates in the G and IN groups; although, the average carbohydrate intake in these groups was only 61 g and 42 g respectively. Interestingly, the blood glucose concentration of the C group was stable through the 2.5 h training session despite consuming no exogenous carbohydrates (Figure 1D). In comparison, trained cyclists working at 74% VO_2max in laboratory conditions experienced a significant decrease in blood glucose after 90 minutes of cycling [30]. Examination of substrate metabolism during 60 minutes of cycling at 70% VO_2max at 0°C revealed almost 60% of energy expenditure was from carbohydrate metabolism [31]. This level was maintained regardless of infused non-esterified fatty acids, suggesting that carbohydrates are a preferred source of energy in cold conditions as fatty acid metabolism has been found to increase based on substrate availability in temperature environments [32]. While the intensity of Laser sailing in conditions similar to CCS reached approximately 65% VO_2max [11], this difference in intensity may have been enough to prevent deleterious changes in blood glucose in the C condition.

In WCS, blood glucose levels were surprisingly unchanged between the drink conditions (Figure 2D). Although a main effect for time was observed ($p = 0.006$), indicating that blood glucose was higher after training, this was largely driven by the G and INW groups. The carbohydrate content in the G drink was 66 $g \cdot L^{-1}$, which is approximately in-line with the current American College of Sports Medicine recommendations [4]. These guidelines were based on the understanding that carbohydrates ingested during exercise could only be oxidized at a maximum rate of 1 $g \cdot min^{-1}$ [33]. However, advances in carbohydrate metabolism research have determined up to 1.75 $g \cdot min^{-1}$ can be oxidized when using multiple transportable carbohydrates, such as glucose and fructose [34]. As such, the carbohydrate content in the INW drink was comprised of glucose and fructose delivered in a 2:1 ratio at 1.3 – 1.5 $g \cdot min^{-1}$ based on a concentration of 90 $g \cdot L^{-1}$. Previous work has determined this ratio of carbohydrate delivered in solution and ingestion at 1.5 $g \cdot min^{-1}$ can improve exogenous carbohydrate metabolism during exercise by 13% [35] to 48% [36] compared to consuming an isocaloric glucose only solution. While carbohydrate oxidation was not measured in this study, consuming a drink with high carbohydrate concentration using multiple transporters has a potentially powerful effect for sailing athletes, as World Cup regattas last 5–7 days with up to three hours of competitions per day. Therefore, reducing endogenous carbohydrate oxidation could potentially preserve stored muscle glycogen energy for later in the competition, which has previously been found to have a performance enhancing effect [37].

During competition, sailors can spend anywhere from two hours to six hours on-water, with time divided between warm-up, racing and waiting for changes in wind and weather and cool-down. Given the length of time on-water, the co-ingestion of carbohydrates and protein is necessary to prevent extended periods of muscle protein breakdown. Research examining the addition of whey protein to carbohydrate electrolyte beverages has revealed inconsistent results for improved athletic performance in both acute exercise [38,39] and cycling time trials [40,41]. In these studies, the addition of protein to an experimental beverage was focused on improving athletic performance in acute exercise. In contrast, the addition of protein to a carbohydrate electrolyte drink used during multi-day competitions may be more appropriate for metabolic reasons and worthy of continued investigation. Saunders et al. [42] found the use of a fluid replacement drink fortified with protein during a two cycle-to-exhaustion tests within the same day was effective in attenuating the nutritional deficit incurred during exercise and helped to reduce skeletal muscle damage compared to a carbohydrate electrolyte drink alone. Therefore, performing multiple bouts of exercise within a day or consecutive days of competition may be necessary to fully observe the nutritional and physiologic effects of protein ingested with a carbohydrate electrolyte beverage during exercise [43].

Limitation

The authors acknowledge there were several limitations to the present study. The sample size for both studies was calculated to detect electrolyte changes. Based on subject variability and the applied nature of this research additional subjects would have been beneficial to detect differences between conditions; however, the maximum number of available participants was recruited.

Conclusion

Participants in the ad libitum design CCS were unable to maintain hydration status in any condition due to inadequate fluid consumption. This may have resulted from a reduced desire to drink and/or poor estimation of individual hydration requirements in cold temperatures. When 11.5 $mL \cdot kg^{-1} \cdot h^{-1}$ of fluid was consumed in the WCS, all conditions improved urinary markers of hydration and prevented a loss of body mass. The C and G conditions were unable to maintain blood electrolyte concentrations while the customized INW condition was effective in maintaining blood sodium concentrations but not potassium. This was the first study to test relative fluid intake based on laboratory sweat rate on the hydration requirements of Olympic class sailors in warm conditions. Therefore, it is important to note that laboratory sweat testing results did not directly correspond with on-water sweat rate. This finding may guide further research of the hydration requirements of sailors in different environmental conditions.

Competing interests

The authors declare that they have no competing interests.

Author contributions

EJHL, SGT and GDW participated in study conception and design. EJHL and SJF performed data collection. EJHL performed statistical analysis and data analysis with SGT and GDW. All authors participated in writing, editing and approval of the final manuscript.

Acknowledgments

The authors would like to thank the athletes and coaches for their participation in this study and the Canadian Yachting Association and CORK for the use of their facilities. Additionally, we would like to thank the Canadian Sport Centre Ontario for the use of their equipment and resources. Evan Lewis was supported by an Ontario Ministry of Health Promotion Research Program in Applied Sport Science Grant and a Mitacs Accelerate Award.

Author details

[1]Department of Nutritional Sciences, University of Toronto, 150 College Street, Toronto, ON M5S 3E2, Canada. [2]Faculty of Life Sciences, McMaster University, 1280 Main Street West, Hamilton, ON L8S 4L8, Canada. [3]Faculty of Kinesiology and Physical Education, The University of Toronto, 55 Harbord Street, Toronto, ON M5R 2W6, Canada. [4]Physiology and Experimental

Medicine, The Hospital for Sick Children, 555 University Avenue, Toronto, ON M5G 1X8, Canada.

References

1. Hargreaves M, Dillo P, Angus D, *et al*: **Effect of fluid ingestionon on muscle metabolism during prolonged exercise.** *J Appl Physiol* 1996, **80:**363–366.
2. D'anci KE, Vibhakar A, Kanter JH, *et al*: **Voluntary dehydration and cognitive performance in trained college athletes.** *Perception and Motor Skills* 2009, **109:**251–269.
3. Coyle E: **Fluid and fuel intake during exercise.** *Journal of Sports Science* 2004, **22:**39–55.
4. ACSM: **Exercise and fluid replacement: Position stand.** *Medicine and Science in Sports and Exercise* 2007, **39:**377–390.
5. Costill D: **Sweating: Its composition and effects on body fluids.** *Annals New York Academy of Science* 1977, **301:**160–174.
6. Coyle E, Montain S: **Benefits of fluid replacement with carbohydrate during exercise.** *Medicine and Science in Sports and Exercise* 1992, **24:**S324–S330.
7. Adam GE, Carter R, Cheuvront SN, *et al*: **Hydration effects on cognitive performance during military tasks in temperate and cold environments.** *Physiology and Behaviour* 2008, **93:**748–756.
8. Allen J, De Jong M: **Sailing and sports medicine: A literature review.** *Br J Sports Med* 2006, **40:**587–593.
9. Slater G, Tan B: **Body mass changes and nutrient intake of dinghy sailors while racing.** *J Sports Sci* 2007, **25:**1129–1135.
10. Legg SJ, Smith P, Slyfield D, *et al*: **Knowledge and reported use of sport science by elite new zealand olympic class sailors.** *J Sports Med Phys Fitness* 1997, **37:**213–217.
11. Castagna O, Brisswalter J: **Assessment of energy demand in laser sailing: Influences of exercise duration and performance level.** *Eur J Appl Physiol* 2007, **99:**95–101.
12. Vogiatzis I, Spurway N, Wilson J, *et al*: **Assessment of aerobic and anaerobic demands of dinghy sailing at different wind velocities.** *J Sports Med Phys Fitness* 1995, **35:**103–107.
13. Neville V, Gant N, Folland J: **Thermoregulatory demands of elite professional america's cup yacht racing.** *Scand J Med Sci Sports* 2009, **20:**475–484.
14. Kurdak S, Shirreffs SM, Maughan R, *et al*: **Hydration and sweating responses to hot-weather football competition.** *Scand J Med Sci Sports* 2010, **20:**133–139.
15. Maughan RJ, Shirreffs SM, Merson SJ, *et al*: **Fluid and electrolyte balance in elite male football (soccer) players training in a cool environment.** *J Sports Sci* 2005, **23:**73–79.
16. Mitchell JB, Voss W: **The influence of volume on gastric emptying and fluid balance during prolong exercise.** *Medicine and Science in Sports and Exercise* 1991, **23:**314–319.
17. Patterson MJ, Galloway SD, Nimmo MA: **Variations in regional sweat composition in normal human males.** *Exp Physiol* 2000, **85:**869–875.
18. Fletcher E, Cunningham P: *Indoor rowing: Sailing guide. Concept 2*. 2007. http://concept2.co.uk/training/sailing.
19. Palmer M, Spriet L: **Sweat rate, salt loss and fluid intake during an intense on-ice practice in elite canadian male junior hockey players.** *Appl Physiol Nutr Metab* 2008, **33:**263–271.
20. Laursen P, Suriano R, Quod M, *et al*: **Core temperature and hydration status during an ironman triathlon.** *Br J Sports Med* 2006, **40:**320–325.
21. Dill DB, Costill DL: **Calculation of percentage changes in volumes of blood, plasma, and red cells in dehydration.** *J Appl Physiol* 1974, **37:**247–248.
22. Casa DJ, Armstrong LE, Hillman SK, *et al*: **National athletic trainer's association position statement: Fluid replacement for athletes.** *Journal of Athlete Training* 2000, **35:**212–224.
23. Hamouti N, Del Coso J, Avila A, *et al*: **Effects of athletes' muscle mass on urinary markers of hydration status.** *Eur J Appl Physiol* 2010, **109:**213–219.
24. Kenefick RW, Hazzard MP, Mahood NV, *et al*: **Thirst sensations and avp responses at rest and during exercise-cold exposure.** *Medicine and Science in Sports and Exercise* 2004, **36:**1528–1534.
25. Passe D, Horn M, Stofan J, *et al*: **Voluntary dehydration in runners despite favorable conditions for fluid intake.** *Int J Sport Nutr Exerc Metab* 2007, **17:**284–295.
26. Noakes TD: **Fluid replacement during exercise.** *Exercise Sport Science Review* 1993, **21:**297–330.
27. Takamata A, Mack GW, Gillen CM, *et al*: **Sodium appetite, thirst and body fluid regulation in humans during rehydration without sodium replacement.** *American Journal of Physiology Regulation and Integrated Comparative Physiology* 1994, **266:**1493–1502.
28. Shirreffs SM, Aragon-Vargas LF, Chamorro M, *et al*: **The sweating response of elite professional soccer players to training in the heat.** *Int J Sports Med* 2005, **26:**90–95.
29. Maughan R, Merson SJ, Broad NP, *et al*: **Fluid and electrolyte intake and loss in elite soccer players during training. International Journal of Nutrition and Exercise.** *Metabolism* 2004, **14:**333–346.
30. Coyle E, Hagberg J, Hurley B, *et al*: **Carbohydrate feeding during prolonged strenuous exercise can delay fatigue.** *J Appl Physiol* 1983, **55:**230–235.
31. Layden J, Malkova D, Nimmo MA: **During exercise in the cold increased availability of plasma nonesterified fatty acids does not affect the pattern of substrate oxidation.** *Metabolism* 2004, **53:**203–208.
32. Hawley JA: **Effect of increased fat availability on metabolism and exercise capacity.** *Medicine and Science in Sports and Exercise* 2002, **34:**1485–1491.
33. Jeukendrup A, Tipton K: **Legal nutritional boosting for cycling.** *Curr Sports Med Rep* 2009, **8:**186–191.
34. Jeukendrup A: **Carbohydrate and exercise performance: The role of multiple transportable carbohydrates.** *Current Opinions in Clinical Nutrition and Metabolic Care* 2010, **13:**452–457.
35. Jeukendrup A, Moseley L, Mainwaring G, *et al*: **Exogenous carbohydrate oxidation during ultra endurance exercise.** *J Appl Physiol* 2006, **100:**1134–1141.
36. Jentjens R, Underwood K, Achten J, *et al*: **Exogenous carbohydrate oxidation rates are elevated after combined ingestion of glucose and fructose during exercise in the heat.** *J Appl Physiol* 2006, **100:**807–816.
37. Coyle E, Coggan AR: **Muscle glycogen utilized during prolonged exercise when fed carbohydrate.** *J Appl Physiol* 1986, **61:**165–172.
38. Ivy JL, Res PT, Sprague RC, *et al*: **Effect of a carbohydrate-protein supplement on endurance performance during exercise of varying intensity.** *Int J Sport Nutr Exerc Metab* 2003, **13:**382–395.
39. Romano-Ely BC, Todd MK, Saunders MJ, *et al*: **Effect of an isocaloric carbohydrate-protein-antioxidant drink on cycling performance.** *Medicine and Science in Sports and Exercise* 2006, **38:**1608–1616.
40. Toone RJ, Betts JA: **Isocaloric carbohydrate versus carbohydrate-protein ingestion and cycling time-trial performance.** *Int J Sport Nutr Exerc Metab* 2010, **20:**34–43.
41. van Essen M, Gibala MJ: **Failure of protein to improve time trial performance when added to a sports drink.** *Medicine and Science in Sports and Exercise* 2006, **38:**1476–1483.
42. Saunders MJ, Kane MD, Todd MK: **Effects of a carbohydrate-protein beverage on cycling endurance and muscle damage.** *Medicine and Science in Sports and Exercise* 2004, **36:**1233–1238.
43. Cathcart AJ, Murgatroyd SR, McNab A, *et al*: **Combined carbohydrate–protein supplementation improves competitive endurance exercise performance in the heat.** *Eur J Appl Physiol* 2011, **111:**2051–2061.

12

Incidence and pattern of injuries among adolescent basketball players in Nigeria

Oluwatoyosi Babatunde Alex Owoeye*, Ashiyat Kehinde Akodu, Bayonle Matt Oladokun and Sunday Rufus Akinwumi Akinbo

Abstract

Background: Basketball is the second most popular sport in Nigeria after football and is commonly played by adolescents. Prospective studies on adolescent basketball players in Nigeria are lacking. Such studies will help to develop injury counter-measures. Hence, this study aimed at determining the incidence and pattern of injuries among adolescent basketball players in Nigeria.

Methods: A prospective observational study involving 141 adolescent basketball players (75 boys and 66 girls; with age range 15 – 18 years) who participated in the 2010 National Finals of the Nigeria Nestlé Milo Basketball Competition. Basketball-related injury data were collected by an assessor during the competition using a standardized basketball injury report form. Data were analyzed using descriptive and inferential statistics.

Results: A total of 32 injuries were recorded with an incidence of 22.7 injuries per 100 participants same for boys and girls. This is equivalent to 1.1 injury per match for boys and 0.9 injuries per match for girls. Jumping/landing was the most common cause of injury (28.1%, N = 9). Most of the injuries were at the lower extremities (75%, N = 24); with majority at the knee joint (40.6%, N = 13). Ligament sprain was the most common types of injury. The pattern of injuries among boys did not significantly differ from that of girls ($P > 0.05$). Most injuries (N = 13, 41%) occurred in the offensive half of the court and cryotherapy was the most frequently used treatment modality.

Conclusion: The overall incidence of match injury among adolescent amateur basketball players during a national competition in Nigeria was 22.7 injuries per 100 participants; equivalence of 1.0 injury per match. The pattern of injuries was similar in both genders and consistent with what has been previously reported in literature for adolescent basketball players. Exercise-based injury prevention programmes aimed at improving core strength and neuromuscular control at the lower limbs may help reduce the incidence of injuries.

Background

Youth sports injury is a public health concern, as it has detrimental effects on the health and well being of young athletes [1]. Increasingly, competitive youth sports around the world require adolescents to undertake more prolonged and intensive training programmes [2]. Increased playing is mirrored by an increased risk of traumatic injury or overuse musculoskeletal injury by young sports participants [1]. It has been established that specific injury pattern occur in different sports and at different levels [3,4]. Basketball continues to increase in popularity at all levels of play, from recreational to professional and remains immensely popular, not just in the United States, but throughout the world [5].

Basketball appears to be the second most popular sport in Nigeria after football (soccer). Most public and private schools in Nigeria have standard basketball courts where students play during break time and after school. Epidemiological studies on basketball injuries in Nigeria are sparsely documented compared to the United States and Europe. Literature review showed that only one study has investigated the pattern of basketball injuries in Nigeria [6]. The study was limited to professional male basketball players only. It reported an injury incidence of 0.7 injury per match. It further revealed that the ankle followed by the knee were the most frequently injured body parts, while sprain and contusion were the most common types of injuries sustained. Most of the injuries occurred in the

* Correspondence: toyosialexowoeye@yahoo.com
Department of Physiotherapy, College of Medicine, University of Lagos, Idi-Araba, Lagos, Nigeria

offensive zone of the court and collision was the most common causes of injuries [6]. In another study focused on several sports, basketball players among other athletes were reported to have the highest injury rate [7].

Overall incidence rate in basketball have been reported to be higher during competitive matches than training sessions [8,9]. Results of the most commonly studied population of adolescent basketball players – American public high school players, revealed that injury incidence vary considerably, from 5.6 – 36.8 per 100 participants for boys and 7.8 – 49.0 per 100 participants for girls [9].

There appears to be a dearth of study on the incidence and pattern of basketball injuries among adolescent players in Nigeria. The study aimed at determining the incidence and pattern of injuries among adolescent male and female basketball players in Nigeria. The study also investigated the types of first aid treatments rendered to the injured players.

Methods

Participants and setting

A cohort of 141 basketball players who were duly registered for the national finals of the Nigeria Nestlé Milo Secondary Schools Basketball Competition participated in the study. A total of 32 matches were played and all the matches were prospectively followed. The competition was held at the indoor sports hall of the National Stadium, Surulere, Lagos State, in October, 2010.

The Nestlé MILO Secondary School Basketball Competition is an annual event sponsored by MILO in partnership with the Nigerian School Sports Federation. The programme is targeted at students aged 13 – 18 years. The 12th edition of the competition had a total of 4,252 schools nationwide who participated from the state preliminary stage to the national finals. These secondary schools across the 6 geopolitical zones/conferences of the country were drawn into groups in the various conferences namely: the Savannah Conference, Central Conference, Atlantic Conference, Western Conference, Sahara Conference and Equatorial Conference. Male and female basketball teams competed in playoffs at the various conferences to produce finalists. Two schools emerged from each of the zones in the boys and girls categories which then made the 12 basketball teams (6 for each gender) that participated in the national finals of the competition.

Instrumentation

A standardized basketball injury report form [6] specifically designed for basketball was used for the study. It contained information regarding demographic data, cause of the injury, type of injury, body part injured, first aid rendered, the zone of the court where injury occurred and whether the player returned to the court of play after treatment. Detailed injury reports describing all the aforementioned were completed by the attending physiotherapist who was also the assessor for each injury.

Procedure for data collection

The physiotherapist (a member of the study group) was present at all matches of the competition to attend to injured players and document injuries. An injury was documented when an injured player required at least minimum on-field (medical) care such as ice, tape, etc. regardless of whether the player was able to continue or not (that is both medical attention and time-loss injuries were recorded). All the participating schools gave their consent before the commencement of the competition and ethical approval to conduct the study was also sought for and obtained from the research and ethics committee of the Lagos University Teaching Hospital.

Data analysis

Descriptive statistics of frequency and percentage were used. Inferential statistics of chi-square was used to determine significant difference between certain variables. Incidence of injuries was calculated per 100 participants thus – total number of injuries divided by the total number of players that participated (separately calculated for boys, girls and overall). Incidence was also calculated per match. For all statistical tests, the level of significance was taken at $P \le 0.05$.

Result

Participants

There were 141 players comprising 75 boys (53.2%) and 66 girls (46.8%) aged 16.3 ± 0.9 years (range of 15 – 18 years).

Incidence

A total of 32 injuries (17 for boys and 15 for girls) were recorded during the competition. The overall incidence of injury was 22.7 injuries per 100 participants for both genders. An incidence of 1.1 injuries per match and 0.9 injuries per match were recorded for boys and girls respectively. The overall incidence was 1.0 injury per match.

Causes of injuries

"Jumping/landing" was found to be the most common cause of injury, accounting for 9 cases (28.1%) while "being hit by a projectile ball" was the least cause of injury (N = 1, 3.1%) (Table 1).

Types of injuries and body parts affected

Sprain was found to be the most common type of injury accounting for 62.5% of all injuries (Table 2). There was no statistically significant difference in the mean percentage difference in the number of boys and girls that were injured ($p = 0.481$) (Table 2). The knee was the most commonly affected body part, accounting for 13 cases (40.6%), followed by the ankle (N = 7, 21.9%). The forearm, wrist

Table 1 Causes of injuries

Causes of injuries	Boys n (%)	Girls n (%)	Total n (%)
Collision/contact with obstacle	3 (60.0)	2 (40.0)	5 (15.6)
Jumping/landing	4 (45.0)	5 (55.0)	9 (28.1)
Hit by a projectile ball	1 (100.0)	- (0.0)	1 (3.1)
Previous injury	5 (71.4)	2 (28.6)	7 (21.9)
Sudden turn, twist or stop	4 (50.0)	4 (50.0)	8 (25.0)
Others	- (0.0)	2 (100.0)	2 (6.3)
Total	17	15	32 (100.0)

$X^2 - 4.49$, $p = 0.481$.

and fingers, hip and thigh, and the leg were the least body parts affected, accounting for 1 case each (3.1%) (Table 3). Injuries to the ankle and knee joints occurred more in boys than girls, although, there was no statistically significant difference between them (p = 0.590) (Table 3).

Zone of the court where injury occurred

Majority of the injuries occurred in the offensive half (N = 13, 41%). The defensive half and key area of the court accounted for 8 (25%) and 11 (34%) injuries respectively.

First aid rendered

Cryotherapy (N = 28, 52.8%) was the most frequently administered first aid treatment, followed by strapping/bandaging (N = 15, 28.3%). Bleeding control was the least administered treatment (N = 2, 3.8%) (Table 4). Regarding further care disposition, 75% of the total injured players continued playing after receiving medical attention while 25% could not continue playing despite being treated.

Discussion

The growth and popularity in secondary school (high school) basketball participation in Nigeria creates an urgent need for injury surveillance to identify potential avenues for injury prevention. The present study investigated the incidence and pattern of injuries in a representative sample of adolescent basketball players in Nigeria as a step towards injury prevention.

Table 2 Types of injuries sustained

Injury	Boys n (%)	Girls n (%)	Total n (%)
Contusion	2 (66.7)	1 (33.3)	3 (9.4)
Dislocation	1 (100.0)	- (0.0)	1 (3.1)
Laceration	1 (50.0)	1 (50.0)	2 (6.3)
Sprain	11 (55.0)	9 (45.0)	20 (62.5)
Strain	2 (40.0)	3 (60.0)	5 (15.6)
Cramp	- (0.0)	1 (100.0)	1 (3.1)
Total	17	15	32 (100.0)

$X^2 - 4.93$, $p = 0.424$.

Table 3 Body parts injured

Body part injured	Boys n (%)	Girls n (%)	Total n (%)
Face	2 (100.0)	- (0.0)	2 (6.3)
Abdomen/Trunk	- (0.0)	1 (100.0)	1 (3.1)
Forearm	1 (100.0)	- (0.0)	1 (3.1)
Wrist & Finger	1 (100.0)	- (0.0)	1 (3.1)
Elbow	1 (33.3)	2 (66.7)	3 (9.4)
Hip & Thigh	- (0.0)	1 (100.0)	1 (3.1)
Leg	- (0.0)	1 (100.0)	1 (3.1)
Knee	7 (53.8)	6 (46.2)	13 (40.6)
Ankle	4 (57.1)	3 (42.9)	7 (21.9)
Toes	1 (50.0)	1 (50.0)	2 (6.3)
Total	17	15	32 (100.0)

$X^2 - 7.46$, $p = 0.590$.

Injury in previous related studies range from any incident evaluated to incidents that result in at least a day absence and the metric of risk include percentage injured, injuries per match or injuries per 100 or 1,000 hours of exposure or per 1,000 athletes/participants [10–16]. It is important to note that no publication presently exist concerning a consensus statement for basketball injury surveillance. This has resulted in differences in injury definitions and methodologies by different authors. Our definition of injury included both medical attention and time loss injuries. Differences in methodology made it difficult to compare with some studies done in Europe. However, an incidence of 22.7 injuries per 100 participants recorded in this study for each gender falls within the range documented for American public high school which varies considerably from 5.6–36.8 per 100 participants for boys, and 7.8–49 per 100 participants for girls [9]. An incidence of 1.0 injury per match recorded in this study is comparable to 0.7 recorded by Akinbo et al. [6]. This suggests that there is a higher risk of injuries among adolescent amateur basketball players than among the professionals in Nigeria.

This study revealed that jumping/landing and sudden turn, twists or stop were the most common causes of injuries in young basketball players in Nigeria. This is in

Table 4 First aid rendered to the injured players

Modalities	Frequency (n)	Percentage (%)
Cryotherapy	28	52.8
Massage	5	9.4
Stretching	3	5.7
Strapping/Bandaging	15	28.3
Bleeding Control	2	3.8
Total	53	100

agreement with other studies on adolescent/youth basketball players [10,14]. However, it contrasts with some other studies [6,16] on professional male and female basketball players in which collision with an obstacle (fellow player or opponent) was documented as the major cause of injuries. This contrast may be due to the difference in the levels of play and skills.

Sprain was predominantly the most common type of injury documented for both genders which was more represented at the knee and ankle joints. This is consistent with other previous epidemiological studies on adolescent and professional basketball players [6,10-14]. Jumping/landing caused majority of the knee and ankle ligament sprains documented in this study. Intervention programs that focus on jumping or balance training in these players could prove to be effective injury prevention strategy [17,18].

The present study revealed that the offensive zone recorded the highest injuries of the three zones followed by the key area and then the defensive half. This agrees with other previous studies [6,9,14]. A high incidence of injuries in this zone is probably because it is a very active area where offensive players try to make shots against their opponents followed by the key area where they struggle to get rebounds in other to make a shot or save the ball from getting into their opponent possession.

Concerning body part affectation, the lower limbs, represented mostly by the knee joint accounted for 75% of all injuries. This is consistent with previous studies on basketball [9–16]. There are still some controversies on the most frequently injured anatomical site in basketball. While some authors [15,16] reported the knee as most commonly injured body part, most other authors [9–14] reported the ankle to be the most commonly injured body site. Repetitive jumping in basketball imposes recurring consistent vertical ground reaction forces of up to four times body weight on the weight-bearing knee joint [19]. The maturing (adolescent) neuromuscular system may be unable to maintain knee stability and around-joint control, leading to forces above the physiological threshold, with inevitable injury to the knee joint structures.

The most frequently used treatment modalities were cryotherapy and bandaging. Cryotherapy in the form of cold compress or cold spray application remains the mainstay first aid treatment for most acute on-field injuries. Over 50% of treatments given during the competition involved Cryotherapy. This corroborates other studies [6,7,20,21]. This is because many of the injuries were minor ligament sprains and muscle strains which did not require any form of special treatment modalities. However, some (25%) of the injuries were time loss injuries. This implies that 1 out of every 4 injuries resulted in a disposition of discontinuity of play during the competition. These time loss injuries were moderate and severe injuries that prevented players from returning to play immediately after a sideline treatment. It is imperative that injury countermeasures that would help prevent such injuries in future competitions are introduced.

The level and intensity of play in high risk sports such as basketball, is one area which may be addressed by sports medicine experts, parents, coaches, sports administrators and injury prevention policy makers. The focus of sports activity by young people should be directed at technique development in order to train their neuromuscular system to control the biomechanical strain imposed by the game of basketball.

Conclusion

The incidence of match injuries in adolescent amateur basketball players during a national competition in Nigeria was 22.7 injuries per 100 participants; equivalence of 1.0 injury per match. The pattern of injuries was similar in both genders and consistent with what has been previously reported in literature for adolescent basketball. Majority of the injuries were to the lower extremities and knee ligament sprains were the most reported injuries.

Continued surveillance of nationally representative samples of Nigeria's young basketball players is essential to fully understand the injuries in this population. The increased quantity of data will aid in the development of precise preventive methods and also help in measuring the impact of any interventions. Exercise-based injury prevention programmes aimed at improving core strength and neuromuscular control at the lower limbs may help reduce the incidence of injuries.

Competing interests

No competing interests.

Authors' contributions

OBA was involved with study concept and design, analysis of data, interpretation of data, and preparation of the manuscript. AK was involved with study design, interpretation of data, and drafting of manuscript. BM was involved in study design, acquisition of data, analysis of data and drafting of manuscript. SRA was involved with study concept and design, and interpretation of data. All authors were involved with critical revision of the manuscript for important intellectual content and approved the final version of the manuscript.

Acknowledgement

The authors appreciate the assistance rendered by Dr. Bukola Ajayi of the National Sports Medicine Centre, Lagos during the competition and the cooperation of all the participants and officials of the 2010 National Finals of the Nigeria Nestle Milo Basketball Competition.

References

1. Yang J, Marshall SW, Bowling JM: **Use of discretionary protective equipment and rate of lower extremity injury in high school athletes.** *Am J Epidemiol* 2005, **161**:511–519.
2. Caine D, DiFiori J, Maffuli N: **Physical injuries in children's and youth sports: reason for concern?** *Br J Sports Med* 2006, **40**:749–760.
3. Bahr R, Krosshaugh T: **Understanding injury mechanisms: a key component of presenting injuries in sport.** *British J Sport Med* 2005, **14**:286–290.

4. Bruce CY: **Injury and disability in matched men's and women's intercollegiate sports.** *Am J Public Health* 1991, **80**:410–504.
5. Cantwell JD: **The physician who invented basketball.** *Am J Cardiology* 2004, **93**:1075–1077.
6. Akinbo S, Odebiyi D, Adebayo A: **Pattern of musculoskeletal injuries in professional basketball league in Nigeria.** *The internet Journal of Rheumatology* 2008, **5**(1):87–88.
7. Owoeye OBA: **Pattern and management of sports injuries presented by Lagos state athletes at the 16th National Sports Festival (KADA games 2009) in Nigeria.** *Sports Med, Arthro, Rehab, Therapy Tech* 2010, **2**:3.
8. Zvijac K, Thompson W: **Epidemiology of sport injuries.** *Am J Sports Med* 1996, **53**:86–97.
9. Harmer PA: **Basketball injuries.** *Med Sports Sci* 2005, **49**:31–61.
10. Messina DF, Farney WC, Delee JC: **The Incidence of Injury in Texas High School Basketball. A prospective study among male and female athletes.** *Am J Sports Med* 1999, **27**:294–296.
11. Powell JW, Barber-Foss KD: **Injury pattern in selected high school sports.** *J Athl Train* 1999, **34**(3):277–284.
12. Prebble TB, Chyou PH, Wittman L, McCormich J, Collins K, Zoch T: **Basketball injuries in a rural area.** *Wis Med J* 1999, **98**:22–24.
13. Meeuwisse WH, Sellmer R, Hagel BE: **Rates and risks of injury during intercollegiate basketball.** *Am J Sports Med* 2003, **31**:379–385.
14. Borowski LA, Yard EE, Fields SK, Comstock RD: **The Epidemiology of US high school: basketball injuries, 2005–2007.** *Am J Sports Med* 2008, **36**:23–28.
15. Hickey GJ, Fricker PA, McDonald WA: **Injuries in young elite female basketball players over a six-year period.** *Clin J Sport Med* 1997, **7**:252–256.
16. Da Silva AS, Abdalla RJ, Fisberg M: **Incidence of musculoskeletal injuries in elite female basketball athletes.** *Acta Ortop Bras* 2007, **15**(1):43–46.
17. Emery CA, Rose MS, McAllister JR, Meeuwisse WH: **A prevention strategy to reduce the incidence of injury in high school basketball: a cluster randomized controlled trial.** *Clin J Sport Med* 2007, **17**(1):17–24.
18. McGuine TA, Keene JS: **The effect of a balance training program on the risk of ankle sprains in high school athletes.** *Am J Sports Med* 2006, **34**(7):1103–1111.
19. Silvers HJ, Giza ER, Mandelbaum BR: **Anterior cruciate ligament tear prevention in the female athlete.** *Curr Sports Med Rep* 2005, **4**:341–343.
20. Awotidebe TO, Onigbinde AT, Mbada CE, Oje OO: **Pattern of sport injuries at the 15th Nigeria national sports festival.** *Medicinal Sportiva* 2009, **20**:1197–1203.
21. Jelsma J, Dawson H, Smith G, Satumba C, Madzivire D: **Provision of physiotherapy services at the sixth all Africa games.** *Br J Sports Med* 1997, **31**:246–248.

13

Sex-dimorphic landing mechanics and their role within the noncontact ACL injury mechanism: evidence, limitations and directions

Mélanie L Beaulieu* and Scott G McLean

Abstract

Anterior cruciate ligament (ACL) injuries continue to present in epidemic-like proportions, carrying significant short- and longer-term debilitative effects. With females suffering these injuries at a higher rate than males, an abundance of research focuses on delineating the sex-specific nature of the underlying injury mechanism. Examinations of sex-dimorphic lower-limb landing mechanics are common since such factors are readily screenable and modifiable. The purpose of this paper was to critically review the published literature that currently exists in this area to gain greater insight into the aetiology of ACL injuries in females and males. Using strict search criteria, 31 articles investigating sex-based differences in explicit knee and/or hip landing biomechanical variables exhibited during vertical landings were selected and subsequently examined. Study outcomes did not support the generally accepted view that significant sex-based differences exist in lower-limb landing mechanics. In fact, a lack of agreement was evident in the literature for the majority of variables examined, with no sex differences evident when consensus was reached. The one exception was that women were typically found to land with greater peak knee abduction angles than males. Considering knee abduction increases ACL loading and prospectively predicts female ACL injury risk, its contribution to sex-specific injury mechanisms and resultant injury rates seems plausible. As for the lack of consensus observed for most variables, it may arise from study-based variations in test populations and landing tasks, in conjunction with the limited ability to accurately measure lower-limb mechanics via standard motion capture methods. Regardless, laboratory-based comparisons of male and female landing mechanics do not appear sufficient to elucidate causes of injury and their potential sex-specificity. Sex-specific *in vivo* joint mechanical data, if collected accurately, may be more beneficial when used to drive models (e.g., cadaveric and computational) that can additionally quantify the resultant ACL load response. Without these steps, sex-dimorphic landing mechanics data will play a limited role in identifying the aetiology of ACL injuries in women and men.

Keywords: Landing, Sex-based differences, Knee, Hip, Biomechanics, ACL, Injury, In vivo

Introduction

Injuries to the anterior cruciate ligament (ACL) continue to occur at an alarming rate, whilst carrying significant short- and long-term morbidity and an enormous financial burden [1,2]. Individuals having ruptured their ACL, for example, have a higher susceptibility to developing, within 10-15 years of injury, osteoarthritis at the knee joint [3,4]–a degenerative joint disease that most often leads to knee arthroplasty. An additional concern is the large sex-disparity in injury rates, with females suffering noncontact ACL injuries 2-5 times more frequently than males [5,6]. Given the potentially severe outcomes of this ligament injury, research efforts remain focused on elucidating its causes. A better understanding of its aetiology will allow for more effective risk screening and prevention methods to be developed, and thus a reduction in injury rate and its associated sex disparity.

As a step toward more effective injury screening and prevention, the manoeuvres during which most ACL injuries occur have been identified and examined. Most non-contact ACL injuries are reported to arise from a

* Correspondence: mbeaulie@umich.edu
School of Kinesiology, University of Michigan, Ann Arbor, MI, USA

sudden deceleration while either running and changing direction or landing from a jump [7]. Due to the difficult and unethical nature of deliberately provoking and analysing actual injury causing episodes, researchers have focused on obtaining joint neuromechanical data within systematic examinations of noninjurious scenarios. In particular, numerous research teams have compared the lower-limb mechanics of women performing landing tasks with those of men to gain insights into sex-dimorphic ACL injury rates [8-14]. Subsequently, those joint mechanical variables for which sex-based differences were revealed have been directly inferred as contributing risk factors for ACL injury and its associated sex-specificity. In spite of an extensive array of research with this specific intent, these variables have been inconsistently identified across studies. Such discrepancies make effective screening and prevention virtually impossible. There is a need, therefore, for a synthesis of the work undertaken thus far to accurately identify the biomechanical variables that differ between men and women during landing manoeuvres.

The purpose of this review was to (1) synthesise the reported sex-based differences in lower-limb mechanics of landing manoeuvres; and (2) critically discuss the impact of this body of literature on our understanding of the aetiology of noncontact ACL injuries. First, we summarise research targeting sex-based differences in explicit biomechanical variables during high-risk landings, whilst simultaneously providing rationale for targeting these variables. Second, we address methodological heterogeneity and concerns of this body of literature and discuss their role in the results of our synthesis. Third, we recommend future research directions that aim to more effectively determine why some individuals, especially women, may be more susceptible to noncontact ACL injury than others.

Sex-based differences in landing mechanics: evidence in the literature?

Whilst a large number of factors have been investigated for sex-specificity pertaining to landing mechanics, the present review focuses on biomechanical variables that have been shown to directly contribute to ACL injury risk (Table 1). These variables have been identified through cadaveric and/or computer modelling studies, during which specific forces are applied to the knee joint (e.g., anterior tibial shear force, tibial internal rotation moment) and resulting ACL loading is measured [15-17]. They have also been identified by observational studies that reported lower-limb joint motion during noncontact ACL injuries [18,19] and by a prospective study that evaluated the knee biomechanical profiles of young girls that went on to rupture their ACL [20].

Table 1 Landing kinematic and kinetic variables considered within the current review*

Joint	Kinematic Variables	Kinetic Variables
Knee	Flexion angle	Flexion moment†
	Abduction angle	Abduction moment†
	Internal rotation angle	Internal rotation moment†
	Anterior translation	
Hip	Flexion angle	Flexion moment†
	Adduction angle	Adduction moment†
	Internal rotation angle	Internal rotation moment†

* Variables were chosen based on previously demonstrated links to ACL injury risk

† External moments

To select the research articles that presented original data on sex-based differences in knee and hip mechanics during landing manoeuvres, a literature search was performed. The PubMed database was searched using the following keywords: (1) "sex" OR "gender"; AND (2) "biomechanics"; AND (3) "land*" OR "jump*". Only the articles that met the following criteria, however, were included in the review: (1) healthy, human subjects; (2) comparison of the pre-determined knee and/or hip mechanical variables between sexes, as listed in Table 1; (3) analysis of landing manoeuvres that comprised primarily of a vertical jump or drop jump (and not a landing from a horizontal jump); (4) original research. In addition, the reference lists of included articles were searched for relevant articles that also met the inclusion criteria aforementioned. Thirty-one articles were found and included in the review [8-14,21-44].

Sagittal plane

Potential links between sagittal-plane knee mechanics and ACL injury are highly touted. This is because the ACL is the primary restraint to anterior tibial translation [45]. In fact, the anterior tibial shear force, which drives this motion, is the most direct way of loading the ACL, particularly when the knee is near full extension [15]. The general line of thinking is that the anterior tibial shear force produced at initial impact during the landing phase translates the tibia anteriorly coinciding with an increase in ACL strain, and thus injury risk. By means of the patella tendon, the quadriceps can produce an anterior tibial shear force, again being largest when the knee is near full extension [46,47]. High quadriceps activation in combination with a small knee flexion angle during a landing is thus viewed as a worst-case scenario for sagittal plane-based ACL injury. An extended hip joint, coupling with the knee joint posture during landings [48], has also been linked to greater anterior tibial shear forces during a landing task [12]. This shear force reported by investigators in this research area, however, must be interpreted with caution. Inconsistencies exist in its definition in the literature (i.e., internal joint reaction shear force vs. external joint shear force), which largely affect its interpretation [49,50]. Recent findings further question the role of anterior tibial shear forces obtained by means of inverse dynamics in estimating ACL loading. It was reported that large shear forces during drop landings do not coincide with high anterior tibial translations, contrary to popular beliefs [49]. Based on the above relations, an examination of knee and hip flexion angles and moments, as well as anterior tibial translation, appears warranted.

A lack of consistency exists in the literature regarding sex differences in knee flexion angles during landings, whilst knee flexion moment data appear to be similar between sexes. Results from most studies indicate that women land with similar knee flexion angles to men [9,10,21,32,33,35-37,42,44]. Several studies, however, did report that women land with a more extended knee than men [8,22,29]. Interestingly, others have observed the opposite outcome [24] (Table 2). With regard to knee flexion moments, consensus among studies suggests that no sex differences exist during landings (Table 2) [10,22,32,36]. Of the two studies to report such differences, however, one found that they were not present across all jump heights tested [40]. Specifically, greater knee flexion moments were evident in female compared to male volleyball players when landing from a 60-cm platform, but not from a 40-cm platform. Further work may be needed into potential height-specific variations in male and female knee flexion moments during landings. Regardless, the body of evidence currently examined does not support the hypothesis that women are at greater risk of ACL rupture during landing tasks due to an extended knee posture.

Findings regarding sex-based differences in anterior tibial translation appear inconclusive. Given that accurately measuring tibial translations *in vivo* is challenging, only one study has attempted to do so, finding no sex differences [35]. This outcome, however, may be biased by limitations inherent to the methodological approach. Specifically, tibial translation was quantified by means of retro-reflective markers affixed to the skin tracked by a motion capture system. Although a technique suggested to minimise calculation errors due to skin movement artefact was utilised [51], its success in providing accurate joint rotational and translational data has been questioned [52]. This appears especially true for the small range of sagittal-plane tibial translation (≈ 2 mm) evident during landings [53], for which movement artefact error likely dominates the outcome [54,55]. By means of the accurate method of biplane fluoroscopy, Torry et al. [53] did acquire similar data, both in terms of the absence of sex-based differences and magnitude of tibial translations. The participants of this study, however, were instructed to land with limited flexion at the hip, knee and ankle joints. These instructions most likely modified the knee mechanics typically adopted by women and men, making this study of limited use for comparison purposes.

As with knee flexion, evidence of sex differences in hip flexion angles is inconclusive, with no apparent differences in hip flexion moments. The majority of studies revealed no significant sex differences in hip flexion angles during vertical landing tasks [21,22,32,34,36]. For instance, 88% (7 out of 8 studies) reported no sex differences in hip flexion angle at initial ground contact–a point in time when lower-leg posture is critical as most noncontact ACL ruptures occur milliseconds post-contact [19]. Some studies, however, reported either lower or greater hip flexion angles in females compared to males [10,26,29] (Table 3). As for hip flexion moment, no significant differences between sexes were found for the five studies that investigated this dependent variable [10,22,32,36,40] (Table 3).

Frontal plane

Frontal-plane knee biomechanics during landings have been investigated extensively as a potential contributor to ACL injury aetiology. This research has been driven primarily by the role of the ACL in restraining motions and loads in this plane, in combination with recent prospective work linking them to injury [15,20]. Markolf et al., for example, found in a cadaveric model that ACL loading increased in the presence of an externally applied knee abduction moment, presenting as a worst-case scenario when combined with an anterior tibial shear force or an internal tibial rotation moment [15]. Also, the work of Hewett and associates [20] demonstrated a prospective link between injury and increased knee abduction angles and moments during landings in young adolescent females [20]. Recent studies have shown that increased knee abduction angles may arise via a transfer of altered hip kinematics during landings, and in particular increased hip adduction angles [56]. Hence, frontal-plane knee and hip mechanics during landings have been compared repetitively between males and females to gain insight into the mechanism of ACL injuries and the sex-biased injury rates.

Evidence in the literature supports greater knee abduction angles in females, whilst that for sex-based differences in frontal-plane moments is inconclusive. Most studies (72%; 13 out of 18 studies) found greater knee abduction angles in females during landings compared to males for at least one variable associated with the ground contact phase (angle at initial contact, peak angle, or total range of motion) [10,11,13,23,25,27,28,30-32,37,38,44] (Table 4). Specifically, females were observed to land with greater peak knee abduction

Table 2 Summary of studies investigating sex differences in knee flexion angles and moments during a vertical landing task

References	Population Category	Mean Age (years)	Landing Task Double-Leg vs. Single Leg	Height (cm)	Result† at IC	peak	RoM
Knee Flexion Angle							
Ford et al. [26]	Adolescent	12-16 (range)	Double	31	0	+	—
Walsh et al. [44]	Adult-Athlete	19.5	Double	30.5	0	0	—
Salci et al. [40]	Adult-Athlete	21.4	Double	40 & 60	—	- (40) 0 (60)	—
Hughes & Watkins [29]	Adult-Athlete	21.4	Double	not specified‡	-	0	+
Hughes et al. [31]	Adult-Athlete	21.4	Double	not specified‡	0	+	+
Russell et al. [39]	Adolescent & Adult	9.5 (youth) 23.9 (adult)	Double	50% of maximum vertical jump height	0	—	—
Cortes et al. [21]	Adult	23.8	Double	30	0	0	—
Chaudhari et al. [9]	Adult	19.9	Double	30.48	0	—	—
Earl et al. [23]	Adult	22.8	Double	31	—	0	—
Huston et al. [8]	Adult	28.0	Double	20, 40 & 60	0 (20) - (40 & 60)	0	0
Shultz et al. [12]	Adult	22.4	Double	45	0	—	+
Gehring et al. [27]	Adult	23.8	Double	52	0	+	—
Decker et al. [22]	Adult	27.5	Double	60	-	—	-
Kernozek et al. [32]	Adult	24.1	Double	60	0	0	0
Pappas et al. [37]	Adult	28.5	Double & Single	40	0	0	—
Kiriyama et al. [33]	Adolescent	17.0	Single	20	—	0	—
Lephart et al. [34]	Adult-Athlete	20.3	Single	20	—	-	—
Fagenbaum & Darling [24]	Adult-Athlete	not specified	Single	25.4 & 50.8	+	+	—
Nagano et al. [35]	Adult-Athlete	19.6	Single	30	0	0[a]	—
Orishimo et al. [36]	Adult-Athlete	26.3	Single	30	0	0	0
Urabe et al. [42]	Adult-Athlete	22.1	Single	maximum vertical jump height	0	—	—
Schmitz et al. [41]	Adult	23.2	Single	30	0	—	-
Kernozek et al. [10]	Adult	23.4	Single	50	—	0	—
TOTAL*				**% (-/+/0)**	**20/5/75**	**11/22/67**	**25/38/38**
Knee Flexion Moment							
Ford et al. [26]	Adolescent	12-16 (range)	Double	31	—	0	—
Salci et al. [40]	Adult-Athlete	21.4	Double	40 & 60	—	0 (40) + (60)	—
Chaudhari et al. [9]	Adult	19.9	Double	30.48	—	0	—
Shultz et al. [12]	Adult	22.4	Double	45	—	+	—
Decker et al. [22]	Adult	27.5	Double	60	—	0	—
Kernozek et al. [32]	Adult	24.1	Double	60	—	0	—
Orishimo et al. [36]	Adult-Athlete	26.3	Single	30	0	0	—
Kernozek et al. [10]	Adult	23.4	Single	50	—	0	—
TOTAL*				**% (-/+/0)**	**0/0/100**	**0/22/78**	—

† +: greater value in female subjects; -: smaller value in female subjects; 0: no differences between sexes; —: not investigated

‡ Landing from a jump to block a volleyball in the presence of a net of standard, sex-specific height

[a] knee flexion angle at peak vertical ground reaction force

* Percentage of studies having found lower (-), greater (+), and similar (0) values in female subjects in comparison with male subjects

IC: initial ground contact; RoM: range of motion

Table 3 Summary of studies investigating sex differences in hip flexion angles and moments during a vertical landing task

References	Population		Landing Task		Result†		
	Category	Mean Age (years)	Double-Leg vs. Single Leg	Height (cm)	at IC	peak	RoM
Hip Flexion Angle							
Ford et al. [26]	Adolescent	12-16	Double	31	-	0	—
Salci et al. [40]	Adult-Athlete	21.4	Double	40 & 60	—	- (40) 0 (60)	—
Hughes & Watkins [29]	Adult-Athlete	21.4	Double	not specified‡	0	+	+
Cortes et al. [21]	Adult	23.8	Double	30	0	0[a]	—
Shultz et al. [12]	Adult	22.4	Double	45	0	—	+
Decker et al. [22]	Adult	27.5	Double	60	0	—	0
Kernozek et al. [32]	Adult	24.1	Double	60	0	0	0
Lephart et al. [34]	Adult-Athlete	20.3	Single	20	—	0	—
Orishimo et al. [36]	Adult-Athlete	26.3	Single	30	0	0[a]	0
Schmitz et al. [41]	Adult	23.2	Single	30	0	—	-
Kernozek et al. [10]	Adult	23.4	Single	50	—	+	—
TOTAL*				**% (-/+/0)**	**13/0/88**	**11/22/67**	**17/33/50**
Hip Flexion Moment							
Salci et al. [40]	Adult-Athlete	21.4	Double	40 & 60	—	0	—
Decker et al. [22]	Adult	27.5	Double	60	—	0	—
Kernozek et al. [32]	Adult	24.1	Double	60	—	0	—
Orishimo et al. [36]	Adult-Athlete	26.3	Single	30	0	0	—
Kernozek et al. [10]	Adult	23.4	Single	50	—	0	—
TOTAL*				**% (-/+/0)**	**0/0/100**	**0/0/100**	**—**

† +: greater value in female subjects; -: smaller value in female subjects; 0: no differences between sexes; —: not investigated

‡ Landing from a jump to block a volleyball in the presence of a net of standard, sex-specific height

[a] hip flexion angle at peak knee flexion angle

* Percentage of studies having found lower (-), greater (+), and similar (0) values in female subjects in comparison with male subjects

IC: initial ground contact; RoM: range of motion

angles in the majority of the studies (71%; 12 out of 17 studies). Most investigations (64%; 7 out of 11 studies), however, did not find sex-based knee abduction differences at initial ground contact [21,25,30-32,35,36]. One could argue that the initial contact abduction angle is more critical to ACL injury risk than the peak angle or range of motion. It is this initial landing posture that governs the frontal plane moment arm magnitude and the resultant external abduction moment, which is known to load the ACL [15]. Also, the knee abduction angle peaks well after the time when ACL injuries are viewed to occur (17-50 milliseconds after initial ground contact [19]). The peak angle, however, may represent a lack of ability in females to control frontal-plane motion of the knee joint. In response to valgus perturbations at the knee, women have shown diminished reflex muscle activation responses in comparison to men [57]. With regards to knee abduction moments during landing manoeuvres, a lack of consistency exists. Whilst 33% of studies (2 out of 6) did find women landed with greater moments [13,14] than men, for example, 17% (1 study) found the exact opposite [32], with the majority (3 studies) reporting no sex differences [9,10,36] (Table 4). Frontal-plane knee mechanics during landings, therefore, may in fact play a role in sex-specific injury risk.

With regard to frontal-plane hip mechanics, the literature does not provide convincing evidence of sex-dependence (Table 5). Differences between men and women were not observed, for example, in hip adduction angle at initial ground contact during drop jump landings [32,36]. Similar outcomes were evident for peak hip adduction angles, with 71% of the studies (5 out of 7) reported no sex-based differences [10,32,34,36,37]. The remaining studies (29%) found women to land with a greater peak hip adduction angles than their male counterparts [23,43]. In addition, all studies investigating hip adduction moments during landing tasks found no sex differences [9,32,36]. Hence, the sex disparity in ACL injury rates does not appear to be explained by sex differences in frontal-plane hip mechanics in landing tasks.

Transverse plane

Although transverse-plane mechanics have received less attention in the literature, they have still been theorised to play an important role in the mechanism of ACL injuries. Krosshaug and colleagues used video footage to

Table 4 Summary of studies investigating sex differences in knee abduction angles and moments during a vertical landing task

References	Population Category	Mean Age (years)	Landing Task Double-Leg vs. Single Leg	Height (cm)	Result† at IC	peak	RoM
Knee Abduction Angle							
Schmitz et al. [11]	Adolescent	14.1	Double	30	—	—	+[a]
Ford et al. [25]	Adolescent	16.0	Double	31	0	+	—
Ford et al. [13]	Adolescent	12-16	Double	31	—	+[b]	—
Hewett et al. [28]	Adolescent	14.1	Double	31	+	+	—
Walsh et al. [44]	Adult-Athlete	19.5	Double	30.5	+	+	—
Hughes et al. [30]	Adult-Athlete	21.4	Double	not specified‡	0	+	+
Hughes et al. [31]	Adult-Athlete	21.4	Double	not specified‡	0	+	+
Wallace et al. [43]	Adult-Athlete	21.6	Double	maximum vertical jump height	—	0	—
Cortes et al. [21]	Adult	23.8	Double	30	0	0[c]	—
Earl et al. [23]	Adult	22.8	Double	31	—	+	—
Gehring et al. [27]	Adult	23.8	Double	52	+	+	—
Kernozek et al. [32]	Adult	24.1	Double	60	0	+	+
Pappas et al. [37]	Adult	28.5	Double & Single	40	—	+[d]	—
Kiriyama et al. [33]	Adolescent	17.0	Single	20	—	0	—
Nagano et al. [35]	Adult-Athlete	19.6	Single	30	0	0[e]	—
Orishimo et al. [36]	Adult-Athlete	26.3	Single	30	0	0[c]	0
Kernozek et al. [10]	Adult	23.4	Single	50	—	+	—
Russell et al. [38]	Adult	22.5	Single	60	+	+[c]	—
TOTAL*				% (-/+/0)	**0/36/64**	**0/71/29**	**0/80/20**
Knee Abduction Moment							
Ford et al. [13]	Adolescent	12-16	Double	31	—	+[b]	—
Sigward et al. [14]	Adolescent	14.7	Double	36	—	+[f]	—
Chaudhari et al. [9]	Adult	19.9	Double	30.48	—	0	—
Kernozek et al. [32]	Adult	24.1	Double	60	—	-	—
Orishimo et al. [36]	Adult-Athlete	26.3	Single	30	0	0	—
Kernozek et al. [10]	Adult	23.4	Single	50	—	0	—
TOTAL*				% (-/+/0)	**0/0/100**	**17/33/50**	**—**

† +: greater value in female subjects; -: smaller value in female subjects; 0: no differences between sexes; —: not investigated

‡ Landing from a jump to block a volleyball in the presence of a net of standard, sex-specific height

[a] frontal-plane angle in two dimensions

[b] in post-pubertal group only (and not pre-pubertal group)

[c] knee abduction angle at peak knee flexion angle

[d] knee abduction angle at 40° knee flexion angle

[e] knee abduction angle at peak vertical ground reaction force

[f] average knee abduction moment

* Percentage of studies having found lower (-), greater (+), and similar (0) values in female subjects in comparison with male subjects

IC: initial ground contact; RoM: range of motion

assess the knee and hip motions of 30 individuals suffering noncontact ACL injuries. They found that in the majority of cases, the knee medially collapsed with combined hip internal rotation, knee abduction, and tibial *external* rotation [19]. Acknowledging the limitations of estimating joint kinematics and the timing of injury from ordinary television footage, the authors recognised that the tibial *external* rotation may have occurred after ligament rupture. In fact, recent cadaveric injury simulations support this tenet, observing *internal* rotation of the tibia before ligament rupture and *external* rotation following ligament failure [17]. Whilst debate exists with regard to which rotation (internal vs. external) is more risky, most evidence supports tibial internal rotation as the primary contributing factor. Markolf et al. [15], for instance, found that a tibial *internal* rotation moment in combination with an anterior tibial shear force applied to an extended knee produced the greatest ACL force. In contrast, the addition of a tibial *external* rotation moment to an anterior tibial shear force reduced ACL force. Most recently, the application of a tibial *internal* moment was reported to increase ACL strain in

Table 5 Summary of studies investigating sex differences in hip adduction angles and moments during a vertical landing task

References	Population		Landing Task		Result†		
	Category	Mean Age (years)	Double-Leg vs. Single Leg	Height (cm)	at IC	peak	RoM
Hip Adduction Angle							
Wallace et al. [43]	Adult-Athlete	21.6	Double	maximum vertical jump height	—	+	—
Earl et al. [23]	Adult	22.8	Double	31	—	+	—
Kernozek et al. [32]	Adult	24.1	Double	60	0	0	0
Pappas et al. [37]	Adult	28.5	Double & Single	40	—	0[b]	—
Lephart et al. [34]	Adult-Athlete	20.3	Single	20	—	0	—
Orishimo et al. [36]	Adult-Athlete	26.3	Single	30	0	0[a]	0
Kernozek et al. [10]	Adult	23.4	Single	50	—	0	—
TOTAL*				**% (-/+/0)**	**0/0/100**	**0/29/71**	**0/0/100**
Hip Adduction Moment							
Chaudhari et al. [9]	Adult	19.9	Double	30.48	—	0	—
Kernozek et al. [32]	Adult	24.1	Double	60	—	0	—
Orishimo et al. [36]	Adult-Athlete	26.3	Single	30	0	0	—
TOTAL*				**% (-/+/0)**	**0/0/100**	**0/0/100**	**—**

† +: greater value in female subjects; -: smaller value in female subjects; 0: no differences between sexes; —: not investigated

[a] hip adduction angle at peak knee flexion angle

[b] hip adduction angle at 40° knee flexion angle

* Percentage of studies having found lower (-), greater (+), and similar (0) values in female subjects in comparison with male subjects

IC: initial ground contact; RoM: range of motion

comparison to an *external* moment or to an absence of an axial moment [58]. Lower-limb transverse-plane joint mechanics evident during landings, and particularly tibial *internal* rotation, therefore, appear to play an important role in ACL loading and resultant ACL injury risk.

There is limited agreement regarding sex-based differences in transverse-plane knee and hip mechanics during landings (Table 6). Although no sex-based differences were found in tibial internal rotation at initial ground contact [35], greater peak tibial rotations were reported in women for 50% of the studies (2 out of 4) [33,35]. The remaining 50%, however, observed no sex differences [23,34]. A similar trend is present for hip internal rotation angles (Table 6). On the other hand, women and men appear to demonstrate similar knee and hip internal rotation moment magnitudes during landings. It should be noted, however, that only one study to date has investigated these kinetic variables [9].

In spite of strong assertions regarding "known" biomechanical risk factors for ACL injury, there is limited evidence to suggest that sex-based differences in ACL injury rates arise from concomitant differences in such factors. The one exception is peak knee abduction angle, where women were found to typically land with greater abduction than men. For most biomechanical variables of interest, however, no consensus among studies was reached. Further, for knee and hip flexion angles, and hip adduction angle, the majority of the evidence in the literature supports a lack of sex-based differences.

Methodological heterogeneity and concerns

When a lack of consistency exists between the results of various studies, investigators have often pointed to methodological discrepancies as the primary cause. The studies investigating sex-based joint mechanical differences within a vertical landing task indeed demonstrate methodological variation in factors such as landing type (single- vs. double-leg landing), height of landing, and population characteristics (adolescents vs. adults, recreational vs. elite athletes). These variations, however, do not appear to govern the lack of consensus observed in most of the variables examined herein. As seen in Tables 2, 3, 4, 5, 6, results did not generally diverge according to the nature of the task or sample population characteristics. Several interesting trends are present, however, indicating that some sex differences may be task- or population-dependent.

First, all of the studies that reported smaller initial contact knee flexion angles in females compared to males examined double-leg landings; whereas the lone study that revealed greater angles investigated a single-leg landing task. This task-dependency is somewhat counterintuitive seeing that single-leg landings appear to be more difficult to execute [37]. During a double-leg landing, both lower-limbs contribute to the deceleration

Table 6 Summary of studies investigating sex differences in knee and hip internal rotation angles and moments during a vertical landing task

References	Population Category	Mean Age (years)	Landing Task Double-Leg vs. Single Leg	Height (cm)	Result† at IC	peak	RoM
Knee Internal Rotation Angle							
Earl et al. [23]	Adult	22.8	Double	31	—	0	—
Kiriyama et al. [33]	Adolescent	17.0	Single	20	—	+	—
Lephart et al. [34]	Adult-Athlete	20.3	Single	20	—	0	—
Nagano et al. [35]	Adult-Athlete	19.6	Single	30	0	+[a]	—
TOTAL*				**% (-/+/0)**	**0/0/100**	**0/50/50**	**—**
Knee Internal Rotation Moment							
Chaudhari et al. [9]	Adult	19.9	Double	30.48	—	0	—
Hip Internal Rotation Angle							
Earl et al. [23]	Adult	22.8	Double	31	—	0	—
Lephart et al. [34]	Adult-Athlete	20.3	Single	20	—	+	—
Hip Internal Rotation Moment							
Chaudhari et al. [9]	Adult	19.9	Double	30.48	—	0	—

† +: greater value in female subjects; -: smaller value in female subjects; 0: no differences between sexes; —: not investigated

[a] knee internal/external rotation angle at peak vertical ground reaction force

* Percentage of studies having found lower (-), greater (+), and similar (0) values in female subjects in comparison with male subjects

IC: initial ground contact; RoM: range of motion

of the centre of mass. It has been suggested, therefore, that a more extended knee posture may be needed to successfully land on a single leg to limit the impact-induced knee flexion moment counteracted by the quadriceps. Given that women are known to have weaker thigh musculature [34], we would expect them to land with an even more extended knee during single-leg landing to minimise this moment. With a stronger musculature, men can afford to perform a single-leg landing with greater initial contact knee flexion angle. Hence, there does not appear to be any logical trend in initial contact knee flexion angle across landing types.

Second, sex differences in frontal- and transverse-plane knee and hip kinematics may also be task-dependent. Both studies that reported greater hip adduction angles in women than men investigated the mechanics of double-leg landings, as oppose to single-leg landings. The increased sensitivity of out-of-plane knee loading to the female 3D hip posture during landings compared to males is well documented [59]. It could thus well be that women have greater difficulty controlling hip motions during double-leg landings. While plausible, evidence supporting this theory of task dependency in frontal-plane hip motion is weak. Only half of the studies assessing hip adduction angles during double-leg landings found women to have greater angles [23,43]. The other studies reported no sex differences [32,37].

Third, greater knee and hip internal rotation angles were present in women during a single-leg landing, whereas double-leg landings did not reveal sex differences in transverse-plane knee and hip mechanics. Given the more challenging nature of the single-leg landing, as stated above, it is plausible that women have a decreased ability to counteract transverse-plane moments produced upon landing, thus leading to greater motion in this plane. In fact, Wojtys et al. [60] have shown women to produce less muscular resistance to internal rotation loading of the tibia, indicative of lower muscular protection of their knee joints.

Lastly, studies reporting greater knee abduction moments in the female group tested adolescent populations, while studies reporting lower female moments or no sex differences tested adults. It is unclear whether an interaction between developmental stage and sex-based knee joint mechanical differences truly exists, or whether it is a coincidence. Only six studies [9,10,13,14,32,36] evaluated sex differences in knee joint abduction moments, and only two tested an adolescent population [13,14]. Across four maturation groups (pre-pubertal, pubertal, post-pubertal, and young adulthood), Sigward et al. [14] found no such interaction. On the other hand, Ford and colleagues [13] reported greater knee abduction moments in post-pubertal girls than boys, whilst no such sex-based differences were observed in the pubertal group. No group of adults, however, were included in their study. Consequently, although a lack of consistency in sex-based knee and hip joint biomechanical differences across studies has often been attributed to concurrent task and age discrepancies, there is limited hard evidence to support such effects.

Some of the discrepancies in results between studies may also stem from anatomical and/or hormonal variations among the participants. None of the studies investigated herein, for example, accounted for potential differences in knee morphology and laxity between participants. Merely two out of the 31 studies controlled for phase of the menstrual cycle during which data collection occurred [9,12]. These factors should not be ignored as they have been shown to influence landing mechanics and ACL injury risk, as well as to be sex-dependent. Knee anatomy, for example, has been reported to differ between ACL-injured patients and uninjured individuals [61-64]. Links have also been found between explicit knee anatomical indices (e.g., posterior-directed slope of the tibial plateau, ACL cross-sectional area) and landing biomechanics (e.g., peak knee abduction, peak knee internal rotation angle, ACL strain) [65-67]. Furthermore, several recent investigations [68,69] consistently support correlations between knee and generalised joint laxity and landing biomechanics, with laxity being dependent on sex [70] and, in women, on menstrual cycle [69,71]. Variations in these additional factors, therefore, may be equally critical to resultant landing biomechanics, thus confounding possible sex-based joint biomechanical differences. Consideration of such factors should be made in future research efforts.

The lack of sex-based differences in knee and hip joint landing biomechanics reported in most studies may be in part due to the means by which joint mechanics are quantified. Typically, joint kinematics are derived from the coordinates (2D or 3D) of retro-reflective markers affixed to the skin that estimate the position of the underlying bones. Whilst skin movement artefact is known to transpire into relatively large errors in the calculation of joint mechanics [54], however, such effects are often disregarded. This can be extremely problematic since errors between 2.2 and 13.1 degrees have been reported in joint rotations for various gait tasks [55,72]. Further, these errors are largest in the frontal and transverse planes, questioning the reliability of sex-based kinematic comparisons in these planes. The validity of these skin marker-derived rotations is thus highly questionable. Given that joint kinetics, such as moments, are also based on data obtained from skin markers, error propagates to these variables as well. Alternatively, dynamic biplane fluoroscopy and x-ray systems offer an accuracy greater than 0.5° for joint rotations and 0.5 mm for joint translations [73]. Such methods, however, afford a limited capture volume, expose participants to radiation, and do not lend well to en-masse testing due to extensive processing time. Despite these shortcomings, future research efforts using such technology as a means toward vast improvements in data accuracy is encouraged.

In addition to error caused by skin movement artefact, data processing techniques are also a common source of error in both kinematic and kinetic data. Overzealous filtering of marker trajectory data may remove critical peaks in joint kinematics and resultant kinetic data. This is particularly problematic if the magnitude of such peaks differs between males and females. Furthermore, discrepancies in kinematic model definitions will also be problematic. Although standards do exist in the biomechanics community [74,75], a wide variety of models are implemented. With regard to joint kinetics, no standards currently exist. This leads to difficulties in reliably comparing both kinematic and kinetic variables across studies. Consequently, collaborative efforts should be made to develop and encourage the adoption of standards with regards to data reduction and processing techniques.

The heterogeneity in the methodologies, the questionable validity of skin marker-based joint mechanics, and potential variations in data processing techniques among studies appears to only partly explain the inconsistencies in reported sex-based joint biomechanical differences. Although some differences appear to be task- or population-dependent, as noted, these trends are generally weak and thus do not seem to explain the lack of consensus in the literature. Also, despite much lower relative error in skin marker-derived joint mechanics in the sagittal plane, evidence of a sex-bias in these examined variables was also inconclusive. Hence, the direct application of the findings of these *in vivo*, laboratory-based studies to elucidate the aetiology of noncontact ACL injury appears to be limited.

Although it was our intention to include all original research that compared knee and hip landing mechanics between healthy females and males, our ability to do so successfully was limited in several ways. As discussed, the studies included in our review demonstrated a diverse range of methodologies, which may have masked commonalities regarding true sex-based differences. Also, we did not systematically quantify the studies' quality. Specifically, we did not report on factors such as adopted methodological standards and techniques, degree of subject proficiency in movement tasks examined, and population sample sizes. Consequently, every study was weighted equally within the review regardless of quality, which may have distorted outcomes. Despite these shortcomings, it is our opinion that our review provides an accurate synthesis of the literature pertaining to sex-based differences in knee and hip landing mechanics.

Moving beyond the status quo

While studies comparing landing mechanics between male and females have provided key baseline information regarding the ACL injury phenomenon, their ability to speak to the aetiology of these injuries may be limited due to the inherent complexity of the injury mechanism. Given that such studies rarely translate findings to the actual ligament load response *in vivo*, for example, we are faced with the challenge of distinguishing which factors truly manifest within the mechanism from those that merely demonstrate sex-dependence. Measurement of the *in vivo* ligament response during such tasks, via implantable gauges similar to those used by Fleming et al. [76,77] and Cerulli et al. [78], may provide valuable knowledge and should be explored further. Critical insights into sex-specific injury causality have also recently been gained through the linking of explicit knee joint mechanical profiles and resultant ACL loading. Mizuno et al. [79], for example, found that sex-based differences in ACL loading arise even when the same external load states are applied to male and female knee joints. They suggested that differences in joint and ligament morphology, rather than mechanical profile, governed sex-biased injury rates. Further, ACL strain measures were found to be higher when female-specific loading patterns were applied to a cadaveric knee simulating a vertical stop-jump task, in comparison with male-specific patterns [80]. "Stiff" landings, characterised by greater knee and hip flexion, also produced greater ACL force than "soft" landings within a musculoskeletal model [81]. In addition, ACL strain was shown to increase by 30% when a knee abduction moment was added to knee compression and flexion loads in a cadaveric simulation of a single-leg landing [82]. These studies highlight that whilst *in vivo* joint biomechanical data in isolation may not elucidate sex-specific injury risk, they are vital in driving studies that can do so. Specifically, they afford valid input data (e.g., cadaveric and computer model simulations) for estimating ACL loading in response to explicit sex-based neuromechanical scenarios. Success of such studies is still dependent on the accuracy with which these biomechanical inputs can be collected. With this in mind, methods geared towards accurate and reliable *in vivo* joint biomechanical data should be actively pursued.

In light of that presented above, we contend that greater insight into the role of joint mechanics within sex-specific injury risk may be obtained by extending analyses beyond the *in vivo* laboratory setting. Such studies for example, do not adequately replicate the mechanical and neuromuscular control strategies typically utilised within the inherently random field setting where injuries do occur. Myers et al. [73] have suggested that within the laboratory environment, subjects can more effectively modify their muscle activation strategies to ensure a safe movement outcomes when presented with "riskier" movement requirements (i.e., extended knee and hip and greater vertical ground reaction forces (GRF)). Such adaptations may not be possible in the field setting, when additional time and movement constraints prevail. It is additionally plausible that noncontact ACL injuries are due, in part, to a neuromuscular "misfire" that occurs infrequently. If this is the case, then neuromechanical assessments derived from the typically limited number of landing trials (e.g., five to ten) are likely insufficient to capture such a rare event. Validated dynamic models of high-risk landing postures can circumvent some of these issues. The impact of systematic and/or random adjustments in the joint mechanical profile on resultant ACL loading can be readily evaluated [83-85]. Innovative body-worn sensor technologies may also allow us to capture lower-limb kinematics within a more realistic movement environment. Miniature, wireless inertial measurement units (IMUs) [86], for example, could be used directly for this purpose, affording ongoing assessments during relevant, unanticipated athletic manoeuvres during gameplay. Research on the aetiology of noncontact ACL injuries and its sex disparity would benefit, therefore, from studies aimed at either replicating, or direct collection within, naturalistic movement and resultant injury scenarios.

Although evidence in the literature supports a multiplanar injury mechanism, most research efforts continue to be aimed at uni-planar injury risk. This is problematic since the ACL injury mechanism is increasingly viewed to arise via a 3D mechanical mechanism [87]. In the sagittal plane, for example, it is unlikely that the force produced by quadriceps activation is the sole contributor to injury. Specifically, it has been shown that in this plane, the rapid deceleration associated with the landing phase creates a posteriorly directed force vector at the shoe-ground interface, which is transferred to the tibia, protecting the ACL [50,88,89]. Due to the moment balance in the sagittal plane following ground contact, increased quadriceps force, therefore, will be countered by the concomitant increase in the posteriorly directed GRF, promoting minimal changes in the net ACL load [90,91]. In addition, bone bruises consequential of noncontact ACL injuries are commonly found on the posterolateral tibial plateau and lateral femoral condyle [92-94]. This suggests an injury mechanism that combines anterior shear, lateral compression and axial rotation components. An isolated frontal-plane injury mechanism is also unlikely. Within a knee model, an abduction moment applied to the knee joint during a simulated single-leg landing was found to increase ACL strain, but not enough to cause rupture [16]. Knee abduction observed during injurious scenarios may also be a consequence of ligament rupture, and not the inciting event. A cadaveric investigation, for example, reported knee abduction only after ACL failure, and not before failure [17]. Future research efforts, therefore, need to consider the injury mechanism as a likely result of forces and moments produced in a combination of planes.

Conclusion

This review revealed that there is limited agreement in the literature as to whether women land differently than their male counterparts. Further, when consensus was reached, a lack of sex differences was reported. The only common difference revealed was that women landed with greater peak knee abduction angles than men. Since knee abduction is known to increase ACL loading, therefore, it is plausible that this variable indeed contributes to observed sex-dimorphic injury rates. Conversely, it may simply demonstrate sex-dependence that is irrelevant to the sex disparity in injury risk. To advance our knowledge of the aetiology of noncontact ACL injuries, as a step toward effective injury screening and prevention, we recommend progressing beyond a sex comparison focus. We recommended adopting a focus that includes additional risk factors and assessments within more realistic and less predictable movement environments. Further utilisation of experimental and modelling techniques that afford quantification of the actual ligament response to realistic joint mechanical inputs also seems imperative. Given that joint biomechanical data measured *in vivo* drive these models, these data, however, should not be discounted. In fact, their accuracy is imperative, which fuels the need for the development of superior methods to quantify biomechanics. Unless these critical steps are taken, progress toward elucidating the aetiology of noncontact ACL injuries will be limited.

Acknowledgements

MLB acknowledges the financial support provided by the Natural Sciences and Engineering Research Council of Canada and by the Bone and Joint Injury Prevention and Rehabilitation Center of the University of Michigan.

Authors' contributions

MLB performed the literature search and summary. MLB and SGM drafted and edited the manuscript, as well as read and approved its final version.

Competing interests

The authors declare that they have no competing interests.

References

1. Griffin LY, Albohm MJ, Arendt EA, Bahr R, Beynnon BD, Demaio M, Dick RW, Engebretsen L, Garrett WE Jr, Hannafin JA, Hewett TE, Huston LJ, Ireland ML, Johnson RJ, Lephart S, Mandelbaum BR, Mann BJ, Marks PH, Marshall SW, Myklebust G, Noyes FR, Powers C, Shields C Jr, Shultz SJ, Silvers H, Slauterbeck J, Taylor DC, Teitz CC, Wojtys EM, Yu B: **Understanding and preventing noncontact anterior cruciate ligament injuries: a review of the Hunt Valley II meeting, January 2005.** *Am J Sports Med* 2006, **34(9)**:1512-1532.
2. Hewett TE, Myer GD, Ford KR: **Anterior cruciate ligament injuries in female athletes: part 1, mechanisms and risk factors.** *Am J Sports Med* 2006, **34(2)**:299-311.
3. Lohmander LS, Englund PM, Dahl LL, Roos EM: **The long-term consequence of anterior cruciate ligament and meniscus injuries: osteoarthritis.** *Am J Sports Med* 2007, **35(10)**:1756-1769.
4. Neuman P, Englund M, Kostogiannis I, Friden T, Roos H, Dahlberg LE: **Prevalence of tibiofemoral osteoarthritis 15 years after nonoperative treatment of anterior cruciate ligament injury: a prospective cohort study.** *Am J Sports Med* 2008, **36(9)**:1717-1725.
5. Walden M, Hagglund M, Werner J, Ekstrand J: **The epidemiology of anterior cruciate ligament injury in football (soccer): a review of the literature from a gender-related perspective.** *Knee Surg Sports Traumatol Arthrosc* 2011, **19(1)**:3-10.
6. Agel J, Arendt EA, Bershadsky B: **Anterior cruciate ligament injury in national collegiate athletic association basketball and soccer: a 13-year review.** *Am J Sports Med* 2005, **33(4)**:524-530.
7. Shimokochi Y, Shultz SJ: **Mechanisms of noncontact anterior cruciate ligament injury.** *J Athl Train* 2008, **43(4)**:396-408.
8. Huston LJ, Vibert B, Ashton-Miller JA, Wojtys EM: **Gender differences in knee angle when landing from a drop-jump.** *Am J Knee Surg* 2001, **14(4)**:215-219, discussion 219-220.
9. Chaudhari AM, Lindenfeld TN, Andriacchi TP, Hewett TE, Riccobene J, Myer GD, Noyes FR: **Knee and hip loading patterns at different phases in the menstrual cycle: implications for the gender difference in anterior cruciate ligament injury rates.** *Am J Sports Med* 2007, **35(5)**:793-800.
10. Kernozek TW, Torry MR, Iwasaki M: **Gender differences in lower extremity landing mechanics caused by neuromuscular fatigue.** *Am J Sports Med* 2008, **36(3)**:554-565.
11. Schmitz RJ, Shultz SJ, Nguyen AD: **Dynamic valgus alignment and functional strength in males and females during maturation.** *J Athl Train* 2009, **44(1)**:26-32.
12. Shultz SJ, Nguyen AD, Leonard MD, Schmitz RJ: **Thigh strength and activation as predictors of knee biomechanics during a drop jump task.** *Med Sci Sports Exerc* 2009, **41(4)**:857-866.
13. Ford KR, Shapiro R, Myer GD, van den Bogert AJ, Hewett TE: **Longitudinal sex differences during landing in knee abduction in young athletes.** *Med Sci Sports Exerc* 2010, **42(10)**:1923-1931.
14. Sigward SM, Pollard CD, Powers CM: **The influence of sex and maturation on landing biomechanics: implications for anterior cruciate ligament injury.** *Scand J Med Sci Sports* 2011.
15. Markolf KL, Burchfield DM, Shapiro MM, Shepard MF, Finerman GA, Slauterbeck JL: **Combined knee loading states that generate high anterior cruciate ligament forces.** *J Orthop Res* 1995, **13(6)**:930-935.
16. Shin CS, Chaudhari AM, Andriacchi TP: **The effect of isolated valgus moments on ACL strain during single-leg landing: a simulation study.** *J Biomech* 2009, **42(3)**:280-285.
17. Meyer EG, Haut RC: **Anterior cruciate ligament injury induced by internal tibial torsion or tibiofemoral compression.** *J Biomech* 2008, **41(16)**:3377-3383.
18. Boden BP, Torg JS, Knowles SB, Hewett TE: **Video analysis of anterior cruciate ligament injury.** *Am J Sports Med* 2009, **37(2)**:252-259.
19. Krosshaug T, Nakamae A, Boden BP, Engebretsen L, Smith G, Slauterbeck JR, Hewett TE, Bahr R: **Mechanisms of anterior cruciate ligament injury in basketball: video analysis of 39 cases.** *Am J Sports Med* 2007, **35(3)**:359-367.
20. Hewett TE, Myer GD, Ford KR, Heidt RS Jr, Colosimo AJ, McLean SG, van den Bogert AJ, Paterno MV, Succop P: **Biomechanical measures of neuromuscular control and valgus loading of the knee predict anterior cruciate ligament injury risk in female athletes: a prospective study.** *Am J Sports Med* 2005, **33(4)**:492-501.
21. Cortes N, Onate J, Abrantes J, Gagen L, Dowling E, Van Lunen B: **Effects of gender and foot-landing techniques on lower extremity kinematics during drop-jump landings.** *J Appl Biomech* 2007, **23(4)**:289-299.
22. Decker MJ, Torry MR, Wyland DJ, Sterett WI, Richard Steadman J: **Gender differences in lower extremity kinematics, kinetics and energy absorption during landing.** *Clin Biomech (Bristol, Avon)* 2003, **18(7)**:662-669.
23. Earl JE, Monteiro SK, Snyder KR: **Differences in lower extremity kinematics between a bilateral drop-vertical jump and a single-leg step-down.** *J Orthop Sports Phys Ther* 2007, **37(5)**:245-252.

24. Fagenbaum R, Darling WG: **Jump landing strategies in male and female college athletes and the implications of such strategies for anterior cruciate ligament injury.** *Am J Sports Med* 2003, **31(2)**:233-240.
25. Ford KR, Myer GD, Hewett TE: **Valgus knee motion during landing in high school female and male basketball players.** *Med Sci Sports Exerc* 2003, **35(10)**:1745-1750.
26. Ford KR, Myer GD, Hewett TE: **Longitudinal effects of maturation on lower extremity joint stiffness in adolescent athletes.** *Am J Sports Med* 2010, **38(9)**:1829-1837.
27. Gehring D, Melnyk M, Gollhofer A: **Gender and fatigue have influence on knee joint control strategies during landing.** *Clin Biomech (Bristol, Avon)* 2009, **24(1)**:82-87.
28. Hewett TE, Myer GD, Ford KR: **Decrease in neuromuscular control about the knee with maturation in female athletes.** *J Bone Joint Surg Am* 2004, **86-A(8)**:1601-1608.
29. Hughes G, Watkins J: **Lower limb coordination and stiffness during landing from volleyball block jumps.** *Res Sports Med* 2008, **16(2)**:138-154.
30. Hughes G, Watkins J, Owen N: **Gender differences in lower limb frontal plane kinematics during landing.** *Sports Biomech* 2008, **7(3)**:333-341.
31. Hughes G, Watkins J, Owen N: **The effects of opposition and gender on knee kinematics and ground reaction force during landing from volleyball block jumps.** *Res Q Exerc Sport* 2010, **81(4)**:384-391.
32. Kernozek TW, Torry MR, VANH H, Cowley H, Tanner S: **Gender differences in frontal and sagittal plane biomechanics during drop landings.** *Med Sci Sports Exerc* 2005, **37(6)**:1003-1012.
33. Kiriyama S, Sato H, Takahira N: **Gender differences in rotation of the shank during single-legged drop landing and its relation to rotational muscle strength of the knee.** *Am J Sports Med* 2009, **37(1)**:168-174.
34. Lephart SM, Ferris CM, Riemann BL, Myers JB, Fu FH: **Gender differences in strength and lower extremity kinematics during landing.** *Clin Orthop Relat Res* 2002, **401**:162-169.
35. Nagano Y, Ida H, Akai M, Fukubayashi T: **Gender differences in knee kinematics and muscle activity during single limb drop landing.** *Knee* 2007, **14(3)**:218-223.
36. Orishimo KF, Kremenic IJ, Pappas E, Hagins M, Liederbach M: **Comparison of landing biomechanics between male and female professional dancers.** *Am J Sports Med* 2009, **37(11)**:2187-2193.
37. Pappas E, Hagins M, Sheikhzadeh A, Nordin M, Rose D: **Biomechanical differences between unilateral and bilateral landings from a jump: gender differences.** *Clin J Sport Med* 2007, **17(4)**:263-268.
38. Russell KA, Palmieri RM, Zinder SM, Ingersoll CD: **Sex differences in valgus knee angle during a single-leg drop jump.** *J Athl Train* 2006, **41(2)**:166-171.
39. Russell PJ, Croce RV, Swartz EE, Decoster LC: **Knee-muscle activation during landings: developmental and gender comparisons.** *Med Sci Sports Exerc* 2007, **39(1)**:159-170.
40. Salci Y, Kentel BB, Heycan C, Akın S, Korkusuz F: **Comparison of landing maneuvers between male and female college volleyball players.** *Clin Biomech (Bristol, Avon)* 2004, **19(6)**:622-628.
41. Schmitz RJ, Kulas AS, Perrin DH, Riemann BL, Shultz SJ: **Sex differences in lower extremity biomechanics during single leg landings.** *Clin Biomech (Bristol, Avon)* 2007, **22(6)**:681-688.
42. Urabe Y, Kobayashi R, Sumida S, Tanaka K, Yoshida N, Nishiwaki GA, Tsutsumi E, Ochi M: **Electromyographic analysis of the knee during jump landing in male and female athletes.** *Knee* 2005, **12(2)**:129-134.
43. Wallace BJ, Kernozek TW, Mikat RP, Wright GA, Simons SZ, Wallace KL: **A comparison between back squat exercise and vertical jump kinematics: implications for determining anterior cruciate ligament injury risk.** *J Strength Cond Res* 2008, **22(4)**:1249-1258.
44. Walsh MS, Waters J, Kersting UG: **Gender bias on the effects of instruction on kinematic and kinetic jump parameters of high-level athletes.** *Res Sports Med* 2007, **15(4)**:283-295.
45. Markolf KL, Mensch JS, Amstutz HC: **Stiffness and laxity of the knee-the contributions of the supporting structures. A quantitative in vitro study.** *J Bone Joint Surg Am* 1976, **58(5)**:583-594.
46. Li G, Rudy TW, Sakane M, Kanamori A, Ma CB, Woo SL: **The importance of quadriceps and hamstring muscle loading on knee kinematics and in-situ forces in the ACL.** *J Biomech* 1999, **32(4)**:395-400.
47. Renstrom P, Arms SW, Stanwyck TS, Johnson RJ, Pope MH: **Strain within the anterior cruciate ligament during hamstring and quadriceps activity.** *Am J Sports Med* 1986, **14(1)**:83-87.
48. McNitt-Gray JL: **Kinematics and impulse characteristics of drop landing from three heights.** *Int J Sport Biomech* 1991, **7(2)**:201-224.
49. Torry MR, Myers C, Shelburne KB, Peterson D, Giphart JE, Pennington WW, Krong JP, Woo SL, Steadman JR: **Relationship of knee shear force and extensor moment on knee translations in females performing drop landings: a biplane fluoroscopy study.** *Clin Biomech (Bristol, Avon)* 2011, **26(10)**:1019-1024.
50. van den Bogert AJ, McLean SG: **Comment: effect of fatigue on knee kinetics and kinematics in stop-jump tasks.** *Am J Sports Med* 2006, **34(2)**:312-315, author reply 313-315.
51. Andriacchi TP, Alexander EJ, Toney MK, Dyrby C, Sum J: **A point cluster method for in vivo motion analysis: applied to a study of knee kinematics.** *J Biomech Eng* 1998, **120(6)**:743-749.
52. Cereatti A, Della Croce U, Cappozzo A: **Reconstruction of skeletal movement using skin markers: comparative assessment of bone pose estimators.** *J Neuroeng Rehabil* 2006, **3**:7.
53. Torry MR, Myers C, Pennington WW, Shelburne KB, Krong JP, Giphart JE, Steadman JR, Woo SL: **Relationship of anterior knee laxity to knee translations during drop landings: a bi-plane fluoroscopy study.** *Knee Surg Sports Traumatol Arthrosc* 2011, **19(4)**:653-662.
54. Leardini A, Chiari L, Della Croce U, Cappozzo A: **Human movement analysis using stereophotogrammetry. Part 3. Soft tissue artifact assessment and compensation.** *Gait Posture* 2005, **21(2)**:212-225.
55. Benoit DL, Ramsey DK, Lamontagne M, Xu L, Wretenberg P, Renstrom P: **Effect of skin movement artifact on knee kinematics during gait and cutting motions measured in vivo.** *Gait Posture* 2006, **24(2)**:152-164.
56. Zeller BL, McCrory JL, Kibler WB, Uhl TL: **Differences in kinematics and electromyographic activity between men and women during the single-legged squat.** *Am J Sports Med* 2003, **31(3)**:449-456.
57. Cammarata ML, Dhaher YY: **Evidence of gender-specific motor templates to resist valgus loading at the knee.** *Muscle Nerve* 2010, **41(5)**:614-623.
58. Fujiya H, Kousa P, Fleming BC, Churchill DL, Beynnon BD: **Effect of muscle loads and torque applied to the tibia on the strain behavior of the anterior cruciate ligament: an in vitro investigation.** *Clin Biomech (Bristol, Avon)* 2011, **26(10)**:1005-1011.
59. McLean SG, Huang X, van den Bogert AJ: **Association between lower extremity posture at contact and peak knee valgus moment during sidestepping: implications for ACL injury.** *Clin Biomech (Bristol, Avon)* 2005, **20(8)**:863-870.
60. Wojtys EM, Huston LJ, Schock HJ, Boylan JP, Ashton-Miller JA: **Gender differences in muscular protection of the knee in torsion in size-matched athletes.** *J Bone Joint Surg Am* 2003, **85-A(5)**:782-789.
61. Hashemi J, Chandrashekar N, Mansouri H, Gill B, Slauterbeck JR, Schutt RC Jr, Dabezies E, Beynnon BD: **Shallow medial tibial plateau and steep medial and lateral tibial slopes: new risk factors for anterior cruciate ligament injuries.** *Am J Sports Med* 2010, **38(1)**:54-62.
62. Simon RA, Everhart JS, Nagaraja HN, Chaudhari AM: **A case-control study of anterior cruciate ligament volume, tibial plateau slopes and intercondylar notch dimensions in ACL-injured knees.** *J Biomech* 2010, **43(9)**:1702-1707.
63. Stijak L, Herzog RF, Schai P: **Is there an influence of the tibial slope of the lateral condyle on the ACL lesion? A case-control study.** *Knee Surg Sports Traumatol Arthrosc* 2008, **16(2)**:112-117.
64. Terauchi M, Hatayama K, Yanagisawa S, Saito K, Takagishi K: **Sagittal alignment of the knee and its relationship to noncontact anterior cruciate ligament injuries.** *Am J Sports Med* 2011, **39(5)**:1090-1094.
65. McLean SG, Lucey SM, Rohrer S, Brandon C: **Knee joint anatomy predicts high-risk in vivo dynamic landing knee biomechanics.** *Clin Biomech (Bristol, Avon)* 2010, **25(8)**:781-788.
66. McLean SG, Oh YK, Palmer ML, Lucey SM, Lucarelli DG, Ashton-Miller JA, Wojtys EM: **The relationship between anterior tibial acceleration, tibial slope and ACL strain during a simulated jump landing task.** *J Bone Joint Surg Am* 2011, **93(14)**:1310-1317.
67. Lipps DB, Oh YK, Ashton-Miller JA, Wojtys EM: **Morphologic characteristics help explain the gender difference in peak anterior cruciate ligament strain during a simulated pivot landing.** *Am J Sports Med* 2012, **40(1)**:32-40.
68. Shultz SJ, Schmitz RJ: **Effects of transverse and frontal plane knee laxity on hip and knee neuromechanics during drop landings.** *Am J Sports Med* 2009, **37(9)**:1821-1830.

69. Shultz SJ, Schmitz RJ, Kong Y, Dudley WN, Beynnon BD, Nguyen AD, Kim H, Montgomery MM: **Cyclic variations in multi-planar knee laxity influence landing biomechanics.** *Med Sci Sports Exerc* 2011.
70. Shultz SJ, Shimokochi Y, Nguyen AD, Schmitz RJ, Beynnon BD, Perrin DH: **Measurement of varus-valgus and internal-external rotational knee laxities in vivo-Part II: relationship with anterior-posterior and general joint laxity in males and females.** *J Orthop Res* 2007, **25(8)**:989-996.
71. Shultz SJ, Schmitz RJ, Beynnon BD: **Variations in varus/valgus and internal/external rotational knee laxity and stiffness across the menstrual cycle.** *J Orthop Res* 2011, **29(3)**:318-325.
72. Reinschmidt C, van den Bogert AJ, Nigg BM, Lundberg A, Murphy N: **Effect of skin movement on the analysis of skeletal knee joint motion during running.** *J Biomech* 1997, **30(7)**:729-732.
73. Myers CA, Torry MR, Peterson DS, Shelburne KB, Giphart JE, Krong JP, Woo SL, Steadman JR: **Measurements of tibiofemoral kinematics during soft and stiff drop landings using biplane fluoroscopy.** *Am J Sports Med* 2011, **39(8)**:1714-1722.
74. Grood ES, Suntay WJ: **A joint coordinate system for the clinical description of three-dimensional motions: application to the knee.** *J Biomech Eng* 1983, **105(2)**:136-144.
75. Wu G, Siegler S, Allard P, Kirtley C, Leardini A, Rosenbaum D, Whittle M, D'Lima DD, Cristofolini L, Witte H, Schmid O, Stokes I: **ISB recommendation on definitions of joint coordinate system of various joints for the reporting of human joint motion–part I: ankle, hip, and spine. International Society of Biomechanics.** *J Biomech* 2002, **35(4)**:543-548.
76. Fleming BC, Renstrom PA, Beynnon BD, Engstrom B, Peura GD, Badger GJ, Johnson RJ: **The effect of weightbearing and external loading on anterior cruciate ligament strain.** *J Biomech* 2001, **34(2)**:163-170.
77. Fleming BC, Renstrom PA, Ohlen G, Johnson RJ, Peura GD, Beynnon BD, Badger GJ: **The gastrocnemius muscle is an antagonist of the anterior cruciate ligament.** *J Orthop Res* 2001, **19(6)**:1178-1184.
78. Cerulli G, Benoit DL, Lamontagne M, Caraffa A, Liti A: **In vivo anterior cruciate ligament strain behaviour during a rapid deceleration movement: case report.** *Knee Surg Sports Traumatol Arthrosc* 2003, **11(5)**:307-311.
79. Mizuno K, Andrish JT, van den Bogert AJ, McLean SG: **Gender dimorphic ACL strain in response to combined dynamic 3D knee joint loading: implications for ACL injury risk.** *Knee* 2009, **16(6)**:432-440.
80. Weinhold PS, Stewart JD, Liu HY, Lin CF, Garrett WE, Yu B: **The influence of gender-specific loading patterns of the stop-jump task on anterior cruciate ligament strain.** *Injury* 2007, **38(8)**:973-978.
81. Laughlin WA, Weinhandl JT, Kernozek TW, Cobb SC, Keenan KG, O'Connor KM: **The effects of single-leg landing technique on ACL loading.** *J Biomech* 2011, **44(10)**:1845-1851.
82. Withrow TJ, Huston LJ, Wojtys EM, Ashton-Miller JA: **The effect of an impulsive knee valgus moment on in vitro relative ACL strain during a simulated jump landing.** *Clin Biomech (Bristol, Avon)* 2006, **21(9)**:977-983.
83. McLean SG, Huang X, van den Bogert AJ: **Investigating isolated neuromuscular control contributions to non-contact anterior cruciate ligament injury risk via computer simulation methods.** *Clin Biomech (Bristol, Avon)* 2008, **23(7)**:926-936.
84. McLean SG, Su A, van den Bogert AJ: **Development and validation of a 3-D model to predict knee joint loading during dynamic movement.** *J Biomech Eng* 2003, **125(6)**:864-874.
85. Wright IC, Neptune RR, van den Bogert AJ, Nigg BM: **The influence of foot positioning on ankle sprains.** *J Biomech* 2000, **33(5)**:513-519.
86. King K, Yoon SW, Perkins NC, Najafi K: **Wireless MEMS inertial sensor system for golf swing dynamics.** *Sens Actuators A* 2008, **141(2)**:619-630.
87. Shultz SJ, Schmitz RJ, Nguyen AD, Chaudhari AM, Padua DA, McLean SG, Sigward SM: **ACL Research Retreat V: an update on ACL injury risk and prevention, March 25-27, 2010, Greensboro, NC.** *J Athl Train* 2010, **45(5)**:499-508.
88. Shin CS, Chaudhari AM, Andriacchi TP: **The influence of deceleration forces on ACL strain during single-leg landing: a simulation study.** *J Biomech* 2007, **40(5)**:1145-1152.
89. Pflum MA, Shelburne KB, Torry MR, Decker MJ, Pandy MG: **Model prediction of anterior cruciate ligament force during drop-landings.** *Med Sci Sports Exerc* 2004, **36(11)**:1949-1958.
90. Domire ZJ, Boros RL, Hashemi J: **An examination of possible quadriceps force at the time of anterior cruciate ligament injury during landing: a simulation study.** *J Biomech* 2011, **44(8)**:1630-1632.
91. McLean SG, Huang X, Su A, van den Bogert AJ: **Sagittal plane biomechanics cannot injure the ACL during sidestep cutting.** *Clin Biomech (Bristol, Avon)* 2004, **19(8)**:828-838.
92. Viskontas DG, Giuffre BM, Duggal N, Graham D, Parker D, Coolican M: **Bone bruises associated with ACL rupture: correlation with injury mechanism.** *Am J Sports Med* 2008, **36(5)**:927-933.
93. Kaplan PA, Walker CW, Kilcoyne RF, Brown DE, Tusek D, Dussault RG: **Occult fracture patterns of the knee associated with anterior cruciate ligament tears: assessment with MR imaging.** *Radiology* 1992, **183(3)**:835-838.
94. Speer KP, Spritzer CE, Bassett FH, Feagin JA Jr, Garrett WE Jr: **Osseous injury associated with acute tears of the anterior cruciate ligament.** *Am J Sports Med* 1992, **20(4)**:382-389.

Biomechanical approaches to understanding the potentially injurious demands of gymnastic-style impact landings

Marianne JR Gittoes* and Gareth Irwin

Abstract

Gymnasts are exposed to a high incidence of impact landings due to the execution of repeated dismount performances. Biomechanical research can help inform recent discussions surrounding a proposed rule change in potentially injurious gymnastic dismounting. The review examines existing understanding of the mechanisms influencing the impact loads incurred in gymnastic-style landings achieved using biomechanical approaches. Laboratory-based and theoretical modelling research of inherent and regulatory mechanisms is appraised. The integration of the existing insights into injury prevention interventions studies is further considered in the appraisals. While laboratory-based studies have traditionally been favoured, the difficulty in controlling and isolating mechanisms of interest has partially restricted the understanding gained. An increase in the use of theoretical approaches has been evident over the past two decades, which has successfully enhanced insight into less readily modified mechanisms. For example, the important contribution of mass compositions and 'tuned' mass coupling responses to impact loading has been evidenced. While theoretical studies have advanced knowledge in impact landing mechanics, restrictions in the availability of laboratory-based input data have suppressed the benefits gained. The advantages of integrating laboratory-based and theoretical approaches in furthering scientific understanding of loading mechanisms have been recognised in the literature. Since a multi-mechanism contribution to impact loading has been evident, a deviation away from studies examining isolated mechanisms may be supported for the future. A further scientific understanding of the use of regulatory mechanisms in alleviating a performer's inherent injury predisposition may subsequently be gained and used to inform potential rule changes in gymnastics. While the use of controlled studies for providing scientific evidence for the effectiveness of gymnastics injury counter measures has been advocated over the past decade, a lack of information based on randomised controlled studies or actual evaluation of counter measures in the field setting has been highlighted. The subsequent integration of insight into biomechanical risk factors of landing with clinical practice interventions has been recently advocated.

Keywords: Impact loading, Laboratory-Based Research, Theoretical Research, Inherent Mechanisms, Regulatory Mechanisms

Review

Introduction

Gymnastic-style landings involving high-velocity impacts and controlled rotation during ground contact are performed regularly in sport e.g. during landing from a vertical jump or in dismounting from a gymnastics apparatus. Gymnasts are naturally exposed to a high frequency of impact landings and may be required to perform dismounts in excess of 200 times a week [1]. Unlike many other sports involving impact landings, gymnastic routines uniquely require a simultaneous address of performance and injury objectives. In dismounting, gymnasts are challenged by the need to modulate a prescribed rotation of the body orientation in flight to ensure the feet contact the ground. For example, when dismounting from the beam apparatus, gymnasts are frequently required to prepare for landing

* Correspondence: magittoes@cardiffmet.ac.uk
Cardiff School of Sport, Cardiff Metropolitan University, Cardiff, Cyncoed Road, Cardiff, UK, CF23 6XD

following a backward or forward somersault (rotation about the transverse axis) performed with high degrees of hip flexion (piked position). The subsequent ground contact or impact landing phase must be achieved using a safe, aesthetic and well-executed, double-foot landing. Although performed less frequently, single-foot impact landings such as performed in a floor routine, require similar performance and injury objectives to be addressed but typically require a succeeding skill to be performed.

Constraints in the ability of a gymnast to satisfy the multiple requirements of competitive landing tasks have subsequently been linked to errors in performance and high injury incidence rates [2]. Performance deductions may, for example be incurred for the execution of an uneven landing involving the use of multiple, single-foot placements during the impact landing phase. A serious problem faced by modern-day gymnasts is however the subsequent injury risks associated with competitive landing tasks. In 1983, Hunter and Torgan [3] questioned the need to re-evaluate gymnastic scoring of dismounts following the high incidence of associated major acute knee injuries e.g. tears to the anterior cruciate ligament. Caine and colleagues [4] highlighted that 36% of all injuries sustained by young competitive females occurred during dismounting. Singh and colleagues [5] more recently confirmed that gymnastics had one of the highest injury rates for all girls' sports between 1999 and 2005 and reported a high proportion of acute strain/sprain (44.5%) and fracture/dislocation (30.4%) diagnoses within the respective cohort. While contemporary epidemiological studies of gymnastic-related injuries have remained sparse, discussions for rule changes to de-emphasise 'sticking' landing routines in the scoring of dismounts have remained evident in the biomechanics literatures [e.g. [6]].

The ability of a performer to resist the collapse of the lower extremities has been suggested to influence the success with which reaction forces are attenuated [2]. Performers are exposed to rapidly occurring and high magnitudes of ground reactions forces during impact landings typically performed in gymnastic. Peak vertical ground reaction forces exceeding nine bodyweights and occurring in less than 0.05 s have been reported by McNitt-Gray and colleagues [2] for drop landings (height: 1.82 m) performed by gymnasts. Biomechanical analyses of the loading mechanisms used in double- and single-foot impact landings provide scientific support for the physical demands incurred on the gymnastic performer. Quantification of the physical demands imposed in landing may subsequently help to inform the respective discussions surrounding a potential rule change in gymnastic dismounting. The aim of this review was to appraise the development of current understanding of the loading mechanisms influencing the potentially injurious demands of gymnastic-style impact landings using biomechanical approaches. The review typically appraised existing insights into double-foot impact landings in order to assist the discussions regarding regulatory changes in commonly performed gymnastics dismounts.

Loading mechanisms

As evidenced in Table 1, biomechanical investigations of commonly-performed gymnastic-style impact landings have endeavoured to enhance insight into the inherent and regulatory mechanisms that can influence loading and the physical demands incurred. Multiple innate mechanisms including a performer's lower leg alignment [7], neuromuscular control [8], knee joint musculature [9-11] and joint laxity [12] have been linked to injury predisposition and have further been accounted for by gender differences. Gender disparities in the incidence of impact landing injuries have additionally been attributed to athletic posture and movement patterns [13], which may be modified or regulated by the performer. As a partial consequence of the voluntary or sub-conscious adaptations that can be achieved and integrated into safe and effective landing protocols, insights into regulatory loading mechanisms have typically been widespread in the literature. Studies of regulatory mechanisms have examined landing experience [14], impact velocity or height [2,14,15], technique [16-18] and the nature of the impacting interface [2]. While some mechanisms have been consistently recognised as contributors to injury predisposition in impact landings, less well documented mechanisms such as a performer's inherent mass composition [19,20] and lower extremity stiffness response, which was defined as the relationship between the deformation of a body and a given force [21], have recently emerged in the literature. The most prominent mechanisms contributing to impact loading have however been difficult to ascertain due to the frequent examination of isolated mechanisms and the use of diverse research approaches and analyses.

Laboratory-based studies of loading mechanisms

The majority of biomechanical investigations of impact landings have utilised laboratory-based approaches that have provided descriptive insights into regulatory loading mechanisms. While the laboratory-based approaches have included, practical hypothesis-driven experimental studies, the majority of studies have been observational in nature. As highlighted by Yeow and colleagues [15], many previous studies had specifically used motion analyses to examine various landing conditions e.g. diverse heights [14,15,22-24], lower extremity landing technique [15,16,25-27], experience [14,22,24] and the nature of

Table 1 Summary of biomechanical studies of loading mechanisms in impact landings

Mechanism	Study	Study type	Load estimation approach	Landing task protocol	Landing height	Key loading response finding(s)
Technique						
Knee joint flexion						
	[15]	Laboratory	Inverse dynamics	Drop (Double-foot)	0.15-1.05 m	Inverse relationship between initial knee flexion & peak GRFr
	[16]	Laboratory	Inverse dynamics	Drop (Double-foot)	0.59 m	Inverse relationship between maximum knee flexion & GRFv
	[23]	Laboratory		Drop (Double-foot)	0.80 m & 1.15 m	Higher (32%) GRFv with stiff than soft knee (0.80 m, hard mat)
	[25]	Laboratory	Inverse dynamics	Drop (Double-foot)	0.32 m, 0.62 m,1.03 m	Direct relationship between knee stiffness & peak GRFv
	[26]	Laboratory	Spring-mass assumption	Drop (Double-foot)	0.30 m (12 inch)	Higher GRFv (55%) with stiff than soft (bent) knee
	[27]	Laboratory	Simulation modelling		0.10 m-0.40 m	Non-linear, inverse relationship between knee flexion & peak GRFv
	[51]	Theoretical		Drop (Double-foot)	0.46 m	Change in peak GRFv (1.5 BW) with modified knee flexion timing
Foot placement						
	[17]	Laboratory	Inverse dynamics & electromyography	Drop (Double-foot)	0.40 m	Higher (3.4 times) GRFv impact peak in HTL than FFL
	[18]	Laboratory		Drop (Double-foot)	0.30 m	Unreported kinetic measures
Gender-specific						
	[11]	Laboratory	Electromyography	Drop (Double-foot)	0.52 m	No gender difference in peak GRFv or IGRF at 50 & 100 ms
	[18]	Laboratory		Drop (Double-foot)	0.30 m	Unreported kinetic measures
	[28]	Laboratory	Inverse dynamics	Drop (Double-foot)	0.60 m	No gender difference in magnitude, time and rate of peak GRFv
	[30]	Laboratory	Inverse dynamics	Stop-jump	Not reported	Higher peak GRFv (24%) in females than males
	[31]	Laboratory	Inverse dynamics	Drop (Single-foot)	0.30 m	Higher peak GRFv (9%) in females than males
	[34]	Laboratory	Inverse dynamics	Stop-jump	Not reported	Higher knee extension & valgus moments in females than males
	[35]	Laboratory	Inverse dynamics	Drop (Double-foot)	0.60 m	Higher peak GRFv (34%) in females than males
Landing height						
	[2]	Laboratory		Drop (Double-foot)	0.69 m, 1.25 m, 1.82 m	Positive relationship between landing height & peak GRFv
	[14]	Laboratory		Drop (Double-foot)	0.32 m, 0.72 m, 1.28 m	Positive relationship between landing height & peak GRFv
	[15]	Laboratory	Inverse dynamics	Drop (Double-foot)	0.15-1.05 m	Exponential relationship between landing height & peak GRFr
	[23]	Laboratory		Drop (Double-foot)	0.80 m & 1.15 m	Unreported kinetic measures
	[24]	Laboratory		Drop (Double-foot)	0.30 m, 0.60 m, 0.90 m	No reported statistical comparison between heights
	[25]	Laboratory	Inverse dynamics	Drop (Double-foot)	0.32 m, 0.62 m,1.03 m	Positive relationship between landing height & peak GRFv

Table 1 Summary of biomechanical studies of loading mechanisms in impact landings *(Continued)*

	[27]	Laboratory	Spring-mass assumption	Jump (Double-foot)	0.10 m-0.40 m	Exponential relationship between landing height & peak GRFv
Impacting interface						
	[2]	Laboratory		Drop (Double-foot)	0.69 m, 1.25 m, 1.82 m	No difference in peak GRFv between mat stiffness
	[23]	Laboratory		Drop (Double-foot)	0.80 m & 1.15 m	No difference in peak GRFv between mat stiffness
	[46]	Theoretical	Simulation modelling	Drop (Double-foot)	0.43 m	Peak GRFv sensitivity to heel pad stiffness
Performer experience						
	[14]	Laboratory		Drop (Double-foot)	0.32 m, 0.72 m, 1.28 m	
	[24]	Laboratory		Drop (Double-foot)	0.30 m, 0.60 m, 0.90 m	Higher GRFv in gymnasts than recreational athletes (0.60 & 0.90 m)
Landing task						
	[32]	Laboratory		Backward rotating tuck & pike (beam)	2.18 m & 2.22 m	Unreported kinetic measures
		Laboratory	Inverse dynamics & electromyography	Drop, front & back tucked salto (beam)	0.72 m	Between task differences in net joint moments after contact
	[48]	Theoretical	Simulation modelling	Backward & forward rotating somersault (vault)	Not reported	Reduced peak GRFv & GRFh in tasks using optimised strategies
Mass composition						
	[19]	Theoretical	Simulation modelling	Drop (Double-foot)	0.43 m	Peak GRFv (24.3 bodyweights) attenuated by soft tissues
	[20]	Theoretical	Simulation modelling	Drop (Double-foot)	0.46 m	Peak GRFv sensitivity to soft & rigid mass composition
	[46]	Theoretical	Simulation modelling	Drop (Double-foot)	0.43 m	Higher peak GRFv (13%) with higher bone mass (20%)
	[49]	Theoretical	Simulation modelling	Drop (Double-foot)	0.46 m	Peak GRFv (8.6 bodyweights) attenuated by soft tissues
Mass coupling						
	[20]	Theoretical	Simulation modelling	Drop (Double-foot)	0.46 m	Subject-specific GRFv response to coupling parameter changes
	[47]	Theoretical	Simulation modelling	Drop (Double-foot)	0.43 m	Insensitivity in peak GRFv to coupling parameters

GRFr: Peak resultant ground reaction force, GRFv: Peak vertical ground reaction force, GRFvh Peak horizontal ground reaction force IGRF: ground reaction force impulse, HTL: heel-toe landing, FFL: forefoot landing

the impacting interface [2,23]. Laboratory-based studies examining regulatory changes to landing technique have been the most evident in the literature. Decker and colleagues [28] reported that it has generally been accepted that the internal and external loads experienced in landing may be manipulated by the lower extremity kinematics (technique). While investigations of self-selected techniques have established a common phasic joint-by-joint reduction in whole body momentum [14,16,19,29], studies identifying individual and marginal ankle, knee and hip joint kinematic adjustments have suggested contradictory effects on the resulting impact loads [2,15,30,31]. Other studies [15,16,23,25-27] examined the effects of diverse degrees of knee joint flexion during ground contact using controlled comparisons of 'stiff' and 'soft' landing techniques, which were typically differentiated by the maximum knee flexion permitted on initial ground contact. As illustrated in Table 1, an inverse relationship between the degree of initial or maximum knee flexion and the resulting peak ground reaction force experienced has been commonly reported in the respective studies. As a consequence of the need to execute prescribed landing techniques to achieve high dismount scores in gymnastics, biomechanical studies implementing a restricted rather than self-selected knee joint motion may better examine the demands of a gymnastic performer.

Further research has examined the associative effects of multiple regulatory loading mechanisms. Studies investigating the interaction of landing height with experience [14,22,24] or the nature of the impacting interface [22,23] have been prominent but a continuing lack of laboratory-based data regarding high landing heights has been reported [15]. As evidenced in Table 1, laboratory-studies involving controlled drop landings have been common and have typically examined landing performed from heights of less than 1.50m without prior flight phase rotation. Studies examining 'real' gymnastic-style landings e. g. Gittoes and colleagues [32], have however highlighted that realistic landing heights for gymnastic dismounts typically exceed 2.00m. While some insight into more complex gymnastic-style landings involving flight phase rotation has been achieved in the literature [32,33] limited understanding of the regulation of loading in more challenging dismounts continues to exist. Since, gymnastic dismounts are typically characterised by: 1. a requirement to gain height in flight; 2. a need to control whole body orientation in landing and 3. an exacerbated lower limb injury risk, extended insight into challenging 'realistic' height conditions and more complex gymnastic landing manoeuvres is warranted.

Within gymnastics routines, females typically have a shorter time in the air and subsequently gain less height than males. In order to achieve higher scores, females continue to attempt similar transverse (somersaulting) and longitudinal (twisting) rotations to their male counterparts, which potentially accentuates the physical demands experienced by females. The heightened injury predisposition of females performing impact landings has primarily been addressed by an extensive body of research examining gender-related mechanical responses [18,28,31,34,35]. Contradictory findings regarding gender-based techniques have however limited understanding of the primary loading mechanisms underpinning impact landings. Gender comparisons of the techniques employed in double-foot drop jump landings have suggested a tendency for the use of a greater range of motion in the knee (20%) [28] and ankle (up to 39%) [28,35] by females compared to males. Cortes and colleagues [18] contrastingly suggested a lack of gender differences in lower extremity joint flexion angles during the ground contact phase of double-foot drop landings performed utilising diverse foot placement strategies.

In contrast to studies examining landing technique, investigations of gender-based loading responses in single- [31] and double-foot [35] have frequently confirmed heightened lower extremity loading in females compared to males. Females have been suggested to be predisposed to larger peak vertical ground reaction forces of between 9% [31] and 34% [35] when compared to their male counterparts. The current lack of consensus regarding the gender-based landing technique and loading responses predisposing females to injury in impact landings inhibits the extent to which gender-based prevention strategies may be developed and implemented. The preference for kinematic analyses alone and diversity in the protocols investigated in gender-based studies may partially contribute to the incomplete insight gained in the literature. Further insight into the gender-disparity may subsequently be achieved by the wider application of more comprehensive biomechanical analyses. As evidenced by Decker and colleagues [28], examinations of internal joint kinetics have been important in quantifying loads for establishing gender-based control strategies during drop landings. Future studies that further examine the interaction of gender-based technique modifications and the resulting internal and external loads may therefore be warranted in the literature.

Quantification of the joint moments of force produced at the ankle, knee and hip have provided a valuable understanding of the internal loads, joint-specific stresses and controlling mechanisms used to decelerate the body in landing [36]. Inverse dynamics, which integrates kinematic, external force and inertia data collected in a laboratory based setting with a linked-segment assumption, has been the preferred tool for the estimation of internal joint loading. While employing inverse dynamic analyses, DeVita and Skelly [16] established a 19% greater absorption of the body's kinetic energy in a soft landing (less than 90° knee flexion) compared to a stiff landing (greater than 90° of knee flexion). While also using inverse dynamic analyses, Kovacs and colleagues [17] reported greater relative knee joint contributions to the total lower extremity torque produced using a heel toe (45%) compared to a forefoot (37%) landing technique. However, Kovacs and colleagues [17] further recognised the need to examine individual muscle contributions, which are precluded in inverse dynamic analyses, through the use of electromyography. More recent laboratory-based studies continue to advocate the use of inverse dynamics [e.g. [15]] and electromyography [e.g. [11]] for the estimation of internal loading in dynamic movements. Although potentially limited by their descriptive nature, laboratory-based studies continue to remain popular in biomechanical investigations of landing and are becoming more evident in a growing body of research examining the influence of applied injury prevention strategies.

Application of laboratory-based studies to injury prevention strategies

As suggested by Daly and colleagues [6] in 2001, controlled trials may provide the best scientific evidence for the effectiveness of gymnastics injury counter measures, but a lack of information based on randomised controlled studies or actual evaluations of counter measures in the field setting existed. While the use of a 'correct technique' had been considered essential to prevent gymnastics injuries in landing [6], an explicit link between adapted landing techniques and an alleviation of the high incidence of gymnastic-style landing injuries had been difficult to ascertain in the literature. As further evidenced by the contradictory outcomes of gender-based studies, establishing common responses to loading mechanisms, that may inform injury prevention programs, has proven difficult. In 2000, Boden and colleagues [13] had however suggested that improved jumping, stopping and turning techniques had shown promising results in injury prevention programs.

A number of recent studies have attempted to identify biomechanical predictors of landing injuries for prevention interventions [37-39]. 'Clinician friendly' approaches for predicting anterior cruciate ligament injuries in impacts using biomechanical measures such as knee flexion range of motion have been identified [37,39]. However, relatively less attention has been given to establishing the short- and long-term effectiveness of injury prevention interventions. As suggested by Daly and colleagues [6] over a decade ago, continuing biomechanical research into the mechanism(s) of gymnastics injury and the influence of different landing techniques on injury prevention should be considered in counter measure research. More recently, the continued need to 'bridge the gap' between laboratory identification of biomechanical risk factors in landing and clinical practice has been recognised by Myer and colleagues [39].

Theoretical studies of loading mechanisms

Despite intense laboratory-based study, the associated descriptive analyses, and control and ethical constraints has precluded a thorough causal insight into the effects of prevalent loading mechanisms in challenging impact landings. As indicated in Table 1, biomechanics studies using a less conventional theoretical approach have emerged in the landing literature. A theoretical approach uses a theory or model to make predictions about the behaviour of a system [40] and permits a non-invasive, systematic manipulation of independent variables or mechanisms of interest through simulation. While a theoretical approach alone offers a solution to the limited control associated with more traditional scientific approaches, caution in using the approach must be taken due to a potential lack of realism to the living human performer. Laboratory-derived data from experimental or observational studies are however frequently used to ensure realistic inputs for a theoretical model, and to check the accuracy and validity of the predicted outcomes.

Until recently, theoretical approaches using rigid body simulation models, which assume the human performer may be represented by a series of single segment rigid components, have been customary for gaining insight into loading mechanisms [41,42]. The frequent presence of uncharacteristic oscillations in the internal joint load estimations derived in numerous kinetic analyses conducted using rigid body and inverse dynamic assumptions [16,22] had however questioned the assumption of whole body rigidity, particularly for dynamic impacts. In 1998, Gruber, and colleagues [43] conducted an innovative theoretical study to specifically examine the potential limitations of inverse dynamic analyses and rigid body assumptions on load estimations during a gymnastic-style drop landing. Gruber and colleagues [43] reported that rigid body assumptions yielded completely incorrect predictions of internal joint loads during the impact phase such that hip joint torques may be three to four times too large. More realistic skeleto-mechanical models of impact landings that incorporate soft tissue properties have subsequently become more evident in the literature over the past decade. The models, which have been termed 'wobbling mass' models, have increasingly been used to investigate the influence of soft and rigid tissue mass compositions on impact loading during simulated running [44,45] and more dynamic gymnastic-style landings [20,46-49]. Simulation studies employing 'wobbling mass' models have reported soft tissue contributions to an external peak impact load reduction of as much as 8.6 [49] and 24.3 [19] bodyweights in double foot drop landings performed with a forefoot- and heel-first ground contact, respectively.

'Wobbling mass' studies have partially attributed soft tissue loading contributions to regulation of the coupling between soft and rigid masses, which has been associated with modified muscle activity levels or muscle tuning [45]. Mass coupling represents the elasticity and damping characteristics of soft tissue (e.g. muscle, skin, subcutaneous fat) motion relative to the underlying rigid mass (e.g. bone) within a human segment e.g. thigh or shank. Liu and Nigg [44] had further supported the notion that through muscle tuning, mass coupling properties may interact with inherent mass distributions to control the forces incurred in simulated running impacts. Reductions in the damping between soft and rigid masses were later found to positively interact with localised rigid mass compositions by providing a 0.13 bodyweight additional external load attenuation during potentially injurious gymnastic-style landings [20]. If the concept of muscle tuning is correct, a subject-specific response to impact loading may be expected [45] and has been supported by the reporting of idiosyncratic responses to peak load attenuation with adapted soft tissue compositions [20]. Insight into prevalent loading mechanisms and injury predisposition in gymnastic-style landings may subsequently warrant more individual performer analyses in the future.

The theoretical support for a link between impact loading and mass compositions advocates the need for extended 'wobbling mass' modelling research into regulatory mechanisms that may alleviate a performer's innate injury predisposition. While high-speed filming of impact situations has provided insight into the complex damped manner of soft tissue motion [43], the general lack of soft and rigid mass information from living subjects currently inhibits the widespread use of 'wobbling mass' models [50]. While evidently beneficial, the increase in model complexity associated with wobbling mass compared to rigid body models is further associated with heightened development and processing demands. Despite the potential increase in simulation run time, Mills and colleagues [47] advocated a continued need to prioritise the selection of a simulation model that determines realistic internal forces when assessing injury risk in gymnastics landing. The continued merger of laboratory information with advances in theoretical modelling may subsequently offer a successful approach to ensuring a sustained enhancement of knowledge in impact biomechanics and injury prevention strategies.

Application of theoretical studies to injury prevention strategies

While recent efforts to integrate laboratory-based findings into injury prevention studies are being made [37-39], the explicit integration of theoretical study insights remains sparse. Unlike laboratory-based studies, theoretical investigations can provide explicit information on the magnitude of impact loading change that may be incurred by systematic changes to a regulatory loading mechanism. The permitted address of 'cause and effect' based research questions can subsequently provide advance knowledge for injury prevention interventions.

Recent theoretical studies [19,49] have explicitly supported the load attenuation benefits of soft tissue properties and marginally adapted mass coupling regulatory mechanisms, which have traditionally been difficult to ascertain in laboratory-based studies. Further studies have acknowledged that while a performer's innate mass compositions may be difficult to alter, tuning of the self-selected landing technique [51] and mass coupling [19,49] responses may alleviate a natural predisposition to high impact loading. As further suggested in the study of Gittoes and colleagues [51], marginal changes (up to 5 ms) to the timing of the ankle and knee joint action could influence external impact loading by as much as 3.9 and 1.5 bodyweights, respectively in gymnastic-style landing protocols.

Due the potential counter effect of internal and external loading [48,51], and idiosyncratic responses [51], caution in considering the explicit influence of regulatory changes on impact loading has been highlighted by the theoretical literature. As recently evidenced by Mills and colleagues [48], using a reduction in external loading (ground reaction force), due to a change in landing technique, as a basis for a reduction in injury potential in gymnastic movements may not be appropriate since internal loading can be heightened. Injury prevention programmes that are customised to specific performers, and assessed following internal and external loading analyses may therefore be warranted when informing prevention strategies developed to alleviate the physical demands incurred in gymnastic-style landings.

Future directions

While the existing body of biomechanical research into gymnastic-style impact landings has traditionally been laboratory-based, theoretical studies, which have offered distinct advancements in knowledge, remain relatively sparse in the literature. In order to benefit from the ecological validity of laboratory studies, and the systematic control and non-invasive testing environment of theoretical investigations, a more widespread use of an approach that integrates data obtained from the field or laboratory with theoretical models may be advocated in future investigations. In particular, the growing number of theoretical studies using 'wobbling mass' models [20,46,47], may be more effectively employed to develop insight into loading in gymnastic-style landings with the availability of increased empirical support regarding soft tissue properties. While the mechanisms predisposing a performer to gymnastic-style impact injuries may be multi-factorial in nature, the majority of existing research continues to favour examination of isolated loading mechanisms. The extent to which regulatory mechanisms can be used to alleviate an innate predisposition remains relatively under-documented. Evidence of performer-specific responses to impact loading [20,31] supports a need to further consider, through the simultaneous examination of multiple mechanisms, the interaction of innate profiles and regulatory mechanisms in understanding injury predisposition. A deviation from the tendency to consider internal and external loading in isolation may be further advocated in future research due to evidential support from theoretical studies [48,51] for a potential antagonistic response in the respective measures.

Considering the likely maintenance of a scoring system for gymnastic dismounting, which requires the achievement of constrained landing techniques, regulatory strategies such as mass coupling tuning, may alleviate a performer's innate predisposition to high physical demands without substantial alterations to technique. Accommodating self-selected landing techniques, which are tailored to the movement conditions and a performer's unique physical composition in the scoring system, may conversely offer substantially greater protection benefits for performers repeatedly executing demanding landings. The success of injury referral schemes and clinical practice is partially reliant on the comprehensive evaluation of injury prevention programmes used in training and competition. While the suggested need for a growing body of scientific evidence remains justified [6], further attempts to fully integrate existing insight in the development and evaluation of tailored injury prevention interventions is also warranted.

Conclusion

The review has appraised the development of current understanding of the loading mechanisms contributing to the physical demands of gymnastic-style impact landings using biomechanical approaches. While current insights have typically been derived from laboratory-based studies, investigations employing theoretical approaches are becoming more widely employed in the literature. As a partial consequence of the tendency to examine isolated mechanisms within the respective laboratory and theoretical studies, the primary loading mechanisms influencing the physical demands of gymnastic-style landings remain difficult to ascertain. While enhanced scientific understanding of the interaction of inherent and regulatory mechanisms is warranted to inform potential scoring changes in gymnastics, increased attempts to inform the development and evaluation of tailored injury prevention interventions using existing insights should also be made.

Authors' contributions

MJRG prepared and compiled the manuscript. MJRG and GI both contributed to the appraisal of the literature and the approval of the final manuscript.

Competing interests

The authors declare that they have no competing interests.

References

1. Özgüven HN, Berme N: **An experimental and analytical study of impact forces during human jumping.** *Journal of Biomechanics* 1988, **21**:1061-1066.
2. McNitt-Gray JL, Yokoi T, Millward C: **Landing strategy adjustments made by female gymnasts in response to drop height and mat composition.** *Journal of Applied Biomechanics* 1993, **9**:173-190.
3. Hunter LY, Torgan C: **Dismounts in gymnastics: Should scoring be reevaluated?** *The American Journal of Sports Medicine* 1983, **11**:208-210.
4. Caine D, Cochrane B, Caine C, Zemper E: **An epidemiologic investigation of injuries affecting young competitive female gymnasts.** *The American Journal of Sports Medicine* 1988, **17**:811-820.
5. Singh S, Smith GA, Fields SK, Mackenzie LB: **Gymnastics-related injuries to children treated in emergency departments in the *United States, 1990 2005*.** *Paediatrics* 2008, **121**:954-960.
6. Daly RM, Bass SL, Finch CP: **Balancing the risk of injury to gymnasts: how effective are countermeasures?** *British Journal of Sports Medicine* 2001, **35**:8-20.
7. Arendt EA: **Common musculo-skeletal injuries in women.** *The Physician and Sports Medicine* 1996, **24**:39-50.
8. Hewett TE, Myer GD, Ford KR, Heidt RS, Colosimo AJ, McLean SG, van den Bogert AJ, Paterno MV, Succop P: **Biomechanical measures of neuromuscular control and valgus loading of the knee predict anterior cruciate ligament injury risk in female athletes: A prospective study.** *The American Journal of Sports Medicine* 2005, **33**:492-501.
9. Hewett TE, Stroupe AL, Nance TA, Noyes FR: **Plyometric training in female athletes - decreased impact forces and increased hamstring torques.** *American Journal of Sports Medicine* 1996, **24**:765-773.
10. Wojtys EM, Huston LJ, Schock HJ, Boylan JP, Ashton-Miller JA: **Gender differences in muscular protection of the knee in torsion in size-matched athletes.** *The Journal of Bone and Joint Surgery* 2003, **84-A**:782-789.
11. Gehring D, Melnyk M, Gollhofer A: **Gender and fatigue have influence on knee joint control strategies during landing.** *Clinical Biomechanics* 2009, **24**:82-87.
12. Myer GD, Ford KR, Paterno MV, Nick TG, Hewett TE: **The effects of generalised joint laxity on risk of anterior cruciate ligament injury in young female athletes.** *The American Journal of Sports Medicine* 2008, **36**:1073-1080.
13. Boden BP, Griffin LY, Garrett WE Jr: **Etiology and prevention of noncontact ACL injury.** *The Physician and Sports Medicine* 2000, **28**:53-60.
14. McNitt-Gray JL: **Kinematics and impulse characteristics of drop landings from three heights.** *International Journal of Sport Biomechanics* 1991, **7**:201-224.
15. Yeow CH, Lee PVS, Goh JCH: **Regression relationships of landing height with ground reaction forces, knee flexion angles, angular velocities and joint powers during double leg-landing.** *The Knee* 2009, **16**:381-386.
16. DeVita P, Skelly WA: **Effect of landing stiffness on joint kinetics and energetics in the lower-extremity.** *Medicine and Science in Sports and Exercise* 1992, **24**:108-115.
17. Kovacs I, Tihanyi J, DeVita P, Racz L, Barrier J, Hortobagyi T: **Foot placement modifies kinematics and kinetics during drop jumping.** *Medicine and Science in Sports and Exercise* 1999, **31**:708-716.
18. Cortes N, Onate J, Abrantes J, Gagen L, Dowling E, Van Lunen B: **Effects of gender and foot-landing techniques on lower extremity kinematics during drop-jump landing.** *Journal of Applied Biomechanics* 2007, **23**:289-299.
19. Pain MTG, Challis JH: **The influence of soft tissue movement on ground reaction forces, joint torques and joint reaction forces in drop landings.** *Journal of Biomechanics* 2006, **39**:119-124.
20. Gittoes MJR, Kerwin DG: **Interactive effects of mass proportions and coupling properties on external loading in simulated forefoot impact landings.** *Journal of Applied Biomechanics* 2009, **25**:238-246.
21. Butler RJ, Crowell HP III, McClay-Davis I: **Lower extremity stiffness: implications for performance and injury.** *Clinical Biomechanics* 2003, **18**:511-517.
22. McNitt-Gray JL: **Kinetics of the lower-extremities during drop landings from 3 heights.** *Journal of Biomechanics* 1993, **26**:1037-1046.
23. Arampatzis A, Brüggemann GP, Klapsing GM: **A three-dimensional shank-foot model to determine the foot motion during landings.** *Medicine and Science in Sports and Exercise* 2002, **34**:130-138.
24. Seegmiller JG, McCaw ST: **Ground reaction forces among gymnasts and recreational athletes in drop landings.** *Journal of Athletic Training* 2003, **38**:311-314.
25. Zhang S, Bates BT, Dufek JS: **Contributions of lower extremity joints to energy dissipation during landings.** *Medicine and Science in Sport and Exercise* 2000, **32**:812-819.
26. Self BP, Paine D: **Ankle Biomechanics during four landing techniques.** *Medicine & Science in Sports and Exercise* 2001, **33**:1338-1344.

27. Elvin NG, Elvin AE, Arnockzy SP, Torry MP: **The correlation of segment angular accelerations and impact forces with knee angle in jump landing.** *Journal of Applied Biomechanics* 2007, **23**:203-212.
28. Decker MJ, Torry MR, Wyland DJ, Sterett WI, Steadman JR: **Gender differences in lower extremity kinematics, kinetics and energy absorption during landings.** *Clinical Biomechanics* 2003, **18**:662-669.
29. Lees A: **Methods of impact absorption when landing from a jump.** *Engineering in Medicine* 1981, **10**:207-211.
30. Yu B, Lin C, Garrett WE: **Lower extremity biomechanics during the landing of a stop-jump task.** *Clinical Biomechanics* 2006, **21**:297-305.
31. Schmitz RJ, Kulas AS, Perrin DH, Riemann BL, Shultz SJ: **Sex differences in lower extremity biomechanics during single leg landings.** *Clinical Biomechanics* 2007, **22**:681-688.
32. Gittoes MJR, Irwin GI, Mullineaux DR, Kerwin DG: **Whole-body and multi-joint kinematic control strategy variability during backward rotating dismounts from beam.** *Journal of Sport Sciences* 2011, **29**:1051-1058.
33. McNitt-Gray JL, Hester DME, Mathiyakom W, Munkasy BA: **Mechanical demand and multijoint control during landing depend on orientation of the body segments relative to the reaction force.** *Journal of Biomechanics* 2001, **34**:1471-1482.
34. Chappell JD, Yu B, Kirkendall DT, Garrett WE: **A comparison of knee kinetics between male and female recreational athletes in stop-jump tasks.** *American Journal of Sports Medicine* 2002, **30**:261-267.
35. Kernozek TW, Torry MR, van Hoof H, Cowley H, Tanner S: **Gender differences in frontal and sagittal plane biomechanics in drop landings.** *Medicine and Science in Sport and Exercise* 2005, **37**:1003-1012.
36. Dufek JS, Bates BT: **Biomechanical factors associated with injury during landing in jump sports.** *Sports Medicine* 1991, **12**:326-337.
37. Myer GD, Ford KR, Khoury J, Succop P, Hewett TE: **Clinical correlates to laboratory measures for use in non-contact anterior cruciate ligament injury risk prediction algorithm.** *Clinical Biomechanics* 2010, **25**:693-699.
38. Padua DA, Boling MC, DiStefano LJ, Onate JA, Beutler AI, Marshall SW: **Reliability of landing error scoring system real-time, a clinical assessment tool of jump-landing biomechanics.** *Journal of Sport Rehabilitation* 2011, **20**:145-156.
39. Myer GD, Ford KR, Hewett TE: **New method to identify athletes at high risk of ACL injury using clinic-based measurements and freeware computer analysis.** *British Journal of Sports Medicine* 2011, **45**:238-244.
40. Yeadon MR, Challis JH: **Review of sports biomechanics research.** *Journal of Sports Sciences* 1994, **12**:3-32.
41. Hatze H: **A comprehensive model for human motion simulation and its application to the take-off phase of the long-jump.** *Journal of Biomechanics* 1981, **14**:135-142.
42. Gerritsen KGM, van den Bogert AJ, Nigg BM: **Direct dynamics simulation of the impact phase in heel-toe running.** *Journal of Biomechanics* 1995, **28**:661-668.
43. Gruber K, Ruder H, Denoth J, Schneider K: **A comparative study of impact dynamics: Wobbling mass model versus rigid body models.** *Journal of Biomechanics* 1998, **31**:439-444.
44. Liu W, Nigg BM: **A mechanical model to determine the influence of masses and mass distribution on the impact force during running.** *Journal of Biomechanics* 2000, **33**:219-224.
45. Nigg BM, Liu W: **The effect of muscle stiffness and damping on simulated impact force peaks during running.** *Journal of Biomechanics* 1999, **32**:849-856.
46. Pain MTG, Challis JH: **Wobbling mass influence on impact ground reaction forces: A simulation model sensitivity analysis.** *Journal of Applied Biomechanics* 2004, **20**:309-316.
47. Mills C, Pain MTG, Yeadon MR: **The influence of simulation model complexity on the estimation of joint loading in gymnastics landings.** *Journal of Biomechanics* 2008, **41**:620-628.
48. Mills C, Pain MTG, Yeadon MR: **Reducing ground reaction forces in gymnastics' landings may increase internal loading.** *Journal of Biomechanics* 2009, **42**:671-678.
49. Gittoes MJR, Brewin MA, Kerwin DG: **Soft tissue contributions to impact forces using a four-segment wobbling mass model of forefoot-heel landings.** *Human Movement Science* 2006, **25**:775-787.
50. Arthurs KL, Andrews DM: **Upper extremity soft and rigid tissue mass prediction using segment anthropometric measures and DXA.** *Journal of Biomechanics* 2009, **42**:389-394.
51. Gittoes MJR, Kerwin DG, Brewin MA: **Sensitivity of loading to the timing of joint kinematic strategies in simulated forefoot impact landings.** *Journal of Applied Biomechanics* 2009, **25**:229-237.

15

The treatment of medial tibial stress syndrome in athletes; a randomized clinical trial

Maarten Hendrik Moen[1*], Leonoor Holtslag[2], Eric Bakker[3], Carl Barten[4], Adam Weir[5], Johannes L Tol[5] and Frank Backx[1]

Abstract

Background: The only three randomized trials on the treatment of MTSS were all performed in military populations. The treatment options investigated in this study were not previously examined in athletes. This study investigated if functional outcome of three common treatment options for medial tibial stress syndrome (MTSS) in athletes in a non-military setting was the same.

Methods: The study design was randomized and multi-centered. Physical therapists and sports physicians referred athletes with MTSS to the hospital for inclusion. 81 athletes were assessed for eligibility of which 74 athletes were included and randomized to three treatment groups. Group one performed a graded running program, group two performed a graded running program with additional stretching and strengthening exercises for the calves, while group three performed a graded running program with an additional sports compression stocking. The primary outcome measure was: time to complete a running program (able to run 18 minutes with high intensity) and secondary outcome was: general satisfaction with treatment.

Results: 74 Athletes were randomized and included of which 14 did not complete the study due a lack of progress (18.9%). The data was analyzed on an intention-to-treat basis. Time to complete a running program and general satisfaction with the treatment were not significantly different between the three treatment groups.

Conclusion: This was the first randomized trial on the treatment of MTSS in athletes in a non-military setting. No differences were found between the groups for the time to complete a running program.

Trial registration: CCMO; NL23471.098.08

Keywords: Running program, Exercises, Compression sleeve, Shin splints

Introduction

One of the most common causes of overuse leg injuries is medial tibial stress syndrome (MTSS) with incidences varying between 4 and 35% in athletic and military populations [1-3]. In the past the etiology of this syndrome was not clear, and several possible causes were described e.g. increased intracompartimental pressure or a traction induced periostitis [4,5]. Recently, different imaging techniques have demonstrated that the tibial cortex is **probably** involved in MTSS. With dual energy x-ray absorptiometry (DEXA) scanning Magnusson et al. showed that decreased bone density was present in the symptomatic part of the tibia [6]. High resolution computer tomography (CT) scans revealed osteopenia in the involved tibial cortex [7]. **However, histological studies are needed in which the bone overload theory is confirmed. Until then, bone overload as a cause of MTSS remains a hypothesis**.

Despite the high incidence of MTSS, a recent systematic review of the literature only identified three randomized controlled trials in the treatment of MTSS, all performed in military population [8]. In the study by Andrish et al. five different interventions (ice application, aspirin and ice application, phenylbutazone and ice application, heel cord stretching and ice application, walking cast) were compared. The outcome measure was being able to run 500 meters comfortably [1]. The study by Nissen et al. studied if the application of gallium-arsenic laser treatment compared to sham laser treatment shortened the time to

* Correspondence: m.moen@umcutrecht.nl
[1]Rehabilitation and Sports Medicine Department, University Medical Center Utrecht, Utrecht, Holland
Full list of author information is available at the end of the article

return to duty [9]. Johnston et al. investigated if a leg brace added to a rehabilitation program influenced the time to complete 800 meters of running pain free [10]. None of these studies found that the intervention group recovered significantly faster than the control group [1,9,10]. Besides these three RCTs there were two non-randomized controlled studies [11,12], and a few lower quality studies found [13-17]. In these treatment studies many different outcome measures were used. There is no recognized validated outcome measure for MTSS.

In clinical practice, graded running, strengthening and stretching exercises for the calf muscles are frequently prescribed for MTSS [18,19]. Graded running in itself could strengthen the tibial cortex [20-22]. Waldorff et al. showed that physiological loading allowed increased remodeling of the tibiae and increased resorption of micro-damage [22]. While very few studies have been published on the effect of stretching for MTSS [1,12], stretching is frequently included in treatment programs. Some research has been published on the effect of muscles in protecting the cortex. Animal and human studies showed that diminished muscle force negatively influences the bone adaptation process. Weaker muscles that oppose tibial bending allow an increase in bending to occur [23-26]. A recent military study showed that tibial strain, measured with strain gauges, increased after performing fatiguing long distance marches [27].

Sports compression stockings are used frequently in the Netherlands to treat MTSS [28]. A sports compression stocking might provide direct compression of the tibia and via the surrounding soft tissues, especially during intermittent loading. Compression of bony tissue has been shown to promote the expression of bone specific genes [29].

The effects of these interventions have not been previously studied in randomized trials in an athletic population. The aim of this study was to study, in a non-military, athletic population, a graded running program alone or with additional strengthening and stretching exercises or while wearing a sport compression stocking for the leg for the treatment of MTSS in a randomized trial.

Methods

Subjects

The design of the study was a randomized multi-center trial with three groups. Each athlete was randomly assigned to a treatment group, and all the athletes in the group received an intervention. The multi-center study was announced to physical therapists, general practitioners, sports medicine physicians and orthopedic surgeons. They informed the athletes about the existence of the study. They could all refer an athlete to a sports physician in one of three participating sports medicine clinics in the Netherlands (two large district and one university hospital). The sports physicians examined the athlete for complaints of MTSS and for suitability for inclusion. If the athlete was suitable for inclusion, the sports physician referred the athlete to one of the investigators for intake. A single sports physician identically trained the investigators for the study. The diagnosis of MTSS was made according to the criteria of Yates et al. (see Table 1) [30]. For exclusion criteria the description of symptoms provided by Edwards et al. in their recent review were used to specify stress fractures of the tibia and chronic exertional compartment syndrome (CECS) [31]. Pain in stress fractures is often focal (clinically and with physical examination) and the start of complaints is usually abrupt. Pain initially occurs as a mild ache after exercise, but as the condition progresses pain can be felt early after starting exercise. Athletes with CECS often complain of burning, cramping or pain over the involved compartment with exercise. Pain is progressive with continued exercise and will disappear after cessation of activities [31].

The athletes had to be involved in sport at least once a week. The inclusion was definitive when the diagnosis MTSS by an instructed sports physician was confirmed according to the Yates et al. criteria [30] and the presence of exclusion criteria [31] was excluded (Table 1) and informed consent was given.

Randomization

For the randomization at each location there were three identical opaque blank envelopes in a box each containing a letter, explaining to which of the three groups the athlete had been allocated. After the athlete had been allocated the letter was returned to the envelope and into the box to be used again by the next athlete.

Intake

At baseline the investigators noted sex, weight, height, body mass index (BMI), kind of sport in which the athlete was involved, centimeters of pain on palpation of the postero-medial border of the tibia, side of the complaints and number of days with complaints. Subsequently, a running test was performed. The running test consisted of running on a treadmill at a fixed speed, while wearing the athlete's own running shoes. Although the running test is not validated for the use in MTSS athletes it has been used previously in a treatment studies on MTSS [32,33].

First, the athlete was shown a visual analogue scale (VAS) for pain by the investigators. Then the athlete was told that when a four (on a 1-10 VAS scale) for MTSS was experienced, defined as an indication that the pain was starting to become annoying, the running test had to be stopped. The running test started at 7,5 km/hour for two minutes. After this initial warming-up phase the distance was noted that could be run at 10 km/hour until a

Table 1 Inclusion and exclusion criteria

Inclusion criteria	Exclusion criteria
Pain induced by exercise and present during or after exercise	Tibial fracture in the past
Pain on the postero-medial border of the tibia	History of paresthesia
Diffuse pain on palpation of the postero-medial tibia **for at least 5 centimeters**	Clinical suspicion of a tibial stress fracture [31]**or stress fracture present on x-ray**
Age > 16 years old	Clinical suspicion of exercise induced compartment syndrome [31]**or increased intra-compartimental pressure**
Active in sport at least once per week	
Complaints for more than 3 weeks	

four on the VAS scale was noted. The distance ran at 7,5 km/hour was subtracted from the total meters run and was called "meters run at 10 km/h".

Graded running program

With the result of the running test the athlete was placed in one of the six phases of the graded running program (see Table 2) [32,33]. When "meters run at 10 km/hour" was between 0-400 meters, the athlete started the running program in phase one. When 401-800 meters could be run, the athlete started in phase two. When 801-1200 meters could be run the athlete started in phase three. When 1201-1600 meters could be run, the athlete started phase four. When 1600 meters or more could be run, athletes started phase five. When pain was present already during walking no running test was performed. Then the athlete was advised about how to avoid complaints by reducing loading of the leg. When in these athletes pain was not present during walking for two consecutive days, phase one of the running program was started. The running program was performed three times per week, with a day off between each session.

A new phase of the running program could be commenced if a phase was finished without a pain score of four or higher on the 1-10 VAS pain scale during the running. When pain (four or more on the VAS scale) was present immediately after the running or the day after the running the program did not progress and running remained in the same phase and the time run was decreased by two minutes.

Graded running program with exercises

In addition to the graded running, which is described above, athletes performed exercises at home five times per week (see addendum). The exercises consisted of stretching and strengthening exercises of the calves. The investigators practiced the exercises with the athletes until they were familiar enough to perform them at home. The exercise schedule consisted of five phases. When a certain phase could be performed without a four on a 0-10 VAS pain scale, the following phase could be started. When phase five was finished, the athlete kept on exercising with a random mix of exercises from different phases.

Graded running program with a sports compression stocking

In addition to the graded running program, which is described above, a sports compression stocking for the leg (Herzog Medical, Woudenberg, the Netherlands) was worn when the athlete was walking or running. The compression stocking could only be taken off when the athlete was seated or laying down for more than 15 minutes. To supply the right size, the investigators measured the circumference of the calf just below the knee fold, the maximal calf circumference and the circumference just above the malleoli. Based on these measurements a size 1-6 of the stockings was supplied.

Follow-up

Follow-up took place at week 2,4,6,8,10,12,16,22, 28,34,42,50. To structure and perform follow-up, the

Table 2 Running program

Running phase	Surface	Minutes	Total	Speed/intensity
1	Treadmill	2 **2** 2 **2** 2 **2** 2 **2**	16 minutes	2 = running at 10 km/hour, **2** = walking at 6 km/hour
2	Treadmill	2 **2** 2 **2** 2 **2** 2 **2**	16 minutes	2 = running at 12 km/hour, **2** = walking at 6 km/hour
3	Concrete	3 **2** 3 **2** 3 **2** 3 **2**	20 minutes	Intensity 1-2 (*)3 = running, **2** = walking
4	Concrete	3 **2** 3 **2** 3 **2** 3 **2**	20 minutes	Intensity 2-3 (*)3 = running, **2** = walking
5	Concrete	Continuous running	16 minutes	Intensity 1-2 (*)
6	Concrete	Continuous running	18 minutes	Intensity 2-3 (*)

(*): Intensity 1; running speed: light jogging. Intensity 2; running speed; jogging while able to speak. Intensity 3; running speed: jogging while speaking becomes difficult investigators were identically trained by one sports physician (MM). Athletes were asked about progress with the running schedule, complaints and compliance with the treatment. Additionally, a physical examination was performed and feedback was provided.

Compliance

A commonly used method to measure compliance is self-reported adherence to the treatment [34,35]. At follow-up athletes were asked to choose from the following sentences: "I stuck to the prescribed activities", "most of the time I stuck to the prescribed activities", "I stuck to the prescribed activities at the beginning, but not anymore", or, "I did not follow the prescription at all" (adapted from Kallings et al., 2009) [34]. The athletes that answered "I stuck to the prescribed activities" and "most of the time I stuck to the prescribed activities", when asked about the adherence of the prescribed activities, formed the group that adhered.

Blinding

The athletes and investigators were not blinded. The data analyst (EB) was blinded to the chosen therapy. The athlete was not blinded to the treatment, because it was not possible to perform blinding. The investigators were not blinded, because the investigators had to give feed-back to the athlete about the intervention. The investigators also asked about compliance of the prescribed treatment.

Outcome measurement

Primary outcome: the number of days from inclusion to the completion of phase six (being able to run 18 consecutive minutes outdoors at a speed in which speech becomes difficult) of the running schedule was used as primary outcome measurement. Although this outcome measurement was used in previous studies on the treatment of MTSS [32,33], this outcome measurement has not been validated. Unfortunately, no validated outcome measurements for MTSS exist.

When an athlete was not able to finish the running program and quit the study, the Likert scale was used to assess the status of the athlete [36]. This scale was scored as: 1 = completely recovered, 2 = much improved, 3 = somewhat improved, 4 = same, 5 = worse and 6 = much worse. When a athlete did not have progress anymore and wanted to quit the study the Likert score was collected. The Likert scale was shown by the investigator and the investigator asked how the athlete was doing at the moment of quitting the study compared to baseline. The athlete chose a number. Satisfaction with the treatment in general on a 1-10 scale was used as secondary outcome measurement, in which 1 = very dissatisfied with treatment and 10 = highly satisfied with the treatment in general.

Data analysis

Data was entered using SPSS 17.0 (SPSS Inc, Chicago, Illinois, USA). To compare the outcome between groups Analysis of Variance (ANOVA) with post-hoc analysis according to Games-Howell was used. For dichotomized variables Chi-Square analysis was used. The athletes were analyzed by intention-to-treat. For athletes that were lost to follow-up a worst and best case scenario was calculated. For athletes that withdrew from the study due to a lack of progress, the time to complete the running program was entered as missing data in the database. Kaplan-Meier analysis was used to obtain reversed survival curves.

The local medical ethical committee agreed with the study beforehand (reference number for the study; NL23471.098.08). The committee agreed to include athletes who were 16 years of age and older. Informed consent was received from each participant.

Power analysis Previous studies on the treatment of MTSS reported a maximum time to recovery of 17.2 days and a standard deviation of 9,5 days [1,9,10]. Based on these findings, we considered a reduction of 50% in time to recovery would be clinically relevant. Sample size calculation indicated that 22 athletes (including an expected 10% lost to follow-up) per treatment group were needed to detect such difference with a power of 80% at a significance level of 0.05.

Results

Between October 2008 and February 2010 athletes were included in the study. 81 athletes were assessed for suitability for inclusion and 74 fitted the criteria and were randomized. The flow of athletes through the study is shown in Figure 1. The baseline characteristics for all athletes groups are presented in Table 3. No significant differences in baseline characteristics were found between the treatment groups. Most athletes (69%) started in phase 1 or 2 of the running program. No significant differences were found for the starting phase between the groups. The follow-up period ended in June 2010. The athletes were involved in different kind of sports. The most prevalent were soccer (24%), running (15%) and field hockey (10%). The mean number of hours that the athletes were involved in sport was 5,1 (SD 3,2) hours/week (range 1-21 hours/week). No significant differences in hours/week involvement in sport were found between the groups.

No differences were found between the groups for primary and secondary outcome measures after intention-to-treat analysis (Table 4). The mean number of days to complete the running program was 105.2 days (SD 54.6)

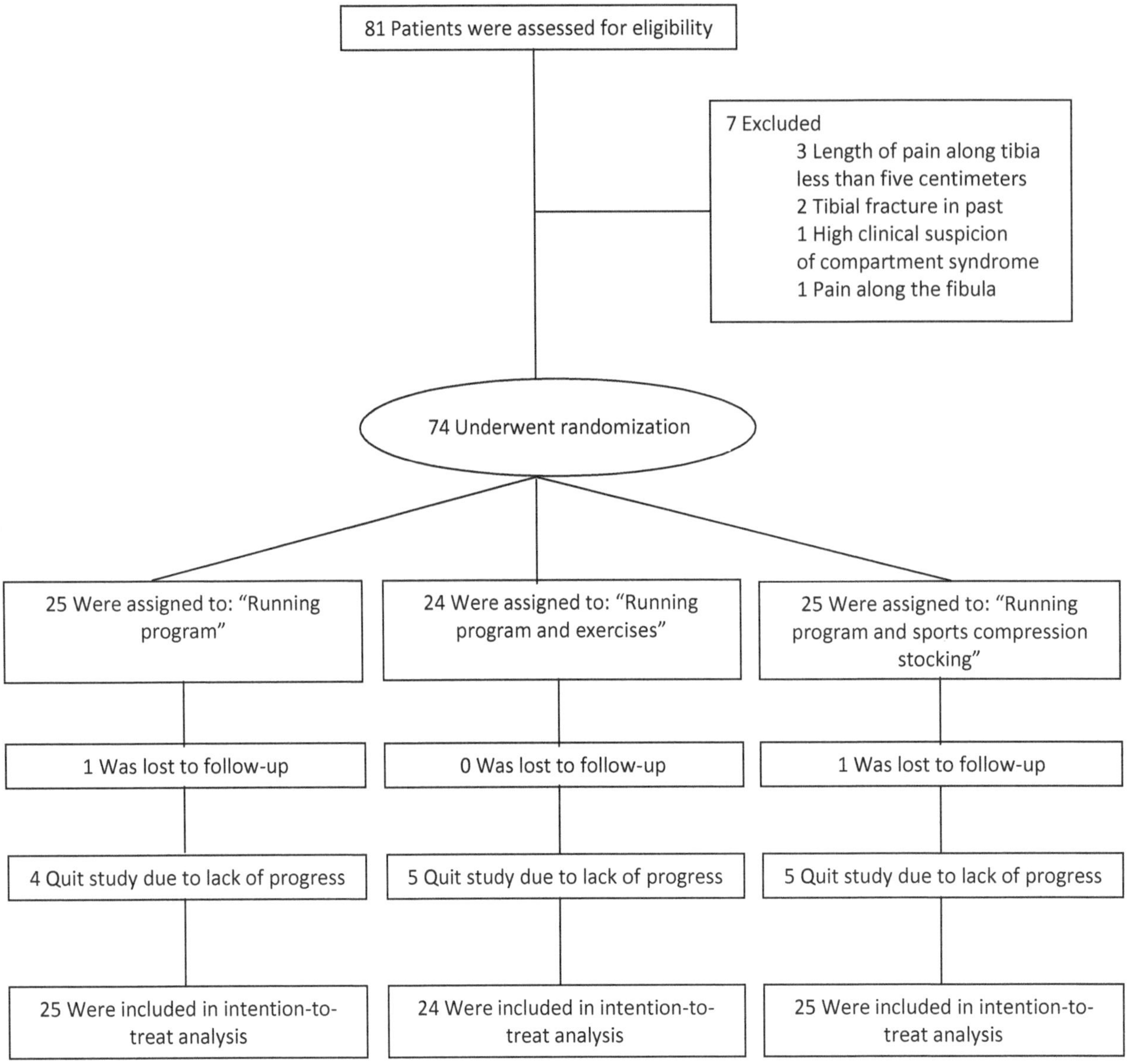

Figure 1 **Flow of patients through the study.**

for the group with the running program, 117.6 days (SD 64.2) for the group with the running program and exercises and 102.1 days (SD 52.3) for the group with the running program and the sports compression stocking ($p > 0.05$). The reversed survival curve is presented in Figure 2. No significant differences were found in the number of meters able to run on quitting the study in athletes that withdrew between the groups.

For satisfaction with the treatment in general (secondary outcome measurement) no differences were found between the groups ($p > 0.05$). Satisfaction in the running program group was 6.5 (SD 1.3), in the running program with exercises group 5.9 (SD 1.6) and 6.8 (SD 2.0) in the running program and sports compression stocking.

No significant differences were found in the number of athletes that quit the study due to subjective lack of progress with the injury or that were lost to follow-up (see Figure 1). The Likert score for these athletes was not significantly different between the groups and ranged from 3 to 4. In a worst case/best-case scenario for the intention-to-treat analysis (the lost athletes were calculated as fastest recovery (17 days) or slowest recovery (278 days)) still no significant differences between groups could be found in days to complete the running program.

No athletes were excluded from the study due to a lack of compliance. All athletes reported, "I have stuck to the prescribed activities" or "most of the time I have stuck to the prescribed activities". No complications were reported after the treatments.

Table 3 Baseline characteristics for the three treatment groups

	Running program (SD) N = 25	Running program + exercises (SD) N = 24	Running program + compression stocking (SD) N = 25	*p*-value
Height (centimeters)	175,4 (4,9)	171,6 (5,1)	177,0 (9,9)	NS
Weight (kilograms)	68,7 (8,1)	68,3 (7,7)	70,4 (11,2)	NS
BMI (kilograms/(length)^2)	22,2 (1,8)	22,9 (2,6)	22,3 (2,6)	NS
Age (years)	22,2 (6,8)	20,7 (6,4)	23,0 (8,2)	NS
Sex (percentage females)	65,2%	72,7%	53,5%	NS
Side with complaints (percentage bilateral complaints)	87,0%	77,3%	96,4%	NS
Centimeters of pain on palpation	12,2 (4,9)	11,6 (5,1)	16,1 (8,8)	NS
Days with complaints	178,0 (319,2)	174,0 (274,1)	213,7 (363,8)	NS
Meters run without pain on treadmill	708,7 (423,9)	572,6 (419,2)	591,8 (427,2)	NS
	Phase 1: 36% Phase 2: 28% Phase 3: 24% Phase 4: 12%	Phase 1: 38% Phase 2: 33% Phase 3: 17% Phase 4: 13%	Phase 1: 44% Phase 2: 28% Phase 3: 16% Phase 4: 20%	NS

Abbreviations: *NS* not significant ($p > 0.05$)

Discussion

This is the first randomized study on the treatment of MTSS in athletes outside the military. No significant differences for time to complete a running program and athlete satisfaction were found between the treatment groups. The interventions in this study were implemented for both sexes, a wide range of different sports and ages between 16-51 years old. This means that the results from this study can be generalized to a broad athletic population. The results from this study are in keeping with the only three other published RCTs on the treatment of MTSS [1,9,10].

Prior to the start of treatment a running test was performed, which is not validated. The running test, although not validated, was used in previous studies on MTSS [32,33]. **The results of the running tests in these studies were more or less comparable to the findings in this study. For the future, the running test should be validated.**

In the literature no validated outcome measure for MTSS is available and therefore several outcome measures are used. The development of validated outcome measures is a priority in this research field **to increase the quality of treatment studies on MTSS**. The previous randomized studies were all conducted in a military population and used different outcome measures. Andrish et al. used no reported tenderness or being able to run 500 consecutive meters as outcome measure [1]. In the study by Nissen et al., days to return to active duty was the primary outcome measurement [9]. The study by Johnston et al. used the time to run 800 meters without pain as outcome measure [10].

This study used time to complete a running program (defined as running continuously at a pace when speech becomes difficult) as the primary outcome measure. This is similar to the studies by Andrish et al. and Johnston et al. [1,10]. In a pilot study conducted by our research group, a lot of athletes were able to run further than 800 meters during the running test at intake. That is why the decision was made to lengthen the running program compared to these studies.

No significant differences between the groups for primary and secondary outcome measures were found. **Therefore, if MTSS is treated with a running program, no large additional effect of the two interventions can be expected**. It should however, be noted that a graded running program has not been compared with a control group that rested in any study. Now, only assumptions can be made that the graded running program improves the density and strength of the tibia, and that rest does not have this effect. This is why no conclusions can be drawn from this or other studies that a graded running program is superior to rest. While setting up the study, it was tried to include a control group that rested. However, several

Table 4 Primary and secondary outcome measures

	Running program (SD, 95% CI)	Running program and exercises (SD, 95% CI)	Running program and compression stocking (SD, 95% CI)	*p*-value
Days to complete the running program	105.2 (54.6, 80.4-130.1)	117.6 (64.2, 86.7-148.6)	102.1 (52.3, 76.9-127.2)	NS
Satisfaction with treatment in general on 1-10 scale	6.5 (1.3, 4,5-8,6)	5.9 (1.6, 4.6-7.3)	6.8 (2.0, 5,7-8,0)	NS

Abbreviations: *NS* not significant ($p > 0.05$), *SD* standard deviation, 95% *CI* 95% confidence interval

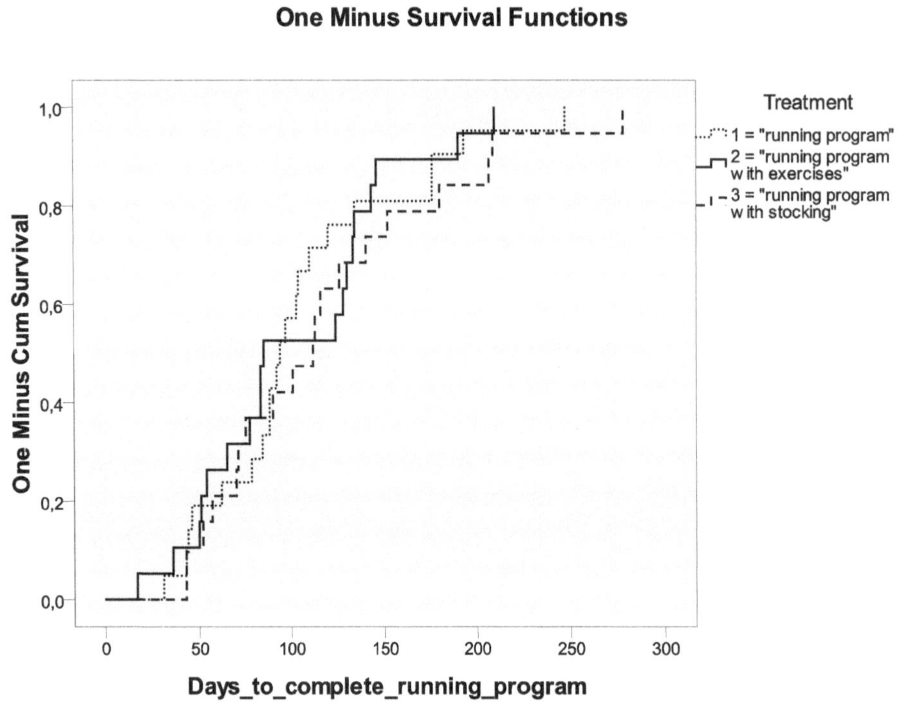

Figure 2 Reversed Kaplan-Meier survival curve for days to complete the running program.

physical therapists, sports physicians and orthopedic surgeons did not want to participate in the study if the control group rested, because they believed then they couldn't offer anything to the athletes. This was the reason that the control group performed a graded running program.

Self- reported adherence to the treatment was used to quantify compliance. This method of quantifying adherence carries a potential risk of bias, including social desirability [34]. Nevertheless, self-reported adherence has been found to be accurate and reliable when compared to objective quantification of physical activity [34,35]. No gold standard for quantifying adherence to physical activity or physical activity levels exist [37].

In all three groups athletes quit the study due to a lack of progress. These athletes were included in the analysis and this did not affect the outcome. With a relatively high dropout percentage (18,9%), this is a shortcoming of the study. The number of athletes that quit was not significantly different, with a dropout percentage varying between 16,0 and 20,8%.

Another limitation of this study is the lack of blinding of the athletes and the investigators. The studied treatment modalities were so different, that it was very hard to apply blinding to the athletes. The investigators were not blinded, as they had to give feedback to the athletes on the treatment received.

One of the weakness of this study is the power analysis used. At the start of the study, based on the available information from military studies [1,9,10], we assumed that 22 athletes per treatment group were needed to find a clinically relevant reduction of 50% in time to recovery, i.e. from 17 days to 8-9 days, with alpha set on 0.05 and a power of 0.8. However, recent studies [12,32,33] indicated that a time to recovery of 60-100 days is likely to be more realistic in athletes with MTSS. The current study was therefore able to detect a large effect of the interventions. For future studies, with the data from these studies and the data from this study a more precise power analysis could be possible [12,32,33].

Conclusion

This is the first randomized controlled study on MTSS in athletes outside a military setting. No significant differences were found between the three treatment groups in days to complete a running program (primary outcome measure) and satisfaction with the treatment (secondary outcome measure). This study does provide insight in recovery of MTSS in athletes with an average time to complete a running program of 102.1 (SD 52.3) - 117.6 days (SD 64.2). Further RCT's should be performed to test the hypothesis that a graded running program leads to a favorable outcome compared with rest. In future studies validated outcome measures should be developed and new interventions can be tested by comparing their effectiveness to a graded running program.

Author details

[1]Rehabilitation and Sports Medicine Department, University Medical Center Utrecht, Utrecht, Holland. [2]Department of Orthopedic Surgery, Academic Medical Center Amsterdam, Amsterdam, Holland. [3]Department of Clinical Epidemiology, Biostatistics and Bioinformatics, Academic Medical Center Amsterdam, Amsterdam, Holland. [4]Department of Physical Therapy, Academy of Physical Education, The Hague, Holland. [5]Department of Sports Medicine, Medical Center Haaglanden, Leidschendam, Holland.

Authors' contributions

MM designed the study and instructed the physical therapists, sports physicians, orthopedic surgeons and investigators. LH was one of the leading investigators and initiated patient contacts at the beginning of the study. EB performed the statistical analysis after the data was obtained. CB was one of the leading physical therapists involved in the study and had a large role in recruiting patients. AW was involved in designing the study methodologically and practically. JT was involved as well in designing the study methodologically and practically. FB coordinated the process of conducting the study. All authors read and approved the final manuscript.

Competing interests

We declare that none of the authors has any financial or non-financial competing interests.

References

1. Andrish JT, Bergfeld JA, Walheim J: **A prospective study on the management of shin splints.** *J Bone Joint Surg Am* 1974, **56A(8)**:1697-1700.
2. Bennett JE, Reinking MF, Pluemer B, Pentel A, Seaton M, Killian C: **Factors contributing to the development of medial tibial stress syndrome in high school runners.** *J Orthop Sports Phys Ther* 2001, **31(9)**:504-510.
3. Clanton TO, Solcher BW: **Chronic leg pain in the athlete.** *Clin Sports Med* 1994, **13(4)**:743-759.
4. Beck BR, Osternig LR, Oregon E: **Medial tibial stress syndrome: the location of muscles in the leg in relation to symptoms.** *J Bone Joint Surg Am* 1994, **76-A(7)**:1057-1061.
5. Detmer DE: **Chronic shin splints: classification and management of medial tibial stress syndrome.** *Sports Med* 1986, **3(6)**:436-446.
6. Magnusson HI, Westlin NE, Nyqvist F, Gardsell P, Seeman E, Karlsson MK: **Abnormally decreased regional bone density in athletes with medial tibial stress syndrome.** *Am J Sports Med* 2001, **29(6)**:712-715.
7. Gaeta M, Minutoli F, Scribano E, *et al*: **CT and MRI imaging findings in athletes with early tibial stress injuries: comparison of bone scintigraphy findings and emphasis on cortical abnormalities.** *Radiology* 2005, **235(2)**:553-561.
8. Moen MH, Tol JL, Weir A, Steunebrink M, de ThC W: **Medial tibial stress syndrome, a critical review.** *Sports Med* 2009, **39(7)**:523-546.
9. Nissen LR, Astvad K, Madsen L: **Low-energy laser treatment of medial tibial stress syndrome.** *Ugeskr Laeger* 1994, **156(49)**:7329-7331.
10. Johnston E, Flynn T, Bean M, *et al*: **A randomised controlled trial of a leg orthosis versus traditional treatment for soldiers with shin splints: a pilot study.** *Mil Med* 2006, **171(1)**:40-44.
11. Callisson M: **Acupuncture and tibial stress syndrome.** *J Chinese Med* 2002, **70**:24-27.
12. Rompe JD, Cacchio A, Furia JP, Maffulli N: **Low energy extracorporeal shock wave therapy as a treatment for medial tibial stress syndrome.** *Am J Sports Med* 2010, **38(1)**:125-132.
13. Eickhoff CA, Hossain SA, Slawski DP: **Effects of prescribed foot orthoses on medial tibial stress syndrome in collegiate cross country runners.** *Clin Kinesiol* 2000, **54(4)**:76-80.
14. Loudon JK, Dolphino MR: **Use of foot orthoses and calf stretching for individuals with medial tibial stress syndrome.** *Foot Ankle Spec* 2010, **3(1)**:15-20.
15. Moen MH, Ratnayake A, Weir A, Suraweera HJ, Backx FJG: **The treatment of medial tibial stress syndrome with bisphosphonates; a report of two cases.** *Dutch J Sports Medicine* 2011, **1**:1-4.
16. Morris RH: **Medial tibial syndrome: a treatment protocol using electric current.** *Chiropractic Sports Med* 1991, **5(1)**:5-8.
17. Schulman RA: **Tibial shin splints treated with a single acupuncture session: case report and review of the literature.** *J Am Med Acupuncture* 2002, **13(1)**:7-9.
18. Andrish JT: **The shin splint syndrome.** In *Orthopaedic sports medicine chapter 29.*. 2 edition. Edited by: DeLee JC, Drez D. Amsterdam: Elsevier; 2003:2155-2158.
19. Kortebein PM, Kaufman KR, Basford JR, Stuart MJ: **Medial tibial stress syndrome.** *Med Sci Sports Exerc* 2000, **32(Suppl. 3)**:S27-S33.
20. Kaspar D, Seidl W, Neidlinger-Wilke C, Claes L: **In vitro effect of dynamic strain on the proliferative and metabolic activity of human osteoblasts.** *J Musculoskel Neuron Interact* 2000, **1(2)**:161-164.
21. Lozupone E, Palumbo C, Favia A, Ferretti M, Palazzini F, Cantatore FP: **Intermittent compressive load stimulates osteogenesis and improves osteocytes viability in bones cultured in vitro.** *Clin Rheumatol* 1996, **15(6)**:563-572.
22. Waldorff EI, Christenson KB, Cooney LA, Goldstein SA: **Microdamage repair and remodeling requires mechanical loading.** *J Bone Miner Res* 2010, **25(4)**:734-745.
23. Hill DB: **Production and absorption of work by muscle.** *Science* 1960, **131(3404)**:897-903.
24. Paul IL, Murno MB, Abernethy PJ, Simon SR, Radin EL, Rose RM: **Musculo-skeletal shock absorption: relative contribution of bone and soft tissues at various frequencies.** *J Biomech* 1978, **11(5)**:237-239.
25. Radin EL: **Role of muscles in protecting athletes from injury.** *Acta Med Scand Suppl* 1986, **711**:143-147.
26. Winter DA: **Moments of force and mechanical power in jogging.** *J Biomech* 1983, **16(1)**:91-97.
27. Milgrom C, Radeva-Petrova DR, Finestone A: **The effect of muscle fatigue on in vivo tibial strains.** *J Biomech* 2007, **40(4)**:845-850.
28. Zimmermann WO, Paantjes MA: **Sport compression stockings: user satisfaction 50 military personnel.** *Dutch J Mil Med* 2009, **62**:209-213.
29. Roelofsen J, Klein-Nulend J, Burger EH: **Mechanical stimulation by intermittent hydrostatic compression promotes bone-specific gene expression in vitro.** *J Biomech* 1995, **33(12)**:1493-1503.
30. Yates B, White S: **The incidence and risk factors in the development of medial tibial stress syndrome among naval recruits.** *Am J Sports Med* 2004, **32(3)**:772-80.
31. Edwards PH Jr, Wright ML, Hartman JF: **A practical approach to the differential diagnosis of chronic leg pain in athletes.** *Am J Sports Med* 2005, **33(8)**:1241-1249.
32. Moen MH, Bongers T, Bakker EW, *et al*: **The additional value of a pneumatic leg brace in the treatment of medial tibial stress syndrome.** *J Royal Army Med Corps* 2010, **156(4)**:236-240.
33. Moen MH, Rayer S, Schipper M, Schmikli S, Weir A, Tol JL, Backx FJG: **Shockwave treatment for medial tibial stress syndrome in athletes; a prospective controlled study.** *Br J Sports Med* 2011.
34. Kallings L, Leijon M, Kowalski J, Hellenius ML, Stahle A: **Self-reported adherence - a method for evaluating prescribed physical activity in primary health care athletes.** *J Phys Act Health* 2009, **6**:483-492.
35. Leijon ME, Bendten P, Stahle A, Ekberg K, Festin K, Nilsen P: **Factors associated with athletes self-reported adherence to prescribed physical activity in routine primary health care.** *BMC Fam Pract* 2010, **11**:38-47.
36. Likert R: **A simple a reliable method of scoring the Thurstone attitude scales.** *J Soc Psychol* 1934, **5(2)**:228-237.
37. World Health Organisation: *Adherence to long-term therapies: evidence from action. Geneva* 2003.

16

Dietary intake and stress fractures among elite male combat recruits

Daniel S Moran[1,2*], Yuval Heled[1], Yael Arbel[1], Eran Israeli[3], Aharon S Finestone[1,4], Rachel K Evans[5] and Ran Yanovich[1]

Abstract

Background: Appropriate and sufficient dietary intake is one of the main requirements for maintaining fitness and health. Inadequate energy intake may have a negative impact on physical performance which may result in injuries among physically active populations. The purpose of this research was to evaluate a possible relationship between dietary intake and stress fracture occurrence among combat recruits during basic training (BT).

Methods: Data was collected from 74 combat recruits (18.2 ± 0.6 yrs) in the Israeli Defense Forces. Data analyses included changes in anthropometric measures, dietary intake, blood iron and calcium levels. Measurements were taken on entry to 4-month BT and at the end of BT. The occurrence of stress reaction injury was followed prospectively during the entire 6-month training period.

Results: Twelve recruits were diagnosed with stress fracture in the tibia or femur (SF group). Sixty two recruits completed BT without stress fractures (NSF). Calcium and vitamin D intakes reported on induction day were lower in the SF group compared to the NSF group-38.9% for calcium (589 ± 92 and 964 ± 373 $mg \cdot d^{-1}$, respectively, $p < 0.001$), and-25.1% for vitamin D (117.9 ± 34.3 and 157.4 ± 93.3 $IU \cdot d^{-1}$, respectively, $p < 0.001$). During BT calcium and vitamin D intake continued to be at the same low values for the SF group but decreased for the NSF group and no significant differences were found between these two groups.

Conclusions: The development of stress fractures in young recruits during combat BT was associated with dietary deficiency before induction and during BT of mainly vitamin D and calcium. For the purpose of intervention, the fact that the main deficiency is before induction will need special consideration.

Keywords: Basic training, Bone, Calcium, Vitamin D, Nutrition

Background

Military personnel represent a unique population exposed to intense physical and cognitive demands during both training and operational missions. Typically, military service commences with basic training (BT) which is characterized by intense physical training, emotional and mental stress [1]. It should be emphasized that such a challenging environment is enhanced during combat recruit training.

Individuals seeking to enhance physical performance through participation in arduous physical activity, particularly athletes and combat soldiers, must adhere to an appropriate and sufficient dietary intake [2,3]. Inadequate energy intake can prolong recovery from illness and injury, depress immune function, and have a negative impact on physical performance in both training and operational activities [4,5]. It has also been reported that inadequate energy intake, especially restrictive dietary patterns, may be associated with the development of stress fractures [4].

The U.S. Army has published regulations which define the nutritional responsibilities of the Surgeon General of the Army, the Navy, and the Air Force. These regulations, referred to as the Military Dietary Reference Intakes (MDRI), evaluate the effects of environmental factors on energy and nutrient requirements and outline nutrition education policy [5]. The MDRI is a quantitative estimate of the recommended dietary intake for healthy military populations based on US national

* Correspondence: dmoran@sheba.health.gov.il
[1]Heller Institute of Medical Research, Sheba Medical Center, Tel Hashomer, ISRAEL
Full list of author information is available at the end of the article

standards [5]. The Nutritional Standards for Operational and Restricted Rations (NSOR) was established to take into account the higher energy expenditure in field exercises and other operational and logistic factors relevant for training [5]. As an example, studies that quantified energy expenditure during military operations report that Special Forces soldiers had up to 45% higher absolute energy expenditure compared to their non-combat counterparts [6,7]. During prolonged training periods, if energy deficits occur, this may endanger the general health of the soldiers and reduce the muscle mass and bone strength needed for optimal performance. Of note, previous reports have found an association between insufficient dietary intake and increased risk for stress fractures among military recruits [8-10].

Bone overuse injuries, also referred to as stress reactions and stress fractures, are the most common overuse injuries among combat soldiers and are observed most frequently among young army recruits who undergo strenuous exercise during basic training [11]. The occurrence of severe cases of stress fracture has even reached rates as high as 64% in the Finnish army [12] and 31% in the Israeli Defense Forces (IDF) [13].

Stress fractures have been found to be related to several risk factors, both intrinsic and extrinsic [14], over most of which we have no control [13]. These include bone geometry parameters (studied thoroughly in the IDF), gender and hormonal factors, and genetic predisposition. Studies on bone density have been contradictory [14], and biochemical markers of bone turnover are also probably not related to stress fractures [15]. Calcium deficiency has been found deterrent to bone quality in animal models [16,17] but studies on athletes and soldiers have been less conclusive. Calcium and vitamin D are probably important in women [18] and in Finnish males (who may be effected by the latitude) [19], but in general, there is not enough data on males. Lappe et al managed to reduce stress fracture incidence in female navy recruits by about 20% [9]. Smoking (present or history) has also been found to be related to stress fractures, particularly in the US [20], and is possibly related to risk taking behavioral patterns. However, this finding has not been reproduced consistently in other militaries [19,21].

The purpose of this study was to evaluate nutritional intake in male combat recruits before induction and during a 4-month BT period. A secondary aim was to determine the possible association between specific nutrient intake, serum markers of nutrition and the occurrence of bone stress reactions.

Methods

Subjects

The study sample consisted of 74 combat male recruits from an elite combat unit in the IDF. Volunteers were recruited at the beginning of a mandatory three year military service program. All volunteers had successfully completed a strenuous 4-day sorting course 3 months prior to their induction. The military training protocol was designed to prepare the soldiers for combat missions, and included general physical fitness, physical work under pressure, hand to hand combat training, direct fire battle, leadership development and stressful combat conditions.

The study was approved by both Institutional Review Board Committees of the IDF and Sheba Medical Center, and the U.S. Army Research Institute of Environmental Medicine at Natick, MA, and all the participants signed informed consent for participation in the study.

Data collection

Data on the soldiers' anthropometric measurements, nutritional habits, iron indices, and serum calcium were collected on induction and again after 4 months. Blood samples were also taken 6 months after induction. A medical evaluation was conducted at baseline and then bi-weekly during the 6-month period by two orthopedic surgeons in order to detect the presence of stress fracture and other overuse injuries.

Anthropometric measurements

Anthropometric measurements included body weight, height, body fat percentage and calculation of body mass index (BMI). Height (cm) was measured using a stadiometer (± 1 cm) and body weight (kg) was determined with a metric scale (± 100 gr). In order to avoid errors, the same researcher completed all anthropometric measurements at each data collection point. Body fat percentage was calculated according to Siri from a 4-site skin fold thickness (biceps, triceps, subscapula, and suprailiac) [22] using Lange skin fold calipers (Beta Technology, Santa Cruz, CA).

Nutritional assessment

Food intake was assessed using the food frequency questionnaire (FFQ), developed and validated for the Israeli population by The S. Daniel Abraham International Center for Health and Nutrition at the Ben-Gurion University, Israel [23,24]. It is a long-term dietary assessment tool consisting of 126 food items divided into nine food groups that can be analyzed for nutrient and food group intake, such as: 1) eggs, milk, and milk products; 2) fats (including sauces); 3) chicken, meat, and fish; 4) bread and baked products; 5) starches and legumes; 6) fruit; 7) vegetables; 8) snacks and cookies; and 9) beverages. Subjects completed the FFQ with the assistance of a dietitian at two time points: on induction, referring specifically to the previous 6 months, and then again 4 months after starting BT, referring to the 4 months of BT. All food input was to be reported [25]. The FFQ analysis produces daily nutritional intake of proteins, carbohydrates, total fat, iron, folate, vitamins (D, B_6, and B_{12}), calcium, zinc, and magnesium. Our study referred to the MDRI and NSOR and we compared both raw data and data normalized for body weight.

Hematology and blood chemistry

Blood samples representing nutritional status were collected at three time points (0, 4, 6 months) and the following components were analyzed: hemoglobin (Hgb), iron, transferrin, ferritin, folic acid, vitamin B_{12}, and calcium. Approximately 30 cc's of venous blood samples were obtained by antecubital venipuncture into tubes (BD Vacutainer; Becton, Dickinson and Company®, 2002 BD) containing the appropriate anticoagulant. All samples were taken during the morning hours (0600-0700 h), in a sitting position after an overnight fast (6-10 h) and no exercise. The samples were placed in ice and sent within four hours to be processed and analyzed at the Sheba Medical Center Laboratories (Hematology and Biochemistry). Blood counts were performed on fresh blood using an automated analyzer (Cell-Dyn® 3000; Abbott Diagnostics, Abbott Park, IL) for measuring Hgb values. Serum ferritin was measured using an electrochemiluminescence immunoassay (Roche Elecsys®, Roche Diagnostics GmbH, Mannheim, Germany, reference: of 16-293 ng/ml). Serum iron was measured with a commercial kit on Olympus (AU2700, reference ranges 60-170 μg/dL). Vitamin B_{12} and folic acid levels were determined with an automated analyzer (Architect Abbott Diagnostics). Serum transferrin was measured with an immunoturbidimetric assay (Tinaquant® with Roche Diagnostics GmbH, Mannheim, Germany, reference ranges 193-378 mg/dL). Transferrin saturation was calculated according to the following formula: transferrin saturation (%) = serum iron/serum transferrin. Blood calcium was measured using a commercial kit on Olympus (AU2700, reference values: 8.5-10.9 mg/dl). Radioimmunoassay (RIA) was used to measure 25 (OH)D levels (DiaSorin, Stillwater, MN, reference range 30.0-74.0 ng/ml). Parathyroid hormone (PTH) was measured by immunoassay with chemiluminescent detection on the Immulite 2000 (Diagnostics Products Corporation, Los Angeles, CA, reference range 12.0-72.0 ng/L).

Hematological deficiencies were established as follows: anemia was diagnosed at Hgb levels of less than 14 g/dl, and ferritin levels (< 20 ng/ml).

Nutrition provided to recruits

The recruits had 3 main meals and 3 snacks a day. Breakfast (7-8 am, about 2 h after awakening), which included porridge, bread, 1-2 eggs, cream cheese, vegetables, olives, jam and additional savory spread for the bread (avocado, chickpea etc, depending on the season). A chocolate drink (200 ml milk) and milk desserts were also served. Dinner (12-1 pm) included soup, a meat/chicken/fish portion (200 grams) 2 salads and a cooked vegetable, a starch (potatoes/rice/macaroni), bread and a fruit desert. Supper (5-6 pm) included a main portion (1-2 eggs/macaroni etc) bread, cream cheese and spreads, hard cheese, and all other components served at breakfast. The three intermediate snacks were usually 1-2 sandwiches with jam or chocolate spread. All food was provided at no cost to the recruits.

Dietary supplements were not given or encouraged, though they were not prohibited and their use was not monitored. Formally, recruits were allowed to get additional snacks at the canteen, but they were not given access to the canteen on a regular basis. They might also have eaten extra food sent by relatives.

Injury assessment

Injury surveillance and bone stress injury diagnosis took place over the course of the entire 6-month training period. We used three sources of data: the unit physicians treating the recruits recorded overuse injuries separately in a personal surveillance table. Two orthopedic surgeons examined the recruits every 2-3 weeks and registered their findings in the recruits' central army Computerized Patient Record (CPR). Stress reactions and fractures were diagnosed by clinical examination and confirmed by radiography or bone scintigraphy [26]. Sixty two recruits without clinical signs of stress reactions and those whose imaging ruled out a stress reaction or fracture were classified as the NSF group. Twelve recruits with stress fractures of the tibia or femur confirmed by imaging were classified as the SF group. Since the mechanism for developing stress fractures in the metatarsals is fatigue and not remodeling, as in the long bones [27], we focused only on stress fractures of long bones.

Statistical analysis

Data analysis was performed using the Statistical Package for the Social Sciences software version 15.1 (SPSS INC., Chicago, IL). Comparisons between study groups over the time points, and at each phase were performed using repeated measures ANOVA (groups and time; $\alpha < 0.05$) followed by pairwise comparisons using Student's t-test with adjustments for multiple comparisons by Tukey-Kramer. Analysis of the nutritional data produced descriptive statistics including mean, standard deviation, standard error, and range.

Results

Out of the seventy four recruits who completed all data collection during the 6-month training program, twelve recruits were diagnosed with stress fractures of the long bones (tibia and femur) by imaging during the 6-months.

The results of the measured variables (i.e., anthropometry, nutritional consumption, and hematology) are presented for a total of 74 soldiers: 12 SF recruits vs. the 62 NSF recruits.

Anthropometric measurements

On induction, body weight was not significantly different between the SF and the NSF groups (68.1 ± 4.5 and 71.5 ± 6.8 kg, respectively) but the two groups' body weight did differ significantly ($p < 0.05$) at the end of BT (68.6 ± 4.7 and 72.6 ± 6.2 kg, respectively). No significant statistical differences were evident among the rest of the anthropometric measurements (height, body fat percentage, BMI) between the two study groups.

Nutritional consumption

On induction the SF group reported lower nutritional intake of most nutrients compared to the NSF group with significant differences ($p < 0.05$) in carbohydrates (272 ± 104 and 369 ± 165 g, respectively), calcium (589 ± 92 and 964 ± 373 $mg{\cdot}d^{-1}$, respectively), and vitamin D (117.9 ± 34.3 and 157.4 ± 93.3 $IU{\cdot}d^{-1}$, respectively), as depicted in Table 1. Notably, carbohydrates, calcium, and vitamin D intakes for the SF group were 55.1%, 67.9%, and 59.6% less than the NSOR requirements, respectively. Normalized nutrient intake (for body weight) was also significantly different ($p < 0.05$) between the SF group and the NSF group for these three nutrients: Carbohydrates (4.00 ± 0.04 and 5.2 ± 0.04 $g{\cdot}kg^{-1}$, respectively), calcium (8.6 ± 0.04 and 13.5 ± 0.02 $mg{\cdot}d^{-1}{\cdot}kg^{-1}$, respectively), and vitamin D (1.73 ± 0.13 and 2.2 ± 0.07 $IU{\cdot}d^{-1}{\cdot}kg^{-1}$, respectively).

Dietary intakes for the NSF group decreased significantly ($p < 0.05$) during BT from pre-induction values for almost all measured variables: carbohydrates by 15.6%, folate by 18.8%, vitamin D by 24.3%, calcium by 29.6%, zinc by 20.9%, and magnesium by 14.2%. No significant changes occurred in any of the measured variables among the SF group.

During BT, the recruits' nutritional intake (both groups) did not meet the NSOR recommendations for total energy and most nutrients, including carbohydrates, total fat, folate, vitamin D, calcium, zinc, and magnesium. Vitamin B_{12}, B_6 and protein values, however, were greater than the NSOR recommendations, both pre and post BT as depicted in Table 1.

Table 1 The Study groups' daily nutritional intake (mean ± SD) at induction and after 4-months basic training (BT)in relation (%) to the Nutritional Standards for Operational and Restricted Rations (NSOR) requirements

	NSF (N = 62)		SF (N = 12)	
	Induction	End BT	Induction	End BT
Energy (kcal)	2824 ± 1086 (78.4%)	2587 ± 879 (71.9%)	2325 ± 974 (64.6%)	2447 ± 879 (68.0%)
Proteins (g)	128.6 ± 62.8 (141%)	114.0 ± 42.4 (125%)	111.7 ± 43.1 (123%)	131.7 ± 48.3 (145%)
Carbohydrates (g)	369 ± 165* (74.7%)	335 ± 178 (67.8%)	272 ± 104 (55.1%)	285 ± 129 (57.7%)
Total Fat (g)	100.3 ± 40.5 (32.0%)	89.7 ± 31.5 (31.2%)	84.5 ± 14.8 (34.5%)	108.0 ± 35.0 (34.4%)
Iron (mg)	18.0 ± 7.7# (120%)	15.2 ± 3.5 (101%)	16.1 ± 5.1 (107%)	14.6 ± 4.8 (97.3%)
Folate (μg DFE)	448 ± 198# (112%)	364 ± 132 (91.0%)	362 ± 108 (90.5%)	332 ± 126 (83.0%)
Vitamin D (IU)	157.4 ± 93.3*# (78.7%)	119.2 ± 53.1 (59.6%)	117.9 ± 34.3 (59.0%)	121.6 ± 46.1 (60.8%)
Vitamin B_6 (mg)	3.0 ± 1.3# (231%)	2.3 ± 0.8 (177%)	2.8 ± 1.1 (215%)	2.3 ± 0.9 (177%)
Vitamin B_{12} (μg)	7.1 ± 4.0# (296%)	4.8 ± 2.3 (200%)	5.9 ± 3.2 (246%)	6.2 ± 3.0 (258%)
Calcium (mg)	964 ± 373*# (96.4%)	679 ± 236 (67.9%)	589 ± 92 (58.9%)	609 ± 171 (60.9%)
Zinc (mg)	15.8 ± 6.6# (105%)	12.5 ± 4.3 (83.3%)	14.7 ± 4.6 (98.0%)	12.4 ± 2.6 (82.9%)
Magnesium (mg)	394 ± 155# (93.8%)	338 ± 118 (80.5%)	320 ± 129 (76.2%)	318 ± 108 (75.7%)

* $p < 0.05$ NSF vs. SF at the same phase

# $p < 0.05$ for the same group at different phases

Blood biochemistry variables

Throughout the study, all subjects from the 2 groups demonstrated mean hematological values in accordance with normal levels for young, healthy males. Nevertheless, mean values of Hgb, folic acid, serum calcium, iron, ferritin and transferrin saturation decreased significantly ($p < 0.05$) during BT for both groups as depicted in Table 2. After 6 months, Hgb, serum calcium, ferritin and transferrin saturation remained lower, whereas folic acid and iron levels increased.

On induction and after 4-months BT no differences were observed in all of the measured variables (Hgb, folic acid, calcium, iron, transferrin, ferritin, 25(OH)D and PTH) between the SF and the NSF groups. However, significant differences ($p < 0.05$) were found after 6 months in serum calcium (9.5 ± 0.2 and 9.8 ± 0.3 $mg{\cdot}dl^{-1}$, respectively) and iron (71.7 ± 27.2 and 130.4 ± 71.5 $\mu g{\cdot}dl^{-1}$, respectively).

Discussion

The aim of this study was to evaluate a possible relationship between nutritional intake before induction and during BT and long bone stress fracture occurrence among male combat recruits. We monitored 74 recruits through a 6-month period (4 months BT and 2 months advanced training) of intense physical and mental training. This period is also characterized by a major change in nutritional habits, partially resulting from eating in mess and rations provided in the field. One of the consequences of these changes in lifestyle and training regime was that 16% of the recruits developed stress fractures in their long bones, similar to previous reports on recruits performing this type of training.

Stress fracture susceptibility is multi-factorial. A main factor in the mechanism of long bone stress fractures is imbalance in osteoclasis and osteogenesis that are over-activated to enable the bone remodeling necessary for the bone strengthening [28-31]. In this milieu of excessive osteogenic needs, it is reasonable to assume that dietary deficiency of calcium and/or vitamin D could contribute to stress fractures, as has previously been implicated in rickets, osteomalacia, osteopenia, osteoporosis, fractures and other cases of excessive bone resorption [32].

In this group of recruits, we found considerable dietary deficiency. First, despite the high energy needs during this period of training, the recruits consumed only 70% of the energy recommendations of the NSOR, with the NSF group reporting an 8.4% decrease in their BT total energy intake compared with the pre-induction total energy intake. This low intake may be explained by the presence of fundamental stressors in the military environment, such as periodic food restrictions, sleep deprivation, mental burden, and constant physical evaluations. These findings are in accordance with previous studies pointing to the fact that military personnel normally consume insufficient energy, whether or not they are provided with an adequate amount of food [33]. In this study, the deficient energy intake was not associated with a weight loss but rather an increase of body weight during BT by 1.5%. This is also in line with previous studies, specifically that in this training program the gained weight was in lean body mass and not in fat [34].

We are concerned that our participants did not meet MDRI requirements. These deficiencies were observed for nearly every nutrient evaluated in the FFQ. The highest deficiencies were for vitamin D and calcium in the SF group, both around 60% of the MDRI before induction and also during BT. Of note, among the NSF group, vitamin D intake was the second most deficient

Table 2 Biochemical and biomarker variables (mean ± SD) at induction (0), after 4-month BT (4), and after 6 months from induction (6)

	NSF (N = 62)			SF (N = 12)		
Month	0	4	6	0	4	6
HGB (g/dl)	15.7 ± 0.9$^{+\Delta}$	14.2 ± 0.9	14.2 ± 0.9	15.6 ± 0.5$^{+\Delta}$	14.6 ± 0.8	13.9 ± 1.0
Folic acid serum (ng/dl)	6.1 ± 2.6$^{+\Delta}$	3.9 ± 1.7	7.1 ± 2.5	7.1 ± 3.7^{+}	3.8 ± 1.9	7.0 ± 2.4
Calcium total (mg/dl)	10.1 ± 0.4$^{+\Delta}$	9.7 ± 0.4	9.8 ± 0.3*	9.9 ± 0.3$^{\Delta}$	9.6 ± 0.4	9.5 ± 0.2
Iron (μg/dl)	118.9 ± 51.4^{+}	65.4 ± 24.1	130.4 ± 71.5*	121.2 ± 53.8^{+}	66.8 ± 22.6	71.7 ± 27.2
Transferrin (mg/dl)	303.9 ± 48.2	306.0 ± 28.5	307.6 ± 41.4	264.0 ± 53.5	302.4 ± 67.5	295.9 ± 50.4
Ferritin (ng/ml)	54.3 ± 30.0$^{+\Delta}$	42.6 ± 22.5	22.8 ± 9.6	57.4 ± 30.2$^{\Delta}$	38.7 ± 19.0	31.9 ± 16.5
Transferrin saturation (%)	39.1 ± 12.7^{+}	21.4 ± 8.5	23.4 ± 9.2	41.1 ± 13.5^{+}	22.1 ± 11.7	24.2 ± 10.8
25(OH)D (nmol/L)	75.3 ± 16.3	64.6 ± 10.2	72.4 ± 13.8	70.5 ± 16.5	63.0 ± 12.4	66.4 ± 16.4
PTH (ng/L)	32.4 ± 14.9	50.2 ± 17.1	32.1 ± 19.9	31.9 ± 18.5	43.8 ± 17.8	37.4 ± 22.7

* $p < 0.05$ NSF vs. SF at the same examination date

$^{+}$ $p < 0.05$ at the same group, between induction and end of BT

$^{\Delta}$ $p < 0.05$ at the same group, between induction and 6-month variable, reported to be consumed at a level of 78.7% from MDRI before induction and at even a lower level of 59.6% during BT. In our study, the SF recruits reported 41.0% less initial calcium and vitamin D intakes on induction day than the MDRI recommendations. Although vitamin D3 (cholecalciferol) is either formed in the skin after exposure to sunlight or obtained from nutritional sources, especially fatty fish [32], most IDF soldiers use sunscreen and wear long-sleeved clothing during military training. This may limit vitamin D3 synthesis, and therefore, the importance of balanced nutritional intake, especially of vitamin D and calcium, should be emphasized, even though we did not actually find low serum levels of vitamin D.

Release of PTH is controlled by the level of calcium in the blood, with low blood calcium levels causing an increase in PTH. The main purpose of this hormone is calcium homeostasis. It is therefore not surprising that in these healthy young recruits, we did not find any pathological PTH or calcium values. A slight trend towards higher levels of PTH in the 4-month BT may represent a lack of dietary calcium. However PTH differences between SF and NSF or between induction values and 4 or 6 month values were not significant.

Furthermore, we found that the SF group compared to NSF had insufficient intake of zinc and magnesium (93.8% to 80.5% and 98.0% to 82.9% of the MDRI, respectively) throughout BT. In addition to calcium, minerals and trace elements such as zinc and magnesium are involved in skeletal growth and are required for normal bone metabolism. An adequate intake of these dietary components is therefore necessary to assure optimal bone quality and prevention of bone loss [35].

It is also evident that during BT, SF soldiers developed iron deficiency and anemia symptoms associated with 39% low transferrin saturation (< 16%), 36.4% ferritin deficiency (< 20 ng/ml), and 37.9% hemoglobin deficiency (< 14 g/dl). Notably, similar findings were observed in previous studies involving elite Israeli male athletes [36,37], and in female combatants [38]. Moreover, it is important to note that iron and ferritin levels are a part of an innovative prediction model for stress fractures in young female recruits during basic training, which managed to correctly predict stress fracture occurrence in 76.5% of a sample population [39].

The study has several limitations. Assessing food consumption based on a person's memory is always problematic. This is more so with recruits in a very intense physical and mental training schedule. We also did not monitor personal initiatives in taking nutritional supplements. Previous surveys have demonstrated this to be negligible, with recruits showing minimal interest in calcium and vitamin D. Another problem is the lack of finding of low vitamin D levels, despite the dietary deficiency. We also did not measure serum zinc levels, however, following these results it would seem beneficial to measure these levels for future research on recruits.

Conclusions

The main conclusion from this study is that, contrary to previous beliefs, male infantry recruits in the IDF are nutritionally deficient, specifically in calcium and vitamin D, and those who were more deficient developed more stress fractures. This directly arouses the debate on supplying supplements, following Lappe et al. in the US Navy female recruits [9]. But it is doubtful whether such an intervention is justified for a 20% decrease in stress fracture incidence in the IDF, and further research would be necessary to prove the efficacy in IDF male combat recruits. Another issue is related to the fact that there was dietary deficiency before induction, making intervention by the military at the most appropriated time more complicated. Based on our findings it might be plausible to perform nutritional screening (e.g., questionnaire) of elite combat recruits on induction and possibly assess the deficient subjects for serum levels. We could then treat those with low levels.

It should therefore be emphasized that while engaging in strenuous physical training, proper nutrient intake may act as a long-term protector against bone resorption and stress fracture development, and is recommended for maintaining healthy bones [40].

Acknowledgements
This study was supported in part by a contract from the MRMC (No. W911QY-08-P-0286). The opinions or assertions contained herein are the private views of the authors and should not be construed as official or reflect the views of the US Department of Defence or the Israel Defence Forces.

Author details
[1]Heller Institute of Medical Research, Sheba Medical Center, Tel Hashomer, ISRAEL. [2]Ariel University Center of Samaria, Ariel, ISRAEL. [3]Division of Medicine, Department of Gastroenterology, Hebrew University-Hadassah Medical Center, Jerusalem, ISRAEL. [4]The, Orthopaedic Department, Assaf Harofeh Medical Center, Zerifin and The Sackler School of Medicine, Tel Aviv University, Zerifin, Tel Aviv, ISRAEL. [5]Military Performance Division, U.S. Army Research Institute of Environmental Medicine, Natick, MA, USA.

Authors' contributions
DSM and RY conceived the study idea and analysed the data. DSM, YA, RKE, and RY designed the study. YA and RY carried out data collection. ASF conducted the orthopaedic examinations. DSM and RY drafted the manuscript. All authors contributed to the interpretation of results, critically reviewed the manuscript for intellectual content, and gave approval of the final version of the manuscript to be published.

Competing interests
The authors declare that they have no competing interests.

References

1. Flakoll PJ, Judy T, Flinn K, Carr C, Flinn S: **Postexercise protein supplementation improves health and muscle soreness during basic military training in Marine recruits.** *J Appl Physiol* 2004, **96**:951-956.
2. Israeli E, Merkel D, Constantini N, Yanovich R, Evans RK, Shahar D, Moran DS: **Iron deficiency and the role of nutrition among female military recruits.** *Med Sci Sports Exerc* 2008, **40**:S685-690.
3. Lukaski HC: **Vitamin and mineral status: effects on physical performance.** *Nutrition* 2004, **20**:632-644.
4. Bennell KL, Malcolm SA, Thomas SA, Ebeling PR, McCrory PR, Wark JD, Brukner PD: **Risk factors for stress fractures in female track-and-field athletes: a retrospective analysis.** *Clin J Sport Med* 1995, **5**:229-235.
5. US Department of the Army N, and Air Force HQ: **Nutrition standards and education. Army regulation 40-25.** *Book Nutrition standards and education. Army regulation 40-25. (Editor ed.^eds.)* City: Department of the Army, Navy, and Air Force; 2001, 1-16.
6. Bovill ME, Backer-Fulco CJ, Thairon WJ, Champagne CM, Allen HR, DeLany JP: **Nutritional requirements of United States Army Special Forces soldiers.** *Federation of Am Soc Exp Biol J* 2002, **16**:A252.
7. Tharion WJ, Lieberman HR, Montain SJ, Young AJ, Baker-Fulco CJ, Delany JP, Hoyt RW: **Energy requirements of military personnel.** *Appetite* 2005, **44**:47-65.
8. Ihle R, Loucks AB: **Dose-response relationships between energy availability and bone turnover in young exercising women.** *J Bone Miner Res* 2004, **19**:1231-1240.
9. Lappe J, Cullen D, Haynatzki G, Recker R, Ahlf R, Thompson K: **Calcium and vitamin d supplementation decreases incidence of stress fractures in female navy recruits.** *J Bone Miner Res* 2008, **23**:741-749.
10. Valimaki VV, Alfthan H, Lehmuskallio E, Loyttyniemi E, Sahi T, Suominen H, Valimaki MJ: **Risk factors for clinical stress fractures in male military recruits: a prospective cohort study.** *Bone* 2005, **37**:267-273.
11. Pester S, Smith PC: **Stress fractures in the lower extremities of soldiers in basic training.** *Orthop Rev* 1992, **21**:297-303.
12. Sahi T: **Stress fractures: epidemiology and control.** *Rev Int Serv Sante Armees* 1984, **57**:311-313.
13. Finestone A, Milgrom C: **How stress fracture incidence was lowered in the Israeli army: a 25-yr struggle.** *Med Sci Sports Exerc* 2008, **40**:S623-629.
14. Bennell K, Matheson G, Meeuwisse W, Brukner P: **Risk factors for stress fractures.** *Sports Med* 1999, **28**:91-122.
15. Bennell KL, Malcolm SA, Brukner PD, Green RM, Hopper JL, Wark JD, Ebeling PR: **A 12-month prospective study of the relationship between stress fractures and bone turnover in athletes.** *Calcif Tissue Int* 1998, **63**:80-85.
16. Ferretti JL, Tessaro RD, Audisio EO, Galassi CD: **Long-term effects of high or low Ca intakes and of lack of parathyroid function on rat femur biomechanics.** *Calcif Tissue Int* 1985, **37**:608-612.
17. Lanyon LE, Rubin CT, Baust G: **Modulation of bone loss during calcium insufficiency by controlled dynamic loading.** *Calcif Tissue Int* 1986, **38**:209-216.
18. Nieves JW, Melsop K, Curtis M, Kelsey JL, Bachrach LK, Greendale G, Sowers MF, Sainani KL: **Nutritional factors that influence change in bone density and stress fracture risk among young female cross-country runners.** *PM R* 2010, **2**:740-750, quiz 794.
19. Ruohola JP, Laaksi I, Ylikomi T, Haataja R, Mattila VM, Sahi T, Tuohimaa P, Pihlajamaki H: **Association between serum 25(OH)D concentrations and bone stress fractures in Finnish young men.** *J Bone Miner Res* 2006, **21**:1483-1488.
20. Lappe JM, Stegman MR, Recker RR: **The impact of lifestyle factors on stress fractures in female Army recruits.** *Osteoporos Int* 2001, **12**:35-42.
21. Giladi M, Milgrom C, Simkin A, Danon Y: **Stress fractures.** *Identifiable risk factors. Am J Sports Med* 1991, **19**:647-652.
22. Siri WE: **The gross composition of the body.** *Adv Biol Med Phys* 1956, **4**:239-280.
23. Shahar D, Shai I, Vardi H, Brener-Azrad A, Fraser D: **Development of a semi-quantitative Food Frequency Questionnaire (FFQ) to assess dietary intake of multiethnic populations.** *Eur J Epidemiol* 2003, **18**:855-861.
24. Shai I, Rosner BA, Shahar DR, Vardi H, Azrad AB, Kanfi A, Schwarzfuchs D, Fraser D: **Dietary evaluation and attenuation of relative risk: multiple comparisons between blood and urinary biomarkers, food frequency, and 24-hour recall questionnaires: the DEARR study.** *J Nutr* 2005, **135**:573-579.
25. Etzion-Daniel Y, Constantini N, Finestone AS, Shahar DR, Israeli E, Yanovich R, Moran DS: **Nutrition consumption of female combat recruits in army basic training.** *Med Sci Sports Exerc* 2008, **40**:S677-684.
26. Milgrom C, Finestone A, Shlamkovitc N: **Stress fracture treatment.** *Orthopedics (Int Ed)* 1995, **3**:363-367.
27. Milgrom C, Finestone A, Sharkey N, Hamel A, Mandes V, Burr D, Arndt A, Ekenman I: **Metatarsal strains are sufficient to cause fatigue fracture during cyclic overloading.** *Foot Ankle Int* 2002, **23**:230-235.
28. Milgrom C, Simkin A, Eldad A, Nyska M, Finestone A: **Using bone's adaptation ability to lower the incidence of stress fractures.** *Am J Sports Med* 2000, **28**:245-251.
29. Milgrom C, Finestone A, Hamel A, Mandes V, Burr D, Sharkey N: **A comparison of bone strain measurements at anatomically relevant sites using surface gauges versus strain gauged bone staples.** *J Biomech* 2004, **37**:947-952.
30. Milgrom C, Finestone A, Novack V, Pereg D, Goldich Y, Kreiss Y, Zimlichman E, Kaufman S, Liebergall M, Burr D: **The effect of prophylactic treatment with risedronate on stress fracture incidence among infantry recruits.** *Bone* 2004, **35**:418-424.
31. Finestone A, Milgrom C, Wolf O, Petrov K, Evans R, Moran D: **The epidemiology of metatarsal stress fractures is different from that of tibia and femoral stress fractures during one year of elite infantry training.** *Foot Ankle* 2011, **32**:16-20.
32. Lips P: **Vitamin D physiology.** *Prog Biophys Mol Biol* 2006, **92**:4-8.
33. Fairbrother B, Shippee R, Kramer T: **Nutritional and immunological assessment of soldiers during the special forces assessment and selection course.** *Book Nutritional and immunological assessment of soldiers during the special forces assessment and selection course (Editor ed.^eds.), vol. Technical Report No. T95-22* City: United States Army Research Institute of Environmental Medicine; 1995.
34. Finestone AS, Eshel A, Milgrom C, Katz G, Constantini N: **Components of weight increase during infantry basic training.** *J Isr Milit Med* 2009, **6**:72-75.
35. Branca F, Valtuena S: **Calcium, physical activity and bone health-building bones for a stronger future.** *Publ Health Nutr* 2001, **4**:117-123.
36. Dubnov G, Constantini NW: **Prevalence of iron depletion and anemia in top-level basketball players.** *Int J Sport Nutr Exerc Metab* 2004, **14**:30-37.
37. Eliakim A, Nemet D, Constantini N: **Screening blood tests in members of the Israeli National Olympic team.** *J Sports Med Phys Fitness* 2002, **42**:250-255.
38. Merkel D, Moran DS, Yanovich R, Evans RK, Finestone AS, Constantini N, Israeli E: **The association between hematological and inflammatory factors and stress fractures among female military recruits.** *Med Sci Sports Exerc* 2008, **40**:S691-697.
39. Moran DS, Israeli E, Evans RK, Yanovich R, Constantini N, Shabshin N, Merkel D, Luria O, Erlich T, Laor A, Finestone A: **Prediction model for stress fracture in young female recruits during basic training.** *Med Sci Sports Exerc* 2008, **40**:S636-644.
40. Heaney RP: **Dairy and bone health.** *J Am Coll Nutr* 2009, **28(Suppl 1)**:82S-90S.

Can pre-season fitness measures predict time to injury in varsity athletes?: a retrospective case control study

Michael D Kennedy[1*†], Robyn Fischer[2†], Kristine Fairbanks[2†], Lauren Lefaivre[2†], Lauren Vickery[2†], Janelle Molzan[2†] and Eric Parent[2,3†]

Abstract

Background: The ability to determine athletic performance in varsity athletes using preseason measures has been established. The ability of pre-season performance measures and athlete's exposure to predict the incidence of injuries is unclear. Thus our purpose was to determine the ability of pre-season measures of athletic performance to predict time to injury in varsity athletes.

Methods: Male and female varsity athletes competing in basketball, volleyball and ice hockey participated in this study. The main outcome measures were injury prevalence, time to injury (based on calculated exposure) and pre-season fitness measures as predictors of time to injury. Fitness measures were Apley's range of motion, push-up, curl-ups, vertical jump, modified Illinois agility, and sit-and-reach. Cox regression models were used to identify which baseline fitness measures were predictors of time to injury.

Results: Seventy-six percent of the athletes reported 1 or more injuries. Mean times to initial injury were significantly different for females and males (40.6% and 66.1% of the total season ($p < 0.05$), respectively). A significant univariate correlation was observed between push-up performance and time to injury (Pearson's $r = 0.332$, $p < 0.01$). No preseason fitness measure impacted the hazard of injury. Regardless of sport, female athletes had significantly shorter time to injury than males (Hazard Ratio = 2.2, $p < 0.01$). Athletes playing volleyball had significantly shorter time to injury (Hazard Ratio = 4.2, $p < 0.01$) compared to those playing hockey or basketball.

Conclusions: When accounting for exposure, gender, sport and fitness measures, prediction of time to injury was influenced most heavily by gender and sport.

Keywords: Exposure, Prognosis, Range of motion, Strength, Vertical jump, Sports injury

Background

Injuries among varsity athletes pose a significant challenge for both teams and individual players as demonstrated by surveillance of injuries in the National Collegiate Athletic Association (NCAA) [1-6]. A reportable injury is defined as one resulting from participation in an organized practice or competition and associated with restriction of participation or performance [1]. The opportunity for athletic injury increases with greater time spent participating [7]. Thus, measuring exposure to the possibility of injury in the greatest detail possible, such as minutes played in both practices and games is an important aspect of injury reporting [7]. Despite the fact that exposure is an important aspect of injury reporting, most studies report only on the occurrence of the injury and ignore quantifying exposure or the time from baseline evaluation to injury occurrence. The NCAA defines exposure as 1 athlete participating in 1 practice, which allows for a rate of injury to be determined (number of injuries / 1000 athlete exposures) [8], but does not account for the different exposure encountered by different athletes during practices and games.

Fitness evaluation and pre-participation evaluations (PPE; medicals) are standard practice in university sport [9]. The goal of these medical evaluations are to screen

* Correspondence: kennedy@ualberta.ca
†Equal contributors
1 Faculty of Physical Education and Recreation, University of Alberta, Edmonton, AB, Canada
Full list of author information is available at the end of the article

athletes for cardiac [10], musculoskeletal [11], and high-risk behaviour concerns [9]. Current standard for the musculoskeletal (MSK) part of the PPE include both medical history and a screening physical exam with history being very important for determining previous injuries [11]. Current evidence indicates that the efficacy of the physical screening exam to determine pathology and abnormalities or predict future injury is limited [11]. However, some tests commonly used to evaluate pre-season fitness may be prognostic factors for injury in varsity athletes [12,13].

Specifically, suboptimal musculoskeletal physical characteristics such as flexibility, muscle strength, muscle endurance, muscle power, and agility have been shown to be risk factors for injury in sports [1,13-18]. For example, flexibility is associated with an enhanced ability to dissipate and absorb forces and accommodate stress, thereby reducing injury [19] and strength/fatigue resistance [20] as well as agility, have been shown to prevent injury [21]. In contrast, vertical jump ability although beneficial to sport performance may increase risk of injury due to landing forces [22-24]. Thus, fitness and screening have been shown to be predictive of injury occurrence, however it is unclear whether pre-season fitness performance influences the time to injury.

Thus, the purpose of this study was to determine the utility of preseason fitness measures to predict risk of injury in varsity athletes when accounting for estimates of athlete's exposure. We hypothesized that suboptimal preseason performance scores would be predictive of the time to injuries during the competitive varsity season.

Methods

Design

All participants (eligibility defined in participants) completed a battery of preseason fitness tests during the month preceding their competitive season starting. Exposure data was estimated retrospectively based on available data and expert assessment to determine the amount of time athletes were exposed to the possibility of injury in practice or competition. Injury data was obtained retrospectively using a self-administered injury report survey completed by participants at post-season team meetings for which attendance of all athletes (injured or not) was mandatory.

Testers were trained exercise specialists with experience conducting fitness testing according to accepted protocols [25]. A certified exercise physiologist with 10 years of experience in fitness testing was present at all test sessions to supervise the standard testing protocol. Fitness tests were administered in the same order specified as follows for all athletes to control for the effects of accumulating fatigue on a subsequent performance test: vertical jump, the sit and reach, the modified Illinois agility, push ups, curl ups and the Apley's range of motion test. Standardized guidelines were followed in the administration of all the tests [21,25,26]. All fitness tests included have shown adequate reliability in order to draw inferences on individuals (ICC > 0.9) [21,27-30].

Participants

The sample consisted of 6 varsity teams including men's hockey (n = 23), women's hockey (n = 18), men's volleyball (n = 14), women's volleyball (n = 10), men's basketball (n = 9) and women's basketball (n = 12). This sample of varsity teams includes sports where sport participation involves use of both the upper and lower extremities where both genders are involved. Descriptive data is presented in Table 1. All 86 participants provided written informed consent to participate in accordance with guidelines from the Research Ethics Board for the Faculty in the spirit of the Helsinki declaration. To be eligible for inclusion, an athlete must have participated in a varsity game or practice during the 2008-2009 season and have data for both the preseason fitness testing and the post-season injury survey. At the time of the preseason fitness testing, all athletes were medically cleared to participate as determined by their Pre-Participation Evaluation (PPE) [31]. Each PPE was completed by the athlete and referring physician, then submitted to the head therapist for review. The head therapist then either cleared each athlete for participation (no flagged issues on PPE) or provided arrangements for additional referrals or evaluations as flagged by specific identified issues on the PPE. Only when subsequent referrals and

Table 1 Descriptive variables of each team (mean ± SD)

Team	Age (yrs)	Height (cm)	Weight (kg)	Body Mass Index (BMI)
Men's Basketball	20.6 ± 1.4	189.9 ± 7.0	91.3 ± 12.1	25.2 ± 2.4
Men's Hockey	22.9 ± 1.4	183.1 ± 4.0	85.9 ± 7.2	25.6 ± 1.6
Men's Volleyball	20.1 ± 1.1	195.9 ± 7.0	90.2 ± 8.8	23.5 ± 1.6
Women's Basketball	20.0 ± 1.9	181.1 ± 6.8	74.3 ± 8.5	22.6 ± 2.0
Women's Hockey	20.0 ± 1.5	170.0 ± 12.1	69.5 ± 6.6	24.4 ± 4.4
Women's Volleyball	20.3 ± 1.8	180.7 ± 6.7	69.3 ± 8.8	21.2 ± 2.0

evaluations were completed in those athletes who required follow up did the head therapist clear that athlete for participation.

Procedures

Preseason fitness measures

The vertical jump test estimated instantaneous anaerobic power and lower body strength. No run-up, step up, or pre-jump was permitted. One familiarization jump was allowed to ensure the participant executed the correct technique. Three testing trials were performed with a rest period of 10-15 seconds between each trial. A vertec device was used to measure jump height. The trial with the greatest jump height was recorded to the nearest 0.5 inch. Maximal jump height was converted to centimetres and the difference between the maximum jump height and an athlete's standing reach height was recorded as the vertical jump height (cm).

The sit and reach test was used to evaluate lower back and hip flexibility [32]. Participants were encouraged to stretch hamstrings prior to testing although no formal warm-up was administered. Participants were asked to sit with their legs fully extended, the ankle at 90° and to reach forward as far as possible with their outstretched arms and fingers by bending their back and hips. The maximal position of flexion had to be held for 2 seconds and 2 trials were performed with a 10-15 second rest between. The maximum sit and reach distance was recorded to the nearest 0.5 cm.

The modified Illinois agility test evaluated the participants' ability to accelerate, decelerate, turn in different directions, and run at different angles [26]. The test was administered as described by Vescovi et al [21],. where four cones were used to mark the rectangular agility area (10 meters long, 5 meters wide). Another 4 cones were placed inside the centre of the area at a distance of 3.3 m apart. Participants began on their own time and the tester started the stopwatch at the participant's initial movement. Participants ran straight to the second cone, zigzagged through the series of cones in the centre and finished by running around the final 2 cones of the course. Time was stopped when the participant crossed the finish line. Two trials were permitted with a 1-2 minute rest period in between and the best time was recorded with a handheld stopwatch to the closest hundredth of a second.

The push up test was used to evaluate upper-body endurance specifically, pectoralis major, anterior deltoids and triceps [32]. No pause was allowed at elbow extension and a self-selected tempo had to be maintained throughout the test. The number of repetitions were counted until fatigue or until the participants were unable to maintain proper technique over 2 consecutive repetitions.

The curl-up test evaluated the endurance of the abdominal musculature that provides a foundation for trunk and spine stability [33]. The test was administered to a metronome beat set at 50 beats per minute (25 curl-ups per minute). One warning about improper form was permitted prior to final termination of the test. The number of curl-ups that met the proper technique criteria was recorded [25]. The partial curl-up test was used because it produces the highest activation of the abdominal musculature (rectus abdominus, external obliques, and lower abdominal stabilizers) with minimal activation of the hip flexors [34].

The Apley's ROM test assessed shoulder flexibility, specifically medial rotation with adduction and lateral rotation with abduction. The test reflects functional capacity at the shoulder [35]. Participants were required to remove their shirt to bare skin or bra top. The tester held a measuring stick (cm) with the 20 cm mark at the level of the inferior angle of the scapula. Participants were instructed to reach into lateral rotation and abduction with palm facing anterior. Second, the participants were asked to reach into medial rotation and adduction with palm facing posterior. Participants repeated the same motions on the other side. Measurements were recorded as a positive (good range) or negative (limited range) value measured from the level of the inferior angle (20 cm mark) to the level of the 3rd digit. Measurements were recorded to the nearest 0.5 cm.

Exposure estimate

Exposure was quantified as the total amount of time participants were exposed to the possibility of injury in practice or competition prior to injury.

Practice exposure time was determined by totalling the amount of team practice time (in minutes) that individual athletes participated in prior to the occurrence of their first injury. Team practice time was calculated using each team's practice schedule throughout the season. Due to the retrospective nature of this analysis and because practices are mandatory, the estimate of practice exposure is based on the assumption that athlete's were exposed in the full duration of scheduled practice up until the day on which injury occurred. The absence from practice due illness or personal reasons was not documented.

Based on the retrospective nature of game exposure estimations, game exposure was determined differently for each sport using the best available data. Individual estimates of game exposure were calculated. This was to account for the significant differences in playing time that a starter or first line player might have compared to a substitute or fourth line player. For ice hockey teams, game exposure was derived from coach-estimated average playing time per game per athlete at the end of the competitive season. Using this estimation, total game exposure time per participant was calculated up to the date of injury using the team game schedule. Game exposure time for basketball players was taken directly from game statistics, which recorded the number of minutes each individual played per game. For volleyball players, game exposure was calculated by multiplying the number of sets each athlete played per game by the number of rallies within those sets, their team's average rally time, and a coach-estimated average percentage of court time per set that each athlete played over the season. The lattermost variable accounts for differences in court time not recorded by game statistics. Set played and numbers of rallies were retrieved from game statistics. Average rally time per team was determined by reviewing 5 rallies from each of 3 randomly chosen videotaped games from both the men's and women's 2008-2009 season games.

Injury surveillance survey

The survey was modified from the National Collegiate Athletic Association (NCAA) Injury Surveillance System [8] to be completed by the athletes and for data capture using the Cardiff Teleform system (New England Survey Systems, Brooklyn, MA). The survey was simplified and re-formatted so that participants may effectively report injuries retrospectively. Face validity of the survey was assessed with 2 men's league soccer teams and 2 women's recreational basketball team. Feedback on readability and time to complete survey was collected and appropriate changes were made. Injury data was not retrieved from the central care training room athlete's records. This is because central care only records injuries of those athletes who make a formal appointment to see an athletic therapist. Using only central care data we could have missed injuries that were treated outside of central care. Our strategy is supported by recent research showing that a self-report internet survey of injury reporting by parents of adolescent soccer players captured more injuries than athletic therapist reported injuries [36]. In addition, calendars of each team's preseason and competitive season were distributed at their respective meetings to help athletes determine the exact date at which the injury occurred. Furthermore, trainers were present to assist athletes in recalling injuries that occurred, the type of injury and when the injury occurred.

Statistical analyses

Descriptive analysis consisted of means and standard deviations for subject preseason performance. Frequencies were estimated for each type and location of injury. Univariate analysis of the ability of the preseason measures to predict time without injury was completed using Pearson Correlation coefficients.

Proportional-hazard (or Cox) multivariate regression analysis was used to determine the predictive ability of each pre-season measures for the hazard of injury while taking into account gender and sport. The primary dependent variable in this study was time to initial injury or to the end of the season for athletes who were not injured. Time to initial injury was reported as the percentage of exposure in games and practices from the total season duration prior to injury. For athletes who were not injured, 100% exposure was assumed. Baseline or time zero was determined as the first official practice for each team. The independent variables in this study were the 5 preseason baseline measures (vertical jump, sit and reach, Apley's ROM test, push up test and modified Illinois agility test). Hazard is defined as the probability of being injured at a given point in time, having remained uninjured up until that point [37]. Cox regression accounts for different amounts of exposure to injury amongst participants. It enables the difference between survival times (or time remaining injury free) of

Table 2 Mean and standard deviation for preseason baseline measures

Preseason Baseline Measure	N	Mean	Standard Deviation
Upper extremity right internal rotation	86	7.80*	6.63
Upper extremity left internal rotation	85	11.37*	5.82
Upper extremity right external rotation	86	−8.24*	3.80
Upper extremity left external rotation	85	−8.29*	3.30
Upper extremity strength (push up)	85	22.44‡	12.45
Lower extremity range of motion (sit and reach)	85	38.68*	7.95
Lower extremity power (vertical jump)	83	53.94*	10.34
Modified Illinois agility	60	11.22†	.70
Curl ups	85	28.22§	16.00

* Indicates measured and recorded in cm.
† Indicates measured and recorded in seconds.
‡ Indicates the number of push ups performed.
§ Indicates the number of curl ups performed.

Table 3 Frequency of body part injured and injury types

Body Part	Injury Type											Total
	Bruise	Tendinitis	Ligament sprain incomplete	Ligament sprain complete	Muscle or tendon strain incomplete	Dislocation partial	Dislocation complete	Fracture	Stress fracture	Herniation	Other	
Upper extremity	3	3	8	1	1	1	2	1	0	0	0	20
Lower extremity	1	4	5	0	6	0	1	0	1	0	4	22
Upper back/ neck/ ribs	2	0	0	0	4	0	0	0	0	0	0	6
Lower back/ pelvis	0	1	0	0	4	1	0	0	0	2	3	11
Head	1	0	0	0	0	0	0	0	0	0	5	6
Total	7	8	13	1	15	2	3	1	1	2	12	65

particular groups of participants to be predicted while allowing for other prognostic factors or covariates to be considered at the same time [38]. The preseason scores were entered into the model as continuous variables. Upper and lower extremity range of motion data was entered in the analysis as a distance from the mean to reflect the hypothesis that too much or too little ROM was hypothesized to be a risk for injury. Hazard ratios were reported with 95% confidence intervals (95% CI). Statistical analysis was completed using SPSS v15.0.1.1 (SPSS) using an alpha level of 0.05.

Results

Participant description and injury survey

A total of 46 male and 40 female athletes completed preseason baseline measures (Table 2) and the post-season injury survey. Seventy six percent of athlete's reported one or more injuries during the 2008-2009 season (Table 3), over half of which were new injuries (63.1%). Twenty nine percent were recurrence of past injuries. Injuries to the lower extremity were the most common with 33.8% of athletes reporting injury to this area. The most common injury type reported was incomplete muscle or tendon strain (23.1%).

Most injuries occurred during the regular season (61.5%); 33.8% occurred during the preseason, and 4.6% during the post season (Table 4). The majority of athletes did not miss any games due to their injury (73.8%); however most missed 1 or more practices due to their injury (55.4%). All but 1 athlete sought some form of medical attention following injury (98.5%).

Injuries occurred in a greater percentage of games (11.8%) than practices (6.9%). Over half of practice injuries occurred during regular season practice (57.9%). The remainder occurred in preseason practice (42.1%). No

Table 4 Number of injuries to occur in pre season, regular season and post season play

Team	Practice			Game		
	Pre season	Regular Season	Post Season	Pre season	Regular Season	Post Season
Female hockey	5	3	0	0	7	0
Female volleyball	3	4	0	3	0	0
Female basketball	3	5	0	0	1	0
Male hockey	0	2	0	2	6	3
Male volleyball	4	8	0	0	1	0
Male basketball	1	0	0	1	3	0
Total	16	22	0	6	18	3
Total full season	38			27		

Table 5 Mean time to initial injury expressed as % of season completed with 95% confidence interval

	Mean Time to Initial Injury (%)	95% Confidence Interval (Lower limit; Upper limit)
Team:		
Female hockey	48.9	33.1-64.8
Female volleyball	19.3	5.0-33.7
Female basketball	45.9	23.5-68.3
Male hockey	83.8	72.2-95.4
Male volleyball	35.7	21.9-49.4
Male basketball	66.8	37.2-96.3
Gender:		
Female	40.6	29.5-51.6
Male	66.1	55.3-76.8
Sport:		
Hockey	68.5	57.7-79.3
Volleyball	27.4	17.4-37.3
Basketball	57.6	39.2-76.0

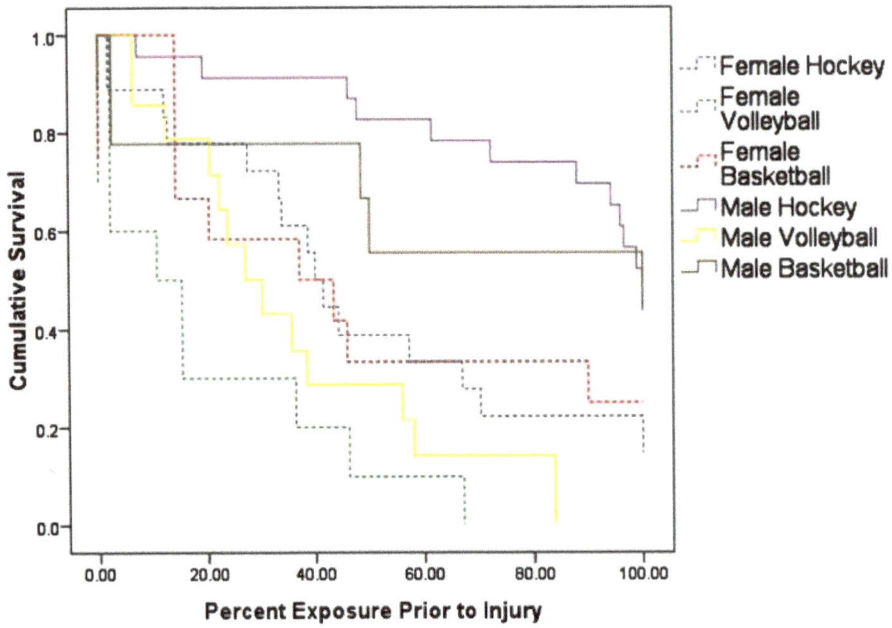

Figure 1 Kaplan Meier survival curves of the time to initial injury for each varsity team.

injuries occurred in post-season practice. Sixty-six percent of game injuries occurred during regular season competition (66.6%). Twenty two percent occurred in pre season games (22.2%), while 11.1% occurred in post-season games (Table 4).

Time to injury in varsity athletes by gender and teams

Mean times to initial injury were significantly shorter for females (40.6% of total season) than for male athletes (66.1%). Mean times to initial injury reported in percent of the total varsity participation were significantly shorter for volleyball players (27.4%) than for hockey players (68.5%) or basketball players 57.6% (Table 5). Kaplan Meier survival curves for each team showing the percent athlete not injured at different percentage of the total varsity participation are presented in Figure 1. Female and male volleyball players had the shortest mean time to injury (19.3% and 35.7%), followed by women's hockey (48.9%) and women's basketball (45.9%). Men's basketball had a mean time to initial injury of 66.8%. Male hockey players had the longest mean time to initial injury at 83.8%.

Correlations between preseason test scores and time to injury

Only 1 significant univariate correlation was observed between preseason test scores and time to injury (Table 6). Weaker upper extremity strength (push ups) was associated with shorter time to injury (Pearson's $r = 0.33$, $p < 0.01$).

Table 6 Pearson correlation of preseason baseline measures and time to initial injury expressed as % of season completed before injury

Preseason Baseline Measure	N	Pearson Correlation	*p*
Right internal rotation deviation from mean	86	−0.14	0.22
Left internal rotation deviation from mean	85	0.07	0.52
Right external rotation deviation from mean	86	0.03	0.76
Left external rotation deviation from mean	85	0.09	0.42
Upper extremity strength (push ups)	85	0.33	<0.01
Lower extremity range of motion deviation from mean (sit and reach)	85	0.15	0.16
Lower extremity power (vertical jump)	83	0.13	0.23
Illinois agility	60	−0.11	0.39
Curl ups	85	−0.08	0.49

Table 7 Cox regression with gender and team acting as covariates

Covariate	Hazard ratio (95% Confidence Interval)	p
Gender		
Female	2.21 (1.34-3.64)	<0.01
Male	1	
Sport		
Volleyball	4.25 (2.05-8.79)	<0.01
Hockey	1.08 (0.55-2.09)	0.83
Basketball	1	

Multivariate prediction of time to injury

Proportional-hazard (Cox) regression was used to determine the effect of each independent variable on the hazard of injury. Cox regression analysis including gender and sport as covariates revealed that none of preseason measures of strength, range of motion, and agility significantly impacted the hazard of injury. Only, vertical jump performance showed a trend toward impacting injury hazard. As vertical jump scores increase, so does the hazard of injury (HR 1.04, $p < 0.10$). The Cox regression model predicting time to injury using only gender and team as predictors is reported in Table 7. Regardless of sport, female athletes had significantly shorter time to injury than males (HR = 2.2, $p < 0.01$). Athletes playing volleyball had significantly shorter time to injury than either basketball or hockey (HR = 4.2, $p < 0.01$).

Discussion

Main findings

This study sought to develop a predictive model for injury in varsity athletes from sports where both upper and lower extremities are used using preseason performance measures. The study accounted for estimated exposure to the risk of injury for male and female basketball, volleyball, and hockey athletes. Overall, the results indicated that female gender is the most predictive factor in determining time to injury in game or practice regardless of preseason performance. Further, volleyball had significantly shorter time to injury than the other sports studied.

Univariate associations suggested that athletes with limited upper extremity endurance as demonstrated by low push up performance had a shorter time to injury. However, when accounting for the relationship between gender and push up performance in the multivariate model, female gender better predicts shorter time to injury. Similarly, Augustsson et al found that males performed significantly more push ups than females and had 44% greater upper body endurance strength [39]. They suggested that females who train upper body endurance may be more likely to avoid injury [39]. In this study, pushups data alone was not sufficient to predict time to injury. However, our results provide some support to investigate the belief that strength and conditioning in athletes may be a good prevention strategy not only for occurrence but also for time to injury.

Vertical jump was the only other pre-season performance measure showing potential to predict time to injury. Athletes who had higher vertical jump scores showed a trend toward being injured earlier. This finding may appear counterintuitive given that greater muscular or aerobic performance scores are typically desirable in sports. However, Martel et al claim that plyometric training of high intensity and high impact to improve vertical jump height increases the possibility for muscle damage and injury [24]. Additionally, Hewett et al identified female athletes with a higher vertical jump performance scores as having higher risk landing profiles and that high jumping females were more likely to incur injuries, especially at the knee [22]. In volleyball and basketball high vertical jumps are desirable, however this research and those previously mentioned [22-24] suggest that this greater performance attribute may be associated with increased risk of injury. Additionally, athletes with the greatest vertical jump height are likely to play more games and thus have greater exposure to injury in competitive situations. Therefore the combination of increased performance and exposure may put athletes in starting positions at higher risk of injury compared to other players.

Of the injuries collected over the 2008/2009 varsity season, injuries occurred in a greater percentage of games (11.8%) than practices (6.9%). This finding is consistent with data from the NCAA where athletes were 3.5 times more likely to sustain an injury during a game than practice [1]. Both our study and the NCAA study found that injuries occurring in games were greatest for athletes involved in contact sports, compared to sports traditionally considered "non-contact" such as volleyball [2]. Contacts are more frequent in game situations [1].

In the present study, lower extremity injury was more prevalent than upper extremity injury in hockey, volleyball, and basketball which is consistent with previous findings [40-43]. The most common types of injuries in the present study across all sports examined were muscle strain (23%), ligament sprain (20%), and tendonitis (12%). These findings are consistent with other studies reporting muscle sprain/strain as the most prevalent injury [41-43]. However, Hootman et al report ligament sprain (14.8%) as the highest injury prevalence [1]. This discrepancy may be due to the difference in injury definition used as Hootman et al [1] only accounted for injuries that resulted in limitation of participation in competition or practice, while we defined injury as one that could have resulted in limited participation, or in the athlete seeking medical attention. In our study, we may have captured more injuries as some participants may have incurred an injury and sought medical treatment but did not restrict themselves from practice.

Gender and sport differences

Our study found that females were more likely to be injured and had a shorter mean time to injury than males. These results are consistent to the majority of studies found in the literature [13,39,44-46]. For example Murphy et al found a discrepancy between male and female injury incidence among diverse populations [13]. They found females to be at greater risk than males when identifying risk factors for lower extremity injury [13]. On the other hand others have found that gender was not an important factor in sport injuries for athletes involved in volleyball, basketball, soccer, wrestling and running [40]. One reason for this difference may be because men are less likely to report injuries [47]. The increased likelihood to report injuries by females may be a cultural bias that may be considered in future studies relying on self-reporting of injuries. For our results, this bias if true likely influenced only injury prevalence reporting and not time to injury in this study.

To our knowledge, no previous studies examined gender differences with respect to mean time to injury thus our finding that female's time to injury was shorter than males is novel. We are confident in the finding that mean time to injury is shorter in females because although our exposure estimate may not be exact the error in estimating exposure in our study should be the same for male and females. Others have identified other female risk factors for increased risk of injury.

Our findings demonstrate that both men's and women's volleyball had the highest rate of injury and the shortest time to injury. Compared to the longitudinal NCAA data our findings are less than the NCAA women' volleyball data which reported 4 injuries per 1000 athlete exposures. The differences might exist due sample size and further longitudinal data collection with Canadian varsity athletes might elucidate any real differences compared to the NCAA data. However, it is noteworthy that we cannot technically compare exposure differences because the NCAA exposure data is a frequency measure defined as 1 athlete participating in 1 practice [8], whereas our exposure is a calculated estimate of exposure in minutes. It has been indicated that a limitation of the NCAA data is the sensitivity of the exposure estimate whereby, "future authors should use a finer level of exposure measurement, such as player-minutes" [1] In this case our estimate of exposure in minutes allows for time to injury to be investigated, with the finding that volleyball has significantly shorter time to injury than basketball or hockey.

Limitations and strengths

Accounting for and documenting practice and game exposure when predicting injury is a novel aspect of this study. The collection of the measurement of the potential predictors of injury was collected before the exposure. However, injury information was collected retrospectively with a risk of recall bias. For feasibility reason, we based the injury data survey on the NCAA Injury Surveillance System modified so that an athlete could complete the survey retrospectively. A member of the research team was present to answer questions or clarify items when the survey was administered. Furthermore, practice and competition schedules were used to help athletes remember injury dates and to reduce any recall bias that may have occurred. Others have shown that retrospective tracking of injuries is sufficiently accurate in athletes [48]. Our injury survey also ensured that we captured all injuries including those that may not have been reported to athletic therapy staff in a prospective injury tracking system because we were asked the athletes themselves.

We combined upper and lower extremity injuries when examining the relationship between preseason performance measures and injury occurrence. This may have reduced the predictive power of the preseason performance measures used in this study because some preseason measures may only be predictive of specific injuries. However, the intent was to assess the ability of the preseason measures to identify athletes at risk of any injuries in sports involving both upper and lower extremity activities.

Missing data may have influenced the results. Due to a scheduling conflict men's hockey did not complete the Modified Illinois Agility test. Other missing fitness measures (<3 per measure) were due to either scheduling conflict or exclusion of invalid result due to instructions not being followed.

Future studies should continue to utilize a comprehensive approach to document time exposed to injury. Larger sample sizes would help confirm if preseason measures are significant predictors of a specific injury in multivariate models when still accounting for gender and sport. Alternatively, because we found differences between genders and between sports, we recommend focussing on only one gender and one sport when planning studies on predictions of shorter time to injuries. Males and females practicing different sports may have different backgrounds in terms of training, and previous injuries. Further, different sports include different activities. Poor scores on fitness measures may predict shorter time to injuries when exposed to risky activities more prevalent in a given sport than another. Nevertheless, our results show that the preseason measures selected in the present study were not strong predictors of short time to injuries over and above gender and sport in sports that were selected because they involved both upper and lower extremity use. Our results provide novel evidence that gender and sports are key predictors of time to injury in out selected varsity sports. To our knowledge this information was lacking from the literature as analyses predicting time to injury are rare in the varsity sport literature.

Likely this means that a different predictor set will be required for different sport even though for simplicity varsity programs may have benefited from using a common dataset for all sports and genders.

In the future, it may be beneficial to examine the predictive ability of more performance measures, however, to ensure the feasibility of preseason screening the added measures should have the ability to be administered rapidly, and require little equipment. Identifying more performance measures with the ability to predict injury is of utmost value for varsity athletics. In the future, collecting injury information and documenting exposure in minutes prospectively should be considered. Future research should consider the impact of other conditions that may influence participation in practice or games when estimating exposure. Also, the modified varsity sport injury survey could be compared to prospective injury recording in order to confirm its validity.

Conclusions

Our study found the prevalence of injury types and location to be similar to those found in other studies. When accounting for exposure, gender and sport, performance measures were not found to be significant predictors of time to injury. Time to injury was influenced most heavily by gender and sport. Our study did not support the hypothesis that baseline performance measures would predict time to injury.

Competing interests

The author(s) declare that they have no competing interests.

Author contributions

MDK contributed to the design, analysis and drafting the manuscript; RF contributed to the design, created the injury surveillance instrument, analyzed and wrote results and helped draft manuscript; KF contributed to the overall design, data collection and manuscript preparation; LL assisted with the conception of the project, collected data and oversaw the development of the methods; LV assisted with the overall design, oversaw data collection and assisted in manuscript preparation; JM assisted in overall design and development of the methods and exposure data collection; EP oversaw the design development, the statistical analysis and assisted in the drafting of the manuscript. All authors read and approved the final manuscript.

Author details

[1]Faculty of Physical Education and Recreation, University of Alberta, Edmonton, AB, Canada. [2]Department of Physical Therapy, Faculty of Rehabilitation Medicine, University of Alberta, Edmonton, AB, Canada. [3]Glenrose Rehabilitation Hospital, Alberta Health Services, Edmonton, AB, Canada.

References

1. Hootman JM, Dick R, Agel J: **Epidemiology of collegiate injuries for 15 sports: summary and recommendations for injury prevention initiatives.** *J Athl Train* 2007, **42**(2):311–319.
2. Agel J, Palmieri-Smith RM, Dick R, Wojtys EM, Marshall SW: **Descriptive epidemiology of collegiate women's volleyball injuries: National Collegiate Athletic Association Injury Surveillance System, 1988-1989 through 2003-2004.** *J Athl Train* 2007, **42**(2):295–302.
3. Agel J, Dick R, Nelson B, Marshall SW, Dompier TP: **Descriptive epidemiology of collegiate women's ice hockey injuries: National Collegiate Athletic Association Injury Surveillance System, 2000-2001 through 2003-2004.** *J Athl Train* 2007, **42**(2):249–254.
4. Agel J, Dompier TP, Dick R, Marshall SW: **Descriptive epidemiology of collegiate men's ice hockey injuries: National Collegiate Athletic Association Injury Surveillance System, 1988-1989 through 2003-2004.** *J Athl Train* 2007, **42**(2):241–248.
5. Agel J, Olson DE, Dick R, Arendt EA, Marshall SW, Sikka RS: **Descriptive epidemiology of collegiate women's basketball injuries: National Collegiate Athletic Association Injury Surveillance System, 1988-1989 through 2003-2004.** *J Athl Train* 2007, **42**(2):202–210.
6. Dick R, Hertel J, Agel J, Grossman J, Marshall SW: **Descriptive epidemiology of collegiate men's basketball injuries: National Collegiate Athletic Association Injury Surveillance System, 1988-1989 through 2003-2004.** *J Athl Train* 2007, **42**(2):194–201.
7. Finch CF: **An overview of some definitional issues for sports injury surveillance.** *Sports Med* 1997, **24**(3):157–163.
8. Dick R, Agel J, Marshall SW: **National Collegiate Athletic Association Injury Surveillance System Commentaries: Introduction and Methods.** *J Athl Train* 2007, **42**(2):173–182. Ref Type: Journal (Full).
9. Joy EA, Paisley TS, Price R Jr, Rassner L, Thiese SM: **Optimizing the collegiate preparticipation physical evaluation.** *Clin J Sport Med* 2004, **14**(3):183–187.
10. Pfister GC, Puffer JC, Maron BJ: **Preparticipation Cardiovascular Screening for US Collegiate Student-Athletes.** *JAMA* 2000 March 22, **283**(12):1597–1599.
11. Garrick JG: **Preparticipation orthopedic screening evaluation.** *Clin J Sport Med* 2004, **14**(3):123–126.
12. Payne KA, Berg K, Latin RW: **Ankle Injuries and Ankle Strength, Flexibility, and Proprioception in College Basketball Players.** *J Athl Train* 1997, **32** (3):221–225.
13. Murphy DF, Connolly DA, Beynnon BD: **Risk factors for lower extremity injury: a review of the literature.** *Br J Sports Med* 2003, **37**(1):13–29.
14. Ekstrand J, Gillquist J: **The frequency of muscle tightness and injuries in soccer players.** *Am J Sports Med* 1982, **10**(2):75–78.
15. Ekstrand J, Gillquist J: **Soccer injuries and their mechanisms: a prospective study.** *Med Sci Sports Exerc* 1983, **15**(3):267–270.
16. Witvrouw E, Danneels L, Asselman P, D'Have T, Cambier D: **Muscle flexibility as a risk factor for developing muscle injuries in male professional soccer players, A prospective study.** *Am J Sports Med* 2003, **31**(1):41–46.
17. Emery CA, Meeuwisse WH, Hartmann SE: **Evaluation of risk factors for injury in adolescent soccer: implementation and validation of an injury surveillance system.** *Am J Sports Med* 2005, **33**(12):1882–1891.
18. Myer GD, Ford KR, Barber Foss KD, Liu C, Nick TG, Hewett TE: **The relationship of hamstrings and quadriceps strength to anterior cruciate ligament injury in female athletes.** *Clin J Sport Med* 2009, **19**(1):3–8.
19. Garrett WE Jr: **Muscle strain injuries: clinical and basic aspects.** *Med Sci Sports Exerc* 1990, **22**(4):436–443.
20. Matzkin E, Zachazewski JE, Garrett WE Jr, Malone TR: *Skeletal muscle: deformation, injury, repair and treatment considerations. Scientific foundations and principles of practice in musculoskeletal rehabilitation.* Missouri: Saunders Elsevier; 2007:107.
21. Vescovi JD, Brown TD, Murray TM: **Positional characteristics of physical performance in Division I college female soccer players.** *J Sports Med Phys Fitness* 2006, **46**(2):221–226.
22. Hewett TE, Myer GD, Ford KR, Slauterbeck JR: **Preparticipation physical examination using a box drop vertical jump test in young athletes: the effects of puberty and sex24.** *Clin J Sport Med* 2006, **16**(4):298–304.

23. Louw Q, Grimmer K, Vaughan C: **Knee movement patterns of injured and uninjured adolescent basketball players when landing from a jump: a case-control study2.** *BMC Musculoskelet Disord* 2006, **7**:22.
24. Martel GF, Harmer ML, Logan JM, Parker CB: **Aquatic plyometric training increases vertical jump in female volleyball players1.** *Med Sci Sports Exerc* 2005, **37**(10):1814–1819.
25. Canadian Society for Exercise Physiology: *Canadian Physical Activity, Fitness, and Lifestyle Approach.*: Canadian Society for Exercise Physiology; 1996. Ref Type: Pamphlet.
26. Roozen M: **Illinois agility test.** *Performance Training Journal* 2004, **3(5)**:5–6. 2004. Ref Type: Journal (Full).
27. Ross M, Paterno G: **Reliability of the Apley`s range of motion test and dominant and nondominant upper extremity differences.** *European Journal Physical Medicine Rehabilitation* 1999, **8**(6):166–169. Ref Type: Journal (Full).
28. Johnson BL, Nelson JK: *Practical measurements for evaluation in physical education*. 2nd edition. Minneapolis, MN: Burgess; 1974.
29. Baumgartner TA, Oh S, Chung H, Hales D: **Objectivity, Reliability, and Validity for a Revised Push-Up Test Protocol.** *Measurement in Phys Education and Exercise Science* 2002, **6**(4):225–242. Ref Type: Journal (Full).
30. Sparling PB, Stafford-Millard M, Snow TK: **Development of a cadence curl-up test for college students.** *Quarterly for Exercise and Sport* 1997, **68**(4):309–316. Ref Type: Journal (Full).
31. Kurowski K, Chandran S: **The preparticipation athletic evaluation.** *Am Fam Physician* 2000, **61**(9):2683–2688.
32. Hoffmann J: *Norms for Fitness, Performance, and Health*. Champaign, Il: Human Kinetics; 2006.
33. Axler CT, McGill SM: **Low back loads over a variety of abdominal exercises: searching for the safest abdominal challenge.** *Med Sci Sports Exerc* 1997, **29**(6):804–811.
34. Parfrey KC, Docherty D, Workman C, Behm DG: **The effects of different sit and curl-up positions on acivation of abdominal and hip flexor musculature.** *Appl Physiol Nutr Metab* 2008, **33**:888–895. Ref Type: Journal (Full).
35. Magee D: *Orthopedic Physical Assessment*. 5th edition. St. Louis, MI: Saunders Elsevier; 2008.
36. Schiff MA, Mack CD, Polissar NL, Levy MR, Dow SP, O'Kane JW: **Soccer Injuries in Female Youth Players: Comparison of Injury Surveillance by Certified Athletic Trainers and Internet.** *J Athl Train* 2010, **45**(3):238–242.
37. Hopkins WG, Marshall SW, Quarrie KL, Hume PA: **Risk factors and risk statistics for sports injuries.** *Clin J Sport Med* 2007, **17**(3):208–210.
38. Bewick V, Cheek L, Ball J: **Statistics review 12: survival analysis.** *Crit Care* 2004, **8**(5):389–394.
39. Augustsson SR, Bersas E, Thomas EM, Sahlberg M, Augustsson J, Svantesson U: **Gender differences and reliability of selected physical performance tests in young women and men.** *Advances in Physiotherapy* 2009, **11**:64–70. 2009. Ref Type: Journal (Full).
40. Dane S, Suleyman C, Gursoy R, Ezirmik N: **Sport Injuries: Relations to Sex, Sport, Injured body region.** *Percept Mot Skills* 2004, **98**:519–524. Ref Type: Journal (Full).
41. Knapik J, Baumin C, Jones B, Harris J, Vaughan L: **Preseason strength and flexibility imbalances associated with athletic injuries in female collegiate athletes.** *Am J Sports Med* 1991, **19(1)**:76–81. Ref Type: Journal (Full).
42. Clarke K, Buckley W: **Women's injuries in collegiate sports.** *Am J Sports Med* 1980, **8**:187–191. Ref Type: Journal (Full).
43. Eisenberg I, Allen W: **Injuries in a women's varsity athletic program.** *Physician Sports Medicine* 1974, **6(3)**:112–120. Ref Type: Journal (Full).
44. Augustsson SR, Augustsson J, Thomee R, Svantesson U: **Injuries and preventive actions in elite Swedish volleyball.** *Scand J Med Sci Sports* 2006, **16**(6):433–440.
45. Myer GD, Ford KR, Hewett TE: **Rationale and Clinical Techniques for Anterior Cruciate Ligament Injury Prevention Among Female Athletes1.** *J Athl Train* 2004, **39**(4):352–364.
46. Arendt E, Dick R: **Knee injury patterns among men and women in collegiate basketball and soccer. NCAA data and review of literature7.** *Am J Sports Med* 1995, **23**(6):694–701.
47. Dick RW: **Is there a gender difference in concussion incidence and outcomes?** *Br J Sports Med* 2009, **43**(Suppl 1):i46–i50.
48. Gabbe BJ, Finch CF, Bennell KL, Wajswelner H: **How valid is a self reported 12 month sports injury history?** *Br J Sports Med* 2003, **37**(6):545–547.

Age-related changes in ultra-triathlon performances

Beat Knechtle[1,2*], Christoph Alexander Rüst[2], Patrizia Knechtle[1], Thomas Rosemann[2] and Romuald Lepers[3]

Abstract

Background: The age-related decline in performance has been investigated in swimmers, runners and triathletes. No study has investigated the age-related performance decline in ultra-triathletes. The purpose of this study was to analyse the age-related declines in swimming, cycling, running and overall race time for both Triple Iron ultra-triathlon (11.4-km swimming, 540-km cycling and 126.6-km running) and Deca Iron ultra-triathlon (38-km swimming, 1,800-km cycling and 420-km running).

Methods: The age and performances of 423 male Triple Iron ultra-triathletes and 119 male Deca Iron ultra-triathletes were analysed from 1992 to 2010 using regression analyses and ANOVA.

Results: The mean age of the finishers was significantly higher for Deca Iron ultra-triathletes (41.3 ± 3.1 years) compared to a Triple Iron ultra-triathletes (38.5 ± 3.3 years) ($P < 0.05$). For both ultra-distances, the fastest overall race times were achieved between the ages of 25 and 44 years. Deca Iron ultra-triathletes achieved the same level of performance in swimming and cycling between 25 and 54 years of age.

Conclusions: The magnitudes of age-related declines in performance in the three disciplines of ultra-triathlon differ slightly between Triple and Deca Iron ultra-triathlon. Although the ages of Triple Iron ultra-triathletes were on average younger compared to Deca Iron ultra-triathletes, the fastest race times were achieved between 25 and 44 years for both distances. Further studies should investigate the motivation and training of ultra-triathletes to gain better insights in ultra-triathlon performance.

Keywords: Swimming, Cycling, Running, Ultra-endurance

Background

In recent years, there has been an increased interest in investigating the effect of aging on endurance running performances [1-6]. Over the last decades, the participation of master athletes (>40 years old) has increased, especially in the longer run distances such as half marathons [2,3], marathons [1-3] and ultra-marathons [7-10]. However, with increasing age, the endurance performance decreases. In general, the peak endurance performance is maintained until the age of 30 to 35 years, followed by a moderate decline until the age of 50 to 60 years, and then a progressively steeper decline after the age of 70 to 75 years, independent of the length of the performance and the kind of the discipline [2-6,11-16].

Considering the age-related decline in male ultra-endurance athletes, Hoffman investigated ultra-marathoners competing over 161 kilometres [7-9]. Beyond the age of 30 to 39 years, the average finishing times increased linearly with increasing age. The 30- to 39-year-old males showed the fastest races times, with athletes in younger and older age groups being slower. The 40- to 49-year age group was approximately 4.0% slower than the 30 to 39 years one [8]. In another study of 161-km ultra-marathoners, performance of the athletes in the 40- to 49-year age group was no different from the performance of the athletes in the < 30 and the 30- to 39-year age groups [9]. Both the moderate decline in running performance and the large number of successful master athletes suggest that master athletes are able to maintain a high degree of physiological performance with increasing

* Correspondence: beat.knechtle@hispeed.ch
[1]Gesundheitszentrum St. Gallen, Vadianstrasse 26, St., Gallen 9011, Switzerland
[2]Institute of General Practice and Health Services Research, University of Zurich, Rämistrasse 71, Zurich 8006, Switzerland
Full list of author information is available at the end of the article

age [17]. For Ironman triathletes, both an increase in participation and an improvement in performance in master athletes have recently been reported [18,19].

The multi-sport discipline triathlon involves successively the three endurance disciplines: swimming, cycling and running. The traditional distances in triathlon vary from the short or Olympic distance, covering 1.5-km swimming, 40-km cycling and 10-km running [20-23], to the Ironman distance covering 3.8-km swimming, 180-km cycling and 42.2-km running [24,25]. Furthermore, ultra-endurance triathlons of longer distances than the Ironman distance do exist such as the Triple Iron ultra-triathlon of 11.4-km swimming, 540-km cycling and 126.6-km running [26,27], and the Deca Iron ultra-triathlon of 38-km swimming, 1,800-km cycling and 420-km running [28,29].

Regarding the performance in a triathlon, the association of different characteristics in physiology [30-33], anthropometry [34-37], training [34,35,38] and previous experience [28,36,37,39,40] with race time has been investigated. Apart from these characteristics, an age-related decline has been described for Olympic distance triathletes [20-23] as well as for Ironman triathletes [22,25]. It seems that the length of an endurance performance has an influence of the age-related performance decline. In short distance triathletes, a significant decline in performance starts at the age of 45 to 50 years [20,23]. In Ironman triathletes, however, the age-related decline in performance starts after the age of 55 years [22].

To date, no study has investigated the age-related decline in performance in an ultra-triathlon longer than the Ironman distance. Therefore, the aim of the present study was to analyse the age-related declines in swimming, cycling, running and total performances for both Triple Iron ultra-triathletes and Deca Iron ultra-triathletes. Since the age-related performance decline occurred later in the longer Ironman triathlons than in the shorter Olympic distance triathlon, we hypothesised that the age-related decline in performance would occur even later for Deca Iron ultra-triathletes than for Triple Iron ultra-triathletes.

Results and Discussion

Participation trends

From 1992 to 2010, there were 423 Triple Iron ultra-triathlon finishers and 119 Deca Iron ultra-triathlon finishers. During this period, the average number of finishers per year was 23 ± 9 (range, 7 to 38) at the Triple Iron ultra-triathlon and 11 ± 5 (range, 2 to 18) at the Deca Iron ultra-triathlon, respectively. From 1992 to 2010, the number of total finishers per age group, for both races, is shown in Table 1. The 5-year age bracket with the largest participation was 35 to 39 years in the Triple Iron ultra-triathlon and 40 to 44 years in the Deca Iron ultra-triathlon.

Age of the ultra-triathletes

The ages of the winners from 1992 to 2010, for both the Triple Iron ultra-triathletes and Deca Iron ultra-triathletes, are shown in Figure 1A. The ages of the winners did not significantly change over this period, in either of these races and, therefore, no differences in the mean age of the winners was found: 35.8 ± 4.5 years (range, 31 to 46 years) in the Triple Iron ultra-triathlon and 38.0 ± 6.8 years (range, 27 to 50 years) in the Deca Iron ultra-triathlon. In contrast, the mean age of the finishers was significantly ($P < 0.05$) higher in the Deca Iron ultra-triathlon compared with the Triple Iron ultra-triathlon; 41.3 ± 3.1 years in the Deca Iron ultra-triathlon and 38.5 ± 3.3 years in the Triple Iron ultra-triathlon (Figure 1B). In addition, the mean age of the finishers significantly increased over this period for both ultra-triathlon distances.

Age-related changes in performance

Total, swimming, cycling and running performances of the top ten triathletes for the different age groups at the Triple Iron triathlon during the 1992 to 2010 period are shown in Table 2. There was a significant age effect for swimming ($F = 62.4$, $P < 0.01$), cycling ($F = 65.7$, $P < 0.01$), running ($F = 209.9$, $P < 0.01$) and the total ($F = 158$, $P < 0.01$) times. No significant difference in time was observed between the age groups 25 to 34 and 35 to 44 years for swimming, cycling, running and total time. The mean best time performances were 176 ± 7 min for swimming (25 to 34 years), 1,030 ± 24 min for cycling (35 to 44 years), 759 ± 38 min for running (35 to 44 years) and 2,069 ± 92 min for the total race time (35 to 44 years).

These are the performances of the different age groups at the Triple Iron ultra-triathlon (data were pooled from 1992 to 2010). [a]Significantly different ($P < 0.01$) from age groups 25 to 34 years and 35 to 44 years. [b]Significantly different ($P < 0.01$) from age groups 25 to 34 years, 35 to 44 years and 45 to 54 years.

Total, swimming, cycling and running performances of the top ten triathletes for the different age groups at the Deca Iron triathlon during the 1992 to 2010 period are shown in Table 3. There was a significant age effect for swimming ($F = 32.2$, $P < 0.01$), cycling ($F = 28.1$, $P < 0.01$), running ($F = 12.7$, $P < 0.01$) and the total ($F = 22.2$, $P < 0.01$) times. No significant difference in running and total times was observed between the age groups 25 to 34 and 35 to 44 years. No significant differences in times were observed for the age groups between 25 and 54 years for swimming and cycling. The mean best time performances were 732 ± 41 min for swimming (35 to 44

Table 1 Total number of finishers per age group in both the Triple and Deca Iron ultra-triathlons (1992 to 2010)

Iron distance	Age groups (years)								
	25 to 29	30 to 34	35 to 39	40 to 44	45 to 49	50 to 54	55 to 59	60 to 64	65 to 69
Triple	12	93	127	102	41	29	12	6	1
Deca	3	19	29	38	11	9	7	2	1

years), 5,758 ± 247 min for cycling (35 to 44 years), 5,055 ± 807 min for running (25 to 34 years) and 12,292 ± 616 min for total performances (35 to 44 years), respectively.

These are the performances of the different age groups at the Deca Iron triathlon (Data were pooled from 1992 to 2010). [a]Significantly different ($P < 0.01$) from age groups 35 to 44 years. [b]Significantly different ($P < 0.01$) from age groups 25 to 34 years and 35 to 44 years. [c]Significantly different ($P < 0.01$) from age groups 25 to 34 years, 35 to 44 years and 45 to 4 years.

The aim of this study was to analyse the age-related declines in swimming, cycling, running and total performances in male Triple and Deca Iron ultra-triathletes. No difference in total performance was found between the ages of 25 and 44 years for both Triple and Deca

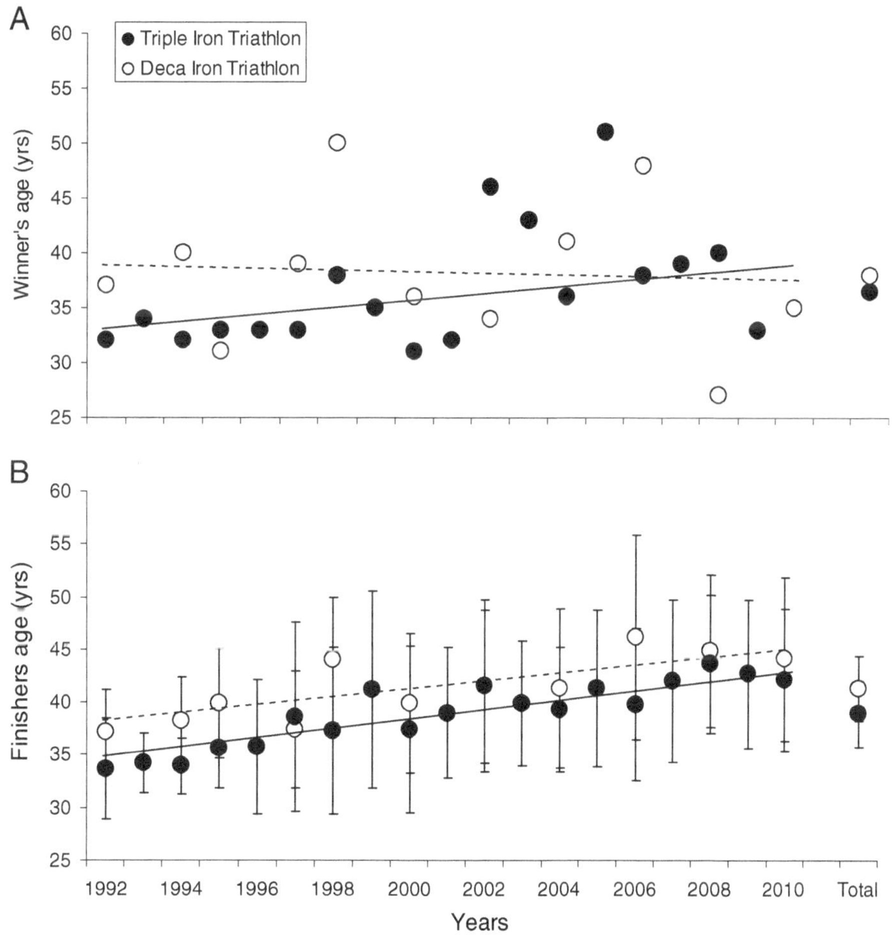

Figure 1 Ages of the winners both in the Triple and Deca Iron triathlons. Covering from 1992 to 2010 (**A**). Mean (±SD) age of the finishers in the Triple and Deca Iron triathlons from 1992 to 2010 (**B**). The years analysed are pooled, and the mean values are shown on the right side of the panels (Total). The dashed lines represent the linear regressions for the Deca Iron triathletes, and the continuous lines represent the linear regressions for the Triple Iron triathletes between 1992 and 2010. For the winners' age, the gradients were not different from zero for both the Deca ($r^2 = 0.01$, $P = 0.07$, $y = -0.141x + 319.9$) and Triple Iron triathletes ($r^2 = 0.18$, $P = 0.07$, $y = 0.409x - 781.4$). In contrast, the age of the finisher gradients increased by 0.4 years per annum ($r^2 = 0.66$, $P = 0.002$, $y = 0.426x - 811.1$) for the Deca Iron triathletes and by 0.5 years per annum ($r^2 = 0.83$, $P = 0.0001$, $y = 0.506x - 974.7$) for the Triple Iron triathletes.

Table 2 Total, swimming, cycling and running performances of the top ten Triple Iron ultra-triathletes

Age groups (years)		Total time (min)	11.4-km swim time (min)	540-km cycle time (min)	126-km run time (min)
25 to 34	Mean	2,091	176	1,037	803
	SD	33	7	27	35
35 to 44	Mean	2,069	180	1,030	759
	SD	92	3	24	38
45 to 54	Mean	2,288[a]	198[a]	1,124[a]	909[a]
	SD	55	6	50	34
55 to 64	Mean	2,828[a,b]	235[a,b]	1,287[a,b]	1,230[a,b]
	SD	137	19	70	69

Iron ultra-triathletes. However, in contrast to Triple Iron ultra-triathletes, Deca Iron ultra-triathletes can achieve the same level of performance in swimming and cycling between 25 and 54 years of age.

The effects of age on the different disciplines of triathlon

A main interesting finding was that the age-related decline occurred later in swimming and cycling compared to running at the Deca Iron ultra-triathlon distance. Previous studies suggested that the age-related decline in triathlon performance was specific to the discipline, with cycling showing fewer declines in performance with age than running in both short distance and Ironman triathletes [20,22]. The present results showed that the swimming and cycling performances were maintained until the age of 54 for the Deca Iron ultra-triathletes but only until the age of 44 for the Triple Iron ultra-triathletes. A potential explanation for this finding could be pre-race experience. It has been shown that previous experience was a strong predictor for a successful finish in an ultra-triathlon [28,39]. Recently, Lepers et al. [41] analysed the performance of 73 triathletes (68 men and 5 women) who finished a Double Iron ultra-triathlon, a Triple Iron ultra-triathlon and a Deca Iron ultra-triathlon. The contribution of swimming to overall ultra-triathlon performance was lower than for cycling and running. Running performance was more important to overall performance for Double Iron ultra-triathlon and Triple Iron ultra-triathlon compared to Deca Iron ultra-triathlon. The Double Iron ultra-triathlon and Triple Iron ultra-triathlon performances were significantly correlated to Deca Iron ultra-triathlon performances for swimming and cycling, but not for running.

The main differences between cycling and running are the change from a nonweight to a weight-bearing activity and the differences in the coordination of the leg muscles with a shift from a predominantly concentric type of muscle action in cycling to a stretch-shortening activity with eccentric contractions in running [42]. Cycling may show differences in the age-related performance decline compared to running due to the contraction types involved. Cycling as a nonweight-bearing activity uses predominantly concentric muscle activation compared with the stretch-shortening activity and eccentric activations during running. As older adults show different rates of decline during fatiguing contractions that involve eccentric as opposed to concentric activations, this may explain the differences in the rate of decline in cycling versus running [43].

The best age to perform in ultra-triathlons

Since the age-related performance started to decline later in an Ironman distance triathlon than in an Olympic distance triathlon, we hypothesised that the age-related decline in performance would occur later for Deca Iron ultra-triathletes than for Triple Iron ultra-

Table 3 Total, swimming, cycling, and running performances of the top 10 Deca Iron triathletes

Age groups		Total time (min)	38-km swim time (min)	1,800-km cycle time (min)	420-km run time (min)
25 to 34 years	Mean	12,954	816	6,403	5,055
	SD	788	91	568	807
35 to 44 years	Mean	12,292	732	5,758	5,134
	SD	616	41	247	388
45 to 54 years	Mean	14,177[a]	855	6,514	6,426[b]
	SD	1,053	81	469	647
55 to 64 years	Mean	16,405[c]	1,213[c]	8,245[c]	6,996[b]
	SD	1,948	194	1,004	1,300

triathletes and the fastest performance in a Deca Iron ultra-triathlon would be achieved at a higher age than in a Triple Iron ultra-triathlon. In contrast to our hypothesis, the age of the best overall performance did not differ between Triple Iron ultra-triathlon and Deca Iron ultra-triathlon and was comprised between 25 and 44 years for both ultra-triathlon distances. However, the group with the largest participation at the Triple Iron ultra-triathlon (35 to 39 years) was younger compared to the Deca Iron ultra-triathletes (40 to 44 years). We analysed in the present study the age-related decline in Triple Iron ultra-triathletes competing for approximately 2,000 min compared to Deca Iron ultra-triathletes racing for approximately 12,000 min. A significant age effect was found for total race time with no difference between the distances. A previous study evidenced that the age-related decline in total performance was less pronounced for the Olympic distance triathlon (approximately 2 to 3 h) than for the Ironman distance triathlon (approximately 9 to 15 h) [22].

The present data showed that, in ultra-triathlons, the athletes were able to maintain their best performances for ages comprised between 25 and 44 years, independent of the distance. In half-marathoners [2], marathoners [2] and short distance triathletes [20-23], generally athletes in the age group 20 to 30 years showed the fastest race times compared to athletes in the other age groups. For longer distances such as the Ironman triathlon, athletes in the age group 30 to 39 years were faster compared to athletes in the age group 20 to 29 years [25]. Apart from training, also the aspect of pre-race experience seems to be important for a successful finish in an ultra-triathlon. It has been demonstrated that the personal best time in a Triple Iron triathlon, not anthropometry or training volume, was associated with total race time in a Triple Iron triathlon [39]. Furthermore, the number of finished Triple Iron triathlons and the personal best time in a Triple Iron triathlon, but not anthropometry, were also related to Deca Iron ultra-triathlon race time [28].

It would be interesting in future studies to perform a longitudinal observation and to compare the age-related decline from cross-sectional and longitudinal data. A short analysis of the present data showed that four ultra-triathletes finished at least eight times the Triple Iron ultra-triathlon between 1992 and 2010. For these four ultra-triathletes, their total performances did not significantly change across the ages (Figure 2). These findings suggest that some exceptional ultra-triathletes are able to perform at the same level of performance during an 8- (subject A) to 16-year (subject D) period.

Physiological considerations

Tanaka and Seals [4] demonstrated that the changes in endurance performance with aging were attributed to reductions in VO_2max and the decline in lactate threshold. Findings for competitive long-distance runners indicated that the decline in running times parallel the age-related reductions in VO_2max and in lactate threshold [15]. For runners, mean VO_2max declined from 71.4 ml · min^{-1} · kg^{-1} in youth to 41.8 ml · min^{-1} · kg^{-1} at a mean age of 56.6 years [44]. The decrease in an ultra-endurance performance may be attributed to an age-related loss in skeletal muscle mass. A large component of lost independence with increasing age is weakness due to a loss of lean muscle mass. Muscle power is lost at a greater rate than is endurance capacity with 3.5% versus 1.8% per year, respectively [6]. The age-related loss of muscle mass is primarily due to a decrease in the size of type II (fast-twitch) muscle fibres and a change in the proportions of fibre types [45,46]. There is an increase in the proportion of type II fibres, which may adapt to high endurance demands [47].

The age-related decline was more pronounced in running compared to cycling for both the Triple Iron ultra-triathletes and the Deca Iron ultra-triathletes. Running involves stretch-shortening cycles with eccentric muscle actions, while cycling is a nonweight-bearing activity with predominant concentric muscle actions. With increasing age, the fast-twitch muscle fibres atrophy more than slow-twitch muscle fibres [48]. Since the fast-twitch fibres seem to be more susceptible to damage than the slow-twitch fibres during stretch-shortening cycles, the greater reduction in running performance compared with cycling could, therefore, be related to muscle typology changes with increasing age [49]. However, the changes in muscle fibre type distribution such as the percentage of type I muscle fibres with advancing age seem to be less pronounced in well-trained master athletes compared to untrained older adults [5].

A further aspect in these ultra-endurance races is the loss of substantial body mass such as skeletal muscle mass and fat mass. In ultra-endurance races, a loss in body mass has been described, contributing to a decrease in solid masses. An ultra-endurance performance leads to a decrease in both skeletal muscle [50-54] and fat masses [55-57]. In Ironman [50], Triple Iron ultra-triathletes [26,55], and Deca Iron ultra-triathletes [28], a significant decrease in skeletal muscle mass has been described. It is, therefore, likely that the more pronounced age-related decline in running performance in the Deca Iron ultra-triathletes was rather due to the considerably longer nature of the race with the corresponding loss in skeletal muscle mass than the effect of age. The decrease in skeletal muscle mass is most probably due to the increased mechanical stress due to the eccentric nature of running. It has been demonstrated that longer distance running in an ultra-marathon induced more impact-stress on the skeletal muscle than a marathon [58].

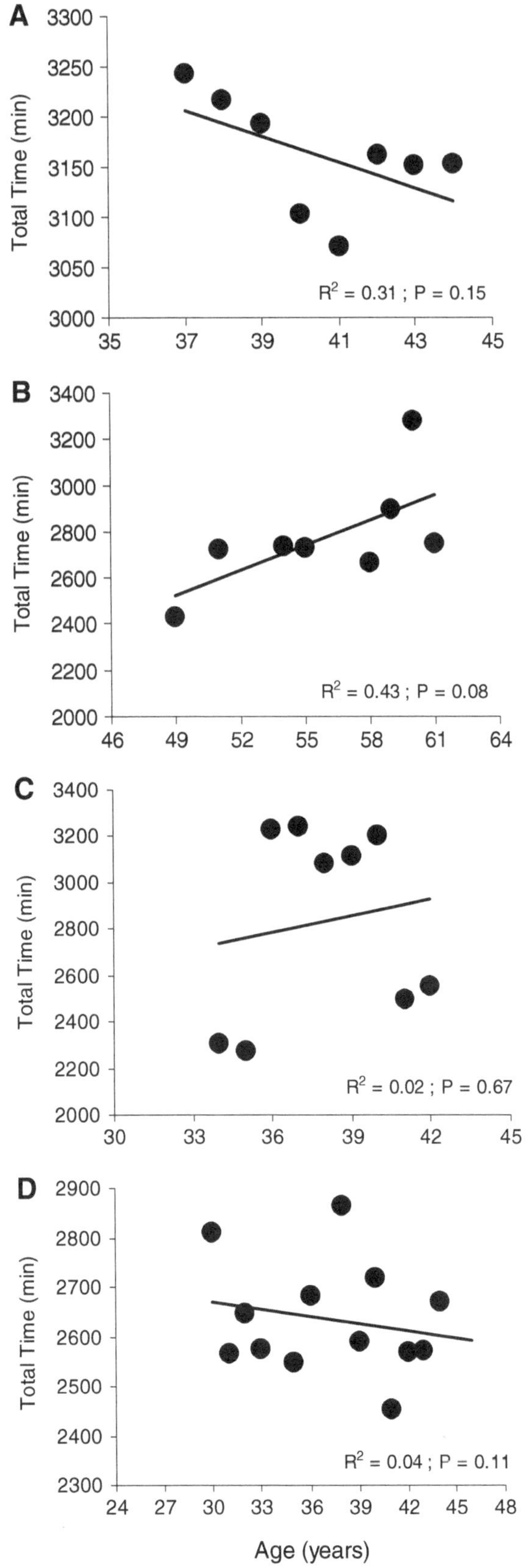

Figure 2 Change in total performance at the Triple Iron ultra-triathlon for four ultra-triathletes. The event was held in Lensahn, Germany. These athletes (**A**, **B**, **C** and **D**) finished at least eight times the event between 1992 and 2010. For all four triathletes, their performances did not significantly change across the age.

Limitations of the present study

The first limitation of this cross-sectional study is the problem arising from the data collection. Firstly, it is not sure at 100% that there are no data errors (age, race time) when taking them from the race websites and the official rankings. Secondly, we cannot assure that the age-related performance decline is not at least partly due to non-participation of older athletes or simply to a self-chosen lower intensity of older athletes. In addition, race participants may represent selected sub-groups of the total population of ultra-triathletes, e.g. some potential participants may have been prevented from participating due to many reasons.

It was not possible to collect other performance-related factors such as characteristics of training [36,37,39], anthropometry [27,29,34,35,39] and previous experience [28,37,38]. Thus, these factors had to be ignored in this study. In addition, we have not included environmental conditions. It has been shown that an ultra-performance [74,75] progressively slows down when the ambient temperature increases [59,60].

Conclusions

This cross sectional study found that the magnitudes of age-related declines in ultra-triathlon performance for Triple Iron and Deca Iron triathlon are quite similar. For both Triple Iron and the Deca Iron ultra-triathletes, the fastest race times were achieved between 25 and 44 years of age, although participants at the Triple Iron triathlon were on average younger compared to the Deca Iron triathlon. Further studies should investigate the motivation and training of ultra-triathletes to gain better insights in ultra-triathlon performance.

Availability of supporting data

The data sets supporting the results of this article are available in http://www.triathlonlensahn.de and http://www.multisport.com.mx.

Methods

This study was approved by the Institutional Review Board of St. Gallen, Switzerland, with a waiver for the requirement of an informed consent given by the subjects since the study involved the analysis of publicly available data. For two annual ultra-triathlons, one Triple Iron triathlon and one Deca Iron triathlon, the age of the athlete in the year of the race together with the swimming, cycling, running and total race times in the year of each race were analysed from 1992 to 2010. During this period, both the Triple Iron triathlons in Lensahn, Germany and the Deca Iron triathlons in Monterrey, Mexico were held regularly. The data set from this study was obtained from the race websites www.triathlonlensahn.de for the Triple Iron triathlon Germany in Lensahn, www.multisport.com.mx for the Deca Iron triathlon in Monterrey, Mexico and from the race directors involved.

Races

The Triple Iron ultra-triathlon in Germany took place in Lensahn, Schleswig-Holstein, Germany, and was comprised of 11.6-km swimming, 540-km cycling and 126.6-km running. The swimming was held in a 50-m heated outdoor pool at a temperature of approximately 25°C, and wetsuits were allowed. After passing through the transition area, the participants cycled 67 laps of 8 km each on a hilly course in the surroundings of the town. At the next transition, the athletes changed and ran 96 laps of a 1.31-km per lap flat run course in the town of Lensahn. The cycling course was nearly free of road traffic, and the run course was completely free of traffic and illuminated during the night. All the athletes had their own support crew to provide nutrition and changes of clothes or equipment. The athletes had to arrive at the finish line within 58 h of the race start. The Deca Iron ultra-triathlon took place in Monterrey, Mexico. The athletes completed a total distance of 38-km swimming, 1,800-km cycling and 422-km running. Swimming commenced in the 50-m outdoor pool in Monterrey in the 'Sociedad Cuauhtemoc & Famosa Park', 3 km away from the cycle and run track in 'Parque Niños Héroes'. The pool was not heated and the water temperature was approximately 27°C. The laps of 100 m were counted by personal lap counters for each athlete. After completing the swimming, the athletes changed in the transition area, and due to the high traffic volume, were transferred by car to 'Parque Niños Héroes'. A period of 30 min was allowed for the transfer from pool to park, which was deducted from the final race time. The park was closed to traffic, completely illuminated and with a 1.915-km cycle/run track that is approximately 95% flat but included an inclination of approximately 5%. After the cycling, the athletes changed and went directly to the run course which was on the same track but in the opposite direction. Drafting in the cycle section was strictly prohibited and controlled by the race director. The laps on both the cycle and run courses were counted electronically using a microchip system. The athletes can be helped by their own support crew for nutrition and changes of equipment and clothes. During the whole race, accommodation is offered in the Sports Village inside the park, about 250 m away from the race site. The athletes and their support crews have a room with bed, toilet and shower. For nutrition, the organiser offered a variety of food in a restaurant, at the race site, that was open 24 h a day.

Data analysis

Age of the participants

In each race year, the age of the winner and the mean age of the male finishers were analysed at both the Triple Iron ultra-triathlons and the Deca Iron ultra-triathlons from 1992 to 2010.

Age-related changes in performance

In order to analyse the age-related changes in swimming, cycling, running and the total race performances, we pooled the data from 1992 to 2010 for both distances. First, in order to evaluate the participation across the ages, we distinguished each age group category as follows: 25 to 29 years, 30 to 34 years, 35 to 39 years, 40 to 44 years, 45 to 49 years, 50 to 54 years, 55 to 59 years, 60 to 64 years and 65 to 69 years, respectively. Because of the small number of subjects per age group, we secondly considered only 4 age-groups for the analysis of performances: 25 to 34 years, 35 to 44 years, 45 to 54 years and 55 to 64 years, respectively. Performance times were converted to minutes. For the Triple and Deca Iron ultra-triathlons, the fastest ten swimming, cycling and running times, together with the total event times for each age group were determined for the 19-year period.

Statistical analysis

Data are reported as means ± standard deviations (±SD) in the text and the figures. Linear regressions were used for estimating the changes in the age of winners and the mean age of finishers *per year*. Pearson's correlation coefficients were used to assess the association between the age and the years. One-way ANOVA was used to compare the ages of the Triple and the Deca Iron ultra-triathlon winners and the mean ages of the finishers. One-way ANOVA was used to compare the swimming, cycling, running and total race times between the different age groups for both distances. Tukey's post hoc analyses were used to test differences within the ANOVA when appropriate. Statistical significance was accepted at $p < 0.05$ (Statsoft, Version 6.1, Statistica, Tulsa, OK, USA).

Competing interests

The authors have no conflict of interest.

Authors' contributions

KB collected the data and drafted the manuscript. RCA added statistical analyses and helped draft the manuscript. KP collected the data. RT participated in the study design and helped draft the manuscript. LR performed the statistical analyses and helped draft the manuscript. All authors read and approved the final manuscript.

Acknowledgements
The authors would like to thank the race directors for providing the race results and Mary Miller for her help in translation.

Author details
[1]Gesundheitszentrum St. Gallen, Vadianstrasse 26, St., Gallen 9011, Switzerland. [2]Institute of General Practice and Health Services Research, University of Zurich, Rämistrasse 71, Zurich 8006, Switzerland. [3]INSERM U1093, Faculty of Sport Sciences, University of Burgundy, Esplanade Erasme, Dijon 21000, France.

References

1. Jokl P, Sethi PM, Cooper AJ: **Master's performance in the New York City Marathon 1983–1999.** *Br J Sports Med* 2004, **38:**408–412.
2. Leyk D, Erley O, Ridder D, Leurs M, Rüther T, Wunderlich M, Sievert A, Baum K, Essfeld D: **Aged-related changes in marathon and half-marathon performances.** *Int J Sports Med* 2007, **28:**513–517.
3. Leyk D, Erley O, Gorges W, Ridder D, Rüther T, Wunderlich M, Sievert A, Essfeld D, Piekarski C, Erren T: **Performance, training and lifestyle parameters of marathon runners aged 20–80 years: results of the PACE-study.** *Int J Sports Med* 2009, **30:**360–365.
4. Tanaka H, Seals DR: **Invited review: dynamic exercise performance in masters athletes: insight into effects of primary human aging on physiological functional capacity.** *J Appl Physiol* 2003, **95:**2152–2162.
5. Tanaka H, Seals DR: **Endurance exercise performance in Masters athletes: age-associated changes and underlying physiological mechanisms.** *J Appl Physiol* 2008, **586:**55–63.
6. Wright VJ, Perricelli BC: **Age-related rates of decline in performance among elite senior athletes.** *Am J Sports Med* 2008, **36:**443–450.
7. Hoffman MD, Ong JC, Wang G: **Historical analysis of participation in 161 km ultramarathons in North America.** *Int J Hist Sport* 2010, **27:**1877–1891.
8. Hoffman MD: **Performance trends in 161-km ultramarathons.** *Int J Sports Med* 2010, **31:**31–37.
9. Hoffman MD, Wegelin JA: **The Western States 100-mile endurance run: participation and performance trends.** *Med Sci Sports Exerc* 2009, **41:**2191–2198.
10. Knechtle B, Rüst CA, Rosemann T, Lepers R: **Age-related changes in 100-km ultra-marathon running performance.** *Age (Dordr)* 2012, **34:**1033–1045.
11. Baker AB, Tang YQ, Turner MJ: **Percentage decline in masters superathlete track and field performance with aging.** *Exp Aging Res* 2003, **29:**47–65.
12. Rüst CA, Knechtle B, Knechtle P, Pfeifer S, Rosemann T, Lepers R, Senn O: **Gender difference and age-related changes in performance at the long distance duathlon World Championsips.** *J Strength Cond Res*, in press.
13. Donato AJ, Tench K, Glueck DH, Seals DR, Eskurza I, Tanaka H: **Declines in physiological functional capacity with age: a longitudinal study in peak swimming performance.** *J Appl Physiol* 2003, **94:**764–769.
14. Fleg JL, Lakatta EG: **Role of muscle loss in the age-associated reduction in VO_2max.** *J Appl Physiol* 1988, **65:**1147–1151.
15. Fuchi T, Iwaoka K, Higuchi M, Kobayashi S: **Cardiovascular changes associated with decreased aerobic capacity and aging in long-distance runners.** *Eur J Appl Physiol* 1989, **58:**884–889.
16. Hunter SK, Stevens AA, Magennis K, Skelton KW, Fauth M: **Is there as sex difference in the age of elite marathon runners?** *Med Sci Sports Exerc* 2011, **43:**656–664.
17. Young BW, Starkes JL: **Career-span analyses of track performance: longitudinal data present a more optimistic view of age-related performance decline.** *Exp Aging Res* 2005, **31:**69–90.
18. Stiefel M, Knechtle B, Lepers R: **Master triathletes have not reached limits in their Ironman triathlon performance.** *Scand J Med Sci Sports* 2012, doi:10.1111/j.1600-0838.2012.01473.x.
19. Lepers R, Rüst CA, Stapley P, Knechtle B: **Relative improvements in endurance performance with age: evidence from 25 years of Hawaii Ironman racing.** *Age*, in press.
20. Bernard T, Sultana F, Lepers R, Hausswirth C, Brisswalter J: **Age-related decline in Olympic triathlon performance: effect of locomotion mode.** *Exp Aging Res* 2010, **36:**64–78.
21. Lepers R, Stapley PJ: **Age-related changes in conventional road versus off-road triathlon performance.** *Eur J Appl Physiol* 2011, **111:**1687–1694.
22. Lepers R, Sultana F, Bernard T, Hausswirth C, Brisswalter J: **Age-related changes in triathlon performances.** *Int J Sports Med* 2010, **31:**251–256.
23. Sultana F, Brisswalter J, Lepers R, Hausswirth C, Bernard T: **Effects of age and gender on Olympic triathlon performances.** *Sci Sports* 2008, **23:**130–135.
24. Lepers R: **Analysis of Hawaii ironman performances in elite triathletes from 1981 to 2007.** *Med Sci Sports Exerc* 2008, **40:**1828–1834.
25. Lepers R, Maffiuletti NA: **Age and gender interactions in ultraendurance performance: insight from the triathlon.** *Med Sci Sports Exerc* 2011, **43:**134–139.
26. Knechtle B, Duff B, Amtmann G, Kohler G: **An ultratriathlon leads to a decrease of body fat and skeletal muscle mass–the Triple Iron Triathlon Austria 2006.** *Res Sports Med* 2008, **16:**97–110.
27. Knechtle B, Kohler G: **Running performance, not anthropometric factors, is associated with race success in a Triple Iron Triathlon.** *Br J Sports Med* 2009, **43:**437–441.
28. Herbst L, Knechtle B, Lopez CL, Andonie JL, Salas Fraire O, Kohler G, Rüst CA, Rosemann T: **Pacing strategy and change in body composition during a Deca Iron triathlon.** *Chin J Physiol* 2011, **54:**255–263.
29. Knechtle B, Knechtle P, Andonie JL, Kohler G: **Influence of anthropometry on race performance in extreme endurance triathletes: World Challenge Deca Iron Triathlon 2006.** *Br J Sports Med* 2007, **41:**644–648.
30. Laursen PB, Knez WL, Shing CM, Langill RH, Rhodes EC, Jenkins DG: **Relationship between laboratory-measured variables and heart rate during an ultra-endurance triathlon.** *J Sports Sci* 2005, **23:**1111–1120.
31. O'Toole ML, Douglas PS, Hiller WD: **Applied physiology of a triathlon.** *Sports Med* 1989, **8:**201–225.
32. O'Toole ML, Douglas PS, Hiller WD: **Lactate, oxygen uptake, and cycling performance in triathletes.** *Int J Sports Med* 1989, **10:**413–438.
33. Whyte G, Lumley S, George K, Gates P, Sharma S, Prasad K, McKenna WJ: **Physiological profile and predictors of cycling performance in ultra-endurance triathletes.** *J Sports Med Phys Fitness* 2000, **40:**103–109.
34. Knechtle B, Knechtle P, Rosemann T: **Similarity of anthropometric measures for male ultra-triathletes and ultra-runners.** *Percept Mot Skills* 2010, **111:**805–818.
35. Knechtle B, Knechtle P, Rosemann T: **Upper body skin-fold thickness is related to race performance in male Ironman triathletes.** *Int J Sports Med* 2010, **32:**20–27.
36. Knechtle B, Wirth A, Rosemann T: **Predictors of race time in male Ironman triathletes: physical characteristics, training or pre race experience?** *Percept Mot Skills* 2010, **111:**437–446.
37. Knechtle B, Wirth A, Baumann B, Knechtle P, Rosemann T: **Personal best time, percent body fat and training volume are differently associated with race time in male and female Ironman triathletes.** *Res Q Exerc Sport* 2010, **81:**62–68.
38. Gulbin JP, Gaffney PT: **Ultraendurance triathlon participation: typical race preparation of lower level triathletes.** *J Sports Med Phys Fitness* 1999, **9:**12–15.
39. Knechtle B, Knechtle P, Rosemann T, Senn O: **Personal best time, not anthropometry or training volume, is associated with total race time in a Triple Iron triathlon.** *J Strength Cond Res* 2011, **25:**1142–1150.
40. Knechtle B, Knechtle P, Lepers R: **Participation and performance trends in ultra-triathlons from 1985 to 2009.** *Scand J Med Sci Sports* 2011, **21:**e82–e90.
41. Lepers R, Knechtle P, Knechtle B, Rosemann T: **Analysis of ultra-triathlon performances.** *Open Access J Sports Med* 2011, **2:**131–136.
42. Bijker KE, de Groot G, Hollander AP: **Differences in leg muscle activity during running and cycling in humans.** *Eur J Appl Physiol* 2002, **7:**556–561.
43. Heiden T, Burnett A: **The effect of cycling on muscle activation in the running leg of an Olympic distance triathlon.** *Sports Biomech* 2003, **2:**35–49.
44. Robinson S, Dill DB, Robinson RD, Tzankoff SP, Wagner JA: **Physiological aging of champion runners.** *J Appl Physiol* 1976, **41:**46–51.
45. Coggan AR, Spina RJ, Rogers MA, King DS, Brown M, Nemeth PM, Holloszy JO: **Histochemical and enzymatic characteristics of skeletal muscle in master athletes.** *J Appl Physiol* 1990, **68:**1896–190.
46. Pyka G, Lindenberger E, Charette S, Marcus R: **Muscle strength and fiber adaptations to a year-long resistance training program in elderly men and women.** *J Gerontol* 1994, **49:**M22–M27.

47. Lexell J, Taylor CC, Sjostrom M: **What is the cause of the ageing atrophy? Total number, size and proportion of different fiber types studied in whole vastus lateralis muscle from 15- to 83-year-old men.** *J Neurol Sci* 1988, **84:**275–294.
48. Faulkner JA, Davis CS, Mendias CL, Brooks SV: **The aging of elite male athletes: age-related changes in performance and skeletal muscle structure and function.** *Clin J Sports Med* 2008, **18:**501–507.
49. Vijayan K, Thompson JL, Norenberg KM, Fitts RH, Riley DA: **Fiber-type susceptibility to eccentric contraction-induced damage of hindlimb unloaded rat AL muscles.** *J Appl Physiol* 2001, **90:**770–776.
50. Knechtle B, Baumann B, Wirth A, Knechtle P, Rosemann T: **Male ironman triathletes lose skeletal muscle mass.** *Asia Pac J Clin Nutr* 2010, **19:**91–97.
51. Knechtle B, Duff B, Schulze I, Kohler G: **A multi-stage ultra-endurance run over 1,200 km leads to a continuous accumulation of total body water.** *J Sports Sci Med* 2008, **7:**357–364.
52. Knechtle B, Knechtle P, Rosemann T, Senn O: **No dehydration in mountain bike ultra-marathoners.** *Clin J Sport Med* 2009, **19:**415–420.
53. Knechtle B, Kohler G: **Running 338 km within 5 days has no effect on body mass and body fat but reduces skeletal muscle mass – the Isarrun 2006.** *J Sports Sci Med* 2007, **6:**401–407.
54. Knechtle B, Wirth A, Knechtle P, Rosemann T: **Increase of total body water with decrease of body mass while running 100 km nonstop–formation of edema?** *Res Q Exerc Sport* 2009, **80:**593–603.
55. Knechtle B, Knechtle P, Rosemann T, Oliver S: **A Triple Iron triathlon leads to a decrease in total body mass but not to dehydration.** *Res Q Exerc Sport* 2010, **81:**319–327.
56. Knechtle B, Wirth A, Knechtle P, Rosemann T, Senn O: **Do ultra-runners in a 24-h run really dehydrate?** *Ir J Med Sci* 2011, **180:**129–134.
57. Knechtle B, Wirth A, Knechtle P, Rosemann T: **An ultra-cycling race leads to no decrease in skeletal muscle mass.** *Int J Sports Med* 2009, **30:**163–167.
58. Kim HJ, Lee YH, Kim CK: **Changes in serum cartilage oligomeric matrix protein (COMP), plasma CPK and plasma hs-CRP in relation to running distance in a marathon (42.195 km) and an ultra-marathon (200 km) race.** *Eur J Appl Physiol* 2009, **105:**765–770.
59. Vihma T: **Effects of weather on the performance of marathon runners.** *Int J Biometeorol* 2010, **54:**297–306.
60. Wegelin JA, Hoffman MD: **Variables associated with odds of finishing and finish time in a 161-km ultramarathon.** *Eur J Appl Physiol* 2011, **111:**145–153.

19

Participation and performance trends in multistage ultramarathons—the 'Marathon des Sables' 2003–2012

Christoph Knoth[1], Beat Knechtle[2,3*], Christoph Alexander Rüst[2], Thomas Rosemann[2] and Romuald Lepers[4]

Abstract

Background: The purpose of this study was to investigate participation and performance changes in the multistage ultramarathon 'Marathon des Sables' from 2003 to 2012.

Methods: Participation and performance trends in the four- or six-stage running event covering approximately 250 km were analyzed with special emphasis on the nationality and age of the athletes. The relations between gender, age, and nationality of finishers and performance were investigated using regression analyses and analysis of variance.

Results: Between 2003 and 2012, a number of 7,275 athletes with 938 women (12.9%) and 6,337 men (87.1%) finished the Marathon des Sables. The finisher rate in both women ($r^2 = 0.62$) and men ($r^2 = 0.60$) increased across years ($p < 0.01$). Men were significantly ($p < 0.01$) faster than women for overall finishers (5.9 ± 1.6 km·h^{-1} versus 5.1 ± 1.3 km·h^{-1}) and for the top three finishers (12.2 ± 0.4 km·h^{-1} versus 8.3 ± 0.6 km·h^{-1}). The gender difference in running speed of the top three athletes decreased ($r^2 = 0.72$; $p < 0.01$) from 39.5% in 2003 to 24.1% in 2012 with a mean gender difference of $31.7 \pm 2.0\%$. In men, Moroccans won nine of ten competitions, and one edition was won by a Jordanian athlete. In women, eight races were won by Europeans (France five, Luxembourg two, and Spain one, respectively), and two events were won by Moroccan runners.

Conclusions: The finisher rate in the Marathon des Sables increased this last decade. Men were significantly faster than women with a higher gender difference in performance compared to previous reports. Social or cultural inhibitions may determine the outcome in this event. Future studies need to investigate participation trends regarding nationalities and socioeconomic background, as well as the motivation to compete in ultramarathons.

Keywords: Ultramarathon, Performance trends, Nationality, Gender difference

Background

Participation in endurance and ultra-endurance events such as running [1-3], triathlon [4,5], and cycling [6,7] is of high popularity. There is an increasing number of ultramarathons, defined as a running race with distance longer than 42 km in every continent [8-10], and more and more athletes from every age and gender participate in these races [1,2,11]. In ultramarathon running, single-stage and multistage races are offered. A single-stage event, such as the 'Western States 100 Mile Endurance Run' [1,2,10], is a non-stop race. In contrast, multistage ultramarathons such as the 'Deutschlandlauf' [12,13] take place over a certain number of days with recovery time overnight [13]. Among the multistage ultramarathons, one of the most challenging events is the 'Marathon des Sables', a multistage ultramarathon in the Moroccan desert with temperatures up to 49°C [14].

Gender differences in endurance performance have been of great interest in the last decades [2,15]. Women run approximately 10–30% slower compared to men [2,16,17]. Hoffman [15] reported no difference in performance between women and men in 80- and 161-km trail ultramarathons when matched for performance in a 50-km trail ultramarathon. However, in anecdotic reports, women

* Correspondence: beat.knechtle@hispeed.ch
[2]Institute of General Practice and for Health Services Research, University of Zurich, Zurich, Switzerland
[3]Gesundheitszentrum St. Gallen, Vadianstrasse 26, St. Gallen 9001, Switzerland
Full list of author information is available at the end of the article

were able to outrun men in ultramarathons [13,17]. A reason for the gender difference might be the higher body fat in women compared to men [18,19], and as core temperature rises, women might therefore not cope with heat as well as men [20]. Other studies suggested that slower runners may have a stronger heat impact on their running performance, which could not be demonstrated in women [21-25].

Previous studies [26-31] suggested that performance in running seemed also to be related to the athletes' origin. Most running races from middle-distance to marathon were dominated by African runners [26]. Several studies reported that East African runners from Kenya [26], Eritrea [27], and Ethiopia [28-30] dominated in long-distance running such as marathon runs worldwide, although the genetic or physiological proof is still missing [31-33]. Demographic characteristics and social and environmental factors such as where they live, which tribe they belong to, and how far the athletes had to run to school seemed to play an important role in the East African runners' performance level and participation in running competitions [26,33]. Onywera et al. [26] reported that East African competitors were very selective in choosing competitions, and a major factor for their participation was the prize money offered in competitions.

To date, little is known about the participation and performance in both single- and multistage ultramarathons regarding the aspect of the nationality of athletes. One study investigated the participation trends concerning nationality or cultural background in ultra-endurance athletes such as triathletes [34]. The authors reported that mainly Europeans competed and won in Double Iron ultra-triathlons. These findings were confirmed for longer distances such as the Triple Iron ultra-triathlon [35] and the Deca Iron ultra-triathlon [36].

The aim of the present study was to investigate the participation and performance trends in the Marathon des Sables in the desert of Morocco from 2003 to 2012. We hypothesized, firstly, that there would be an increase in participation for both sexes, secondly, that runners originating from Northern Africa would dominate the race, and, thirdly, that male ultramarathoners would be faster than female ultramarathoners.

Methods

All finishers in the Marathon des Sables between 2003 and 2012 were analyzed regarding gender, running speed, and nationality. The data set from this study was obtained from DUV ultramarathon statistics [37] and the race website [14]. This study was approved by the institutional review board of St. Gallen, Switzerland, with waiver of the requirement for informed consent given that the study involved the analysis of publicly available data.

The race

The Marathon des Sables is considered to be one of the most challenging ultra-running events worldwide [14]. Organized since 1986 by Frenchman Patrik Bauer, the race takes place in the Moroccan desert where multiple stages of different lengths have to be completed within 7 days. There is a four- and a six-stage setup of the course varying every year. The stages are between 20 and 40 km, and one single stage is approximately 80 km. The runners are supported with daily water rations and a tent to sleep at night but have to carry their own nutrition of at least 2,000 kcal and daily needs such as sleeping bags in backpacks. The stages and the total number of kilometers run differ every year. The course leads the participants through dry river beds, over sand dunes, and stony and rocky surfaces at temperatures up to 40°C. The number of contestants from all over the world is restricted to approximately 800 participants every year.

Data analysis

In total, data were available from 7,275 athletes, consisting of 938 women and 6,337 men. The 7,275 athletes originated from 74 different countries and participated at least once in the Marathon des Sables. The running speed and gender difference in performance of the top three overall male and female athletes were analyzed for each year. For the aspects of nationality, such as development of running speed per country and year or difference in running speed between different countries, only the countries providing at least five finishers per year in at least nine out of the ten regarded years were considered. For women, athletes from France and Great Britain fulfilled these criteria. For men, athletes from France, Great Britain, Spain, Italy, Germany, USA, Morocco, and Switzerland were considered. From all these countries, the both running speeds of the annual top three women and annual top three men were analyzed. In women, the two nationalities that could be included had a total of 547 athletes and thus 58.3% of all female finishers. In men, the eight countries that fulfilled the inclusion criteria provided a total of 5,337 athletes and thus 84.2% of all male finishers. Since the number of stages and the total race distance varied within these years, we calculated running speed to express running performance of the athletes.

The gender difference in percent was calculated using the following formula: (Running speed [men] − Running speed [women]) / Running speed [men] × 100. In order to increase the readability of the data, the gender difference was transformed to absolute values. As a last step, we analyzed for the eight above-mentioned countries the coherence of development in population, gross national income per head, and number of finisher.

Statistical analysis

In order to increase the reliability of data analyses, each set of data was tested for normal distribution as well as for homogeneity of variances in advance of statistical analyses. Normal distribution was tested using a D'Agostino and Pearson omnibus normality test, and homogeneity of variances was tested using a Levene's test in cases of two groups and with a Bartlett's test in cases of more than two groups. To find significant changes in the development of running speed, participation, and gender across years, linear regression was used. Correlation analyses were performed using Pearson's correlation in cases of normal distributed data and Spearman's correlation in cases of not normal distributed data. Statistical analyses were performed using IBM SPSS Statistics (Version 19, IBM SPSS, Chicago, IL, USA) and GraphPad Prism (Version 5, GraphPad Software, LA Jolla, CA, USA). Significance was accepted at $p < 0.05$ (two-sided for t tests). Data in the text are given as mean ± standard deviation.

Results

Participation trends

Between 2003 and 2012, a total of 938 women and 6,337 men finished in the Marathon des Sables during that period, leading to a mean number of 104 female (12.8%) and 704 male (87.1%) finishers per year. Women (r^2 = 0.62) and men (r^2 = 0.60) showed a significant ($p < 0.01$) increase in the number of finishers (Figure 1A). More than half of the competitors of both genders (women 58.3%, men 62.9%) originated from Europe, mainly from France (women 33.2%, men 33.2%) and Great Britain (women 25.1%, men 29.7%) (Figure 1B).

Overall performances

On average, overall men were running significantly faster than overall women ($p < 0.01$). Men were running at 5.9 ± 1.6 km·h^{-1} and women at 5.1 ± 1.3 km·h^{-1} with no change in running speed across years ($p > 0.05$) (Figure 2).

Running performance and gender difference of the top three males and females

During the studied time period, the top three men became slower (r^2 = 0.47; p = 0.03) with a mean running speed of 12.5 ± 0.5 km·h^{-1} in 2003 to 12.1 ± 0.5 km·h^{-1} in 2012 (Figure 3). The top three women showed no change in running speed across years with a mean running speed of 8.3 ± 0.3 km·h^{-1} (r^2 = 0.37; $p > 0.05$). The gender difference in running speed of the top three athletes decreased (r^2 = 0.72; $p < 0.01$) from 39.5% in 2003 to 24.1% in 2012 with a mean gender difference of 31.7 ± 2.0% across years.

Running speed of the top three athletes per nation and year

Figure 4 presents the trend of running speeds by the origin of the athletes for women (Figure 4A) and men (Figure 4B). For women, the annual top three British runners improved their running speed from 6.2 ± 0.6 km·h^{-1} in 2003 to 7.7 ± 1.0 km·h^{-1} in 2012 (r^2 = 0.66; $p < 0.01$). For French women, running speed showed no changes ($p > 0.05$). For men (Figure 4B), the annual top three Spanish runners improved their running speed from 8.7 ± 0.4 km·h^{-1} in 2003 to 10.2 ± 0.7 km·h^{-1} in 2012 (r^2 = 0.58; $p < 0.01$). Moroccan runners became slower across years with a mean running speed of 12.5 ± 0.5 km·h^{-1} in 2003 to 11.5 ± 0.8 km·h^{-1} in 2012 (r^2 = 0.55; $p < 0.01$). Top three runners from France, Italy, Great Britain, USA, Switzerland, and Germany showed no changes in running speed across years ($p > 0.05$). Figure 5 presents the mean running speed of the ever fastest three runners per country for women (Figure 5A) and men (Figure 5B). For women, the top three athletes from Morocco achieved the fastest running speed (9.0 ± 0.3 km·h^{-1}), followed by the top three athletes from France (9.0 ± 0.9 km·h^{-1}), and the top three athletes from Spain (8.3 ± 0.7 km·h^{-1}). For men, the fastest running speed ever was achieved by the top three runners from Morocco (12.3 ± 0.3 km·h^{-1}), Jordan (12.0 ± 0.3 km·h^{-1}), and Spain (11.1 ± 0.7 km·h^{-1}). In men, Moroccans won nine of ten competitions, and one edition was won by a Jordanian. In women, Europeans (France five, Luxembourg two, and Spain one) won most of the events, and two events were won by Moroccan runners.

The aspect of age

In women, the mean age of the overall top three finishers was 39 ± 7 years. Japanese women were the youngest participants with 33 ± 2 years of age in average, and Mexican women are the oldest competitors with 52 ± 15 years of age in average (Figure 6A). For the fastest athletes, Moroccan women were 38 ± 2 years, French women 37 ± 2 years, and Spanish women 37 ± 7 years old. In men (Figure 6B), the overall average was 37 ± 8 years of age. Irish men were the youngest with 24 ± 22 years, followed by runners from Korea (26 ± 23 years), and Japan (29 ± 4 years). Polish athletes were the oldest runners with 47 ± 14 years in average. For the fastest men, Moroccan runners were 37 ± 3 years; Jordan runners were 38 ± 2 years, and Spanish runners were 41 ± 1 years old.

Considering the changes in the age of the annual top three runners across years (Figure 7), the age of peak performance remained unchanged for women at 39.0 ± 6.3 years (r^2 = 0.10; $p > 0.05$). For men, however, the age of the fastest running speed increased from 30.3 ± 1.5 years in 2003 to 41.7 ± 2.5 years in 2012 (r^2 = 0.78; $p < 0.01$).

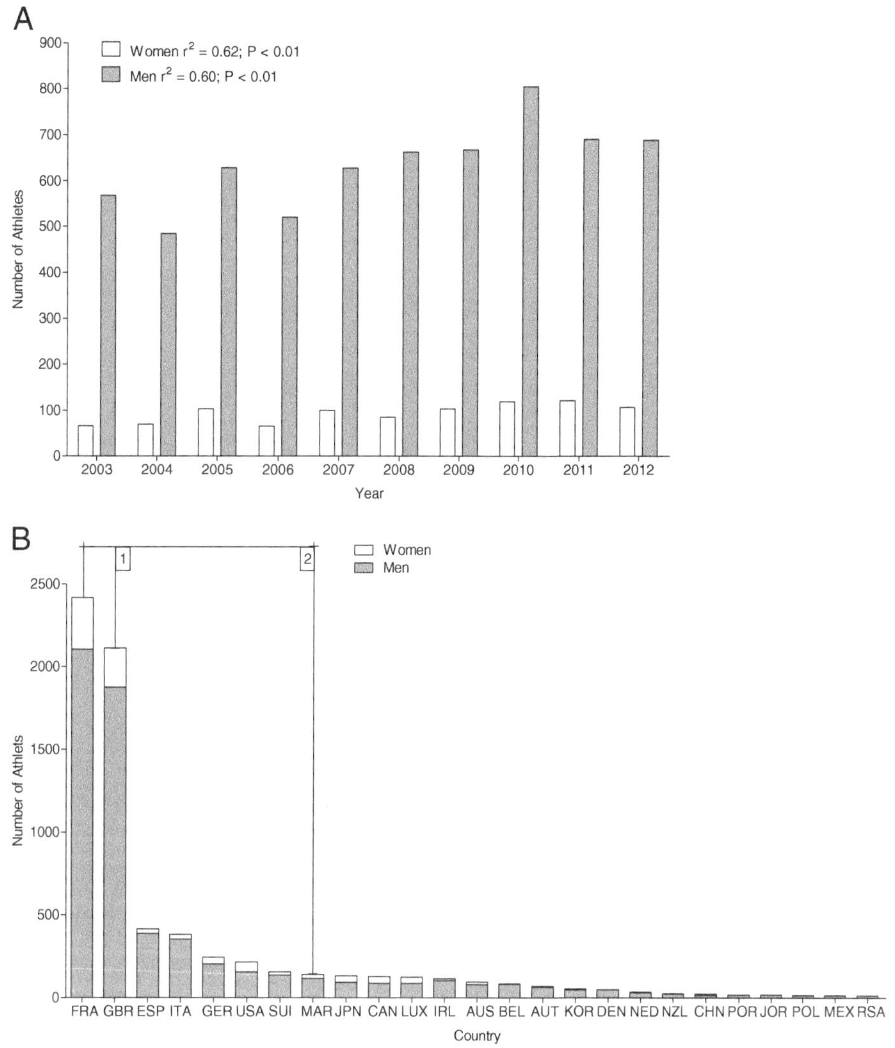

Figure 1 Total number of male and female finishers (A) and number of female and male finishers in the Marathon des Sables per country (B). Countries providing five or more finishers per year and gender are indicated with *1* for women and with *2* for men, respectively. The *frame* indicates the 25 countries with the total highest number of finishers including women and men. *FRA* France, *GBR* Great Britain, *ESP* Spain, *ITA* Italy, *GER* Germany, *USA* United States of America, *SUI* Switzerland, *MAR* Morocco, *JPN* Japan, *CAN* Canada, *LUX* Luxembourg, *IRL* Ireland, *AUS* Australia, *BEL* Belgium, *AUT* Austria, *KOR* Korea, *DEN* Denmark, *NED* Netherlands, *NZL* New Zealand, *CHN* China, *POR* Portugal, *JOR* Jordan, *POL* Poland, *MEX* Mexico, *RSA* Republic of South Africa.

Discussion

This is the first study to describe the participation and performance trends in a multistage ultramarathon in extreme environment such as the Marathon des Sables. The main results were (1) a significant increase in male and female finishers this last decade, (2) most finishers in both sexes originated from Europe, and (3) men were significantly faster for overall and in the top three compared to women with a higher gender difference as reported in previous studies.

Increasing participation across years

A first important finding was the significant increase in the number of finishers for both women and men. When the Marathon des Sables started in 1986, only 23 runners participated and finished, whereas in 2012, already 795 runners finished the race. The present findings confirm the increase in participation in ultra-endurance running races as previously described for 100-km ultramarathoners [38]. Similarly, an analysis of participation in 161-km ultramarathons in North America showed that the number of both competitors and competitions significantly increased over the last decades [1,2].

Most finishers in the Marathon des Sables originated from Europe

A second important finding was that half of the finishers of both genders originated from Europe, mainly from

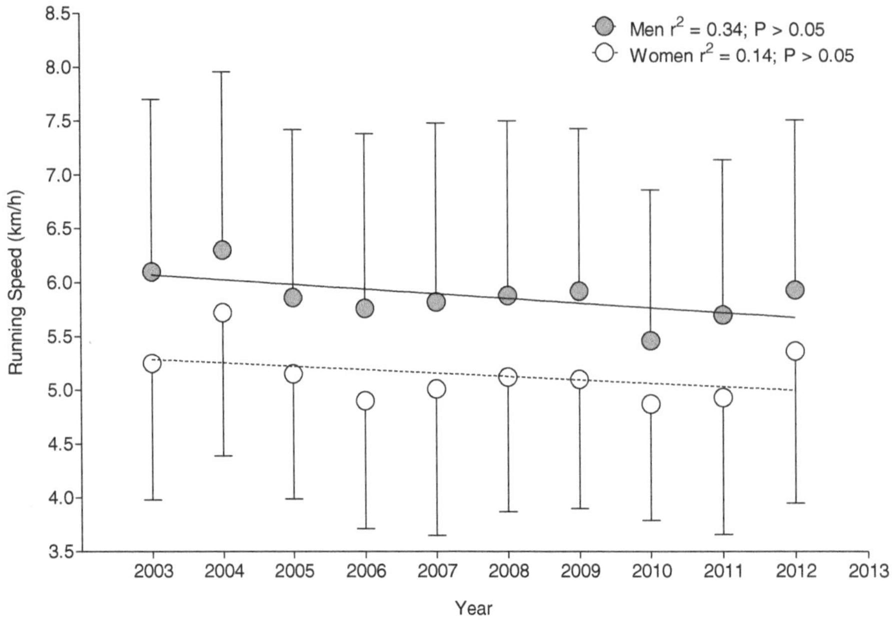

Figure 2 Annual running speed for women and men overall.

France and Great Britain. By comparison, Rüst et al. [34] reported that most finishers in a Double Iron ultra-triathlon originated from Europe. We assume that there is a higher interest of competitors out of 'first world countries' [39] to compete in extreme endurance challenges. With a high inscription fee and a low prize money of 5,000 euros for the overall winner, the Marathon des Sables is expensive for participants. The inscription fee for the Marathon des Sables is approximately 2,800 euros [14]. In contrast, participation in the 'Boston Marathon' costs US$180 for residents and US$200 for international competitors [40], whereas the prize money is approximately ten times higher [41]. We assume that European competitors, as the largest group of finishers in both sexes,

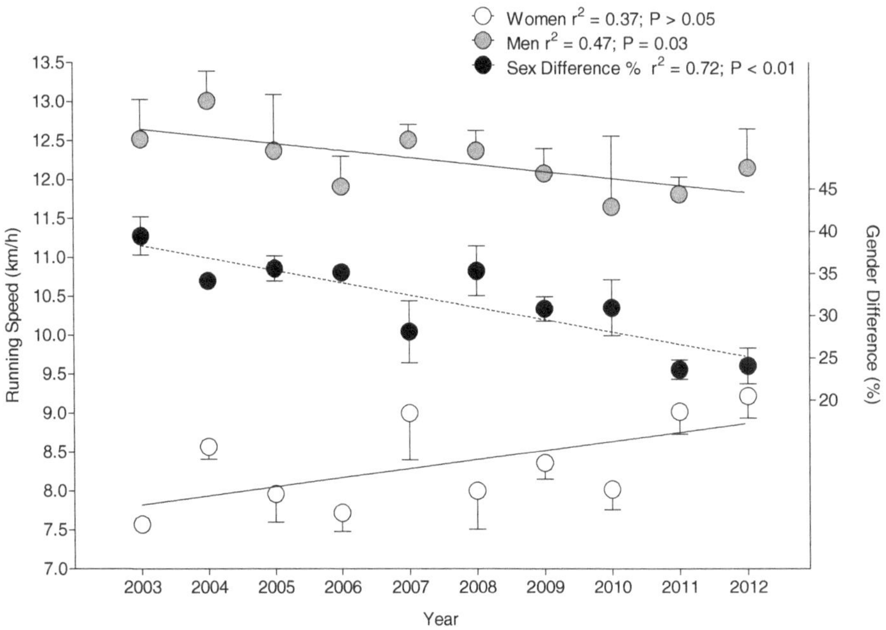

Figure 3 Change in running speed of the annual top three women and annual top three men and gender difference in performance across years.

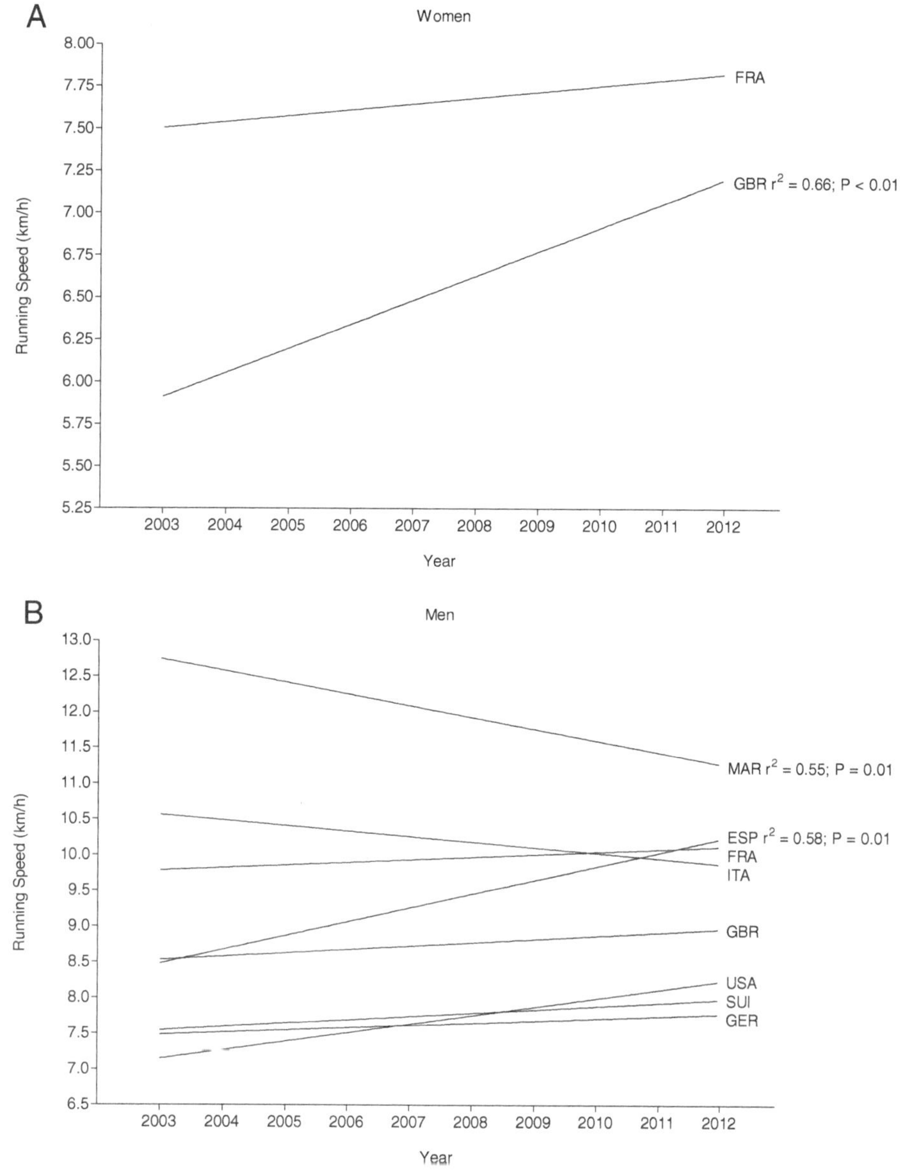

Figure 4 Change in running speed in the annual top three athletes per nation during the 2003–2012 time period for women (A) and men (B). *FRA* France, *GBR* Great Britain, *ESP* Spain, *ITA* Italy, *MAR* Morocco. In case of a significant change in running speed over time, r^2 and as *p* value are inserted.

have the economic background to take part in most ultramarathon events worldwide; competitors from second or third world countries are not able to pay for the dispenses and are reliant on sponsors or prize money to be able to compete all over the world - a reason that East African runners do not dominate in economically less interesting ultra-endurance events. The cultural background might be of importance as well: France has a long history and a close relationship with Morocco, and the Marathon des Sables is organized by a Frenchman. This could be one of the reasons why many French runners compete in the Marathon des Sables.

Participation trends, population growth, and gross national income per capita

We investigated the participation trends, population growth and gross national income per head of the eight countries that could be analyzed from 2003 to 2011 (Table 1). Although all countries showed a significant growth of their population ($p < 0.01$) between 2003 and 2011 and a significant increase in income per head ($p < 0.01$), only Great Britain ($r^2 = 0.65$), Spain ($r^2 = 0.97$), and Switzerland ($r^2 = 0.74$) showed a significant increase in finishers relative to the change in population ($p < 0.01$). Spain and Switzerland showed also a significant correlation between the increase

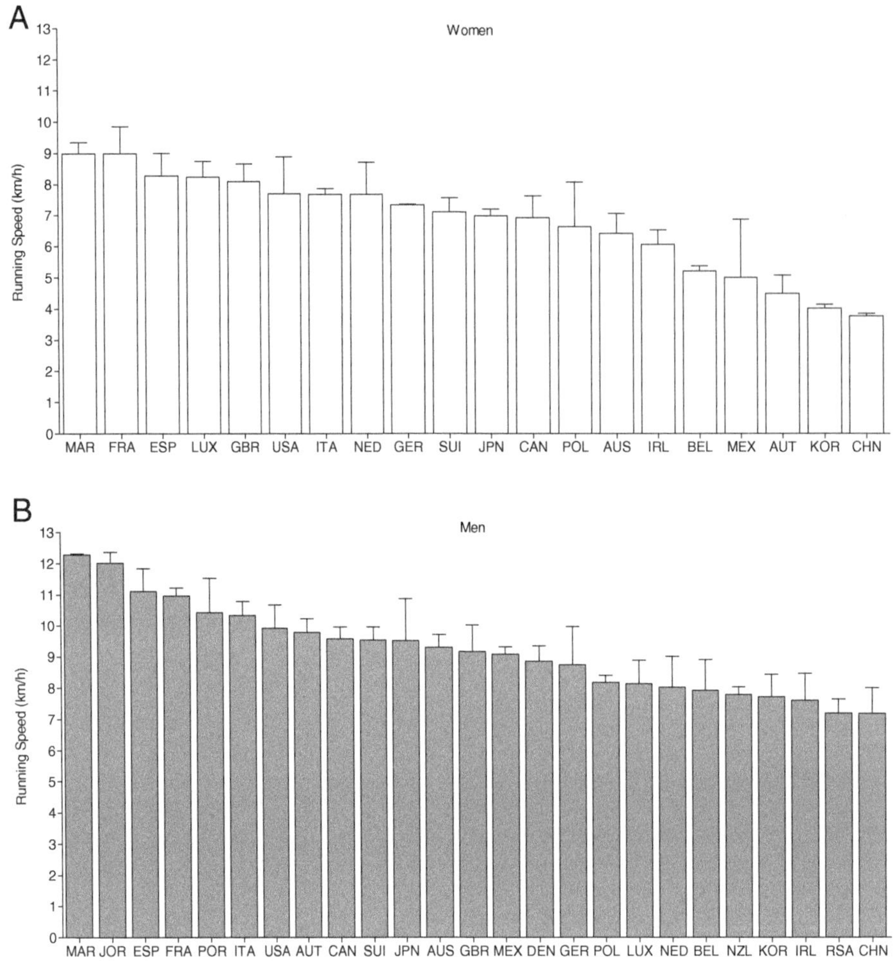

Figure 5 Running speed of the overall top three female (A) and male (B) athletes per country. The *frame* indicates the 25 countries with the total (women and men) highest number of finishers. *FRA* France, *GBR* Great Britain, *ESP* Spain, *ITA* Italy, *JOR* Jordan, *GER* Germany, *USA* United States of America, *SUI* Switzerland, *MAR* Morocco, *JPN* Japan, *CAN* Canada, *LUX* Luxembourg, *IRL* Ireland, *AUS* Australia, *BEL* Belgium, *AUT* Austria, *KOR* Korea, *DEN* Denmark, *NED* Netherlands, *NZL* New Zealand, *CHN* China, *POR* Portugal, *POL* Poland, *MEX* Mexico, *RSA* Republic of South Africa.

in gross national income per head and the increase in participants ($p < 0.01$). Most probably, the economic situation of an athlete decides whether he will be able to participate in the Marathon des Sables. Although Moroccan men won almost every competition, in women, European runners won eight out of ten competitions; only two events were won by female Moroccan runners. No East African runner even participated in the Marathon des Sables in the last 10 years. According to Onywera [26,33], the social background of African runners was very important for their success and that their participation in endurance events was triggered by economic reasons and social background. Onywera et al. [26] showed that East African competitors were very selective in choosing competitions, and a major factor for participation was the prize money available in competitions. Recent studies suggested a mental advantage of African runners because of the nimbus of winning [29] and the psychological atmosphere that could have significant consequences on performance [42], because no genetic advantages have been found. East African runners differed largely in their demographic characteristics. Factors, such as how far the athletes had to run to school and their socio-economic background, seemed to play a great role in later success [26,33]. According to the results of Onywera's findings [26], there would be a lower participation of East African runners in economically less interesting events such as the Marathon des Sables. Furthermore, we expected wealthier competitors with less interest in earning money and more interest in the challenge of ultramarathon participation. Hofmann and Fogard [43] showed that participants in a 161-km ultramarathon were largely well-educated, middle-aged, and married men who rarely missed work due to illness or injury, generally used vitamins and/or supplements, and maintained appropriate body mass with aging. Their findings may confirm our investigations as we found a significant increase in the gross national income

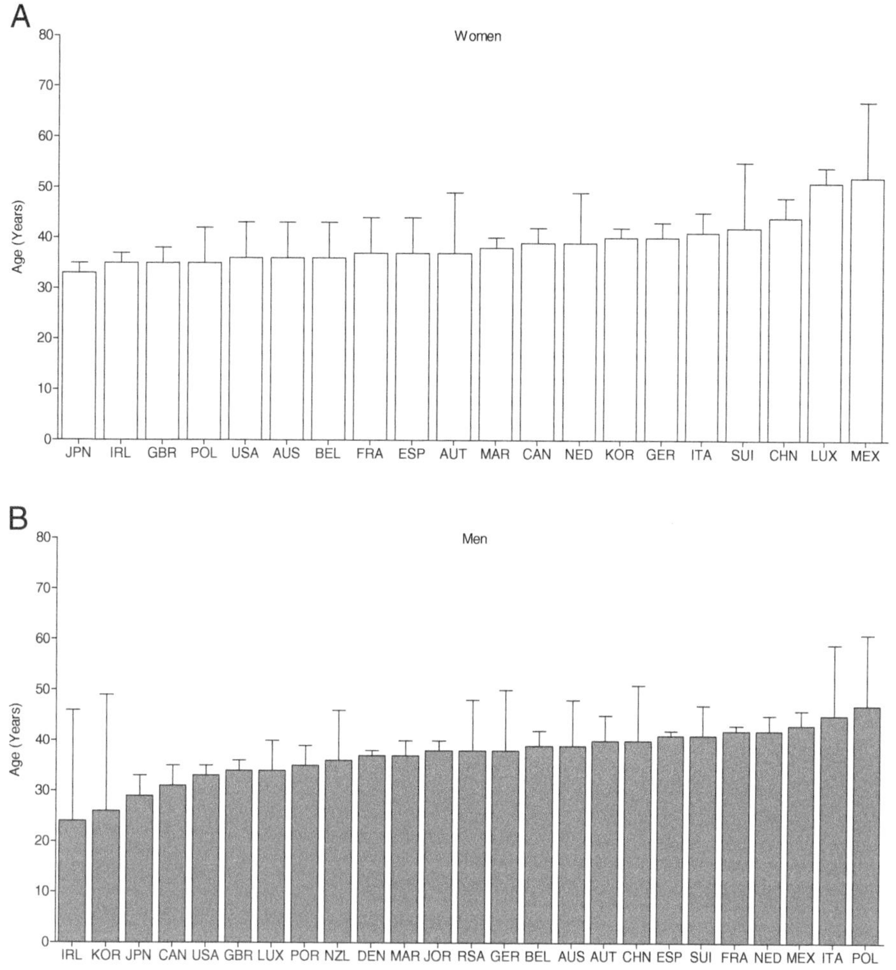

Figure 6 Age of the overall top three female (A) and male athletes (B) per country. *FRA* France, *GBR* Great Britain, *ESP* Spain, *ITA* Italy, *GER* Germany, *USA* United States of America, *SUI* Switzerland, *MAR* Morocco, *JPN* Japan, *JOR* Jordan, *CAN* Canada, *LUX* Luxembourg, *IRL* Ireland, *AUS* Australia, *BEL* Belgium, *AUT* Austria, *KOR* Korea, *DEN* Denmark, *NED* Netherlands, *NZL* New Zealand, *CHN* China, *POR* Portugal, *POL* Poland, *MEX* Mexico, *RSA* Republic of South Africa.

per head from 2003 to 2011 in the eight countries included in the analysis. Also, a significant correlation between participation and income per head for Spanish and Swiss competitors could be seen (Table 1, [44-46]). Similar to Hoffman and Fogard's work [43], most competitors were middle-aged with an average age of 39 years in women and 37 years in men. This demonstrates that older runners with the financial background and the will to prove themselves instead of younger runners with economic interests participate in ultramarathons such as the Marathon des Sables.

Who is winning, and why are there gender differences?

The fastest performance was attained by Moroccan competitors, winning nine of ten editions from 2003 to 2012, although most male finishers in the Marathon des Sables originated from France and Great Britain. We expected the same outcome in women, but only two out of ten competitions were won by Moroccans, eight races were won by Europeans (France five, Luxembourg two, and Spain one). Moroccan women achieved the fastest running speeds, followed by French and Spanish women. The dominance of European females might be due to cultural and religious inhibitions. In Islamic countries, females seem to participate less in competitive sports; therefore, fewer females from Morocco might be competing in the Marathon des Sables [47]. Between 2003 and 2012, only 24 Moroccan women and one Pakistani woman competed, which is only approximately 3% of the female competitors. Another reason might be the high inscription fees and costs to participate in such an event. Most probably, North African women were not as wealthy as European competitors, and the financial backgrounds as well as social or religious reasons were limiting female participation in the Marathon des Sables.

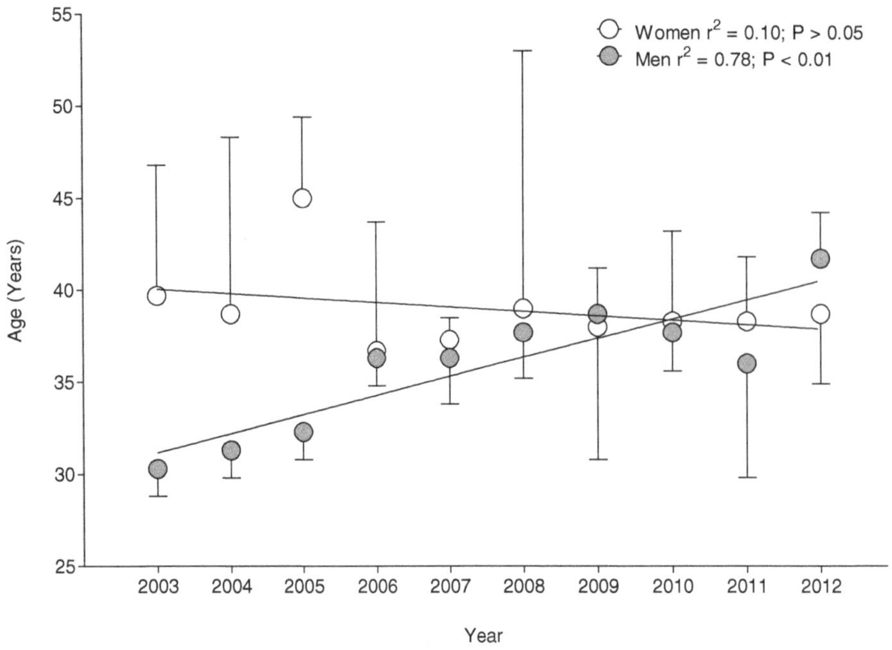

Figure 7 Change in the age of peak performance of the annual top three women and men across years.

Running performance and gender difference

A third important finding was that the top three men became slower across years, whereas the top three women showed no change in running speed across years. The gender difference in running speed of the top three athletes decreased (r^2 = 0.72; $p < 0.01$) from 39.5% in 2003 to 24.1% in 2012 with a mean gender difference of 31.7 ± 2.0% across years. In endurance performance, the gender difference varied largely from 10% to 30% [15,17]. According to previous findings, running performance might be impaired by a higher core temperature [21]. This could be due to higher body fat levels in females [19,48] as well as the stronger heat impact on slower runners, although the effect could not be shown for women [22-25].

An interesting finding was that men became slower and that women showed no change in running speed across years. The decrease in running speed in men could be due to the increase in age in men. The increasing popularity of the Marathon des Sables and the concurrent increase of amateur competitors of all levels might be a reason for the decrease in overall running speed in men. Most probably, more men seek the adventure and thrill a competition like the Marathon des Sables provides and that the competitors in the beginning of the Marathon des Sables were

Table 1 Increase in finishers, population and GNI per capita, PPP, and correlation between finishers and population and participants and GNI per capita 2003–2011

	Finishers				Population (in 1,000)				Finishers / Population						Finishers / Income	
	2003	2011	r^2	*p*	2003	2011	r^2	*p*	2003	2011	r^2	*p*	r^2	*p*	r^2	*p*
FRA	240	230	0.09	>0.05	59,765	63,126	0.96	<0.01	27,460	35,860	0.92	<0.01	0.32	>0.05	0.26	>0.05
GBR	180	228	0.65	<0.01	59,554	62,417	1.0	<0.01	30,250	36,970	0.74	<0.01	0.82	<0.01	0.65	>0.05
ESP	9	76	0.97	<0.01	41,875	46,452	0.96	<0.01	24,470	31,930	0.80	<0.01	0.92	<0.01	0.79	<0.01
ITA	37	46	0.0	>0.05	57,604	60,789	1.0	<0.01	27,080	32,350	0.77	<0.01	0.05	>0.05	0.30	>0.05
GER	33	17	0.09	>0.05	82,533	82,163	0.74	<0.01	28,110	40,170	0.94	<0.01	0.02	>0.05	0.27	>0.05
USA	20	20	0.31	>0.05	290,810	313,085	1.0	<0.01	38,400	48,490	0.81	<0.01	0.54	>0.05	0.41	>0.05
SUI	8	24	0.74	<0.01	7,284	7,702	0.91	<0.01	36,100	50,900	0.96	<0.01	0.78	<0.01	0.85	<0.01
MAR	11	13	0.00	>0.05	30,088	32,644	0.92	<0.01	3,060	4,910	1.0	<0.01	0.07	>0.05	0.06	>0.05

Increase in finishers per country, population per country (in thousands) [44,45] and gross national income per capita, purchasing power parity (PPP) (current international dollar) [46], correlation between finishers and population and participants and gross national income per capita from 2003 to 2011. *FRA* France, *GBR* Great Britain, *ESP* Spain, *ITA* Italy, *GER* Germany, *USA* United States of America, *SUI* Switzerland, MAR Morocco.

prepared better and in a better shape overall as there were only few competitors and the event was not as popular as today [14]. For the unchanged performance in women, the increase in participation in women in ultramarathon might be a potential reason [1]. With a general increase in participation of women, more concurrence occurs, and the level of running speed may rise. Another aspect might be that the running speed rises with the popularity of the Marathon des Sables as more women were participating and training more specifically to compete in this event. In men, Spanish runners were the only ones who were becoming faster across years. Most probably, athletes from countries improving their performance might have had special training programs or national support for their matter [49]. Another reason might be that competing and winning in ultramarathons are more prestigious in certain countries. Because of the similarity of the Mediterranean climates with hot summer temperatures in southern Europe, Spanish competitors might adapt to the heat and extreme conditions easier. Interestingly, Moroccans became slower across years although they would be able to train in the same environment and might therefore have an advantage.

Master runners dominate the Marathon des Sables

The fastest women achieved their best performances at the age between 35 and 40 years (Moroccan women with 38 ± 2 years, French women with 37 ± 2 years, and Spanish women with 37 ± 7 years). Also for men, the fastest runners were between 35 and 40 years old (Moroccan men with 37 ± 3 years, Jordanian men with 38 ± 2 years, and Spanish men with 41 ± 1 years). In addition, the age of the top three runners in 2012 was 41.7 ± 2.5 years for men and 38.7 ± 3.8 years for women. Reaburn and Dascombe [50] described that master athletes were typically older than 35 years of age, were systematically trained, and competed in organized forms of sport specifically designed for older adults. This was due to the observed age-related decline in endurance performance in different sport disciplines such as running, orienteering, rowing, and swimming. Following the definition of Reaburn and Dascombe [50], the top runners in the Marathon des Sables were all master runners. However, the present findings suggest that ultramarathoners do not fall within this definition of master athletes after the age of 35 years since the annual fastest runners in recent years and the fastest runners by country were between 35 and 40 years old.

Limitations

This study is limited because physiological [24], nutritional [51] or environmental [23], and medical [52] influences were not considered. Additionally, the different course and changing numbers of stages might play a role in running speed. These factors may as well have an influence on the outcome of a multistage ultra-endurance race. A questionnaire for income, job, and social background to investigate the socioeconomic influence on participation is missing. The influence of training and equipment [53] might well be a substantial factor for performance, and there might be a correlation between wealth of a nation and the equipment and nutrition the competitors can afford. That may be of importance especially in competitions under extreme circumstances, and further investigations should be done on these parameters.

Conclusions

The number in finishers in the Marathon des Sables increased in the last decade. Most finishers originated from Europe, mainly from France and Great Britain. Moroccan men were the fastest runners, winning nine of ten competitions between 2003 and 2012. We assume that the socioeconomic and religious background plays an important role in participation and running speed in the Marathon des Sables. Men were significantly faster than women, and the mean gender difference of 31.7 ± 2.0% in the top three was rather high compared with previous studies. Moreover, the fastest runners were master athletes. Further studies need to investigate the gender differences in running speed in very hot climates and participation trends concerning nationalities and socioeconomic background, by questionnaire related to participation in ultra-endurance events. The age of peak performance in other ultra-endurance races needs to be determined, and the definition of master athlete as athletes aged > 35 years and competing in sports specifically designed for older adults needs to be questioned.

Competing interests
The authors declare that they have no competing interests.

Authors' contributions
All authors—CK, BK, CAR, TR, and RL—designed the study. The manuscript was written by all authors. All authors read and approved the final manuscript.

Author details
[1]Department of Orthopaedics and Traumatology, Kantonsspital St. Gallen, St. Gallen, Switzerland. [2]Institute of General Practice and for Health Services Research, University of Zurich, Zurich, Switzerland. [3]Gesundheitszentrum St. Gallen, Vadianstrasse 26, St. Gallen 9001, Switzerland. [4]INSERM U1093, Faculty of Sport Sciences, University of Burgundy, Dijon, France.

References

1. Hoffman MD, Ong JC, Wang G: **Historical analysis of participation in 161 km ultramarathons in North America.** *Int J Hist Sport* 2010, **27**:1877–1891.
2. Hoffman MD, Wegelin JA: **The Western States 100-Mile Endurance Run: participation and performance trends.** *Med Sci Sports Exerc* 2009, **41**:2191–2198.
3. Lepers R, Cattagni T: **Do older athletes reach limits in their performance during marathon running?** *Age (Dordr)* 2012, **34**:773–781.
4. Lepers R: **Analysis of Hawaii ironman performances in elite triathletes from 1981 to 2007.** *Med Sci Sports Exerc* 2008, **40**:1828–1834.

5. Knechtle B, Knechtle P, Lepers R: **Participation and performance trends in ultra-triathlons from 1985 to 2009.** *Scand J Med Sci Sports* 2011, **21**:e82–e90.
6. Bescós R, Rodríguez F, Iglesias X, Knechtle B, Marina M, Padullés JM, Torrado P, Vazquez J, Rosemann T: **Nutritional behavior of cyclists during a 24-hour team relay race: a field study report.** *J Int Soc Sports Nutr* 2012, **9**:3.
7. Black KE, Skidmore PM, Brown RC: **Energy intakes of ultraendurance cyclists during competition, an observational study.** *Int J Sport Nutr Exerc Metab* 2012, **22**:19–23.
8. **Deutsche Ultramarathon Vereinigung e.V. Ultra Marathon Statistics.** http://statistik.d-u-v.org/.
9. **Ultramarathon running resource.** http://www.ultramarathonrunning.com/.
10. **The Western States Endurance Run.** http://ws100.com/.
11. Lynch SL, Hoch AZ: **The female runner: gender specifics.** *Clin Sports Med* 2010, **29**:477–498.
12. **Deutschlandlauf.** http://www.deutschlandlauf.org.
13. Knechtle B, Duff B, Schulze I, Kohler G: **The effects of running 1,200 km within 17 days on body composition in a female ultrarunner-Deutschlandlauf 2007.** *Res Sports Med* 2008, **16**:167–188.
14. **27th Sultan Marathon des Sables.** http://www.darbaroud.com/resultats/resultats.php?langue=fr&epreuve_id=2012&simple=1&etape=GENERAL&nom=&dossard=&Submit=Envoyer.
15. Hoffman MD: **Ultramarathon trail running comparison of performance-matched men and women.** *Med Sci Sports Exerc* 2008, **40**:1681–1686.
16. Sparling PB, E. O'Donnell EM, Snow TK: **The gender difference in distance running performance has plateaued: an analysis of world rankings from 1980 to 1996.** *Med Sci Sports Exerc* 1998, **30**:1725–1729.
17. Coast JR, Blevins JS, Wilson BA: **Do gender differences in running performance disappear with distance?** *Can J Appl Physiol* 2004, **29**:139–145.
18. Knechtle B, Knechtle P, Rosemann T, Senn O: **Sex differences in association of race performance, skin-fold thicknesses, and training variables for recreational half-marathon runners.** *Percept Mot Skills* 2010, **111**:653–668.
19. Hoffman MD: **Anthropometric characteristics of ultramarathoners.** *Int J Sports Med* 2008, **29**:808–811.
20. Yokota M, Berglund LG, Bathalon GP: **Female anthropometric variability and their effects on predicted thermoregulatory responses to work in the heat.** *Int J Biometeorol* 2012, **56**:379–385.
21. Cheuvront SN, Haymes EM: **Thermoregulation and marathon running: biological and environmental influences.** *Sports Med* 2001, **31**:743–762.
22. Stearns RL, Casa Lopez RM, McDermott BP, Ganio MS, Decher NR, Scruggs IC, West AE, Armstrong LE, Maresh CM: **Influence of hydration status on pacing during trail running in the heat.** *J Strength Cond Res* 2009, **23**:2533–2541.
23. Vihma T: **Effects of weather on the performance of marathon runners.** *Int J Biometeorol* 2010, **54**:297–306.
24. Lopez RM, Casa DJ, Jensen KA, DeMartini JK, Pagnotta KD, Ruiz RC, Roti MW, Stearns RL, Armstrong LE, Maresh CM: **Examining the influence of hydration status on physiological responses and running speed during trail running in the heat with controlled exercise intensity.** *J Strength Cond Res* 2011, **25**:2944–2954.
25. Parise CA, Hoffman MD: **Influence of temperature and performance level on pacing a 161 km trail ultramarathon.** *Int J Sports Physiol Perform* 2011, **6**:243–251.
26. Onywera VO, Scott RA, Boit MK, Pitsiladis YP: **Demographic characteristics of elite Kenyan endurance runners.** *J Sports Sci* 2006, **24**:415–422.
27. Lucia A, Esteve-Lanao J, Oliván J, Gómez-Gallego F, San Juan AF, Santiago C, Pérez M, Chamorro-Viña C, Foster C: **Physiological characteristics of the best Eritrean runners-exceptional running economy.** *Appl Physiol Nutr Metab* 2006, **31**:530–540.
28. Scott RA, Georgiades E, Wilson RH, Goodwin WH, Wolde B, Pitsiladis YP: **Demographic characteristics of elite Ethiopian endurance runners.** *Med Sci Sports Exerc* 2003, **35**:1727–1732.
29. Scott RA, Pitsiladis YP: **Genotypes and distance running: clues from Africa.** *Sports Med* 2007, **37**:424–427.
30. Legaz-Arrese A, Kinfu H, Munguía-Izquierdo D, Carranza-Garcia LE, Calderón FJ: **Basic physiological measures determine fitness and are associated with running performance in elite young male and female Ethiopian runners.** *J Sports Med Phys Fitness* 2009, **49**:358–363.
31. Ash GI, Scott RA, Deason M, Dawson TA, Wolde B, Bekele Z, Teka S, Pitsiladis YP: **No association between ACE gene variation and endurance athlete status in Ethiopians.** *Med Sci Sports Exerc* 2011, **43**:590–597.
32. Scott RA, Wilson RH, Goodwin WH, Moran CN, Georgiades E, Wolde B, Pitsiladis YP: **Mitochondrial DNA lineages of elite Ethiopian athletes.** *Comp Biochem Physiol B Biochem Mol Biol* 2005, **140**:497–503.
33. Onywera VO: **East African runners: their genetics, lifestyle and athletic prowess.** *Med Sport Sci* 2009, **54**:102–109.
34. Rüst CA, Knechtle B, Knechtle P, Lepers R, Rosemann T, Onywera V: **European athletes dominate performances in Double Iron ultra-triathlons—a retrospective data analysis from 1985 to 2010.** *Eur J Sport Sci* 2012. doi:10.1080/17461391.2011.641033.
35. Jeffery S, Knechtle B, Rüst CA, Knechtle P, Lepers R, Rosemann T: **European dominance in Triple Iron ultra-triathlons from 1988 to 2011.** *J Sci Cycling* 2012, **1**:30–38.
36. Lenherr R, Knechtle B, Rüst CA, Rosemann T, Lepers R: **From Double Iron to Double Deca Iron ultra-triathlon—a retrospective data analysis from 1985 to 2011.** *Phys Cult and Sport. Stud and Rese* 2012, **54**:55–67.
37. **Deutsche Ultramarathon Vereinigung e.V. Ultra Marathon Statistics: results database 2012.** http://statistik.d-u-v.org/geteventlist.php.
38. Knechtle B, Rust CA, Rosemann T, Lepers R: **Age-related changes in 100-km ultra-marathon running performance.** *Age (Dordr)* 2012, **34**:1033–1045.
39. **UNDP: human development reports.** http://hdr.undp.org/en/statistics/.
40. **Boston Marathon.** http://www.baa.org/Races/Boston-Marathon.aspx.
41. **MarathonGuide.** http://www.marathonguide.com/.
42. Baker J, Horton S: **East African running dominance revisited: a role for stereotype threat?** *Br J Sports Med* 2003, **37**:553–555.
43. Hoffman MD, Fogard K: **Factors related to successful completion of a 161-km ultramarathon.** *Int J Sports Physiol Perform* 2011, **6**:25–37.
44. **United Nations Statistics Division - statistics and indicators on women and men.** http://unstats.un.org/unsd/demographic/products/indwm/default.htm.
45. **United Nations Statistics Division - demographic yearbook.** http://unstats.un.org/unsd/demographic/products/dyb/dyb2009-2010.htm.
46. **The World Bank: indicators.** http://data.worldbank.org/indicator.
47. Pollard TM, Guell C: **Assessing physical activity in Muslim women of South Asian origin.** *J Phys Act Health* 2012, **9**(7):970–976.
48. Hoffman MD, Lebus DK, Ganong AC, Casazza GA, Van Loan M: **Body composition of 161-km ultramarathoners.** *Int J Sports Med* 2010, **31**:106–109.
49. **Trail Run Spain.** http://www.trailrunspain.com/.
50. Reaburn P, Dascombe B: **Endurance performance in Masters athletes.** *Eur Rev Aging Phys Act* 2008, **5**:31–42.
51. Getzin AR, Milner C, LaFace KM: **Nutrition update for the ultraendurance athlete.** *Curr Sports Med Rep* 2011, **10**:330–339.
52. Krabak BJ, Waite B, Schiff MA: **Study of injury and illness rates in multiday ultramarathon runners.** *Med Sci Sports Exerc* 2011, **43**:2314–2320.
53. Zaryski C, Smith DJ: **Training principles and issues for ultra-endurance athletes.** *Curr Sports Med Rep* 2005, **4**:165–170.

Skeletal muscle volume following dehydration induced by exercise in heat

Kyle J Hackney[1,2*], Summer B Cook[3], Timothy J Fairchild[4] and Lori L Ploutz-Snyder[5]

Abstract

Background: Intracellular skeletal muscle water is redistributed into the extracellular compartment during periods of dehydration, suggesting an associated decline in muscle volume. The purpose of this study was to evaluate skeletal muscle volume in active (knee extensors (KE)) and less active (biceps/triceps brachii, deltoid) musculature following dehydration induced by exercise in heat.

Methods: Twelve participants (seven men, five women) cycled in the heat under two conditions: (1) dehydration (DHYD) resulting in 3% and 5% losses of estimated total body water ($_{E}$TBW), which was assessed by changes in body mass, and (2) fluid replacement (FR) where 3% and 5% losses of $_{E}$TBW were counteracted by intermittent (20 to 30 min) fluid ingestion via a carbohydrate-electrolyte beverage. During both conditions, serum osmolality and skeletal muscle volume (assessed by magnetic resonance imaging) were measured at baseline and at the 3% and 5% $_{E}$TBW loss measurement points.

Results: In DHYD, serum osmolality increased at 3% ($p = 0.005$) and 5% ($p < 0.001$) $_{E}$TBW losses, while FR decreased serum osmolality at the 5% loss of $_{E}$TBW time point ($p = 0.009$). In DHYD, KE muscle volume declined from 1,464 ± 446 ml to 1,406 ± 425 ml (3.9%, $p < 0.001$) at 3% $_{E}$TBW loss and to 1,378 ± 421 ml (5.9%, $p < 0.001$) at 5% $_{E}$TBW loss. The largest decline in KE volume in DYHD occurred in the mid-belly (31 ml, p = 0.001) and proximal (24 ml, $p = 0.001$) regions of the grouped vasti muscles. There were no changes in volume for the biceps/triceps ($p = 0.35$) or deltoid ($p = 0.92$) during DHYD. FR prevented the loss of KE muscle volume at 3% (1,430 ± 435 ml, $p = 0.074$) and 5% (1,431 ± 439 ml, $p = 0.156$) $_{E}$TBW loss time points compared to baseline (1,445 ± 436 ml).

Conclusions: Following exercise in the heat, the actively contracting muscles lost volume, while replacing lost fluids intermittently during exercise in heat prevented this decline. These results support the use of muscle volume as a marker of water loss.

Keywords: Dehydration, Skeletal muscle, MRI, Cycling, Total body water, Fluid shift

Background

Water accounts for 50% to 60% of the total body mass [1] and approximately 75% of the muscle mass [2]. A loss of total body water (TBW) equivalent or greater than 2% of body mass can significantly reduce performance on prolonged submaximal tasks [2,3] and impaired muscular strength and power [4]. Interestingly, the extent of water loss from specific tissue compartments including the skeletal muscle is not well understood and may depend on the means through which dehydration is induced. In thermally dehydrated (approximately 10% body weight) rats, approximately 40% of the decline in TBW was attributed to intracellular stores within the skeletal muscle tissue [5]. This redistribution of water across the muscle cell membrane during dehydration is primarily dependent on the osmotic gradient [2] and the activity of ionic pumps [6]. However, when exercise is combined with heat to induce dehydration, the physiological and metabolic changes are likely to affect the mobilization of water from the skeletal muscle tissue. For example, the redistribution of blood flow to the active muscle during exercise [7] may account for up to 50% of the change in muscle size [8]. The

* Correspondence: kjhackne@syr.edu
[1]Department of Exercise Science, Syracuse University, 820 Comstock Ave, Room 201Women's Building, Syracuse, NY 13244, USA
[2]Present address: Wyle Integrated Science and Engineering, Exercise Physiology and Countermeasures Project, Houston, TX 77058, USA
Full list of author information is available at the end of the article

accumulation of metabolites associated with energy-yielding pathways is known to alter the osmotic gradient [9] and will therefore result in water movement across tissue compartments, including both active and inactive muscle tissue compartments. Additionally, during prolonged exercise in the heat, there is an increase in plasma and serum osmolality [10,11], which resulted from a greater net loss of water as compared with sodium (Na+). This elevation in osmolality is the primary hypothesized mechanism for the mobilization of water across the muscle cell membrane [12]. Consumption of water or a carbohydrate-electrolyte beverage during prolonged exercise counteracts this increase in serum osmolality [10,11], thus negating one of the primary mechanisms whereby water is sequestered across the muscle cell membrane. The implications of fluid replacement via water or carbohydrate-electrolyte beverages on muscle water during exercise in heat are currently not known.

Storage of glycogen is also associated with water storage, and therefore, the concentration of glycogen will directly influence total muscle water [13]. Approximately 2.7 g of water are bound per gram of glycogen [14], and as glycogen concentration decreases, the water bound to glycogen is released [15]. Indeed, Costill et al. [16] demonstrated that both glycogen and water content in muscle fibers from the vastus lateralis were significantly reduced approximately 30 min after exhaustive cycling in heat. This corresponded to a rate of active skeletal muscle water decline of 1.2% for each 1% decrease in body weight. While no comparisons with less active muscles (e.g., upper body) were available in the study of Costill et al. [16], findings from others suggest that there is some glycogen breakdown occurring in less active tissues during exhaustive bouts of exercise [17].

Magnetic resonance imaging (MRI) offers outstanding spatial resolution of muscle anatomy including the ability to noninvasively evaluate the volume of individual muscles and/or muscle groups [18,19]. The application of MRI to assess changes in hydration status within the skeletal muscle tissue has not previously been reported in the exercise literature. Therefore, the purpose of this study was to evaluate the skeletal muscle volume in active and less active musculature during dehydration induced by exercise in heat. We hypothesized that (1) skeletal muscle volume would decline in both active and less active muscles during dehydration and (2) fluid replacement during exercise in heat would prevent a loss of skeletal muscle volume.

Methods

Participants

Twelve recreationally active men ($n = 7$) and women ($n = 5$) were recruited for the investigation (mean ± standard deviation (SD): body mass = 69.8 ± 16.4 kg, body fat = 17.2 ± 7.9%, estimated TBW ($_E$TBW) = 40.0 ± 10.1 kg). Prior to participation, all subjects were screened for sickle cell trait (AccuBase A1c^{TM}, Diabetes Technologies, Inc, Thomasville, GA, USA) due to the risk of microvascular occlusion during physical exertion [20]. Pregnant females were also excluded from participation due to possible risk of severe dehydration, and for this reason, a urine pregnancy test was adminstered to all female participants on the day of testing. Study participation was supervised and approved by a physician. The project was approved by the Institutional Review Boards from Syracuse University, SUNY Upstate Medical University, and the US Army Surgeon General. All participants provided their written informed consent prior to participating in the study.

Preliminary testing

Prior to experimental testing, an estimate of stable baseline euhydrated body mass (nearest hundredth of 1 kg) was determined for each subject from mean values obtained over consecutive days (9.3 ± 0.8 days). Each measurements were obtained semi-nude using a calibrated digital scale (WeighSouth WSI-600, Mettler-Toledo, Inc, Worthington, OH, USA). These measurements were conducted at the same time of day in the laboratory after voiding and prior to eating. Fat and fat-free body mass were also determined via Dual Energy X-ray Absorptiometry (DEXA) (Lunar DPX; GE Medical Systems, Waukesha, WI, USA). Using the fat and fat-free mass from DEXA, $_E$TBW was calculated using the following equation: $_E\text{TBW} = 0.10\,\text{kg (DEXA fat mass)} + 0.73\,\text{kg (DEXA fat – free mass)}$ [13,21]. During this time period, subjects also completed three to six acute, submaximal heat familiarization sessions (20 to 30 min) on a cycle ergometer in the climate chamber. Subjects performed familiarization sessions until a stable steady state heart rate was observed during submaximal exercise in the heat (data not shown) and until they felt they were comfortable with the testing protocol. Following stable body weight assessment and familiarization, subjects completed an experimental exercise in heat testing sessions under two conditions: (1) dehydration (DHYD) and (2) fluid replacement (FR).

Baseline testing

Both DHYD and FR testing sessions were counterbalanced and began the morning (0700 hours) following an overnight fast (>8 h). On arrival to the laboratory, subjects voided their bladders for assessment urine specific gravity via a refractometer (PAL-10S, Atago, Belevue, WA, USA). Urine specific gravity was only evaluated at baseline to document that subjects were not dehydrated prior to baseline data collection. Body mass was measured using the digital scale previously described (0715 hours), and participants rested in the supine position of 30 min. Blood samples (approximately 5 ml) were obtained via arm venipuncture using Vacutainer® (BD, Franklin Lakes, NJ, USA) containing a clot activator and gel for serum separation (0745 hours). All blood samples were immediately transported to SUNY Medical University Hospital for clinical analysis of serum osmolality (Advanced® Model 330 Micro-Osmometer, Advanced Instruments, Inc., Norwood, MA, USA). Once blood samples were obtained, subjects were transported to the MRI scanner in the supine position using a gurney to avoid fluid shifts [22]. Once correctly positioned in the MRI scanner (0800 hours), 5-mm-thick transaxial images (2,122-ms repetition time, 0.5-mm slice-to-slice interval) were acquired using a 1.5-T Phillips Intera whole body scanner with the software Release 11 (Phillips Medical Systems, Bothell, WA, USA). MRI scans were obtained along the length of the right upper leg from the head of the femur to the knee and along the right upper arm between the head of the humerus to the elbow. Once baseline data collection was completed (0900 hours), participants walked to the climate chamber to complete one of the counterbalanced exercise and heat testing sessions.

DHYD protocol

During the DHYD testing condition, participants cycled at 60 rpm on a Monark cycle ergometer in a climate chamber at 38°C, 32% humidity, and 13 km/h wind. Participants began pedaling at 1 kp but were allowed to change the cycle load if needed to achieve the desired $_E$TBW loss. Rectal temperature (YSI 402AC, YSI Inc., Dayton, OH, USA) and heart rate (Polar A5, Polar Electro Inc., Lake Success, NY, USA) were monitored throughout the exercise sessions. During the DHYD exercise in heat session, no fluids were provided. Participants exercised in heat and were weighed every 20 to 30 min until $_E$TBW loss reached 3% as assessed by body mass. At this time, subjects were allowed to void their bladders and walk to the resting area where a final weight was recorded. Subjects rested in the supine position until a blood sample and MRI scan was obtained 45 min and 60 min, respectively, after exercise. After dependent measures were obtained, the participants went back to the climate chamber for additional exercise in heat. No fluids were provided during acquisition of dependent measures; therefore, participants cycled in heat and were weighed until an additional 2% $_E$TBW was lost (which equaled 5% $_E$TBW loss total for the condition). Once 5% $_E$TBW loss was achieved, the dependent measures (body mass, blood sample, and MRI) were obtained as described previously.

FR protocol

The FR condition was identical to the DHYD condition except that all fluids lost during exercise and heat were intermittently (20 to 30 min) replaced at 1.5 times the rate they were lost using a carbohydrate-electrolyte beverage (14 g carbohydrate, 200 mg sodium, 90 mg potassium/8 oz; Gatorade® Endurance, Chicago, IL,USA) [23]. Replacement of 1.5 times the rate of fluid loss was selected in order to account for continuous sweat and urine production while dependent measures were assessed. Participants began by cycling in heat under the same intensity and thermal conditions previously described. Following 20 to 30 min of exercise in heat, the participants were removed from the thermal chamber and weighed to determine $_E$TBW. This amount was recorded, and fluids were provided. Participants were then re-weighed with the consumed fluid and returned to the thermal chamber for an additional 20 to 30 min of exercise in heat. This process was repeated until the total amount of fluid lost after being removed from the thermal chamber totaled 3% $_E$TBW loss. At this point, our goal was to have adequately replaced the 3%$_E$TBW fluid, so there was no change in body mass. Participants were allowed to void their bladders and walk to the resting area where a final weight was recorded and dependent measures were assessed. Participants then returned to the heat chamber and exercised, and every 20 to 30 min, they were then weighed and given the appropriate amount of fluids. This process continued until an additional 2% $_E$TBW was lost (then replaced); hence, the total amount of fluid lost then replaced was equivalent to 5% $_E$TBW. At this point, the goal was to have no change in body mass from the baseline despite sweating out 5% $_E$TBW during the exercise and heat session. After the 5% $_E$TBW loss, time point was reached in FR, a final body mass was recorded, and dependent measures were reassessed.

MRI analysis

Following both DHYD and FR conditions, MRI images were transferred to a computer for tracing, and skeletal muscle volume was calculated using the NIH ImageJ analysis software (NIH, Bethesda, MD, USA) [24]. Knee extensor muscle volume was determined by adding the volumes from the rectus femoris and vasti muscles, which were analyzed between the appearances of the distal portion of the rectus femoris and the femoral neck. The number of slices analyzed across the distance of the knee extensors was subsequently divided into three sections to determine regional changes in volume. The distal region was characterized by the first third of slices (toward the knee), the mid-belly represented the middle third of slices (mid-thigh), and the proximal region comprised the upper third of slices (toward the hip).

Shoulder muscle volume was determined from the sum of five to six axial slices superior to the appearance of the anterior deltoid. Elbow flexor and extensor muscles were evaluated from the combined area of the biceps brachii and triceps brachii using the sum of five to six axial slices distal to the appearance of the anterior deltoid. The same number of slices was measured for each subject at each of the testing time points, and great care was taken to ensure within-subject measurement replication. Three investigators were responsible for MRI analysis (one for each muscle/group: knee extensors, biceps/triceps, deltoid). All MRI analyzers had previously demonstrated test-retest reliability of <1% in the laboratory and were blinded to condition and time point of the images.

Statistical analysis

Urine specific gravity, chamber temperature, relative humidity, duration of chamber exposure, exercise workload, exercise heart rate, and core body temperature were compared between DHYD and FR conditions using paired *t* tests. Dependent measures of body mass, serum osmolality, and skeletal muscle volume were analyzed using within-subject analysis of variance (ANOVAs) with repeated measures on condition (DHYD, FR) and time (baseline, 3% $_{E}$TBW loss, 5% $_{E}$TBW loss). When significant condition × time interactions were determined, differences within and between conditions were evaluated using Bonferroni corrected Student's *t* tests. Regional (distal, mid-belly, proximal) changes in muscle volume were also evaluated *post hoc* using ANOVA with repeated measures on the muscle (grouped vasti muscles, rectus femoris) and time (baseline, 5% $_{E}$TBW loss) with follow-up Bonferroni corrected Student's *t* tests. Associations among dependent variables were further explored using Pearson's correlations. MRI image quality (motion artifact) at one time point prevented the analysis of muscle volume on one male subject for the knee extensors and one female subject for the arm muscles. Therefore, both leg and arm MRI statistical analyses were performed using $n = 11$. Significance was determined at $p < 0.05$. All values are mean ± SD.

Results

Baseline urine specific gravity did not differ statistically ($p = 0.42$) and were 1.016 ± 0.01 and 1.018 ± 0.01 for DHYD and FR conditions, respectively. Chamber temperature, humidity, exercise workload, and core temperature were closely matched between conditions (Table 1). In DHYD, the total climate chamber exposure time was significantly less, and heart rate was elevated compared with that in FR (Table 1).

There was a significant condition × time interaction for body mass ($p < 0.001$, Table 2). At baseline, there were no differences between conditions ($p = 0.16$). Body mass was significantly lower in the DHYD compared with that in the FR at 3% ($p = 0.007$) and 5% ($p < 0.001$) $_{E}$TBW loss measurement time points. Overall, $_{E}$TBW loss at 3% and 5% measurement points were 3.45 ± 0.73% ($p < 0.001$) and 5.75 ± 0.86% ($p < 0.001$) in DHYD and 0.78 ± 0.81% ($p < 0.05$) and 0.64 ± 0.79% ($p < 0.05$) in FR, respectively.

There was a significant condition × time interaction for serum osmolality ($p < 0.001$, Table 2). At baseline, serum osmolality was similar between conditions ($p = 0.76$). In DHYD, osmolality increased at the 3% ($p = 0.005$) and 5% ($p < 0.001$) $_{E}$TBW loss. In FR, serum osmolality decreased only at the 5% ($p = 0.009$) $_{E}$TBW loss measurement time point. Serum osmolality was significantly greater in the DHYD condition compared with that in FR at both the 3% ($p < 0.001$) and 5% ($p < 0.001$) $_{E}$TBW losses.

There was a significant condition × time interaction for the knee extensor muscle volume (grouped rectus femoris and vasti muscles); $p < 0.001$, Figure 1). At baseline, there were no differences in knee extensor muscle volumes between DHYD (1,464 ± 446 ml) and FR (1,445 ± 436 ml, $p = 0.14$). In FR, there were no changes in knee extensor volume at 3% (1,430 ± 435 ml, $p = 0.74$) or 5% (1,431 ± 439 ml, $p = 0.156$) $_{E}$TBW loss compared to that in the baseline. However, during DHYD, knee extensor volume decreased significantly at both 3% (1,406 ± 425 ml, $p < 0.001$) and 5% (1,378 ± 421 ml, $p < 0.001$) $_{E}$TBW loss measurement points, which represented reductions of 3.96 ± 1.31% and 5.87 ± 1.97%, respectively. Knee extensor volume was lower in the DHYD compared with that in the FR at 3% ($p = 0.005$)

Table 1 Environmental conditions and physiological responses

Variable	DHYD	FR	*p* value
Chamber temperature (°C)	36.9 ± 0.6	37.3 ± 1.0	0.20
Chamber relative humidity (%)	32.4 ± 5.9	30.5 ± 5.9	0.22
Chamber exposure (min)	134 ± 31[†]	154 ± 29	0.02
Exercise workload (W)	96 ± 39	98 ± 40	0.67
Heart rate (beats min^{-1})	147 ± 11[†]	137 ± 7	0.01
Core body temperature (°C)	38.1 ± 0.6	38.2 ± 0.4	0.14

[†]Significantly different from FR, $p < 0.05$. $n = 12$; mean ± SD.

Table 2 Body mass (kilograms) and serum osmolality (milliosmolar per kilogram)

Variable	Condition	Baseline	↓3% $_{E}$TBW	↓5% $_{E}$TBW
Body mass	DHYD	69.4 ± 16.2	67.9 ± 15.8*[†]	67.1 ± 15.6*[†]
	FR	69.1 ± 16.1	68.7 ± 15.8*	68.8 ± 15.9*
Serum osmolality	DHYD	291 ± 7	304 ± 6*[†]	301 ± 4*[†]
	FR	296 ± 7	292 ± 4	290 ± 5*

*Significantly different within condition vs baseline, $p < 0.05$; [†]significantly different from FR, $p < 0.01$. $n = 12$; mean ± SD.

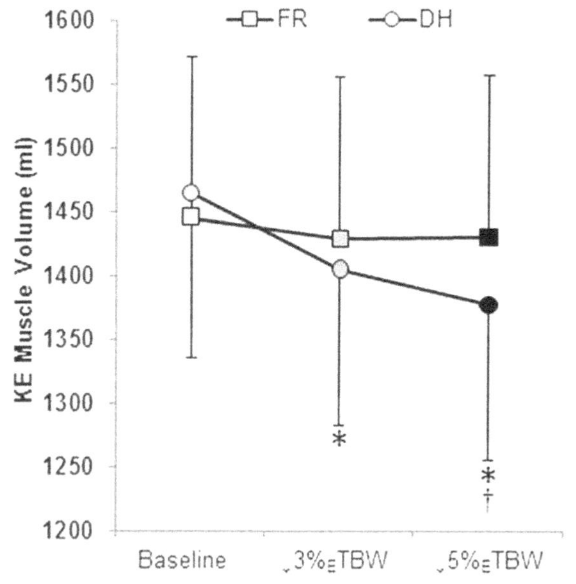

Figure 1 Knee extensor muscle volume (in milliliters) in DHYD and FR. *Significantly different from the baseline ($p < 0.05$); †significantly different from FR ($p < 0.05$). FR, *squares*; DHYD, *circles*; baseline, *white fill*; ↓3% $_E$TBW, *gray fill*; ↓5% $_E$TBW, *black fill*.

and 5% ($p < 0.001$) $_E$TBW losses. An example MRI slice from DHYD and FR conditions at each time point is shown in Figure 2. Overall, there was a significant correlation ($R = 0.57$, $R^2 = 0.39$, $p = 0.006$) between the loss of body mass (fluid loss via sweat) and the loss of knee extensor volume during the DHYD condition. The delta change in body mass relative to the delta change in knee extensor muscle volume is displayed in DHYD (Figure 3A) and FR (Figure 3B).

When the knee extensor muscles (rectus femoris and vasti muscles) were evaluated by region across the distance of the leg in DHYD only, there were significant muscle × time point interactions in the distal ($p < 0.001$), mid-belly ($p = 0.002$), and proximal ($p = 0.02$) regions (Table 3). The volumes of the pooled vasti muscles were significantly greater than those of the rectus femoris in all regions (all p values < 0.001). The volume of the vasti muscles also declined significantly from the baseline to the 5% $_E$TBW measurement point in the distal ($p < 0.001$), mid-belly, ($p = 0.001$), and proximal ($p = 0.001$) regions. There were no significant changes from the baseline to the 5% $_E$TBW measurement point in any region of the rectus femoris (Table 3). There were no significant condition × time interactions for the biceps/triceps ($p = 0.35$) or deltoid ($p = 0.92$) muscle volumes. In addition, no main effects were observed at these sites (all p values > 0.05; Table 4).

Discussion

The main finding of this investigation was dehydration induced through the combination of exercise and heat, which resulted in a significant reduction in skeletal muscle volume in active muscles (knee extensors). The dehydration-related loss of the knee extensor muscle volume as a result of exercise in heat was counteracted by intermitted fluid replacement. We also show for the first time that less active upper body muscles (biceps/ triceps

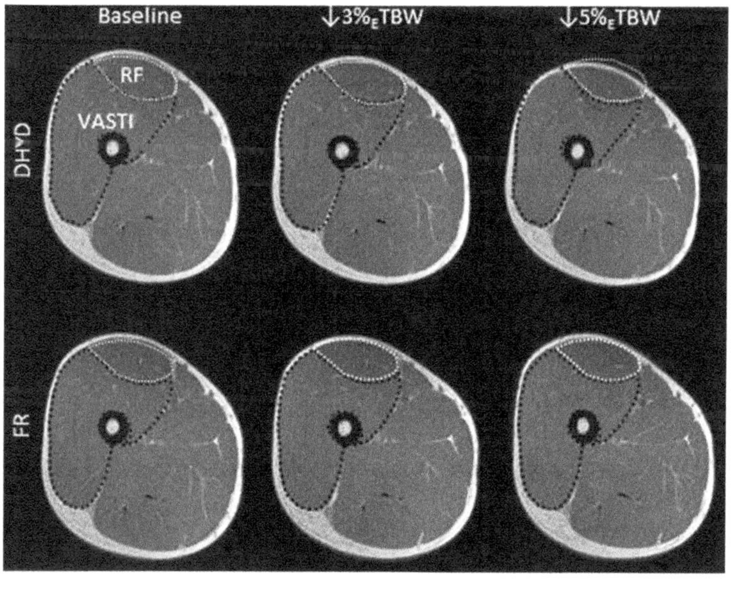

Figure 2 Sample MRI slice depicting knee extensor muscle volume for DHYD and FR conditions. RF, rectus femoris; VASTI, grouped volume of vastus lateralis, vastus intermedius, and vastus medialis. The baseline tracing of proximal muscle size is shown at ↓3% $_E$TBW and ↓5% $_E$TBW losses in DHYD and FR.

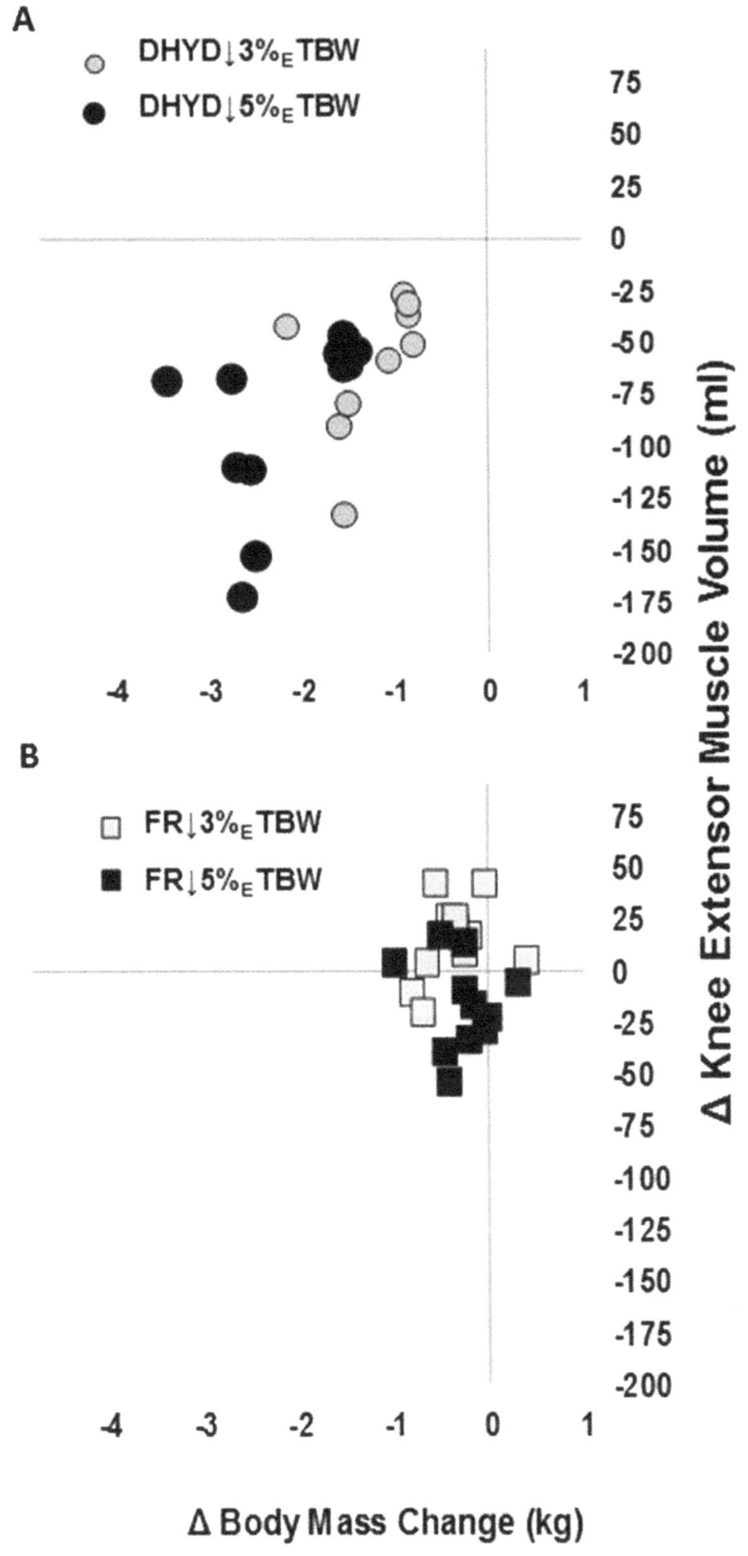

Figure 3 Association between Δ body mass and Δ knee extensor volume for (A) DHYD and (B) FR. FR, *squares*; DHYD, *circles*; ↓3% $_E$TBW, *gray fill*; ↓5% $_E$TBW, *black fil.*

Table 3 Regional changes in knee extensor muscle volume (milliliters) during dehydration

Muscle(s)	Distal		Mid-belly		Proximal	
	Baseline	↓5% $_{E}$TBW	Baseline	↓5% $_{E}$TBW	Baseline	↓5% $_{E}$TBW
Vasti[1]	439 ± 144[†]	419 ± 139*[†]	491 ± 149[†]	460 ± 138*[†]	336 ± 110[†]	312 ± 102*[†]
RF	26 ± 9	25 ± 9	77 ± 29	73 ± 29	94 ± 33	87 ± 29*

*Significantly different vs baseline; [†]significantly different vs RF; $p < 0.05$. [1]Vasti, volume of the vastus lateralis, vastus intermedius, and vastus medialis; RF, rectus femoris. $n = 11$; mean ± SD.

or deltoid) maintain volume when dehydration is induced by exercise in heat.

By the end of the dehydration protocol (5.75 ± 0.86% loss of $_{E}$TBW), the decline in knee extensor muscle volume was 5.89 ±1.9%. The association ($R^2 = 0.32$) between the change in body mass and the change in knee extensor volume suggests that muscle water was sequestered from intracellular stores of the active muscle tissue to the extracellular space. The most notable comparison to the present study is the investigation of Costill et al. [16], wherein the intracellular muscle water loss during dehydration occurred at the rate of approximately 1.20% for each 1% decrease in body mass [16]. This rate was calculated from analysis of the water content from muscle biopsies extracted from the vastus lateralis 30 min following exercise and heat dehydration protocol resulting in approximately 9% TBW loss. Applying the calculated rate established by Costill et al. [16] to the present results, yields predicted losses of knee extensor skeletal muscle water of approximately 3.31% and approximately 5.07% at each measurement point, which compares favorably to the 3.96% and 5.87% loss of knee extensor volume observed using MRI.

The knee extensors were defined as the combined volume of the vasti muscles and the rectus femoris. The vasti muscles were analyzed as a group due to the difficulty of reliably separating the vastus lateralis, vastus intermedius, and vastus medialis along the length of the leg using MRI. At baseline, the pooled vasti muscles accounted for approximately 87% of the overall knee extensor volume, and several studies suggest that these three muscles are slightly more active than the rectus femoris during cycling [25,26]. Hence, it is justifiable that larger losses (−5.89%) in volume occurred in vasti muscles compared with the rectus femoris (−5.51%). In addition, the mid-belly (−6.31%, −31 ml) and proximal regions (−7.14%, −24 ml) of the vasti muscles showed greater changes in volume compared with the distal region (−4.65%, −20 ml), which suggests differential loss of water across the length of the leg. Although this study was not designed to determine the mechanism leading to the observed loss of skeletal muscle volume, it is estimated (although debated) that 2.7 g of water are bound to each 1 g of muscle glycogen [14]. During exercise in heat, muscle glycogenolysis in the actively contracting skeletal muscle tissue is accelerated [27]; hence, water from decomplexing and that produced from metabolic pathways [28] may be free to move from intracellular into extracellular compartments.

Table 4 Muscle volume (milliliters) in less active musculature

Muscle (s)	Condition	Baseline	↓3% $_{E}$TBW	↓5% $_{E}$TBW
Biceps/triceps[1]	DHYD	251 ± 98	247 ± 93	249 ± 100
	FR	254 ±105	251 ± 99	259 ± 108
Deltoid	DHYD	17 ± 8	17 ± 6	17 ± 7
	FR	18 ± 7	17 ± 7	17 ± 7

[1]Combined volume of the biceps brachii and triceps. $n = 11$; mean ± SD. No significant differences were determined, $p > 0.05$.

Consistent with our hypothesis, replacement of lost fluids during exercise in heat prevented a loss of skeletal muscle volume. It was our intent to replace all fluids that were lost throughout the prolonged submaximal exercise in heat session in order to negate changes in body mass. On average, participants consumed 2,800 ± 862 ml of fluids that consisted of 164 ± 50 g of carbohydrate, 2,340 ± 718 mg sodium, 1,050 ± 323 mg potassium, and water during the FR condition. Despite our fluid replacement strategy (1.5 times fluid loss via sweat), there was a small but significant decline in body mass from the baseline at both testing time points (approximated average 0.30 kg). However, knee extensor skeletal muscle volume was preserved, suggesting no change in muscle water content when fluids are replaced during exercise in heat. Participants had a greater total exposure time in the heat chamber in FR and performed exercise at the same workload albeit at a lower heart rate. These data are in agreement with previous studies demonstrating the benefits of maintaining adequate hydration during physical exertion [29-31].

Contrary to our hypothesis, there were no changes in muscle volume in less active muscles (deltoids, biceps/triceps) during the exercise protocols. Our representation of deltoid muscle volume was small (approximately 17 ml) as it consisted five to six MRI slices superior from its appearance. Therefore, it is plausible that greater muscle volumes are required to accurately detect change via MRI. We speculate that vasoconstriction to less active muscle groups and the absence of any significant metabolic perturbations in these muscles [32] are likely to have contributed to the lack of significant change observed in the muscle volume at these sites. However, since specific physiological and metabolic measures were not conducted in this study, the contribution of intramuscular water among less active muscles during dehydration cannot be definitively established.

The time course of the changes observed during our study is worth noting. MRI scanning occurred 60 min following completion of the exercise in heat sessions to allow for equilibration of fluids across compartments [22] and to bring the metabolic rate back to near resting conditions. As a consequence to the dynamic movement of fluids between compartments during physical activity [6], it would be very difficult to accurately assess muscle water during task performance. Another limitation of the study is that water and glycogen content was not directly measured via the skeletal muscle biopsy technique. Although this would quantify water loss in both active and less actives skeletal muscles following exercise in heat, the number of muscle biopsies required from different muscles/groups would have ethical concerns. The noninvasive MRI technique used in the present study quantified muscle volume and assumed the changes of represented muscle water loss given in previous published data using the muscle biopsy technique [16].

Dehydration reduces physical work capacity, lowers tolerance to heat, and remains a significant health risk [3]. Assessment of dehydration still relies heavily on body fluid chemistry, which is impractical in many athletic or occupational settings. While compartmental fluid shifts are fundamentally important to physiological function, our findings may also have direct application to development of sensor technology aimed at detecting water content within specific tissue compartments. For instance, ultra wideband radar [33] is an emerging technology that uses relative permittivity to detect water among different tissues (muscle, fat, skin, etc) [34]. These types of sensors could play an important role in various settings including mining, space flight, and defense services.

Conclusions

In summary, this study evaluated changes in skeletal muscle volume using MRI following exercise in heat, with or without fluid replacement. There was a significant decline in knee extensor (active muscles) volume following dehydration induced by prolonged, submaximal cycling in the heat, wherein the greatest loss of muscle volume occurred in the mid and proximal regions of the knee extensor musculature. This loss of knee extensor volume was prevented through provision of a carbohydrate-electrolyte beverage. No changes in muscle volume in the bicep/triceps brachii or deltoid (less active muscles) were detected with dehydration. The results from this study indicate that skeletal muscle volume assessed by MRI is a useful application to dehydration-related research and warrants further investigation.

Competing interests

The authors declare that they have no competing interests.

Authors' contributions

KJH participated in data acquisition, completed MRI and statistical analysis, and drafted the manuscript. SBC assisted with the coordination of the study, participated in data acquisition, completed MRI analysis, and provided edits to drafts of the manuscript. TJF assisted with the coordination of the study, participated in data acquisition, and provided edits to the manuscript. LPS designed the study, secured funding, assisted with the coordination of the study, participated in data acquisition, and provided edits to drafts of the manuscript. All authors read and approved the final manuscript.

Acknowledgments

We would like to thank Michael Sawka for his contribution to the study design and Vincent Frechette, Gwen Tillapaugh-Fay, Andrew Kelleher, and Patrick Cowley for their contribution to data collection. Funding for this investigation was provided by a grant from the US Army Medical Research and Materiel Command. This study was conducted in collaboration with Intelligent Automation, Inc., Rockville, MD, USA.

Author details

[1]Department of Exercise Science, Syracuse University, 820 Comstock Ave, Room 201Women's Building, Syracuse, NY 13244, USA. [2]Present address: Wyle Integrated Science and Engineering, Exercise Physiology and Countermeasures Project, Houston, TX 77058, USA. [3]Department of Kinesiology, University of New Hampshire, 124 Main Street, Durham, NH 03824, USA. [4]School of Chiropractic and Sports Science, Murdoch University, 90 South Street, Murdoch, WA 6150, Australia. [5]Universities Space and Research Association, Exercise Physiology and Countermeasures Project, NASA Lyndon B Johnson Space Center, 2101 NASA Parkway, SK/261, Houston, TX 77058, USA.

References

1. Maughan RJ: **Impact of mild dehydration on wellness and on exercise performance.** *Eur J Clin Nutr* 2003, **57**(Suppl 2):S19–23.
2. Sawka MN: **Physiological consequences of hypohydration: exercise performance and thermoregulation.** *Med Sci Sports Exerc* 1992, **24**:657–670.
3. Barreca T, Franceschini R, Siani C, Cataldi A, Francaviglia N, Silvestro C, Rolandi E: **Metoclopramide increases plasma but not cerebrospinal fluid vasopressin levels in man: study in hydrocephalic patients.** *Horm Res* 1991, **35**:239–241.
4. Judelson DA, Maresh CM, Anderson JM, Armstrong LE, Casa DJ, Kraemer WJ, Volek JS: **Hydration and muscular performance: does fluid balance affect strength, power and high-intensity endurance?** *Sports Med* 2007, **37**:907–921.
5. Nose H, Morimoto T, Ogura K: **Distribution of water losses among fluid compartments of tissues under thermal dehydration in the rat.** *Jpn J Physiol* 1983, **33**:1019–1029.
6. Senay LC Jr, Pivarnik JM: **Fluid shifts during exercise.** *Exerc Sport Sci Rev* 1985, **13**:335–387.
7. Hudlicka O, Zweifach BW, Tyler KR: **Capillary recruitment and flow velocity in skeletal muscle after contractions.** *Microvasc Res* 1982, **23**:201–213.
8. Nygren AT, Greitz D, Kaijser L: **Changes in cross-sectional area in human exercising and non-exercising skeletal muscles.** *Eur J Appl Physiol* 2000, **81**:210–213.
9. Poortmans JR, Delescaille-Vanden BJ, Leclercq R: **Lactate uptake by inactive forearm during progressive leg exercise.** *J Appl Physiol* 1978, **45**:835–839.
10. Barr SI, Costill DL, Fink WJ: **Fluid replacement during prolonged exercise: effects of water, saline, or no fluid.** *Med Sci Sports Exerc* 1991, **23**:811–817.
11. Sanders B, Noakes TD, Dennis SC: **Sodium replacement and fluid shifts during prolonged exercise in humans.** *Eur J Appl Physiol* 2001, **84**:419–425.
12. Nose H, Mack GW, Shi XR, Nadel ER: **Shift in body fluid compartments after dehydration in humans.** *J Appl Physiol* 1988, **65**:318–324.
13. Sawka MN, Cheuvront SN, Carter R III: **Human water needs.** *Nutr Rev* 2005, **63**:S30–S39.

14. Sherman WM, Plyley MJ, Sharp RL, Van Handel PJ, McAllister RM, Fink WJ, Costill DL: **Muscle glycogen storage and its relationship with water.** *Int J Sports Med* 1982, **3:**22–24.
15. Olsson KE, Saltin B: **Variation in total body water with muscle glycogen changes in man.** *Acta Physiol Scand* 1970, **80:**11–18.
16. Costill DL, Cote R, Fink W: **Muscle water and electrolytes following varied levels of dehydration in man.** *J Appl Physiol* 1976, **40:**6–11.
17. Rauch HG, Hawley JA, Noakes TD, Dennis SC: **Fuel metabolism during ultra-endurance exercise.** *Pflugers Arch* 1998, **436:**211–219.
18. Ploutz-Snyder LL, Convertino VA, Dudley GA: **Resistance exercise-induced fluid shifts: change in active muscle size and plasma volume.** *Am J Physiol* 1995, **38:**R536–R543.
19. Lund H, Christensen L, Savnik A, Boesen J, Danneskiold-Samsoe B, Bliddal H: **Volume estimation of extensor muscles of the lower leg based on MR imaging.** *Eur Radiol* 2002, **12:**2982–2987.
20. Wirthwein DP, Spotswood SD, Barnard JJ, Prahlow JA: **Death due to microvascular occlusion in sickle-cell trait following physical exertion.** *J Forensic Sci* 2001, **46:**399–401.
21. Keys A, Brozek J: **Body fat in adult man.** *Physiol Rev* 1953, **33:**245–325.
22. Conley MS, Foley JM, Ploutz-Snyder LL, Meyer RA, Dudley GA: **Effect of acute head-down tilt on skeletal muscle cross-sectional area and proton transverse relaxation time.** *J Appl Physiol* 1996, **81:**1572–1577.
23. Convertino VA, Armstrong LE, Coyle EF, Mack GW, Sawka MN, Senay LC Jr, Sherman WM: **American College of Sports Medicine position stand. Exercise and fluid replacement.** *Med Sci Sports Exerc* 1996, **28:**i–vii.
24. Abramoff MD, Magelhaes PJ, Ram SJ: **Image processing with ImageJ.** *Biophot Intl* 2004, **11:**36–42.
25. Endo MY, Kobayakawa M, Kinugasa R, Kuno S, Akima H, Rossiter HB, Miura A, Fukuba Y: **Thigh muscle activation distribution and pulmonary VO2 kinetics during moderate, heavy, and very heavy intensity cycling exercise in humans.** *Am J Physiol Regul Integr Comp Physiol* 2007, **293:**R812–R820.
26. Richardson RS, Frank LR, Haseler LJ: **Dynamic knee-extensor and cycle exercise: functional MRI of muscular activity.** *Int J Sports Med* 1998, **19:**182–187.
27. Febbraio MA, Snow RJ, Stathis CG, Hargreaves M, Carey MF: **Effect of heat stress on muscle energy metabolism during exercise.** *J Appl Physiol* 1994, **77:**2827–2831.
28. Pastene J, Germain M, Allevard AM, Gharib C, Lacour JR: **Water balance during and after marathon running.** *Eur J Appl Physiol Occup Physiol* 1996, **73:**49–55.
29. Cheung SS, McLellan TM: **Influence of hydration status and fluid replacement on heat tolerance while wearing NBC protective clothing.** *Eur J Appl Physiol Occup Physiol* 1998, **77:**139–148.
30. McLellan TM, Cheung SS, Latzka WA, Sawka MN, Pandolf KB, Millard CE, Withey WR: **Effects of dehydration, hypohydration, and hyperhydration on tolerance during uncompensable heat stress.** *Can J Appl Physiol* 1999, **24:**349–361.
31. Hargreaves M, Dillo P, Angus D, Febbraio M: **Effect of fluid ingestion on muscle metabolism during prolonged exercise.** *J Appl Physiol* 1996, **80:**363–366.
32. Bergstrom J, Hultman E: **A study of the glycogen metabolism during exercise in man.** *Scand J Clin Lab Invest* 1967, **19:**218–228.
33. Li X, Pancera E, Zwirello L, Wu H, Zwick T: **Ultra wideband radar for water detection in the human body.** In *German Microwave Conference: 15-17 March 2010*. Berlin, NewYork: IEEE; 2010:150–153.
34. Gabriel S, Lau RW, Gabriel C: **The dielectric properties of biological tissues: III. Parametric models for the dielectric spectrum of tissues.** *Phys Med Biol* 1996, **41:**2271–2293.

Participation and performance trends in 'Ultraman Hawaii' from 1983 to 2012

Dimirela Meili[1], Beat Knechtle[1,2*], Christoph Alexander Rüst[1], Thomas Rosemann[1] and Romuald Lepers[3]

Abstract

Background: Participation and performance trends have been investigated in a single stage Ironman triathlon such as the 'Ironman Hawaii,' but not for a multi-stage ultra-triathlon such as the 'Ultraman Hawaii' covering a total distance of 515 km. The aims of this study were to analyze (1) changes in participation and performance, (2) sex-related differences in overall and split time performances, and (3) the age of peak performance in Ultraman Hawaii.

Methods: Age and race times including split times for 98 women and 570 men who successfully finished Ultraman Hawaii (day 1 with 10-km swimming and 145-km cycling, day 2 with 276-km cycling, and day 3 with 84-km running) between 1983 and 2012 were analyzed. Changes in variables over time of annual winners and annual top three women and men were investigated using simple linear regression analyses.

Results: The number of female finishers increased ($r^2 = 0.26$, $p < 0.01$), while the number of male finishers remained stable ($r^2 = 0.03$, $p > 0.05$). Overall race times decreased for both female ($r^2 = 0.28$, $p < 0.01$) and male ($r^2 = 0.14$, $p < 0.05$) winners and for both the annual top three women ($r^2 = 0.36$, $p < 0.01$) and men ($r^2 = 0.14$, $p = 0.02$). The sex difference in performance decreased over time from 24.3% to 11.5% ($r^2 = 0.39$, $p < 0.01$). For the split disciplines, the time performance in cycling on day 1 ($r^2 = 0.20$, $p < 0.01$) and day 2 decreased significantly for men ($r^2 = 0.41$, $p < 0.01$) but for women only on day 2 ($r^2 = 0.45$, $p < 0.01$). Split times showed no changes in swimming and running. The age of the annual winners increased from 28 to 47 years for men ($r^2 = 0.35$, $p < 0.01$) while it remained stable at 32 ± 6 years for women ($r^2 < 0.01$, $p > 0.05$). The age of the annual top three finishers increased from 33 ± 6 years to 48 ± 3 years for men ($p < 0.01$) and from 29 ± 7 years to 49 ± 2 years for women ($p < 0.01$).

Conclusions: Both the annual top three women and men improved performance in Ultraman Hawaii during the 1983–2012 period although the age of the annual top three women and men increased. The sex-related difference in performance decreased over time to reach approximately 12% similar to the reports of other endurance and ultra-endurance events. Further investigations are required to better understand the limiting factors of the multi-activities ultra-endurance events taking place over several days.

Keywords: Ultra-endurance, Swimming, Cycling, Running, Sex difference, Age, Triathlete

Background

Triathlon is an endurance athletic competition consisting of sequential and continuous swimming, cycling, and running events. Triathlon races commonly range from short-distance races such as the 'Olympic distance' of 1.5-km swimming, 40-km cycling, and 10-km running to long-distance races such as the 'Ironman distance' of 3.8-km swimming, 180-km cycling, and 42.2-km running [1]. Ultra-triathlons are of longer distances than the Ironman, such as the Double Iron ultra-triathlon distance of 7.6-km swimming, 360-km cycling, and 84.4-km running, the Triple Iron ultra-triathlon distance of 11.4-km swimming, 540-km cycling, and 126.6-km running, and the Deca Iron ultra-triathlon distance of 38-km swimming, 1,800-km cycling, and 420-km running [2].

During the past decade, participation increased in ultra-endurance races such as ultra-marathons [3,4] and ultra-triathlons [2,5]. Hoffman and Wegelin [3] reported an increase in starters between 1974 and 1986 in the

* Correspondence: beat.knechtle@hispeed.ch
[1]Institute of General Practice and for Health Services Research, University of Zurich, Pestalozzistrasse 24, Zurich 8091, Switzerland
[2]Facharzt FMH für Allgemeinmedizin, Gesundheitszentrum St. Gallen, Vadianstrasse 26, St. Gallen 9001, Switzerland
Full list of author information is available at the end of the article

'Western States 100-Mile Endurance Run,' with stable entries thereafter. Among the overall increase in participation, female participation increased from 10–12% in the late 1980s to 20–22% in 2001, where it remained to the present. Similar findings have been observed for 'Ironman Hawaii' [6]. Each year, more than 1,700 triathletes with approximately 27% women were participating in Ironman Hawaii, the Ironman triathlon World Championship held each year [6]. In triathlons longer than the Ironman distance, the percentage of women is lower. The number of female starters in Double Iron ultra-triathlon slightly increased in the last 10 years and counted for approximately 10%. For the Triple Iron ultra-triathlon distance and the Deca Iron ultra-triathlon distance, women starters were, from the beginning of the events, at 8% and 10%, respectively [2].

It has been suggested that women might outrun men with increasing length of an endurance performance [7-9]. Female ultra-marathoners improved performance over time [3]; however, a sex-related difference in performance still remained [10]. Indeed, men were faster than women, and longer distances were associated with greater sex-related differences in performance [8]. For example, men were approximately 19% faster than women in both a Double and Triple Iron ultra-triathlon, and approximately 30% faster in a Deca Iron ultra-triathlon [2]. Furthermore, the sex-related difference in overall race time for winners in a Triple Iron ultra-triathlon increased from 10% in 1992 to 42% in 2011 [11]. In triathlon, the sex-related difference in performance varied among the three locomotion modes. For example, the overall race times of the top ten men in Ironman Hawaii averaged 12.6% faster than those of the top ten women, but average swimming, cycling, and running times differed by 9.8%, 12.7%, and 13.3%, respectively [6]. Race distance might differentially affect the sex gap in the three locomotion modes [12].

Age has been reported as a limiting variable in endurance performance. Performance in endurance competitions such as marathon running decreased with increasing age [13]. Previous studies reported that peak endurance performance was maintained until the age of 30–35 years, followed by a moderate decline until the age of 50–60 years and then a progressively steeper decline after the age of 70–75 years, independent of the discipline and the length of the event [14,15]. The age of peak triathlon performance seemed to depend on the race distance. For example, in 'Ironman Switzerland' as a qualifier for Ironman Hawaii, the age of the top ten finishers was 25–39 years for women and 18–39 years for men [16]. Furthermore, in Ironman Hawaii, the age of the overall top ten finishers increased between 1983 and 2012 from 26 ± 5 years to 35 ± 5 years for women and from 27 ± 2 years to 34 ± 3 years for men [17]. In Triple Iron and Deca Iron ultra-triathlons, the age of peak performance has been found between 25 years and 44 years for men [18]. In addition, the mean age of male finishers appeared significantly higher for Deca Iron ultra-triathletes with 41.3 ± 3.1 years than for Triple Iron ultra-triathletes with 38.5 ± 3.3 years [18].

A few studies investigated participation and performance trends in ultra-endurance events held over different stages during several days, i.e., with rest between stages [19-21]. Apart of multi-stage races consisting in single disciplines such as the 'Tour de France' or the 'Vuelta a Espana' [22,23], a new kind of multi-stage ultra-endurance race was launched in 2006 for ultra-distance triathlon, the 'World Challenge Deca Iron Triathlon' [19,20] where athletes have to perform the daily distance of one Ironman triathlon of 3.8-km swimming, 180-km cycling, and 42.2-km running for ten consecutive days [21]. It was concluded that performance in a Deca Iron ultra-triathlon decreased throughout the competition, with the fastest race on day 1 and the slowest on day 10 [21].

In contrast to conventional ultra-triathlons held without stops between the three disciplines [2], the 'Ultraman' triathlon taking place in Hawaii as 'Ultraman Hawaii' is divided into three stages and is held over three days with a total distance close to a Double Iron ultra-triathlon distance [2] with 10-km swimming and 145-km cycling on day 1, 276-km cycling on day 2, and 84-km running on day 3. The first Ultraman Hawaii was held in 1983 [24]. The 'Ultraman Triathlon' is unique in the field and provides therefore an intriguing opportunity to examine the sex-related effects on performance in a multi-stage ultra-endurance event. Previous studies analyzed participation and performance trends in the Ironman distance triathlon [5,6], but no studies examined these trends in multi-stage ultra triathlons such as Ultraman Hawaii. Since both Ironman Hawaii and Ultraman Hawaii are of high interest for ultra-endurance athletes, participation and performance trends in Ultraman Hawaii need to be investigated and compared to existing findings for Ironman Hawaii.

Therefore, the aims of the present study were to examine (1) the participation and performance trends, (2) the sex-related difference in performance, and (3) the age of peak performance in Ultraman Hawaii during its 20 years of history. Race results from 1983–2012 were analyzed to test the hypotheses whether (1) the participation in women would increase over time, (2) the performance of both sexes would improve over time, (3) the sex-related differences in overall performance would decrease over time, and (4) the age of peak performance would increase over time.

Methods

The present study included all athletes who successfully finished Ultraman Hawaii between 1983 and 2012, excluding the years 1987 and 1991, where no races were held. Sex, age, and overall race time were obtained from the event website [24]. Data were available for a total of 671 athletes including 98 women (14.6%) and 573 men (85.4%). No information was given for the age for three men who started in 1998; therefore, they were excluded from the analysis. Ultimately, complete data with age and overall race times including split times for 98 women and 570 men who successfully finished Ultraman Hawaii between 1983 and 2012 were included in the analysis. All procedures used in the study met the ethical standards of the Swiss Academy of Medical Sciences [25] and were approved by the Institutional Review Board of Kanton St. Gallen, Switzerland (decision letter of 1 June 2010), with a waiver of the requirement for informed consent of the participants given the fact that the study involved the analysis of publicly available data.

The race

The annual edition of Ultraman Hawaii is limited to 40 athletes on an invitation-only basis and attracts participants from around the world. Participants must complete a 10-km open ocean swim, a 421-km cross-country non-drafting cycling, and an 84-km ultra-marathon. Each athlete has to be accompanied over the entire course by a support team of at least two persons. The events start around sunrise on each day. The swimming and first cycling events are held on day 1. Average water temperature for the open ocean swim is 21°C, and wetsuits are allowed. Following the swimming event, the participants have to cycle 145 km, with an elevation gain of approximately 2,500 m. On day 2, the participants cycle 276 km, with an elevation gain of approximately 2,600 m. On day 3, the athletes need to complete an 84-km ultra-marathon with an elevation gain of approximately 168.5 m. Each stage must be completed within 12 h.

Data analysis

Annual female and male winners (i.e., athletes with the fastest overall race time) and the annual overall top three women and men were analyzed to determine changes in the fastest overall race times and in the age of the fastest finishers during the 1983–2012 period. Participation and performance trends in the three split disciplines were analyzed only between 2001 and 2012 due to insufficient data in earlier years. The sex-related difference in performance was calculated using the equation ([race time in women] – [race time in men]) / [race time in men] × 100. The sex-related differences were transformed into absolute values prior to analysis. To calculate the mean sex-related difference in performance between the annual top three women and women, the differences for each pair (e.g., first man and first woman, second man and second woman, third man and third woman) were calculated separately and averaged. The age of the athletes was calculated by year of race – year of birth.

Statistical analysis

To optimize the reliability of data analysis, each set of data was tested for homogeneity of variances prior to statistical analysis, using Levene's test in cases of two groups and Bartlett's test in cases of more than two groups. Linear regression was used to determine the significance of changes in a variable (speed, age) across years. The variables between two groups were compared using unpaired *t* test. Statistical analyses were performed using IBM SPSS Statistics (Version 19, IBM SPSS, Chicago, IL, USA) and GraphPad Prism (Version 5, GraphPad Software, La Jolla, CA, USA). Statistical significance was accepted at $p < 0.05$ (two-sided for *t* tests). Data in the text are given as mean ± standard deviation (SD).

Results

Participation trends

Between 1983 and 2012, the annual number of male finishers in Ultraman Hawaii remained unchanged ($r^2 = 0.03$, $p > 0.05$), while the number of female finishers increased over time ($r^2 = 0.26$, $p < 0.01$) (Figure 1). The number of female finishers increased from three women (14% of the total field) in 1984 to seven women (26% of the total field) in 2012. The largest number of female finishers (26.5%) was in the age group of 35–39 years, while the largest number of male finishers (24%) was in the age group of 40–44 years. Athletes from 15 countries accounted for 93% of all finishes. The largest number of male finishers was achieved by participants from USA (48%), followed by participants from Japan, Germany, Canada, and Brazil (Figure 2). Most of the female finishers (54.7%) originated from the USA, followed by athletes from Puerto Rico, Japan, Canada, and Brazil.

Performance trends and sex difference in performance

For the annual winners, the overall race time decreased across years for both women ($r^2 = 0.28$, $p < 0.01$) and men ($r^2 = 0.14$, $p < 0.05$) (Figure 3). The sex-related difference in overall race time decreased from 24.3% in 1983 to 11.5% in 2012 ($r^2 = 0.16$, $p = 0.04$). When the top three finishers of each sex were considered, performance improved for both women ($r^2 = 0.36$, $p < 0.01$) and men ($r^2 = 0.14$, $p = 0.02$) (Figure 4). The sex-related difference in race time decreased over time ($r^2 = 0.39$, $p < 0.01$). Figure 5 presents the change in performance for swimming on day 1 (Figure 5A), cycling on day 1 (Figure 5B), cycling on day 2 (Figure 5C), and running on day 3 (Figure 5D). During the 2001–2012 period, the

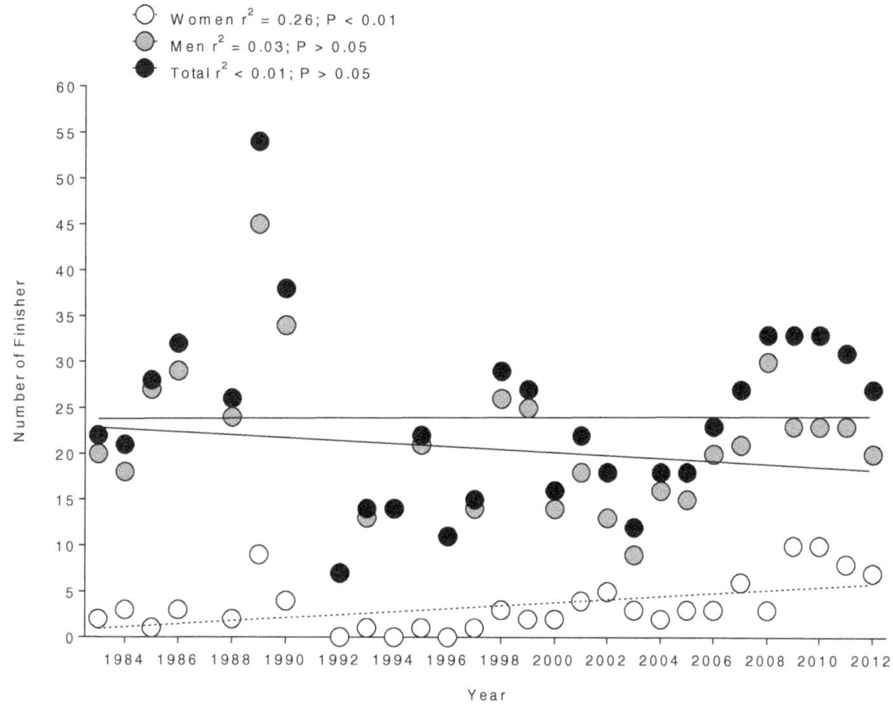

Figure 1 Changes in the annual number of male, female, and overall finishes in Ultraman Hawaii. From 1983 to 2012.

swim time on day 1 (Figure 5A) remained unchanged for the annual top three women (r^2 = 0.11, p > 0.05) and men (r^2 = 0.02, p > 0.05). However, the sex difference in swimming performance decreased (r^2 = 0.13, p = 0.04). The cycling time on day 1 (Figure 5B) showed no change for women (r^2 = 0.02, p > 0.05) but decreased in men (r^2 = 0.20, p < 0.01). The sex difference in cycling performance decreased significantly by 1.4% *per annum* (r^2 = 0.28, p < 0.01). In contrast, the cycling time on day 2 (Figure 5C) decreased over time from 632 ± 50 min to

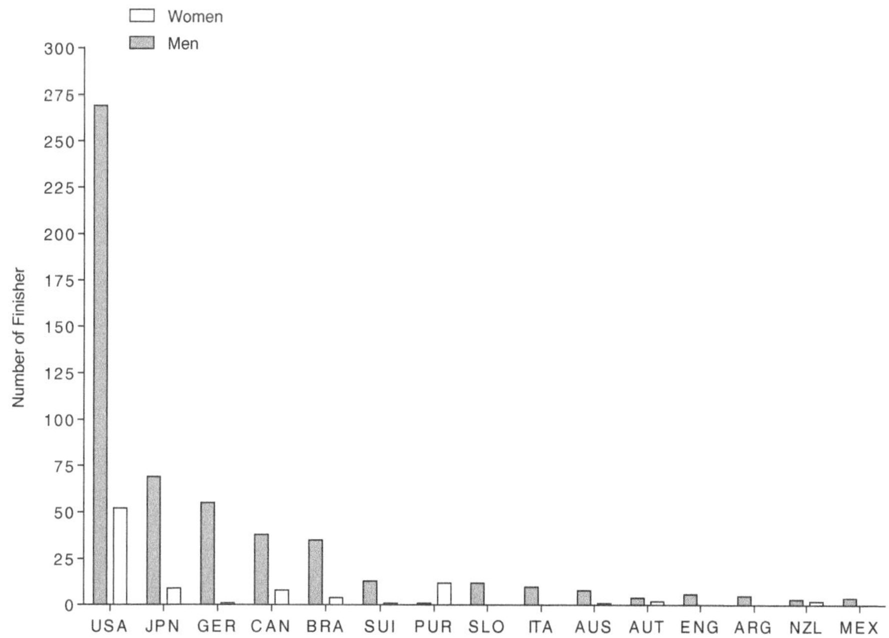

Figure 2 Number of male and female finishes per country in Ultraman Hawaii between 1983 and 2012. The frame indicates the 15 countries with the highest number of male and female finishes. Athletes from these 15 countries accounted for 92.7% of all finishers.

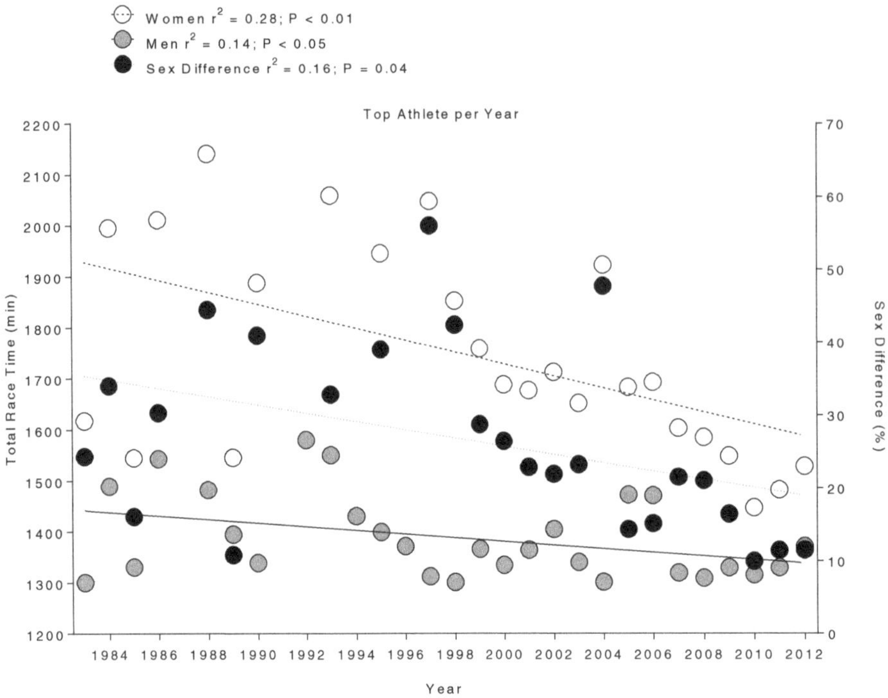

Figure 3 **Changes in overall race time with sex difference of the annual top women and men from 1983 to 2012.**

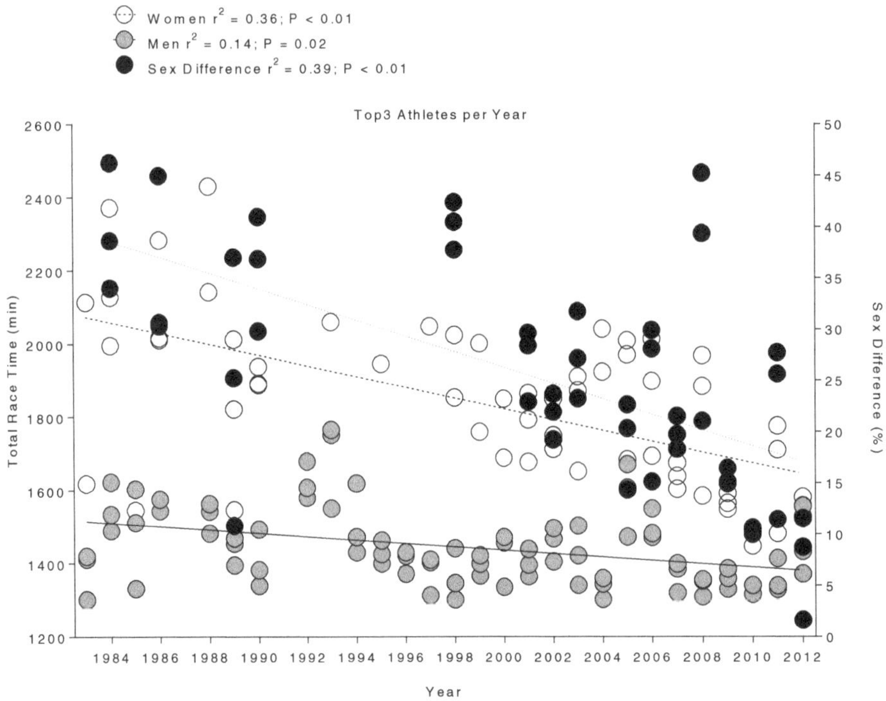

Figure 4 **Changes in overall race time with sex difference of the annual top three women and men from 1983 to 2012.** Values are means ± SD.

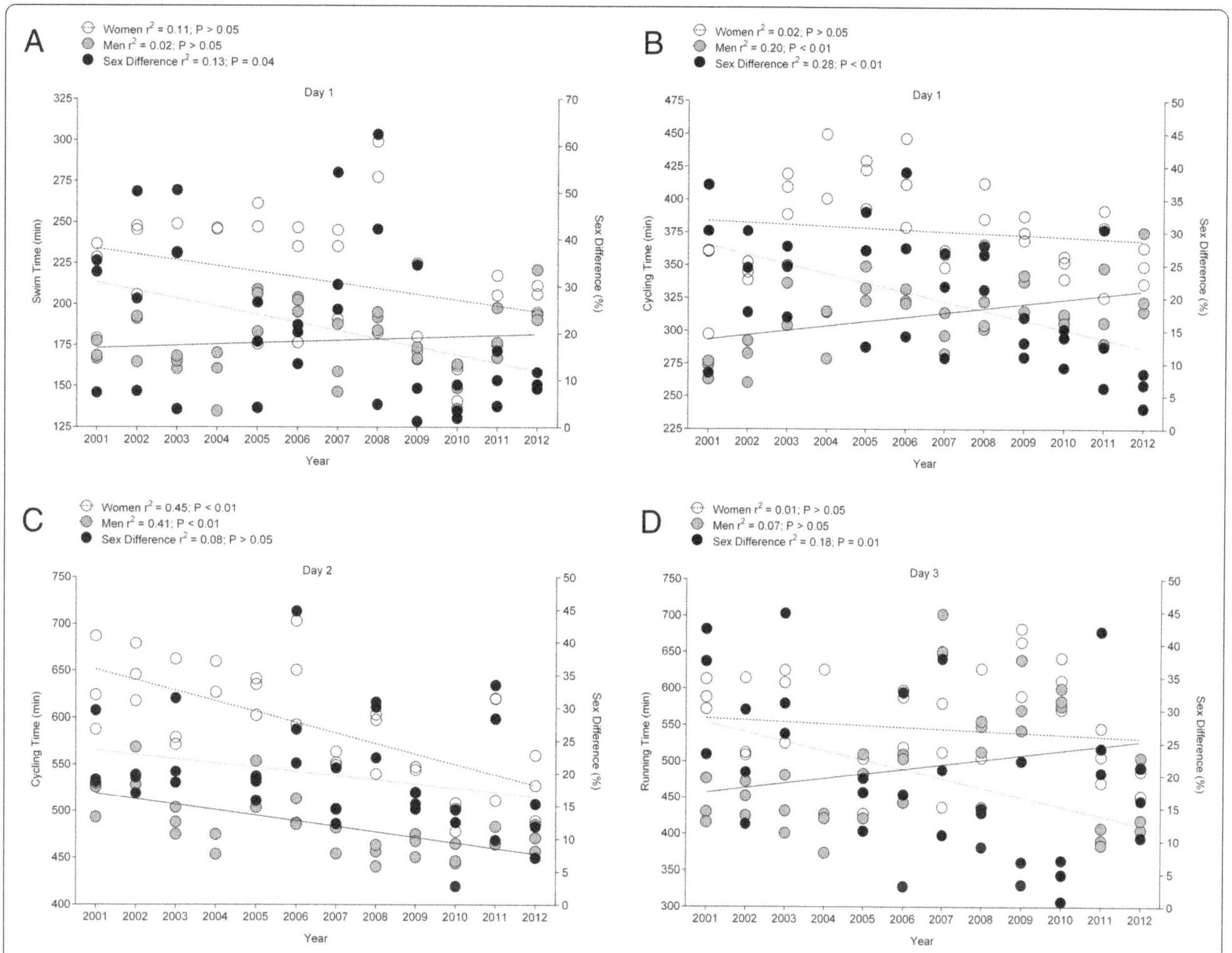

Figure 5 Changes in performance during the three days. Panel **A**: Swim time on Day 1, Panel **B**: Cycling time on Day 1, Panel **C**: Cycling time on Day 2, Panel **D**: Running time on Day 3 and corresponding sex difference of the annual top three women and men from 2001 to 2012. Values are means ± SD.

525 ± 35 min for women (r^2 = 0.45, $p < 0.01$) and from 516 ± 20 min to 471 ± 14 min for men (r^2 = 0.41, $p < 0.01$), while the sex differences remained stable (r^2 = 0.08, $p > 0.05$). On day 2, women improved cycling performance by 11 min and men by 6 min *per annum*. For the marathon on day 3 (Figure 5D), sex difference decreased (r^2 = 0.18, p = 0.01), but running time showed no change for both women (r^2 = 0.01, $p > 0.05$) and men (r^2 = 0.07, $p > 0.05$).

Age of peak performance

The mean age of overall finishers was lower for women with 32 ± 5 years compared to men with 35 ± 6 years ($p < 0.001$). The age of the annual winners increased from 28 to 47 years (r^2 = 0.35, $p < 0.01$) for men, while it remained stable at 32 ± 6 years ($r^2 < 0.01$, $p > 0.05$) for women (Figure 6). The age of the annual top three finishers increased from 33 ± 6 years to 48 ± 3 years for men (r^2 = 0.32, $p < 0.01$) and from 29 ± 7 years to 49 ± 2 years for women (r^2 = 0.11, $p < 0.01$) (Figure 7).

Discussion

The aims of the present study were to examine (1) trends in participation and performance, (2) the sex-related differences in performance, and (3) the age of peak performance in Ultraman Hawaii between 1983 and 2012. The main findings were (1) the number of female finishers increased over time, (2) overall race times of the annual winners and the annual three fastest finishers decreased over time for both women and men, (3) the sex-related difference in performance decreased over time, and (4) the age of the annual three fastest women and men increased over time.

Participation trends

The results of the present study supported the hypothesis that the number of female finishers in Ultraman Hawaii increased during 1983–2012, while the number of male finishers remained relatively constant. The number of female finishers in ultra-endurance events generally

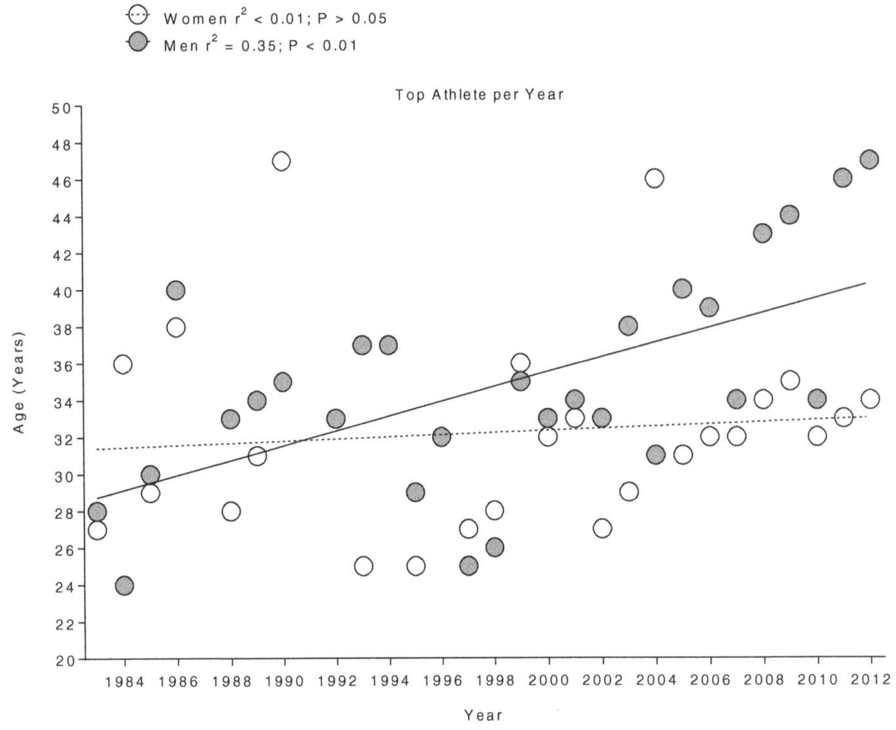

Figure 6 Changes in the age of the annual top women and men from 1983 to 2012.

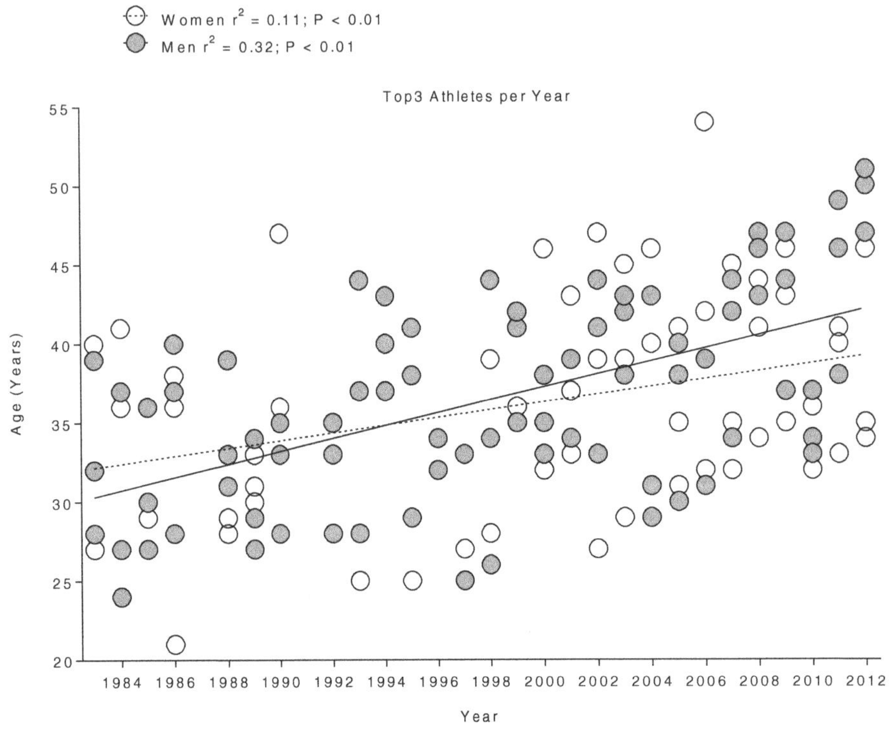

Figure 7 Changes in the age of the annual top three women and men from 1983 to 2012. Values are means ± SD.

increased over time, as is evident in Ultraman Hawaii with two female participants in 1983 and seven in 2012, as well as in Ironman Hawaii with 20 female participants in 1981 and more than 450 in 2007, respectively [6]. The reasons for the increase in female participation are not clear, but sociological phenomena such as an increased focus on physical fitness and on the positive influence of healthy living on longevity might be potential explanations [26]. For female ultra-marathoners, the strongest sources of motivation were health and personal achievement [27]. Men, on the other side, rather search for competition and try to reach high rankings. Lombardo suggested that sport began as a way for men to develop the skills needed in primitive hunting and warfare, then developed to act primarily as a competition where athletes display and male spectators evaluate the qualities of potential allies and rivals [28]. Successful ultra-endurance performance is characterized by the ability to sustain a higher absolute speed for a given distance than other competitors [29]. Hunter and Stevens [30] reported for marathoners that the greater sex difference in velocity occurring with age and lower performance was primarily explained by the lower number of female finishers compared to male finishers. These data provided evidence that a lower participation among female competitors could amplify the sex difference in running velocity above that due to physiological sex difference alone. In Ultraman Hawaii, the largest number of finishers originated from the USA, probably because long triathlons offered worldwide provide athletes from Europe and other parts of the world the opportunity to participate without having to travel such long distances [31].

Changes in overall performance

Overall race time for both sexes decreased significantly during 1983–2012, supporting our second hypothesis. The improvement in performance over time by both sexes in Ultraman Hawaii might be related to an increase in participation in ultra-triathlon events. The increasing number of athletes was probably due to improvements in training, nutrition, and experience-related pacing strategies [6]. During the last century, there has been a continuous decrease in performance times in different sports disciplines such as track and field and swimming [32,33]. Previous experience seemed to play an important role in ultra-endurance performance. Overall race time in a Triple Iron ultra-triathlon was more closely associated with personal best time in previous ultra-triathlons than with anthropometry or training [34]. Race time in a Deca Iron ultra-triathlon was also more closely related to the number of finished Triple Iron ultra-triathlons and personal best time than to anthropometric characteristics [21]. Considering these findings, the number of successfully finished Triple Iron ultra-triathlons and a fast personal best time in Triple Iron ultra-triathlon might reflect pre-race training volume and experience, where athletes with a higher training volume might compete faster in a longer ultra-triathlon than athletes with a lower training volume and less experience.

Changes in sex-related differences in performance

The sex-related difference in overall performance for both the top three athletes and the annual winners decreased over time. The annual top three women and men improved cycling time. The sex difference in performance decreased for day 1 annually by 1.4%. On day 2, both women and men became faster over time, but the sex difference in performance remained unchanged. Female athletes performed by 11 min faster *per annum*, while male by 6 min *per annum*. One third of the Ultraman Hawaii distance consists of cycling, so this mode of locomotion has a strong influence on overall race time. Cycling technology has improved consistently since 1981 [35], probably contributing to improved performance by both sexes in the cycling portion of the race. Based on the single top finishers and the top three finishers of each sex, men consistently performed better than women in Ultraman Hawaii.

Long-distance events were generally associated with large sex-related differences in performance [4,8,11,36]. Men were physically stronger and had greater aerobic capacity than women [37]. Men also tended to have stronger ego involvement in athletic competitions than women [38]. Female ultra-marathoners were more task-orientated than ego-orientated and set goals other than winning [27]. Deaner [39] and Deaner and Mitchell [40] argued that the ultimate benefit of studying sex differences in enduring competitiveness from an evolutionary perspective is not to support an essentialist position. The payoff, instead, should be improved in the understanding of the various factors that affect long-term achievement motivation. Deaner showed the importance of sex but also highlighted that motivation should be modulated by whether achievement in the domain yields status or resources and whether one perceives that they possess talent in the domain [39]. In particular, men should be relatively more motivated to achieve in context where their talent allows them to compete for status whereas women would be relatively more likely to compete for resources.

Previous studies investigating performance in ultra-triathlons showed that changes in male and female performance varied among the three locomotion modes. In Ironman Hawaii, for example, the sex-related difference remained stable in swimming (+0.1% per decade), increased slightly in cycling (+0.8% per decade), and decreased in running (−2.8% per decade) between 1981 and 2007 [6]. Rüst et al. showed that for Ironman Hawaii from 1983 to 2012, the sex differences decreased over years for overall race time and running but not for swimming and cycling [17]. Sex-related differences in running were predicted to diminish as distance increases beyond the marathon [7] because women have greater fat stores and an improved fat metabolism compared to men and should be more fatigue-resistant than male athletes during ultra distances [41]. In Ultraman Hawaii, running performance during day 3 is the last part of this multi-stage event. During the day, the temperature may increase up to 30°C in Hawaii [42]. Presumably, the athletes might have had only little reserves left for the run after two races of racing. The training and previous experience might provide the athletes with the empirical knowledge to select the optimal pacing strategy with the ability to maintain race pace [21]. During multi-stage races such as Tour the France and Vuelta de Espana [22,23], race intensity is rather high. Rodríguez-Marroyo et al. showed that experienced athletes modulated the intensity of each stage due to the total race duration [23]. Ironman triathletes have a special strategy during the cycling phase dependent upon the wind [43]. In a multi-stage triathlon such as Ultraman Hawaii, a specific pacing strategy is needed including also the aspect of recovery and nutrition between the stages [20,21].

The age of peak performance

The results of the present study only partly supported the hypothesis that the average age of finishers increased over time. The age of the annual top male finishers increased, while the age of annual top female finishers showed no changes. It must be stated that the increase in the age of the male winner across years was not due to the same athlete. Several different athletes were able to win Ultraman Hawaii [24]. Considering the annual top three finishers, age increased in both women and men. Participation in master athletes in triathlons [44] and ultra-triathlons [5,44,45] increased over the last two decades, so it was not surprising that the mean age increased in finishers. Master athletes were generally defined by the age at which the world record in open elite sport peaks, typically older than 35–40 years [46]. The lack of a comparable increase in the age of female finishers over time might be attributable to the small number of female finishers over 40 years of age or to a low number of female master athletes in general. Overall, the decline in athletic performance with age was greater in women than in men [47]. The age-related decrease in maximal oxygen uptake seemed to be the most consistent contributor to the decline in endurance performance with advancing age, and age-related reduction in lactate threshold might also be important [48]. One reason for the increase in the age of peak performance could be the increasing importance in training and competition strategies [49] as the number of competitors was growing in endurance sport events [2-6,50]. Another reason for the increasing age of peak performance might be the popularity of Ultraman Hawaii, which attracted more athletes and especially more master athletes in recent years.

Limitations of the present study and practical applications

The major limitation of the present study is the small number of participants (maximum of 40 invited athletes per year) and finishers in the Ultraman Hawaii. This is especially true for female participants who have never made up more than 26% of the total group. The inclusion of individual participants who finished in more than 1 year probably did not strongly influence the results. Another limitation was the lack of information about performance-related factors such as training [34,37], motivation [27], nutrition [20,51,52], fluid metabolism [53,54], previous experience [21,34], weather [55], equipment [35,56], and anthropometry [57,58] of individual participants, which could significantly affect individual performance and overall strength of the athlete. We did not check for disqualification of athletes due to doping. One athlete was disqualified in 1998 due to unsportsmanlike conduct. For practical applications, the fastest finishers improved performance, and the age of the fastest finishers increased in Ultraman Hawaii as has also been found in Ironman Hawaii [59]. However, the fastest finishers in Ironman Hawaii seemed younger than the fastest finishers in Ultraman Hawaii [59]. The upper limits in the age of peak performance in both Ironman Hawaii and Ultraman Hawaii seemed not reached for both women and men.

Conclusions

The number of female finishers in Ultraman Hawaii increased, while the number of male finishers remained unchanged between 1983 and 2012. Performance by both sexes improved over time, but men remained faster than women. The sex-related difference in overall performance decreased over time from 24.3% to 11.5%. The age of peak performance was higher for men than for women and it increased for both the fastest women and the fastest men. Further investigations are required to better understand the limiting factors of the multi-activities ultra-endurance events taking place over several days.

Competing interests
The authors declare that they have no competing interests.

Authors' contributions

All authors designed the study. The manuscript was written by all authors. All authors read and approved the final manuscript.

Acknowledgement

The authors thank the race director of Ultraman Hawaii for providing all race data. This research received no grant from any funding agency in the public, commercial, or not-for-profit sectors.

Author details

[1]Institute of General Practice and for Health Services Research, University of Zurich, Pestalozzistrasse 24, Zurich 8091, Switzerland. [2]Facharzt FMH für Allgemeinmedizin, Gesundheitszentrum St. Gallen, Vadianstrasse 26, St. Gallen 9001, Switzerland. [3]INSERM U1093, Faculty of Sport Sciences, University of Burgundy, UFR STAPS, BP 27877, Dijon Cedex 21078, France.

References

1. Bentley DJ, Millet GP, Vleck VE, McNaughton LR: **Specific aspects of contemporary triathlon: implications for physiological analysis and performance.** *Sports Med* 2002, **32**:345–359.
2. Knechtle B, Knechtle P, Lepers R: **Participation and performance trends in ultra-triathlons from 1985 to 2009.** *Scand J Med Sci Sports* 2011, **21**:e82–e90.
3. Hoffman MD, Wegelin JA: **The Western States 100-mile endurance run: participation and performance trends.** *Med Sci Sports Exerc* 2009, **41**:2191–2198.
4. Hoffman MD: **Performance trends in 161-km ultramarathons.** *Int J Sports Med* 2010, **31**:31–37.
5. Lepers R, Rüst CA, Stapley PJ, Knechtle B: **Relative improvements in endurance performance with age: evidence from 25 years of Hawaii Ironman racing.** *Age (Dordr)* 2013, **35**(3):953–962.
6. Lepers R: **Analysis of Hawaii ironman performances in elite triathletes from 1981 to 2007.** *Med Sci Sports Exerc* 2008, **40**:1828–1834.
7. Bam J, Noakes TD, Juritz J, Dennis SC: **Could women outrun men in ultramarathon races?** *Med Sci Sports Exerc* 1997, **29**:244–247.
8. Coast JR, Blevins JS, Wilson BA: **Do gender differences in running performance disappear with distance?** *Can J Appl Physiol* 2004, **29**:139–145.
9. Beneke R, Leithauser RM, Doppelmayr M: **Women will do it in the long run.** *Br J Sports Med* 2005, **39**:410.
10. Knechtle B, Rüst CA, Rosemann T, Lepers R: **Age-related changes in 100-km ultra-marathon running performance.** *Age (Dordr)* 2012, **34**:1033–1045.
11. Lepers R, Maffluletti NA: **Age and gender interactions in ultraendurance performance: insight from the triathlon.** *Med Sci Sports Exerc* 2011, **43**:134–139.
12. Rüst CA, Knechtle B, Knechtle P, Rosemann T, Lepers R: **Participation and performance trends in triple iron ultra-triathlon-a cross-sectional and longitudinal data analysis.** *Asian J Sports Med* 2012, **3**:145–152.
13. Leyk D, Erley O, Ridder D, Leurs M, Ruther T, Wunderlich M, Sievert A, Baum K, Essfeld D: **Age-related changes in marathon and half-marathon performances.** *Int J Sports Med* 2007, **28**:513–517.
14. Wright VJ, Perricelli BC: **Age-related rates of decline in performance among elite senior athletes.** *Am J Sports Med* 2008, **36**:443–450.
15. Baker AB, Tang YQ, Turner MJ: **Percentage decline in masters superathlete track and field performance with aging.** *Exp Aging Res* 2003, **29**:47–65.
16. Knechtle B, Rüst, Rosemann T, Lepers R: **Age and gender differences in half-ironman triathlon performances-the ironman 70.3 Switzerland from 2007 to 2010.** *Open Access J Sports Med* 2012, **3**:59–66.
17. Rüst C, Knechtle B, Rosemann T, Lepers R: **Sex difference in race performance and age of peak performance in the ironman triathlon world championship from 1983 to 2012.** *Extreme Physiology & Med* 2012, **1**:15.
18. Knechtle B, Rust C, Knechtle P, Rosemann T, Lepers R: **Age-related changes in ultra-triathlon performances.** *Extreme Physiology & Med* 2012, **1**:5.
19. Knechtle B, Knechtle P, Andonie JL, Kohler G: **Influence of anthropometry on race performance in extreme endurance triathletes: world challenge deca iron triathlon 2006.** *Br J Sports Med* 2007, **41**:644–648.
20. Knechtle B, Knechtle P, Schèck R, Andonie JL, Kohler G: **Effects of a deca iron triathlon on body composition: a case study.** *Int J Sports Med* 2008, **29**:343–351.
21. Herbst L, Knechtle B, Lopez CL, Andonie JL, Fraire OS, Kohler G, Rüst CA, Rosemann T: **Pacing strategy and change in body composition during a deca iron triathlon.** *Chin J Physiol* 2011, **54**:255–263.
22. Lucia A, Hoyos J, Santalla A, Earnest C, Chicharro JL: **Tour de France versus Vuelta a Espana: which is harder?** *Med Sci Sports Exerc* 2003, **35**:872–878.
23. Rodríguez-Marroyo JA, García-López J, Juneau C-É, Villa JG: **Workload demands in professional multi-stage cycling races of varying duration.** *Br J Sports Med* 2009, **43**:180–185.
24. Ultraman World Championships Hawaii: http://ultramanlive.com.
25. Swiss Academy of Medical Sciences: www.samw.ch/en/Ethics/Guidelines/Currently-valid-guidelines.html.
26. Lee MS, Tanaka K: **Significance of health fitness appraisal in an aging society.** *Appl Human Sci* 1997, **16**:123–131.
27. Krouse RZ, Ransdell LB, Lucas SM, Pritchard ME: **Motivation, goal orientation, coaching, and training habits of women ultrarunners.** *J Strength Cond Res* 2011, **25**:2835–2842.
28. Lombardo MP: **On the evolution of sport.** *Evol Psychol* 2012, **10**:1–28.
29. Zaryski C, Smith DJ: **Training principles and issues for ultra-endurance athletes.** *Curr Sports Med Rep* 2005, **4**:165–170.
30. Hunter SK, Stevens AA: **Sex differences in marathon running with advanced age: physiology or participation?** *Med Sci Sports Exerc* 2012, **45**:148–156.
31. Jeffery S, Knechtle B, Rüst CA, Knechtle P, Rosemann T, Lepers R: **European dominance in Triple Iron ultra-triathlons from 1988 to 2011.** *J Sci Cycling* 2012, **1**:30–38.
32. Berthelot G, Len S, Hellard P, Tafflet M, Guillaume M, Vollmer JC, Gager B, Quinquis L, Marc A, Toussaint JF: **Exponential growth combined with exponential decline explains lifetime performance evolution in individual and human species.** *Age (Dordr)* 2012, **34**:1001–1009.
33. Schulz R, Curnow C: **Peak performance and age among superathletes: track and field, swimming, baseball, tennis, and golf.** *J Gerontol* 1988, **43**:P113–P120.
34. Knechtle B, Knechtle P, Rosemann T, Senn O: **Personal best time, not anthropometry or training volume, is associated with total race time in a triple iron triathlon.** *J Strength Cond Res* 2011, **25**:1142–1150.
35. Faria EW, Parker DL, Faria IE: **The science of cycling: factors affecting performance - part 2.** *Sports Med* 2005, **35**:313–337.
36. Knoth C, Knechtle B, Rust CA, Rosemann T, Lepers R: **Participation and performance trends in multistage ultramarathons–the 'Marathon des Sables' 2003–2012.** *Extreme Physiology & Med* 2012, **1**:13.
37. Knechtle B, Wirth A, Baumann B, Knechtle P, Rosemann T, Oliver S: **Differential correlations between anthropometry, training volume, and performance in male and female Ironman triathletes.** *J Strength Cond Res* 2010, **24**:2785–2793.
38. Hanrahan SJ, Cerin E: **Gender, level of participation, and type of sport: differences in achievement goal orientation and attributional style.** *J Sci Med Sport* 2009, **12**:508–512.
39. Deaner RO. **Distance running as an ideal domain for showing a sex difference in competitiveness.** *Arch Sex Behav* 2013, **42**(3):413-28.
40. Deaner RO, Mitchell D: **More men run relatively fast in U.S. road races, 1981–2006: a stable sex difference in non-elite runners.** *Evol Psychol* 2011, **9**:600–621.
41. Tarnopolsky MA: **Gender differences in substrate metabolism during endurance exercise.** *Can J Appl Physiol* 2000, **25**:312–327.
42. Hawaii Weather Today: www.hawaiiweathertoday.com.
43. Abbiss CR, Quod MJ, Martin DT, Netto KJ, Nosaka K, Lee H, Surriano R, Bishop D, Laursen PB: **Dynamic pacing strategies during the cycle phase of an ironman triathlon.** *Med Sci Sports Exerc* 2006, **38**:726–734.
44. Lepers R, Sultana F, Bernard T, Hausswirth C, Brisswalter J: **Age-related changes in triathlon performances.** *Int J Sports Med* 2010, **31**:251–256.
45. Stiefel M, Knechtle B, Lepers R: **Master triathletes have not reached limits in their Ironman triathlon performance.** *Scand J Med Sci Sports* 2012. 10.1111/j.1600-0838.2012.01473.x.
46. Ransdell LB, Vener J, Huberty J: **Masters athletes: an analysis of running, swimming and cycling performance by age and gender.** *J Exerc Sci Fit* 2009, **7**:S61–S73.
47. Tanaka H, Seals DR: **Invited review: dynamic exercise performance in masters athletes: insight into the effects of primary human aging on physiological functional capacity.** *J Appl Physiol* 2003, **95**:2152–2162.

48. Tanaka H, Seals DR: **Endurance exercise performance in masters athletes: age-associated changes and underlying physiological mechanisms.** *J Physiol* 2008, **586:**55–63.
49. Knechtle B, Wirth A, Rosemann T: **Predictors of race time in male ironman triathletes: physical characteristics, training, or prerace experience?** *Percept Mot Skills* 2010, **111:**437–446.
50. Lepers R, Cattagni T: **Do older athletes reach limits in their performance during marathon running?** *Age (Dordr)* 2012, **34:**773–781.
51. Robins A: **Nutritional recommendations for competing in the ironman triathlon.** *Curr Sports Med Rep* 2007, **6:**241–248.
52. Jeukendrup AE, Jentjens RL, Moseley L: **Nutritional considerations in triathlon.** *Sports Med* 2005, **35:**163–181.
53. Rüst CA, Knechtle B, Knechtle P, Rosemann T: **Higher prevalence of exercise-associated hyponatremia in triple iron ultra-triathletes than reported for ironman triathletes.** *Chin J Physiol* 2012, **55:**147–155.
54. Knechtle B, Knechtle P, Rosemann T, Oliver S: **A triple iron triathlon leads to a decrease in total body mass but not to dehydration.** *Res Q Exerc Sport* 2010, **81:**319–327.
55. Wegelin JA, Hoffman MD: **Variables associated with odds of finishing and finish time in a 161-km ultramarathon.** *Eur J Appl Phyiol* 2011, **111:**145–153.
56. O'Connor LM, Vozenilek JA: **Is it the athlete or the equipment? An analysis of the top swim performances from 1990 to 2010.** *J Strength Cond Res* 2011, **25:**3239–3241.
57. Knechtle B, Knechtle P, Rosemann T, Senn O: **Personal best time and training volume, not anthropometry, is related to race performance in the 'Swiss Bike Masters' mountain bike ultramarathon.** *J Strength Cond Res* 2011, **25:**1312–1317.
58. Knechtle B, Wirth A, Baumann B, Knechtle P, Rosemann T: **Personal best time, percent body fat, and training are differently associated with race time for male and female ironman triathletes.** *Res Q Exerc Sport* 2010, **81:**62–68.
59. Gallmann D, Knechtle B, Rüst CA, Rosemann T, Lepers R: **Elite triathletes in 'Ironman Hawaii' get older but faster.** *Age (Dordr)* 2013. 10.1007/s11357-013-9534-y.

Participation and performance trends in ultra-endurance running races under extreme conditions - 'Spartathlon' versus 'Badwater'

Kristina da Fonseca-Engelhardt[1], Beat Knechtle[2,4*], Christoph Alexander Rüst[1], Patrizia Knechtle[2], Romuald Lepers[3] and Thomas Rosemann[1]

Abstract

Background: The aim of the present study was to compare the trends in participation, performance and age of finishers in 'Badwater' and 'Spartathlon' as two of the toughest ultramarathons in the world of more than 200 km of distance.

Methods: Running speed and age of male and female finishers in Badwater and Spartathlon were analyzed from 2000 to 2012. Age of peak performance and sex difference in running speed were investigated during the studied period.

Results: The number of female and male finishes increased in Badwater and Spartathlon. Women accounted on average for 21.5% ± 6.9% in Badwater and 10.8% ± 2.3% in Spartathlon. There was a significant increase in female participation in Badwater from 18.4% to 19.1% ($p < 0.01$) and in Spartathlon from 11.9% to 12.5% ($p = 0.02$). In men, the age of finishers was higher in Badwater (46.5 ± 9.3 years) compared to Spartathlon (44.8 ± 8.2 years) ($p < 0.01$). The age of female finishers of both races was similar with 43.0 ± 7.5 years in Badwater and 44.5 ± 7.8 years in Spartathlon ($p > 0.05$). Over the years, the age of the annual five fastest men decreased in Badwater from 42.4 ± 4.2 to 39.8 ± 5.7 years ($p < 0.05$). For women, the age remained unchanged at 42.3 ± 3.8 years in Badwater ($p > 0.05$). In Spartathlon, the age was unchanged at 39.7 ± 2.4 years for men and 44.6 ± 3.2 years for women ($p > 0.05$). In Badwater, women and men became faster over the years. The running speed increased from 7.9 ± 0.7 to 8.7 ± 0.6 km/h ($p < 0.01$) in men and from 5.4 ± 1.1 to 6.6 ± 0.5 km/h ($p < 0.01$) in women. The sex difference in running speed remained unchanged at 19.8% ± 4.8% ($p > 0.05$). In Spartathlon, the running speed was stable over time at 10.8 ± 0.7 km/h for men and 8.7 ± 0.5 km/h for women ($p > 0.05$). The sex difference remained unchanged at 19.6% ± 2.5% ($p > 0.05$).

Conclusions: These results suggest that for both Badwater and Spartathlon, (a) female participation increased, (b) the fastest finishers were approximately 40 to 45 years, and (c) the sex difference was at approximately 20% Women will not outrun men in both Badwater and Spartathlon races. Master ultramarathoners can achieve a high level of performance in ultramarathons greater than 200 km under extreme conditions.

Keywords: Running, Ultra-endurance, Extreme conditions, Age, Sex differences

* Correspondence: beat.knechtle@hispeed.ch
[2]Gesundheitszentrum St. Gallen, St. Gallen 9000, Switzerland
[4]Facharzt FMH für Allgemeinmedizin, Gesundheitszentrum St. Gallen, Vadianstrasse 26, St. Gallen 9001, Switzerland
Full list of author information is available at the end of the article

Background

In the past two decades, the field of ultra-endurance events defined as performance exceeding 6 h [1] has widened to a new arena in the sport of long-distance performances in particular ultra-running [2-4] and ultra-triathlon [5-7]. Today, more than a hundred thousand of ultramarathoners compete in more than a thousand races held annually around the world [8].

In recent years, the growth of ultra-endurance sports has drawn increased attention to investigate participation and performance trends [2,9,10]. A major focus of research in endurance sports was the sex difference in performance [11]. In the analysis of the world's best times of female marathoners from 1980 to 1996, women were approximately 11% slower than men, although there was initially a considerable improvement in female running speed in the 1980s [12]. A similar sex difference for running speed has been found when running times between 100 m and 200 km were compared. Women were generally running approximately 12.4% slower than men [13]. In 160-km ultramarathons, the performance of the fastest women remained approximately 20% slower than that of the fastest men after an initial improvement relative to men throughout the 1980s [2]. In the shorter 100-km distance in the '100 km Lauf Biel', the running times of the annual top ten finishers remained stable from 1998 to 2010 for women, while running times significantly increased for the annual top ten men [10]. The trend in sex difference was narrowing over time and averaged to 22% [10].

In both endurance and ultra-endurance events, a high-level performance seemed to be maintained until the age of 30 to 40 years, followed by a modest decrease until the age of 50 to 60 years, with a progressively accelerated decline after the age of 70 to 75 years [14-22]. The study of Hoffman [9] showed that peak running speed of the top performers in a 161-km ultramarathon was achieved by athletes in the age of upper 30 to 40 years. These results suggested an age shift into higher age in elite ultramarathon running in comparison with elite marathon running, where the fastest running speed were achieved by athletes of approximately 30 years of age [19].

Among the ultra-running events, the 'Badwater' [23] in the USA and the 'Spartathlon' [24] in Greece, Europe are recognized as two of the toughest running events worldwide. The common feature of both nonstop races is the distance of more than 200 km. The Badwater is characterized by its environmental conditions with extreme high temperatures and large altitude differences to overcome, while the Spartathlon is well known for its cut-off regulations with strict time limitations, apart from its unique historical background. To date, no study investigated the participation and running speed of female and male ultramarathoners competing in races longer than 200 km under extreme conditions such as heat and time limit. Therefore, the aims of the present study were to investigate (1) participation and performance trends and (2) the age of peak running speed in ultramarathons of more than 200-km race distance. Based upon present findings, we hypothesized (1) an increase in participation and an improvement in performance and (2) an age of peak ultramarathon performance between 30 and 40 years.

Methods

The data set for this study was obtained from the race websites of Badwater [23] and Spartathlon [24]. Running speed and age of all female and male finishers in Badwater and Spartathlon between 2000 and 2012 were analyzed. The study was approved by the Institutional Review Board of St. Gallen, Switzerland, with waiver of the requirement for informed consent given that the study involved the analysis of publicly available data.

Badwater

The event was established as an official foot race in 1987 with five successful US participants. Since 1989, the race starts at Badwater, the lowest elevation in the Western Hemisphere at 85 m below sea level and finishes at the Mt. Whitney Portals at nearly 2,530 m. Badwater covers a total distance of 217 km (135 miles) of highway non-stop across the Death Valley in California, USA. The course includes a total of 3,962 m of cumulative vertical ascent and 1,433 m of cumulative descent. During the race in Death Valley in mid-July, the average daily high temperature reaches 46.9°C, and temperatures over 50°C are common [25]. No aid stations are provided along the Badwater course, so runners rely on their own support crew to pass across the Death Valley. The number of participants is limited to 90 competitors.

Spartathlon

The Spartathlon starting in 1982 is a nonstop foot race covering a total distance of 246 km (152 miles) from Athens to Sparta in Greece, Europe. Since 1983, the race has been continuously held each September. The course includes elevations which range from sea level to 1,200 m. The cumulative gain of elevations is approximately 1,650 m and the route runs on tarmac road, trail, or mountain footpath. The weather conditions during the race are typically changing between warm temperatures with about 27°C during the day and cold temperatures with about 5°C during the night. Aid stations are placed every 3 to 5 km, providing competitors with water and food. Each of the 75 race control points has its own time limitations and runners arriving later than the official closing time will be eliminated from the race. Nowadays, the number of applicants for the Spartathlon exceeds the limit of 350.

Data analysis

Due to overall low participation and partially missing data in earlier years, only data between 2000 and 2012 were included for data analysis. In order to increase comparability of data, running times were converted to running speed prior to analysis. Converting was done using the equation running speed (km/h) = running distance (km) / running time (h). The changes in the performance and in the age of peak performance across years for both men and women were analyzed by examining the running speed and age of the annual top five female and male finishers from 2000 to 2012. The sex difference in performance between women and men was calculated using the equation sex difference (%) = [running speed in women (km/h) – running speed in men (km/h)] / running speed in men (km/h) × 100.

Statistical analysis

In order to increase the reliability of the data analyses, each set of data was tested for normal distribution and for homogeneity of variances prior to statistical analyses. Normal distribution was tested using a D'Agostino and Pearson omnibus normality test, and homogeneity of variances was tested using a Levene's test in case of two groups and with a Bartlett's test in case of more than two groups. To find the significant changes in the development of a variable across the years, linear regression was used. To find significant differences between two groups, a Student's t test was used in case of normal distributed data with additional Welch's correction in case of significantly different variances between the analyzed groups and a Mann–Whitney test was used in case of not normal distributed data. To compare performance of men and women between the two races, a year-by-year analysis was performed using a two-way-analysis of variance with subsequent Bonferroni *post hoc* analysis. Also the interaction between the type of competition and time (years) on performance in genders was analyzed using a two-way-ANOVA (competition × time). Statistical analyses were performed using IBM SPSS Statistics (Version 19, IBM SPSS, Chicago, IL, USA) and GraphPad Prism (Version 5, GraphPad Software, La Jolla, CA, USA). Significance was accepted at $p < 0.05$ (two-sided for t tests). Data in the text are given as mean ± standard deviation or SD.

Results

Between 2000 and 2012, data were available from 663 men and 183 women finishing Badwater and from 1,157 men and 141 women finishing Spartathlon.

Participation trends

During the 13-year period, the annual overall percent finishes averaged 79% (ranging from 62% to 93%) for Badwater and 43% (ranging from 39% to 50%) for Spartathlon. Between 2000 and 2012, the number of both female and male finishes increased in both Badwater (Figure 1A) and Spartathlon (Figure 1B). A mean of 51 ± 11 men finished annually in Badwater and 89 ± 23 men in Spartathlon. In women, the mean number of annual finishers was on average 14 ± 5 athletes in Badwater and 11 ± 4 in Spartathlon. There was a significant increase in female participation in Badwater from 18.4% to 19.1% (maximum of 30.9% in 2011) and in Spartathlon from 11.9% to 12.5% (maximum of 14.5% in 2007). Women accounted on average for 21.5% ± 6.9% in Badwater and 10.8% ± 2.3% in Spartathlon of the overall finishes.

Age of finishers in Badwater and Spartathlon

In men, the mean age of all finishers was higher in Badwater (46.5 ± 9.3 years) compared to Spartathlon (44.8 ± 8.2 years) ($p < 0.01$). The mean age of female finishers in both races was similar with 43.0 ± 7.5 years in Badwater and 44.5 ± 7.8 years in Spartathlon ($p > 0.05$).

The age distribution of finishers is presented in Figure 2 for Badwater (Figure 2A) and Spartathlon (Figure 2B). In men, the largest participation was in athletes in the age group of 45 to 49 years in both races. For women, the largest participation was in age groups of 40 to 44 and 45 to 49 years in Badwater; while in Spartathlon, the largest participation was in the age group of 50 to 54 years. Master athletes (>40 years of age) represented 76% (642/846) of the total field in Badwater and 71% (899/1,262) in Spartathlon.

Over the years, the age of the annual five fastest men decreased in Badwater from 42.4 ± 4.2 years in 2002 to 39.8 ± 5.7 years in 2012 (Figure 3A). For women, the mean age of the annual five fastest finishers remained unchanged at 42.3 ± 3.8 years in Badwater. In Spartathlon (Figure 3B), the age of the annual five fastest finishers was unchanged at 39.7 ± 2.4 years for men and 44.6 ± 3.2 years for women.

Running speed of the annual top five finishers

Regarding the annual top five finishers, the mean running speed was lower in Badwater compared to Spartathlon ($p < 0.001$). In Badwater, both women and men became faster over years (Figure 4A). Running speed in men increased from 7.9 ± 0.7 km/h in 2000 to 8.7 ± 0.6 km/h in 2012. In women, running speed increased from 5.4 ± 1.1 km/h to 6.6 ± 0.5 km/h. The sex difference in running speed remained stable at 19.8% ± 4.8%. In Spartathlon running speed remained unchanged at 10.8 ± 0.7 km/h for men and 8.7 ± 0.5 km/h for women (Figure 4B). The sex difference in running speed remained unaltered at 19.6% ± 2.5%.

The running speed of the annual top five finishers was significantly ($p < 0.01$) faster in Spartathlon compared to

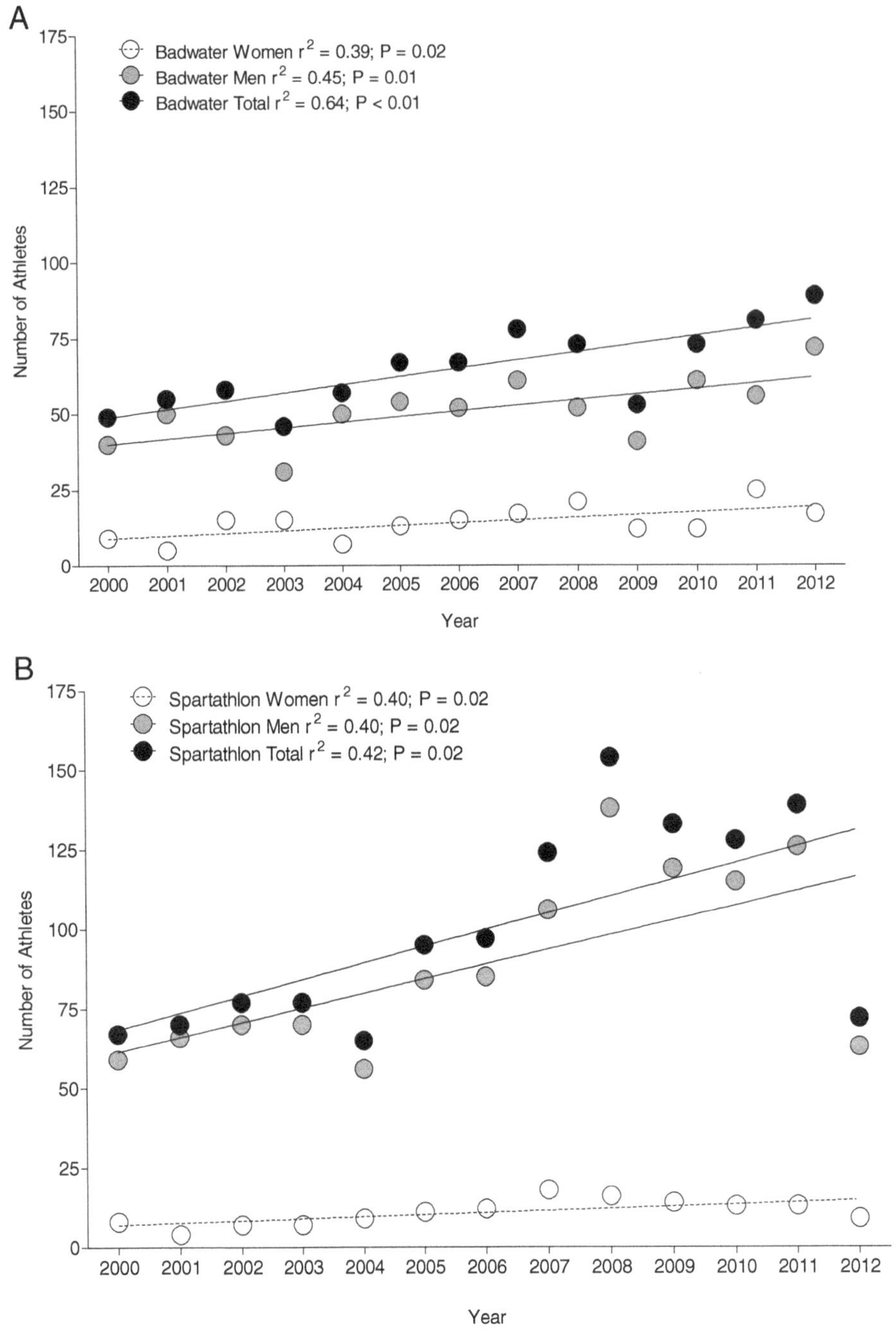

Figure 1 Annual number of female, male and overall finishes in Badwater (A) and Spartathlon (B).

Badwater for women and men, with the exception of 2011 in women (Figure 5A) and 2012 in men (Figure 5B). The analysis of interaction between type of competition and time (years) on running speed showed for women a highly significant ($F = 4.1$; $p < 0.01$) interaction between type of competition and time accounting for 7.8% of the total variance, whereas the type of competition accounted for 69.2% ($F = 436$; $p < 0.01$) and time accounted for 6.7% ($F = 3.5$; $p < 0.01$) of the total variance. In men, the interaction between the type of competition and time accounted for 9.9% of the total variance ($F = 7.4$; $p < 0.01$), whereas type of competition accounted for 71.6% ($F = 642.1$; $p < 0.01$) and time accounted for 7.0% ($F = 5.2$; $p < 0.01$) of the total variance.

Discussion

This study intended to investigate participation and performance trends and to determine the age of peak

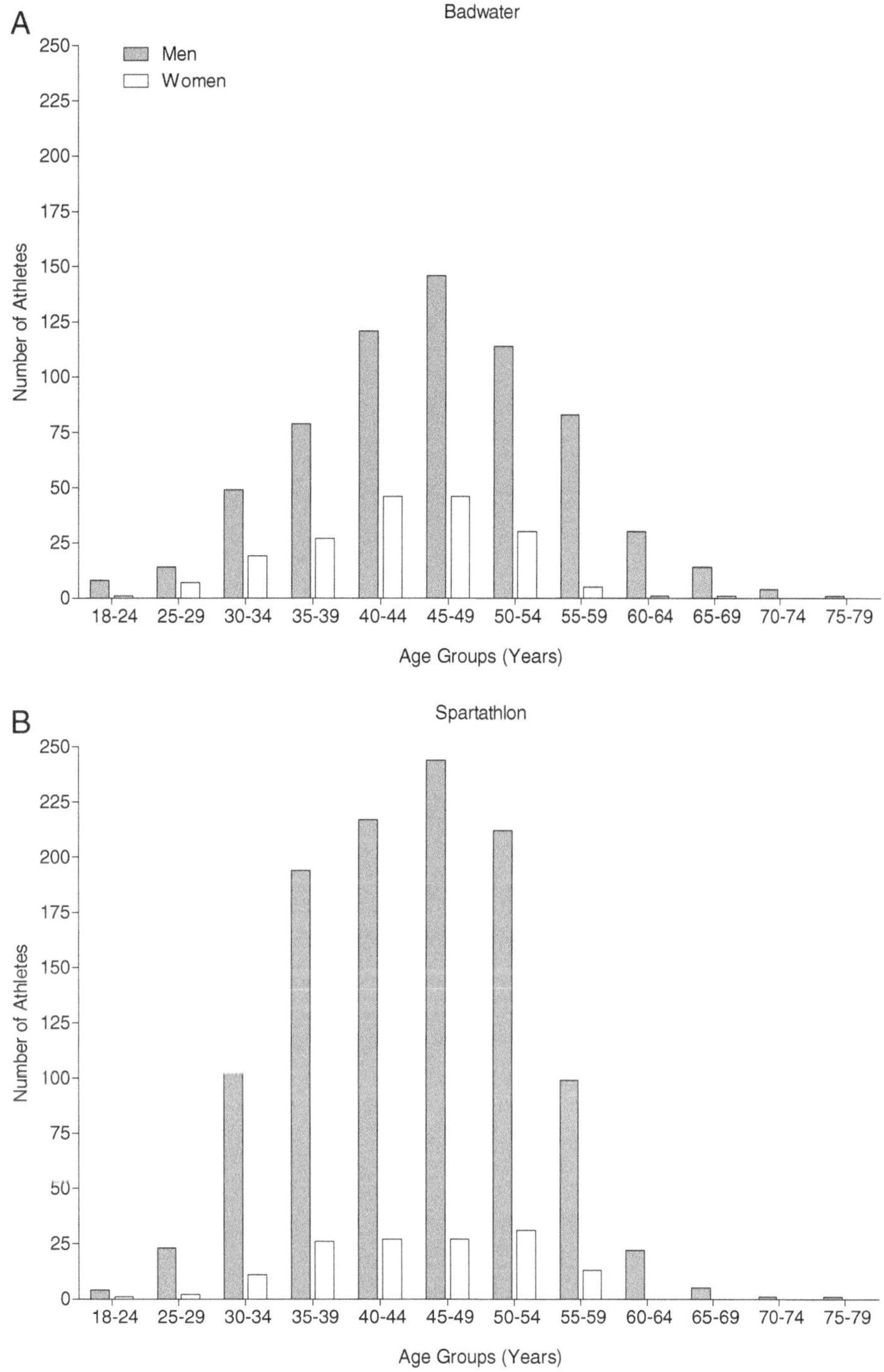

Figure 2 Male and female finishes in Badwater (A) and Spartathlon (B) per age group.

running speed in ultramarathons of more than 200-km race distance. Based upon existing literature, an increase in participation, an improvement in performance, and an age of peak ultramarathon performance between 30 and 40 years were hypothesized. The main findings for both races were that (1) the female participation increased over time, (2) the fastest finishers were approximately 40 to 45 years of age, and (3) the sex difference was at approximately 20% unchanged over years.

Participation trends

Concerning the total numbers of finishes over the history, it appears reasonable that in Badwater considerably fewer athletes competed since the qualifying standards were

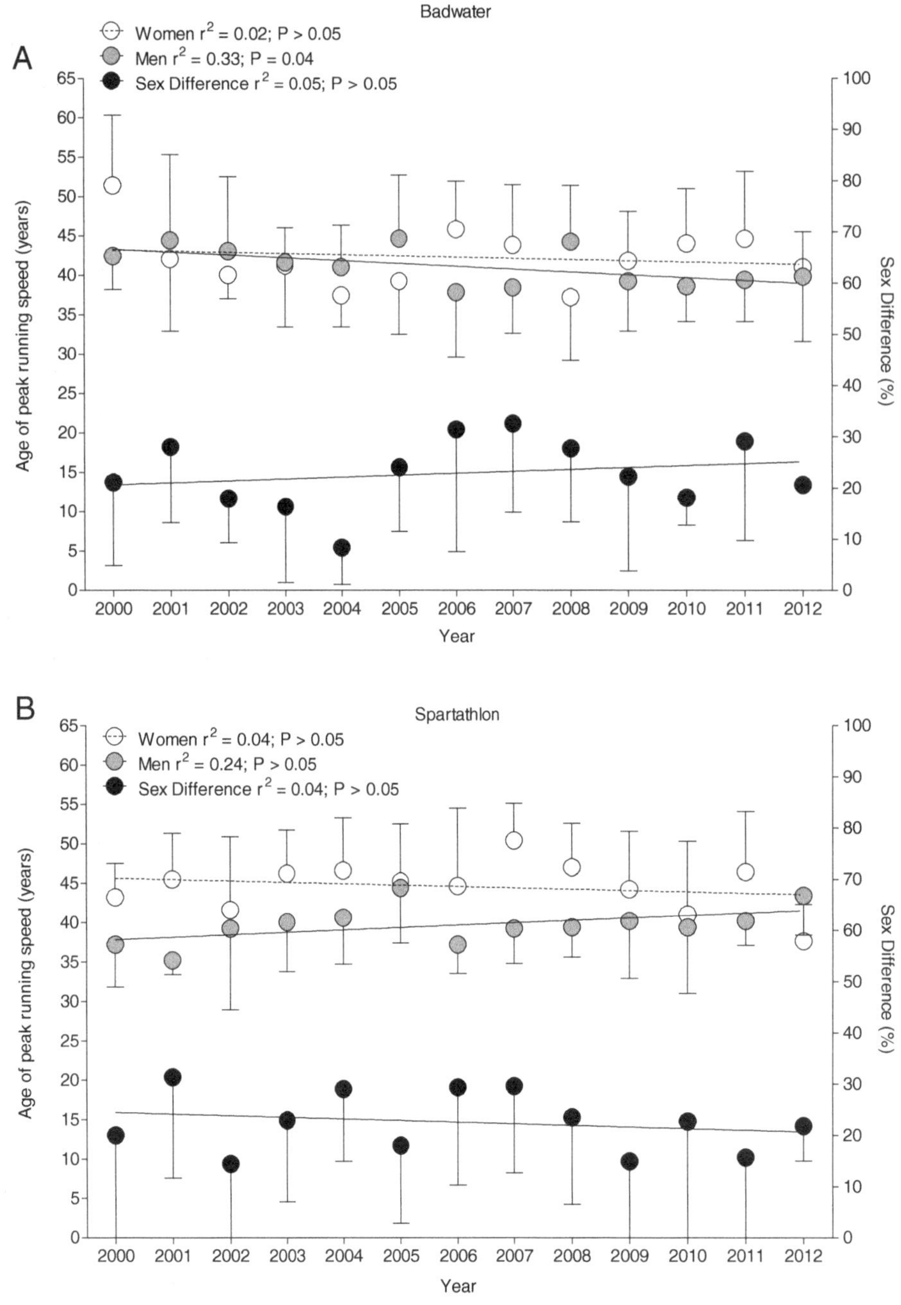

Figure 3 Age of the annual top five women and men in Badwater (A) and Spartathlon (B).

higher [23] than in Spartathlon [24]. Another limiting factor may be attributed to the greater financial expenses to participate in the Badwater because there are high additional costs for logistics and the necessity of a supporting team [23]. Across the history of Badwater race, the annual percentage of finishes averaged to 79% versus 43% in the Spartathlon. This relative low percentage of finishes in the Spartathlon may reflect the extraordinary demands on running speed due to rigorous cut-off limits in the Spartathlon.

Regarding the sex-specific participation, female ultramarathoners accounted on average for approximately 22% in Badwater versus approximately 11% in Spartathlon. Since women were generally slower in ultramarathon running than men [2-4], the cut-off limits in the Spartathlon could have a greater influence on women for a successful finish. Present findings were in accordance with other studies regarding the fact of a relatively low female participation in ultramarathon in comparison to shorter running events such as a marathon [3,4,9,10]. For instance, in the

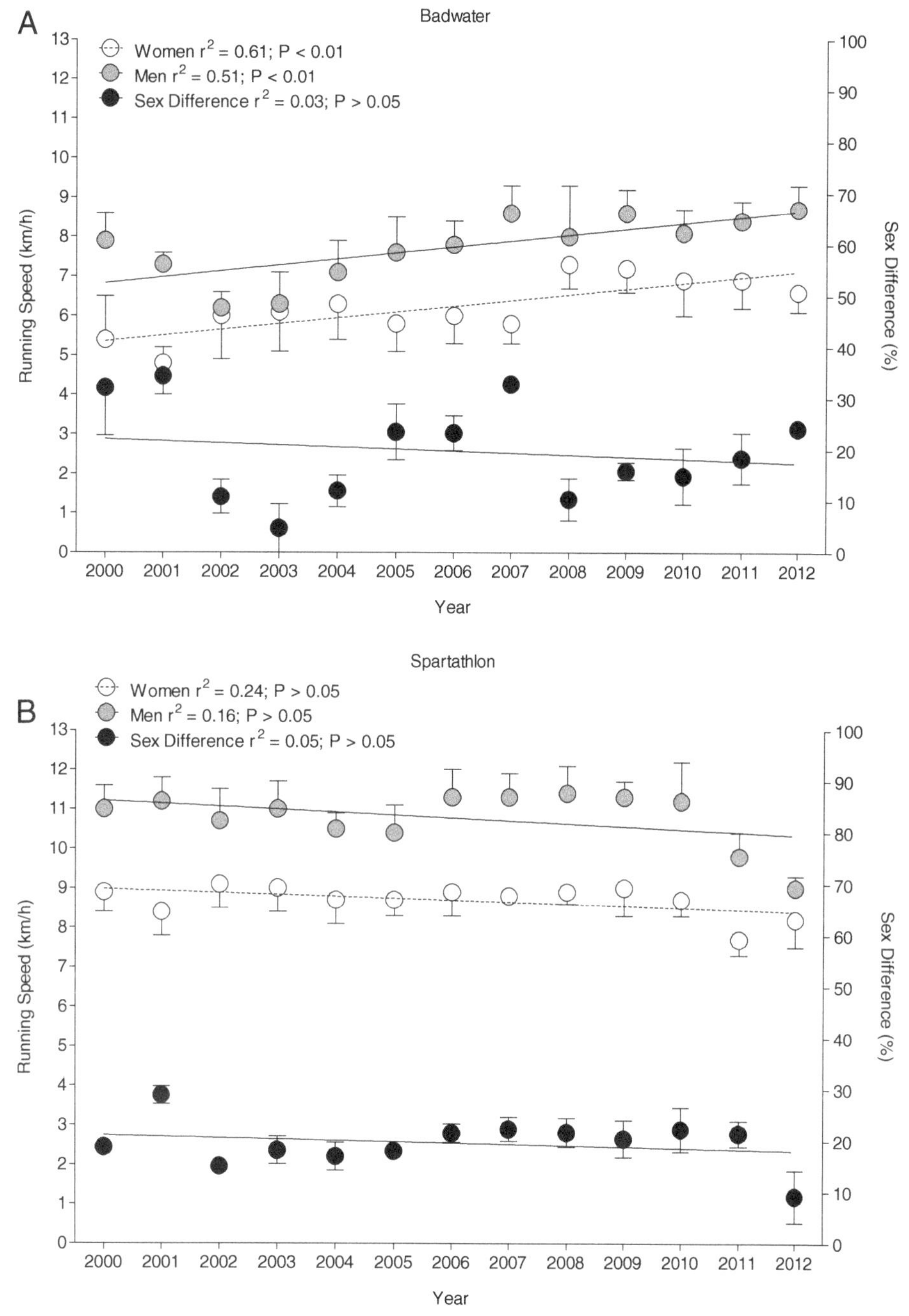

Figure 4 Running speeds of the annual top five women and men in Badwater (A) and Spartathlon (B).

100 km Lauf Biel in Switzerland, female participation was at approximately 13%. Hoffman reported a female participation of approximately 20 to 22% in 161-km ultramarathon events held in North America, which comes close to the female participation in Badwater. Men are over-represented in sports [26]. Generally, men were running faster than women [27], and the sex difference in relative performance can partially be attributed to men's greater training motivation [26]. The motivation to train and compete seems different between women and men. The most popular modern male sports require the skills needed for success in male-male physical competition [28]. In contrast, female ultramarathoners were described as task-oriented, internally motivated, healthy, and financially conscious individuals [29].

The three five-year age groups between 40 and 54 years accounted for the largest participation regardless of sex and race location. This age-related finding, together with the fact of numerous finishes from athletes aged 40 years and older in Badwater (76%) and in Spartathlon (71%), is

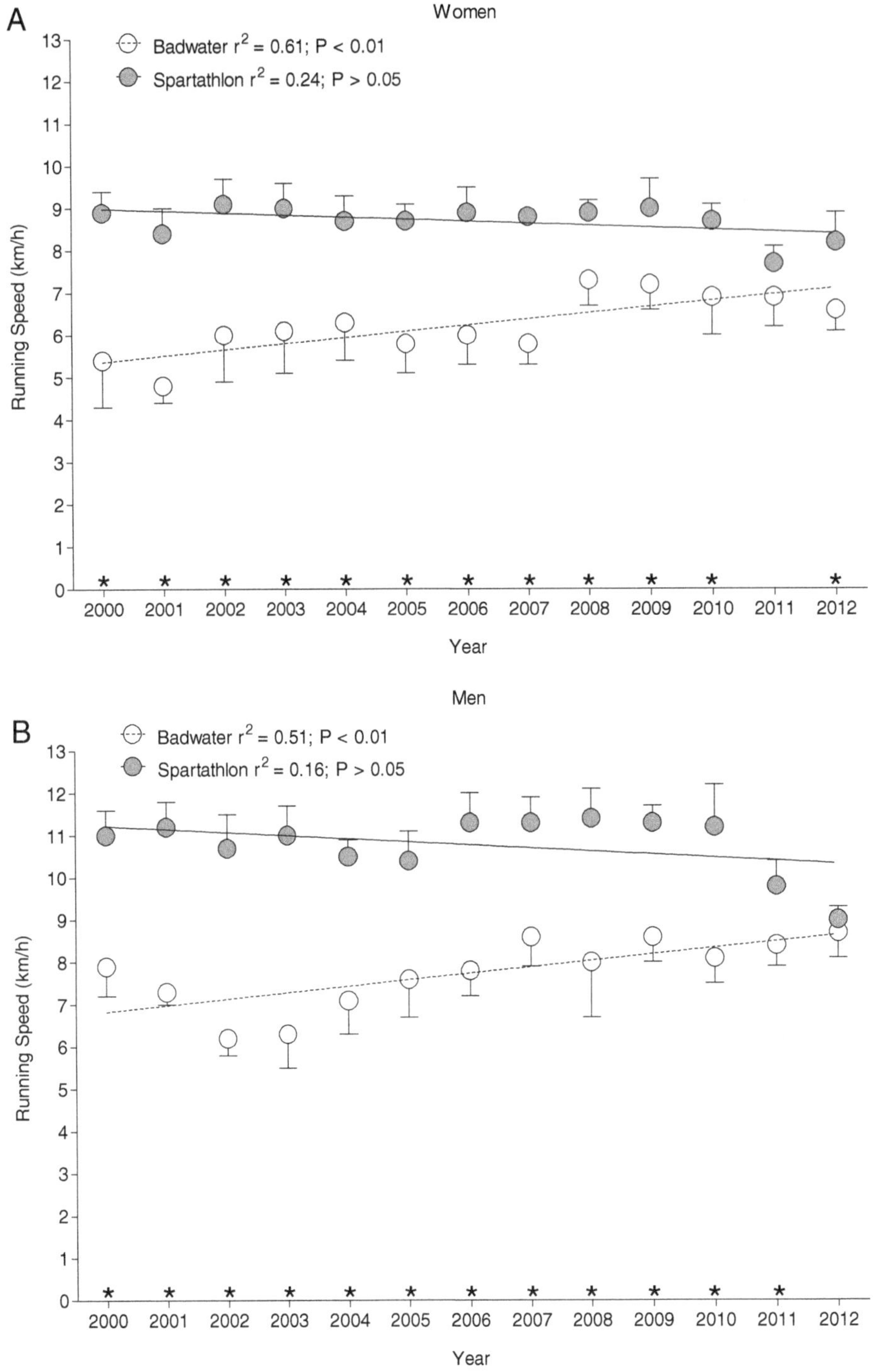

Figure 5 Comparison of running speed between Badwater and Spartathlon for annual top five. Comparison of running speed between Badwater and Spartathlon for the annual top five women (**A**) and men (**B**). An *asterisk* indicates years in which the running speed in Badwater was significantly different ($p < 0.01$) from the running speed in Spartathlon.

comparable with the results of other studies investigating the age distribution in ultra-running events [4,9,10]. Our data may reflect a lifestyle trend in sports activities towards ultramarathon. Younger athletes are increasingly more attracted by technical sports with higher intensity [10,30,31]. The higher participation of elderly athletes may be due to social and psychological factors such as spare time resources connected with an increase in the competitive spirit [32]. Hoffman and Fogard [4] described 161-km ultramarathoners as master runners at a mean age of 44.5 ± 9.8 years with a range between 20 and 72 years. These runners were generally men (80.2%), married (70.1%), and had higher education with bachelor's (43.6%) or graduate (37.2%) degrees. A further reason for the high percentage of older finishers across the studied history of both races could be related to the logistic demands, particularly of Badwater. The extraordinary distance over 200 km of both events may require an enormous volume of training over years. In ultramarathoners, previous experience is of importance for a successful race outcome [5].

Performance trends

The present study adds valuable results considering the change in demographic aspects of participation and performance in two extraordinary strenuous ultramarathons of more than 200 km in length. The improvement in running speed in Badwater might be attributed to a progress in the supporting teams and to an accumulation of pre-race experience [33,34]. The increase in the number of competitors and finishers might reflect that faster and more experienced runners enter this race [35-37].

In Spartathlon, however, athletes were not able to improve running speed. The stable running speeds in Spartathlon over the same time span could be attributed to the character of this race which is more a pure running event and has not to rely so much on external support in comparison to the Badwater [23]. Analyses of Hoffman and Wegelin [9] and Knechtle et al. [10] could not detect a clear improving or declining performance trend for the top ultramarathoners in terms of running speeds. Concerning Badwater, our data give a different impression due to a significant improvement of race speed regardless of sex. On the whole, independent of sex, considerably faster running speeds were achieved by the annual top five finishers in Spartathlon in comparison to the annual top five runners in Badwater. Different speed levels reflect the different physical demands of either race. Interestingly, in 2011 the running speeds in women narrowed. One possible explanation for this finding could be a lower top five elite field in the Spartathlon in that year. Further adverse race conditions may slow down women running speed in the Spartathlon in 2011.

Sex difference in ultra-running performance

In both Badwater and Spartathlon, the sex difference in running performance was at approximately 20%. Generally, the sex difference in endurance performance is at approximately 11 to 12% [12,13]. The analysis of world best times in 1,500 m and marathon running from 1980 to 1996 revealed that men were approximately 11% faster than women [12]. In a further widespread investigation of running distances between 100 m and 200 km, men were approximately 12% faster compared to women accompanied by the tendency that longer distances were associated with greater sex differences in endurance performance [13].

Regarding the sex difference in elite ultramarathon running, our data are in accordance with the previous studies. Hoffman [2] reported for 161-km ultramarathoners that the fastest women were approximately 20% slower than the fastest men. In a comparable race, the 100 km Lauf Biel in Switzerland, the top ten women were approximately 22% slower than the top ten men [10]. In the current discussion about sex difference in ultramarathon running, exceptional findings do exist supporting the assumption that women could outperform men in ultra-endurance sports. For instances, Bam et al. [38] compared long-distance performances in both men and women and observed that men were faster over distances up to marathon, but this was not evident in a 90-km ultramarathon. Also Knechtle et al. [39] described a female overall winner in a multi-stage ultramarathon.

Looking upon the sex-related running speed difference between the top elite runners over the 2000 to 2012 period, it is notable that in the 2002 and 2003 Badwater races, the sex difference in top five running speed was close to zero. Moreover, female winners even outperformed male winners in these years. In 2003, the hottest climate conditions have ever been registered in Death Valley with the highest drop off rate of 37% was published for this year [23]. Thus, these results from 2002 to 2003 appeared to reflect a possible better coping against heat among women. Jacob et al. [40] reported that increasing ambient temperatures had less adverse effects on running speed for women than for men in 161-km ultramarathons. Our findings do underline the assumption that top running speed of women does not converge with or even surpass those of men apart from exceptional women top running speed as seen in the Badwater in 2002 and 2003.

The higher sex difference in performance in these ultramarathoners might be explained by differences in anthropometry, physiology, training, and motivation between women and men. Ultramarathon running leads to a decrease in skeletal muscle mass [41]. Since male ultramarathoners [42] have a higher skeletal muscle mass compared to female ultramarathoners [43], the lower muscle mass in women might be a limiting factor for ultramarathon performance. However, physiology still plays an inevitable roll that sex differences probably will continue in the future. Sex difference in performance is considered due primarily to inherent gender-specific differences in body composition and oxygen transport capacity [12,44-46]. Considering training and motivation, female and male ultra-endurance athletes were trained for about the same weekly hours, but men were training faster than women [47,48]. Furthermore, men pay closer attention to male sports than women do and male champion athletes obtain a higher status [28].

The age of peak ultra-running performance

From 2000 to 2012, for both men and women, the age of the annual top five finishers remained at 39 to 45 years in Badwater and Spartathlon. Women achieved their peak running speed at higher age than men in either event. Our data were comparable with other studies in ultramarathon running events. By investigating the top ten runners in the 100 km Lauf Biel, the age of the best performance was found at approximately 39 to 40 years [10]. Across the history of the 161-km 'Western State Endurance Run' in North America, the average age of the top five finishers gradually increased from the early 30s to the upper 30s [9].

Furthermore, existing literature and our findings suggest that with the increasing length of running events, athletes achieved their peak of running speed at higher age than in shorter running events [9,49,50]. The analysis of the 'New York City Marathon' [51] documented that among the top fifty performers, no runner was older than 39 years independent of gender. The present data of Badwater and Spartathlon are also consistent with the findings of Schulz and Curnow [50], reporting a relationship between the age of peak performance and specific events already in the 1980s. Taken as a whole, the present and previous findings [9,10] evidenced that among the top ultramarathon, elite runners were master athletes defined as participants older than 35 years of age [52]. Usually, however, these older athletes are considered to have either finished their formal competitive careers, to be 'weekend warriors' who sporadically train and compete, or to have start again dynamic exercises after a long time span of physical inactivity [53]. Thus, present and other findings appear to suggest that the definition of master runners need to be revised for ultramarathoners.

Limitations

This cross-sectional data analysis is limited since aspects such as anthropometry [35-37], the physiology [54,55], and the training [35-37] of the runners, their previous experience [34-37], their pacing strategy [56], the environmental conditions [57], and both nutrition [58-60] and fluid intake [61,62] were not considered.

Conclusions

To summarize, female participation increased in ultramarathons of more than 200 km such as Badwater and Spartathlon; the fastest finishers were approximately 40 to 45 years of age, and the sex difference was at approximately 20%. These results suggest that women will not outrun men in the near future in ultramarathons of greater than 200 km in length such as Badwater and Spartathlon. Master ultramarathoners can achieve high level of performance in ultramarathons greater than 200 km under extreme conditions such as heat and time limit. Apart from the influence of other limiting factors on the running speed in ultramarathon such as physiological and anthropometric characteristics, further studies need to investigate what motivates female and male master ultramarathoners to compete in these extreme races. The definition of master runners as athletes aged 35 years and older needs to be revised for ultramarathoners competing in races of greater than 200 km. Future studies need to investigate the age of peak ultramarathon performance in longer running distances.

Availability of supporting data

The data sets supporting the results of this article are available in http://spartathlon.gr/ and http://badwater.com/.

Competing interests

The authors declare that they have no competing interests.

Authors' contributions

KFE drafted the manuscript. BK participated in the conception and design of the study, helped to draft the manuscript, and participated in the analysis and interpretation of data. CAR performed the analysis of data and participated in the interpretation of data. PK helped in the acquisition of data. RL and TR performed the interpretation of data and manuscript preparation. All authors read and approved the final manuscript.

Acknowledgments

We thank Matthias Knechtle for his help in the translation.

Author details

[1]Institute of General Practice and for Health Services Research, University of Zurich, Zurich 8091, Switzerland. [2]Gesundheitszentrum St. Gallen, St. Gallen 9000, Switzerland. [3]INSERM U1093, Faculty of Sport Sciences, University of Burgundy, Dijon 21078Cedex, France. [4]Facharzt FMH für Allgemeinmedizin, Gesundheitszentrum St. Gallen, Vadianstrasse 26, St. Gallen 9001, Switzerland.

References

1. Zaryski C, Smith DJ: **Training principles and issues for ultra-endurance athletes.** *Curr Sports Med Rep* 2005, **43:**165–170.
2. Hoffman MD: **Performance trends in 161-km ultramarathons.** *Int J Sports Med* 2010, **31:**31–37.
3. Hoffman MD, Ong JC, Wang G: **Historical analysis of participation in 161-km ultramarathons in North America.** *Int J Hist Sport* 2010, **27:**1877–1891.
4. Hoffman MD, Fogard K: **Demographic characteristics of 161-km ultramarathon runners.** *Res Sports Med* 2012, **20:**59–69.
5. Knechtle B, Knechtle P, Rosemann T, Lepers R: **Predictor variables for a 100-km race time in male ultra-marathoners.** *Percept Mot Skill* 2010, **111:**681–693.
6. Lepers R: **Analysis of Hawaii Ironman performance in elite triathletes from 1981 to 2007.** *Med Sci Sports Exerc* 2008, **40:**1828–1834.
7. Lepers R, Sultana F, Thierry B, Hausswirth C, Brisswalter J: **Age-related changes in triathlon performance.** *Int J Sports Med* 2010, **31:**251–256.
8. IAU Ultra Marathon: http://iau-ultramarathon.org.
9. Hoffman MD, Wegelin JA: **The western states 100-mile endurance run: participation and performance trends.** *Med Sci Sports Exerc* 2009, **41:**2191–2198.
10. Knechtle B, Rüst CA, Rosemann T, Lepers R: **Age-related changes in 100-km ultra-marathon running performance.** *Age* 2012, **34:**1033–1045.
11. Lepers R, Maffiuletti NA: **Age and gender interactions in ultraendurance performance: insight from the triathlon.** *Med Sci Sports Exerc* 2011, **43:**134–139.
12. Sparling PB, O'D EM, Snow TK: **The gender difference in distance running performance has plateaued: an analysis of world rankings from 1980 to 1996.** *Med Sci Sports Exerc* 1998, **30:**1725–1729.

13. Coast JR, Blevins JS, Wilson BA: **Do gender differences in running performance disappear with distance?** *Can J Appl Physiol* 2004, **29**:139–145.
14. Baker AB, Tang YQ, Turner MJ: **Percentage decline in masters superathlete track and field performance with aging.** *Exp Aging Res* 2003, **29**:47–65.
15. Balmer J, Bird S, Davison R: **Indoor 16.1-km time-trial performance in cyclists aged 25–63 years.** *J Sports Sci* 2008, **26**:57–62.
16. Donato AJ, Tench K, Glueck DH, Seals DR, Eskurza I, Tanaka H: **Declines in physiological functional capacity with age: a longitudinal study in peak swimming performance.** *J Appl Physiol* 2003, **94**:764–769.
17. Fleg JL, Lakatta EG: **Role of muscle loss in the age-associated reduction in VO_2 max.** *J Appl Physiol* 1988, **65**:1147–1151.
18. Fuchi T, Iwaoka K, Higuchi M, Kobayashi S: **Cardiovascular changes associated with decreased aerobic capacity and aging in long-distance runners.** *Eur J Appl Physiol* 1989, **58**:884–889.
19. Hunter SK, Stevens AA, Magennis K, Skelton KW, Fauth M: **Is there a sex difference in the age of elite marathon runners?** *Med Sci Sports Exerc* 2011, **443**:656–664.
20. Leyk D, Erley O, Ridder D, Leurs M, Rüther T, Wunderlich M, Sievert A, Baum K, Essfeld D: **Age-related changes in marathon and half-marathon performances.** *Int J Sports Med* 2007, **28**:513–527.
21. Leyk D, Erley O, Gorge W, Ridder D, Rüther T, Wunderlich M, Sievert A, Essfeld D, Pierkarski C, Erren T: **Performance, training and lifestyle parameters of marathon runners aged 20–80 years: result of the PACE-study.** *Int J Sports Med* 2009, **30**:360–365.
22. Tanaka H, Seals DR: **Invited review: dynamic exercise performance in master athletes: insight into effects of primary human aging on physiological function capacity.** *J Appl Physiol* 2003, **95**:2152–2162.
23. Adventure CORPS Presents the Badwater Ultramarathon Official Website. http://badwater.com.
24. ΣΠΑΡΤΑΘΛΟΝ: http://spartathlon.gr.
25. Western U.S. Climate Historical Summaries Weather: Desert Research Institute: [http://wrcc.dri.edu/cgi-bin/cliMAIN.pl?ca2319]. Retrieved 29 May 2009.
26. Deaner RO: **Distance running as an ideal domain for showing a sex difference in competitiveness.** *Arch Sex Behav* 2012, doi:10.1007/s10508-012-9965-z.
27. Deaner RO, Mitchell D: **More men run relatively fast in U.S. road races, 1981–2006: a stable sex difference in non-elite runners.** *Evol Psychol* 2011, **9**:600–621.
28. Lombardo MP: **On the evolution of sport.** *Evol Psychol* 2012, **10**:1–28.
29. Krouse RZ, Ransdell LB, Lucas SM, Pritchard ME: **Motivation, goal orientation, coaching, and training habits of women ultrarunners.** *J Strength Cond Res* 2011, **25**:2835–2842.
30. Baker AB, Tang YQ: **Aging performance for masters records in athletics, swimming, rowing, cycling, triathlon and weightlifting.** *Exp Aging Res* 2010, **36**:453–477.
31. Bernard T, Sultana F, Lepers R, Hausswirth C, Brisswalter J: **Age related decline in Olympic triathlon performance: effect of locomotion mode.** *Exp Aging Res* 2010, **36**:64–78.
32. Lepers R, Cattagni T: **Do older athletes reach limits in their performance during marathon running?** *Age (Dordr)* 2012, **34**:773–781.
33. Knechtle B, Knechtle P, Lepers R: **Participation and performance trends in ultra-triathlons from 1985 to 2009.** *Scand J Med Sci Sports* 2011, **21**:e82–e90.
34. Knechtle B, Knechtle P, Rosemann T, Senn O: **Personal best time, not anthropometry or training volume, is associated with total race time in a Triple Iron triathlon.** *J Strength Cond Res* 2011, **25**:1142–1150.
35. Knechtle B, Knechtle P, Rosemann T, Senn O: **What is associated with race performance in male 100-km ultra-marathoners - anthropometry, training or marathon best time?** *J Sports Sci* 2011, **29**:571–577.
36. Knechtle B, Knechtle P, Rosemann T, Lepers R: **Predictor variables for a 100-km race time in male ultra-marathoners.** *Percept Mot Skills* 2010, **111**:681–693.
37. Knechtle B, Knechtle P, Rosemann T, Lepers R: **Personal best marathon time and longest training run, not anthropometry, predict performance in recreational 24-hour ultrarunners.** *J Strength Cond Res* 2011, **25**:2212–2218.
38. Bam J, Noakes TD, Juritz J, Dennis SC: **Could women outrun men in ultramarathon races?** *Med Sci Sports Exerc* 1997, **29**:244–247.
39. Knechtle B, Duff B, Schulze I, Kohler G: **The effects of running 1,200 km within 17 days on body composition in a female ultrarunner - Deutschlandlauf 2007.** *Res Sports Med* 2008, **16**:167–188.
40. Jacob A, Wegelin M, Hoffman MD: **Variables associated with odds of finishing and finish time in a 161-km ultramarathon.** *Eur J Appl Physiol* 2011, **111**:145–153.
41. Knechtle B, Knechtle P, Wirth A, Alexander Rüst C, Rosemann T: **A faster running speed is associated with a greater body weight loss in 100-km ultra-marathoners.** *J Sports Sci* 2012, **30**:1131–1140.
42. Knechtle B, Senn O, Imoberdorf R, Joleska I, Wirth A, Knechtle P, Rosemann T: **No fluid overload in male ultra-runners during a 100 km ultra-run.** *Res Sports Med* 2011, **19**:14–27.
43. Knechtle B, Senn O, Imoberdorf R, Joleska I, Wirth A, Knechtle P, Rosemann T: **Maintained total body water content and serum sodium concentrations despite body mass loss in female ultra-runners drinking *ad libitum* during a 100 km race.** *Asia Pac J Clin Nutr* 2010, **19**:83–90.
44. Cureton KJ, Bishop P, Hutchinson P, Newland H, Vickery S, Zwiren L: **Sex difference in maximal oxygen: effect of equating haemoglobin concentration.** *Eur J Appl Physiol* 1986, **54**:656–660.
45. Joyner MJ: **Physiological limiting factors and distance running: influence of gender and age on record performances.** *Exerc Sport Sci Rev* 1993, **21**:103–133.
46. Sparling PB, Cureton KJ: **Biological determinants of the sex difference in 12-min run performance.** *Med Sci Sports Exerc* 1983, **15**:218–223.
47. Knechtle B, Wirth A, Baumann B, Knechtle P, Rosemann T, Oliver S: **Differential correlations between anthropometry, training volume, and performance in male and female Ironman triathletes.** *J Strength Cond Res* 2010, **24**:2785–2793.
48. Knechtle B, Wirth A, Baumann B, Knechtle P, Rosemann T: **Personal best time, percent body fat, and training are differently associated with race time for male and female ironman triathletes.** *Res Q Exerc Sport* 2010, **81**:62–68.
49. Lepers R, Rüst CA, Stapley PJ, Knechtle B: **Relative improvements in endurance with age: evidence from 25 years of Hawaii Ironman racing.** *Age (Dordr)* 2012, doi:10.1007/s11357-012-9392-z.
50. Schulz R, Curnow C: **Peak performance and age among superathletes: track and field, swimming, baseball, tennis and golf.** *J Gerontol* 1988, **43**:113–120.
51. Jokl P, Sethi PM, Cooper AJ: **Master's performance in the New York City Marathon 1983–1999.** *Br J Sports Med* 2004, **38**:408–412.
52. Reaburn P, Dascombe B: **Endurance performance in masters athletes.** *Eur Rev Aging Phys Act* 2008, **5**:31–42.
53. Maron BJ, Araújo CG, Thompson PD, Fletcher GF, de Luna AB, Fleg JL, Pelliccia A, Balady GJ, Furlanello F, Van Camp SP, Elosua R, Chaitman BR, Bazzarre TL: **Recommendations for preparticipation screening and the assessment of cardiovascular diseases in masters athletes.** *Circ* 2001, **103**:327–334.
54. Davies CT, Thompson MW: **Aerobic performance of female marathon and male ultramarathon athletes.** *Eur J Appl Physiol Occup Physiol* 1979, **41**:233–245.
55. Landman ZC, Landman GO, Fatehi P: **Physiologic alterations and predictors of performance in a 160-km ultramarathon.** *Clin J Sport Med* 2012, **22**:146–151.
56. March DS, Vanderburgh PM, Titlebaum PJ, Hoops ML: **Age, sex, and finish time as determinants of pacing in the marathon.** *J Strength Cond Res* 2011, **25**:386–391.
57. Wegelin JA, Hoffman MD: **Variables associated with odds of finishing and finish time in a 161-km ultramarathon.** *Eur J Appl Physiol* 2011, **111**:145–153.
58. Onywera VO, Kiplamai FK, Boit MK, Pitsiladis YP: **Food and macronutrient intake of elite Kenyan distance runners.** *Int J Sport Nutr Exerc Metab* 2004, **14**:709–719.
59. Glace BW, Murphy CA, McHugh MP: **Food intake and electrolyte status of ultramarathoners competing in extreme heat.** *J Am Coll Nutr* 2002, **21**:553–559.
60. Knechtle B, Knechtle P, Schulze I, Kohler G: **Vitamins, minerals and race performance in ultra-endurance runners - Deutschlandlauf 2006.** *Asia Pac J Clin Nutr* 2008, **17**:194–198.
61. Knechtle B, Knechtle P, Rosemann T: **Low prevalence of exercise-associated hyponatremia in male 100-km ultra-marathon runners in Switzerland.** *Eur J Appl Physiol* 2011, **111**:1007–1016.
62. Knechtle B, Knechtle P, Rosemann T: **Do male 100-km ultra-marathoners overdrink?** *Int J Sports Physiol Perform* 2011, **6**:195–207.

23

Control and sensation of breathing during cycling exercise in hypoxia under naloxone: a randomised controlled crossover trial

Laurent Koglin[1] and Bengt Kayser[2*]

Abstract

Background: Opioid receptors are possibly involved in the perception of exertion and the ventilatory response to exercise. We compared incremental cycling exercise in conditions of normoxia and hypoxia (11% O_2) after injection of the opioid receptor antagonist naloxone (30 mg i.v.) or placebo. Naloxone was expected to increase sensation of breathing and cycling and to curtail exercise performance more in hypoxia.

Methods: Ten healthy subjects (29 ± 2 years, 183 ± 6 cm, 75 ± 7 kg, mean ± SD) cycled in normoxia and hypoxia until voluntary exhaustion, receiving naloxone or placebo in a balanced double-blind crossover design.

Results: Hypoxia decreased peak power output by 37%–39% with placebo and naloxone ($P < 0.001$, no effect of naloxone). Switching to normoxia at exhaustion in hypoxia allowed continuing up to 97%–100% of power developed in normoxia with placebo and naloxone ($P < 0.001$, no effect of naloxone). Perceived exertion increased in hypoxia, dropped upon switching to normoxia and increased again towards exhaustion, no effect of naloxone. SpO_2 (earlobe oximetry) was lower in hypoxia, dropping to 64%–68% with naloxone and placebo. The ventilatory response to exercise in normoxia and hypoxia was not changed by naloxone.

Conclusions: It follows that in healthy subjects the ventilatory response and the perception of exertion in hypoxia as compared to normoxia do not involve the endogenous opioid system, and the latter does not play a role in limiting maximum exercise capacity in hypoxia.

Keywords: Altitude, Exercise, Human, Opioid, Hypoxia

Background

In both healthy subjects and patients, dyspnoea and leg fatigue are the main symptoms limiting exercise capacity [1-4]. Dyspnoea is accompanied by activation of cortico-limbic structures implicated in interoceptive awareness and nociceptive sensations, such as pain, and involves the opioid system [5]. In patients with dyspnoea, exogenous opioids can alleviate breathing-related discomfort and improve exercise performance [5-8], while injection of naloxone hydrochloride, a non-specific opioid antagonist that crosses the blood–brain barrier, can decrease performance [5]. Opioids can relieve dyspnoea by altering central processing of efferent and afferent sensory information [5]. Sgherza et al. [9] found that in normoxia, in healthy trained subjects, naloxone compared to placebo decreased incremental exercise performance and suggested that sensation of exertion is under influence of endogenous opioids and may be a limiting factor for maximum aerobic exercise capacity.

Acute hypoxia is a potent stressor, especially when combined with an exercise challenge, changing the perceived level of exertion [10]. Acute exposure to hypoxia increases ventilation and cardiac output in order to minimise the reduction in arterial oxygen content and systemic mass oxygen transport. Despite these acute adaptations, incremental exercise testing in such conditions (e.g. an FiO_2 equivalent to an altitude of 5,000 m or higher, hereafter referred to as severe hypoxia) invariably results in compromised aerobic exercise capacity. The mechanisms behind this limitation of exercise

* Correspondence: bengt.kayser@unige.ch
[2]Institute of Movement Sciences and Sports Medicine, Faculty of medicine, University of Geneva, 10, rue du Conseil Général, Genève 4 1205, Switzerland
Full list of author information is available at the end of the article

capacity in hypoxia are still poorly understood [11-13]. A puzzling observation is that despite maximum effort in severe hypoxia, cardiac output remains submaximal, suggesting early motor drive withdrawal [11,12]. However, while the locomotor muscles are not driven as hard during large muscle volume effort in such conditions, the contrary is the case for the respiratory muscles. Ventilation is higher for any given level of oxygen consumption during exercise in hypoxia, as compared to normoxia, and is accompanied by a concomitant increase in the sensation of breathing effort [10]. Since blocking the effect of endogenous opioids on the sensation of exertion can increase symptom intensity and curtail performance in normoxia [9], it is possible that such an effect would be exacerbated in hypoxia. We therefore hypothesised that blocking opioid receptors may decrease aerobic exercise performance more in hypoxia than in normoxia. To test this hypothesis, we compared incremental cycling exercise in conditions of normoxia and hypoxia (11% O_2) after injection of the opioid antagonist naloxone in comparison to a placebo. Our expectations were that under naloxone the sensation of breathing effort and that of cycling would increase and curtail exercise performance more in hypoxia as compared to normoxia.

Methods

Subjects

Thirteen healthy trained men volunteered to participate in the study. Inclusion criteria were an age between 18 and 30 years and >4 h/week of endurance training. Exclusion criteria were presence of any relevant chronic or acute disease, having done a maximal capacity training or a race during the last 48 h, symptoms/signs of viral illness in the week preceding the experiments or exposure to altitude in the 2 months before the study. The study was approved by the research ethics commission of the Geneva University Hospitals and SwissMedic and complied with the principles of the Declaration of Helsinki. All subjects were screened by a physician, were fully informed of the nature and risks of the experiments, knew of their right to withdraw at any time and signed an informed consent form.

Exercise protocol

After inclusion, the subjects first performed two habituation experiments, identical to the real experiments except for the injection, to get used to the equipment and to experience cycling in acute hypoxia. They were instructed not to do any heavy training on the days preceding the experiments and to refrain from caffeine in the 4 h preceding a test. To control for circadian rhythm, for a given subject, all experiments were performed at similar times of the day. After the habituation tests, the subjects came to the lab on four different occasions at least 24 h apart to perform incremental cycling exercise until voluntary exhaustion, twice in normoxia and twice in acute normobaric hypoxia (FIO_2 = 10.65% O_2, in Geneva the equivalent of an altitude of approximately 5,000 m). The subjects cycled at 80 rpm on a mechanically braked ergometer (Monark 282E, Varberg, Sweden). After 3 min of resting baseline measurements, the subjects would warm up at 40 watt for 3 min. In order to obtain similar durations of exercise times between subjects and between conditions of normoxia and hypoxia, the duration of steps was adapted between conditions and stages. After warm-up, the subjects incremented by 3-min steps of 40 up to 200 watt in normoxia and then by 20 watt up to voluntary exhaustion, while in hypoxia, they incremented by 40 up to 120 watt and then by 20 watt up to voluntary exhaustion. When reaching exhaustion in hypoxia, the subjects were switched to room air ('normoxia switch') and strongly encouraged to continue cycling while the load was increased by 20 watt every 90 s until reaching secondary voluntary exhaustion.

Intervention

In each condition, they did this once after immediate pre-exercise intravenous injection of naloxone (30 mg naloxone HCl in 30 ml saline) and once after placebo (30 ml saline). The conditions normoxia and hypoxia were in a randomised order. Naloxone and placebo were administered in a balanced double-blind crossover design. The research support section of the Geneva University Hospitals pharmacy prepared the vials, the numbering scheme and the randomization envelopes and released the randomization key after data analysis was completed. The subjects started exercising within 5 min after injection and reached exhaustion within 30 min, approximately one half of the serum half-life of naloxone reported in humans [14]

Normoxia and hypoxia

Normobaric hypoxia was obtained by mixing N_2 into ambient air under control of FIO_2 (Altitrainer, SMTec, Nyon, Switzerland). The gas-mixing system was attached via a piece of large-bore low-resistance tubing to the inspiratory valve of a low-resistance three-way valve (Hans Rudolph 2700, Shawnee, KS, USA) mounted in series with a turbine flow measurement set-up (Vmax 29c, Sensormedics, Loma Linda, CA, USA) attached to a tightly fitted face mask (Hans Rudolph). The subjects always breathed through the same set-up, also in normoxia. The gas-mixing device was set to room air for the normoxia experiments and to a simulated altitude of 5,000 m for the hypoxia experiments.

Material and measurements

Gas exchange and breathing parameters were measured breath-by-breath with a metabolic cart (Vmax 29c, Sensormedics). Prior to each experiment, the system was calibrated with a 3-L syringe and gas mixtures of known composition. Heart rate was measured by telemetry with a thoracic belt (Polar, Tampere, Finland). Arterial blood haemoglobin saturation (SpO_2) was measured on an earlobe with a pulse oximeter (Ohmeda, Helsinki, Finland) connected to the metabolic cart. Arterialized blood from a hyperaemic earlobe (Trafuril Cream, Ciba-Geigy, Basel, Switzerland) was used to measure lactate (Accutrend, Roche, West Sussex, UK).

To quantify locomotor muscle activation, a surface electromyogram (EMG) was obtained from the right vastus lateralis muscle. After cleaning with ether and light abrading of the skin, two electrodes (Kendall H59P, Mansfield, OH, USA) were applied directly next to each other on the distal part of the muscle. In addition to marking the skin with indelible ink, we used transparent foil to mark the sites of the electrodes together with skin marks such as moles and scars to reposition the electrodes on the same sites between sessions. Inter-electrode resistance was measured and considered acceptable if <3 kΩ. A reference electrode was placed over a bony area near the knee. The signal was amplified, filtered with a Butterworth band pass between 10 and 200 Hz (BMA-830, CWE, Ardmore, OK, USA), digitised at 1,000 Hz with an AD-board (NI-Daqcard, National Instruments, Austin, TX, USA) and stored on a computer. The data were analysed *post hoc* with custom routines in Matlab (Matlab, Natick, MA, USA) to obtain, for each single contraction, the integrated rectified EMG (iEMG) and, after a fast-Fourier transformation, the median (i.e. centroid, CPF) and mean power (MPF) frequencies, as described before [15]. iEMG was normalised with the signal obtained at 80 watt.

Perception of exertion

The subjects were asked to rate the rate of perceived exertion (RPE) on a 0–10-point CR-10 Borg ratio scale [2]. At the end of each exercise level, the subjects rated their perception of exertion separately for their legs (How hard is it to cycle?), breathing (How hard is it to breathe?) and overall (How hard is the overall effort?). The anchors were 0 for no exertion at all and 10 for the maximum imaginable. When prompted, the subject would point to the scale and nod when the experimenter called the correct corresponding number out loud.

Analysis and statistics

For each subject and each condition, the data were averaged over the last 30 s of each workload with the exception of the maximum when a mean over 15 s was used. The data were analysed with SPSS version 18 (IBM, Chicago, IL, USA). Repeated measures ANOVA was used to test for within-group effects across time. Following significant main effects, planned pairwise comparisons were made using Holm's sequential Bonferroni procedure. Results are expressed as mean ± SD. Statistical significance was set at $P < 0.05$.

Results

Of the 13 recruited subjects, 1 dropped out after the first habituation test (no reason given), 2 subjects were excluded for a vagal reaction to hypoxia at rest, and 10 completed the study (age 29 ± 2 years (mean ± SD), height 183 ± 6 cm, weight 75 ± 7 kg, maximum aerobic capacity ($V'O_2max$) 50 ± 8 ml/kg/min). The injection of naloxone was well tolerated. Table 1 shows the results observed at exhaustion in the different conditions.

Hypoxia decreased power output by 39% in the placebo condition ($P < 0.001$) and by 37% in the naloxone condition ($P < 0.001$, no significant difference between conditions). Switching to normoxia at exhaustion in hypoxia allowed continuing up to 97% of power developed in normoxic control under placebo ($P < 0.001$) and to almost 100% under naloxone ($P < 0.001$, no significant difference between conditions).

$V'O_2$ peak was 3.77 ± 0.80 L/min (placebo) and 3.85 ± 0.76 L/min (naloxone) in normoxia, reached 2.39 ± 0.4 L/min in hypoxia (both placebo and naloxone) and increased again to 94% (placebo) and 95% (naloxone) of normoxia values after the normoxia switch at exhaustion from hypoxia (no significant difference between conditions). Time to exhaustion was similar in normoxia and hypoxia (22 ± 3 min) and reached a total of 27 ± 4 min for hypoxia when adding the additional exercise time after the normoxia switch (no effects of naloxone).

Figure 1 shows the overall levels of perceived exertion and those pertaining to breathing and leg effort separately. In normoxia, perceived exertion increased in a curvilinear way, and there was no effect of naloxone. The rate of increase was greater in hypoxia, dropped upon switching to acute normoxia at exhaustion, and increased again towards exhaustion (no effect of naloxone).

The top panel of Figure 2 shows the increase in minute ventilation (V'_E) with exercise intensity and its more pronounced increase in hypoxia. After the normoxia switch, ventilation dropped but not completely to the normoxic level. There was no effect of naloxone. The second panel of Figure 2 shows the evolution of $P_{ET}CO_2$. In conditions of normoxia, the typical pattern of a slight increase followed by a drop beyond the ventilatory threshold was observed. Conversely, hypoxia immediately induced hyperventilation and reduced $P_{ET}CO_2$ values, which were not restored upon the normoxia switch. There was no effect of naloxone. The third panel

Table 1 Peak values at exhaustion in normoxia, hypoxia and after the normoxia switch at exhaustion in hypoxia

	Normoxia		Hypoxia		Normoxia switch after hypoxia	
	Placebo	Naloxone	Placebo	Naloxone	Placebo	Naloxone
Power (watt)	296 ± 48	292 ± 52	182 ± 36*	184 ± 34*	282 ± 51	291 ± 49
Time (min)	22.5 ± 2.6	22.3 ± 2.4	22.0 ± 3.8	22.4 ± 3.7	27.1 ± 4.2	27.6 ± 3.9
HR (/min)	184 ± 5	181 ± 7	169 ± 7*	168 ± 7*	173 ± 5	170 ± 6
Lactate (mM)	11.3 ± 3.7	10.5 ± 2.4	10.4 ± 2.9	10.3 ± 3.7	11.3 ± 3.0	10.9 ± 5.1
RPE global (a.u.)	9.7 ± 0.5	9.6 ± 0.5	9.4 ± 0.7	9.7 ± 0.5	9.3 ± 0.9	9.4 ± 0.5
RPE resp (a.u.)	9.5 ± 0.7	9.4 ± 0.9	9.5 ± 0.6	9.5 ± 0.7	9.0 ± 1.1	8.9 ± 0.4
RPE legs (a.u.)	9.9 ± 0.3	9.7 ± 0.7	9.6 ± 0.5	9.8 ± 0.4	10.0 ± 0.0	10.0 ± 0.0
SaO_2 (%)	91.7 ± 4.1	93.3 ± 6.4	67.5 ± 8.9*	63.6 ± 8.8*	90.55±	95.70±
$P_{ET}CO_2$ (kPa)	4.44 ± 0.70	4.56 ± 0.48	3.50 ± 0.18*	3.49 ± 0.26*	4.48 ± 0.32	4.42 ± 0.40
$V'O_2$ (L/min)	3.77 ± 0.8	3.85 ± 0.76	2.39 ± 0.40*	2.39 ± 0.40*	3.53 ± 0.71	3.64 ± 0.63
$V'CO_2$(L/min)	4.92 ± 1.1	4.86 ± 0.80	3.19 ± 0.53*	3.30 ± 0.57*	3.86 ± 0.78	4.05 ± 0.85
V'_E (L/min)	150 ± 33	146 ± 21	128 ± 20*	133 ± 24*	123 ± 21	132 ± 28
V'_A (L/min)	159 ± 43	154 ± 27	133 ± 26*	137 ± 37*	126 ± 27	138 ± 37
Vt (L)	2.98 ± 0.39	3.16 ± 0.41	2.89 ± 0.51	2.97 ± 0.72	2.91 ± 0.45	3.09±
RR (/min)	50 ± 8	47 ± 7	45 ± 7	44 ± 7	42 ± 6	43 ± 5
MEFR (L/sec)	5.1 ± 1.2	5.0 ± 0.8	4.2 ± 0.7	4.3 ± 0.9	4.1 ± 0.8	4.4 ± 1.0

Naloxone had no effect on any of these parameters in either condition. Power, mechanical power output on cycle ergometer; time, time to exhaustion; HR, heart rate; lactate, arterialized lactate concentration; RPE, rate of perceived exertion (overall, respiratory, legs); SaO_2, earlobe oximetry; $P_{ET}CO_2$, end-tidal CO_2; $V'O_2$, oxygen consumption; $V'CO_2$, expired CO_2; V'_E, minute ventilation; V'_A, alveolar ventilation; Vt, tidal volume; RR, respiratory frequency; MEFR, peak expiratory flow.
*Significantly different from normoxia.

of Figure 2 shows the evolution of respiratory frequency, which followed a similar pattern as that of ventilation and tidal volume (not shown), without any effect of naloxone.

iEMG was higher during hypoxia (Figure 3). No differences were observed in CPF or MPF (not shown). At exhaustion in hypoxia, after the hypoxia switch, iEMG increased and reached higher values at exhaustion compared to normoxia. There were no effects of naloxone.

Blood lactate levels (Figure 3) increased in a typical curvilinear manner both in normoxia and hypoxia, with an early onset of the exponential increase in hypoxia. There was no effect of naloxone.

SpO_2 showed a slight drop at higher intensities in conditions of normoxia, whereas it dropped right from the start of exercise in hypoxia. Upon the normoxia switch, it normalised rapidly. There was no effect of naloxone. SpO_2 reached lower values in hypoxia, dropping to 68% with placebo and 64% with naloxone (no significant difference), and increased after the normoxia switch. Heart rate response to exercise showed the typical linear increase with a steeper slope in hypoxia, a drop at the normoxia switch and similar maximum heart rates at exhaustion (no effects of naloxone; data not shown).

Figure 4 shows the relationship between ventilation and RPE breathing, and iEMG and RPE legs. Both relationships were slightly displaced to the left in hypoxia compared to normoxia, but there was no effect of naloxone.

Discussion

Contrary to our expectations naloxone had no effect on any of the investigated variables, neither in normoxia nor in hypoxia. It follows that, at least in trained healthy young male subjects, during incremental exercise tests, in normoxia and normobaric hypoxia with an FIO_2 of 10.65 (equivalent to approximately 5,000 m), endogenous opioid receptors are not involved in the ventilatory and heart rate responses to exercise nor in the sensation of overall levels of perceived exertion or those pertaining to breathing or cycling effort specifically.

Naloxone dosage

Could it be that there was insufficient blockade of opioid receptors? This seems unlikely. The 'normal' dose for clinical use of naloxone is 1–4 mg, largely sufficient for full reversal of the effects of exogenously administered opioids and to trigger withdrawal symptoms [16]. Naloxone hydrochloride is partly actively transported through the blood–brain barrier and reaches higher central nervous system (CNS) concentrations than in the plasma [17]. Positron emission tomography studies showed that with 1 mg naloxone, 50% of opioid receptors in the CNS were blocked [18]. Santiago and Edelman [19] recommended a minimal dose of 0.1 mg/kg for peripheral and central receptor blockade. We used 30 mg, i.e. 0.40 ± 0.04 mg/kg, a dose that is four times in excess, to compare our results to those of a previous study [9]. Naloxone has a half-life of about 1 h [14]. Our subjects started exercising within 5 min

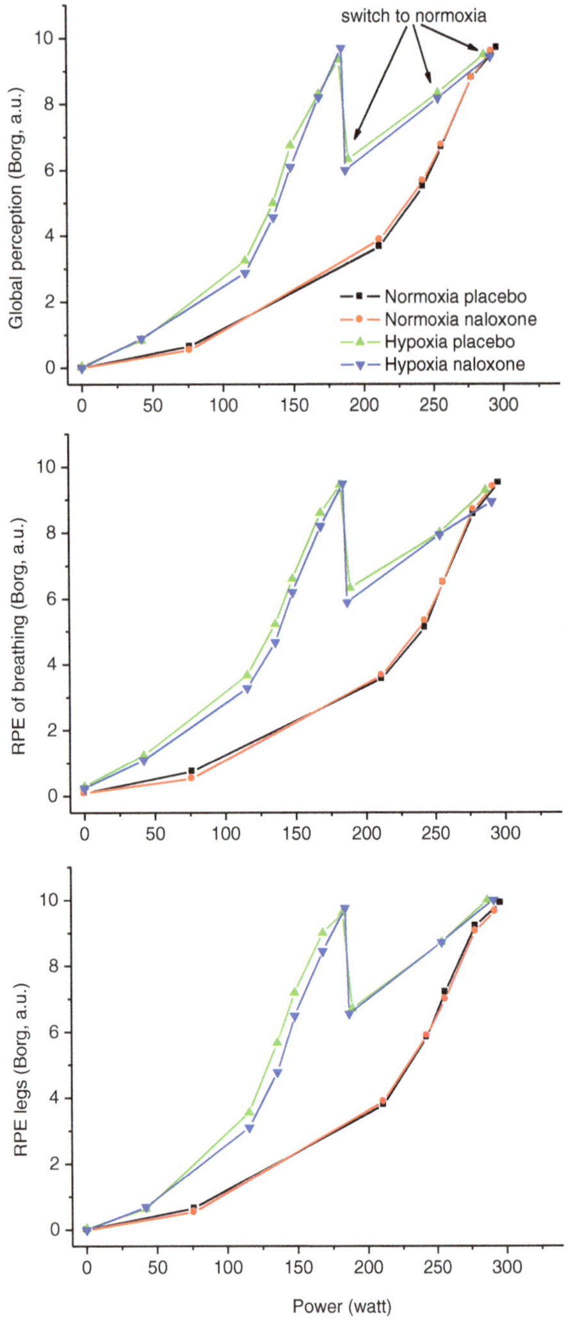

Figure 1 The *top panel* shows the overall RPE vs. power output. At exhaustion from exercise in hypoxia, the subjects were switched to room air and strongly encouraged to continue pedalling until reaching secondary exhaustion. The *arrows* indicate the measurements after the switch; for reasons of legibility, the *arrows* are not shown on the other graphs. The *middle panel* shows the RPE breathing vs. power output. The *bottom panel* shows the RPE legs vs. power output. Error bars were omitted for clarity. The coloured symbols and lines represent the same conditions for all figures.

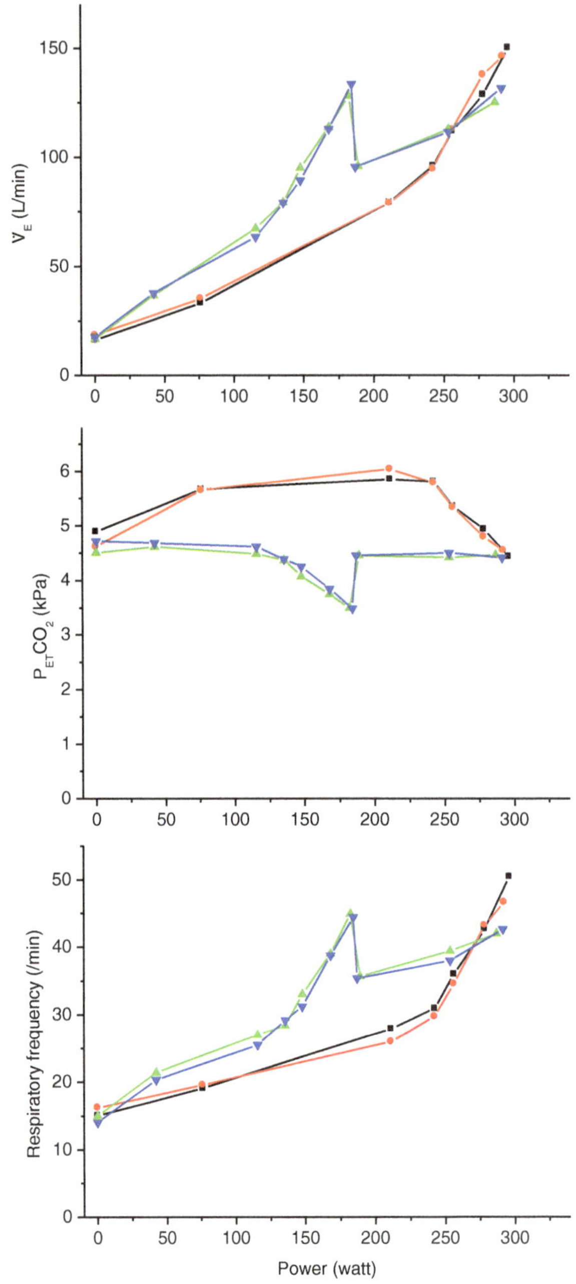

Figure 2 The *top panel* shows the total ventilation (V'E) vs. power output. The *middle panel* shows the end-tidal CO_2 tension ($P_{ET}CO_2$) vs. power output. The *bottom panel* shows the respiratory frequency vs. power output.

after injection and reached exhaustion in less than 30 min, largely inside the therapeutic time window. Finally, even though admittedly anecdotal, several subjects indicated missing their habitual post-exercise 'high' and feeling somewhat 'bland' instead, which after the breaking of the randomization key appeared to correspond to the naloxone experiments, suggestive of naloxone blocking the

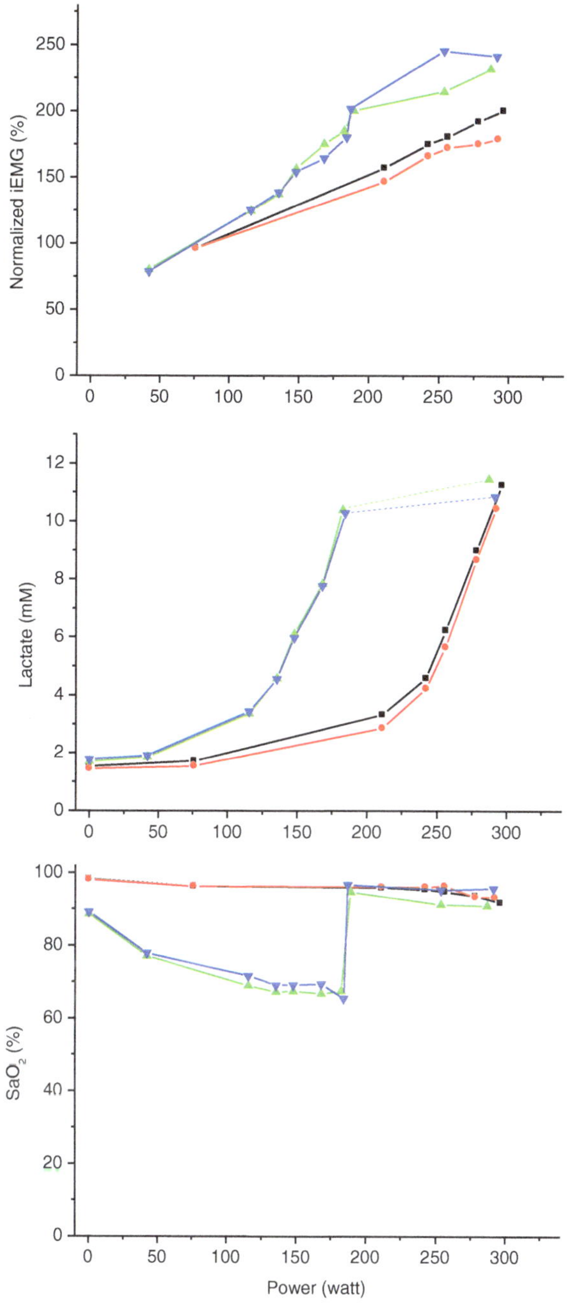

Figure 3 The *top panel* shows normalised integrated vastus lateralis surface electromyogram (iEMG) vs. power output. The *middle panel* presents the arterialized blood lactate concentration [La] vs. power output. The *bottom panel* presents the arterial oxygen saturation (earlobe oximetry) vs. power output.

effect of endogenous opioid release post-exercise, possibly related to the 'feeling good' after a workout [20,21].

Opioids and dyspnoea

What can explain the difference between our findings and the repeated finding of a role for opioids in patients with dyspnoea? For example, naloxone increased dyspnoea sensation in asthmatics when challenged with metacholine, and similar findings were reported for chronic obstructive pulmonary disease (COPD) patients during exercise [22,23]. Jensen et al. [7] compared inhaled nebulized fentanyl citrate (an opioid analogue) to placebo in COPD patients and found dyspnoea attenuation and improved exercise performance. Both sensations of intensity and unpleasantness were affected. There are similar observations in patients with terminal cancer-related dyspnoea [24], and opioids have a role as therapeutic means in dealing with dyspnoeic patients in general [5,6,25].

One explanation for an absence of effect in our study may reside in the complexity of what is covered by the term dyspnoea. The American Thoracic Society defined dyspnoea as 'a subjective experience of breathing discomfort that consists of qualitatively distinct sensations that vary in intensity' [5,26]. Dyspnoea includes both sensory (intensity) and affective (unpleasantness) components [26]. Distinct mechanisms and afferent pathways are associated with different sensory qualities (notably work/effort, tightness and air hunger/unsatisfied inspiration); distinct sensations most often do not occur in isolation, and dyspnoea sensations also vary in their unpleasantness and in their emotional and behavioural significance [5]. In patients, the affective component is often of great importance [27], whereas it is of less significance in a healthy athletic subject during a non-threatening challenge like an exercise test limited in time. A patient with COPD associates the difficulty to breathe during an exercise test with fear to suffocate, whereas a healthy subject will not [28]. Nevertheless, in healthy subjects, intravenous morphine sulphate reduces the discomfort ('air hunger') induced by hypercapnia to a similar extent as observed during clinical studies [25].

Breathing during heavy exercise in severe hypoxia is accompanied by dyspnoea with affective aspects [29]. In the present study, the subjects quantified the rate of perceived exertion in the classic sense originally proposed by Borg [2], i.e. the central generated sensation of effort [30]. Affective components of unpleasant sensations related to the exercise like leg pain or air hunger were not explicitly quantified. There are two different dimensions of exercise-related sensations: (1) one reflecting the sensation of effort, likely centrally generated and unrelated to afferent feedback and (2) one related to afferent feedback from various tissues involved in the effort [30]. Aliverti et al. [10] reported that breathing RPE was uniquely related to total respiratory power output at low and high altitudes (hypobaric hypoxia, 4,559 m). In the present study, in conditions of normobaric hypoxia, the tendency for a leftward shift of the curve relating breathing RPE to V'_E (see Figure 1) suggests that breathing RPE may have been influenced by other parameters but that the endogenous opioid system was not involved. However, even if an

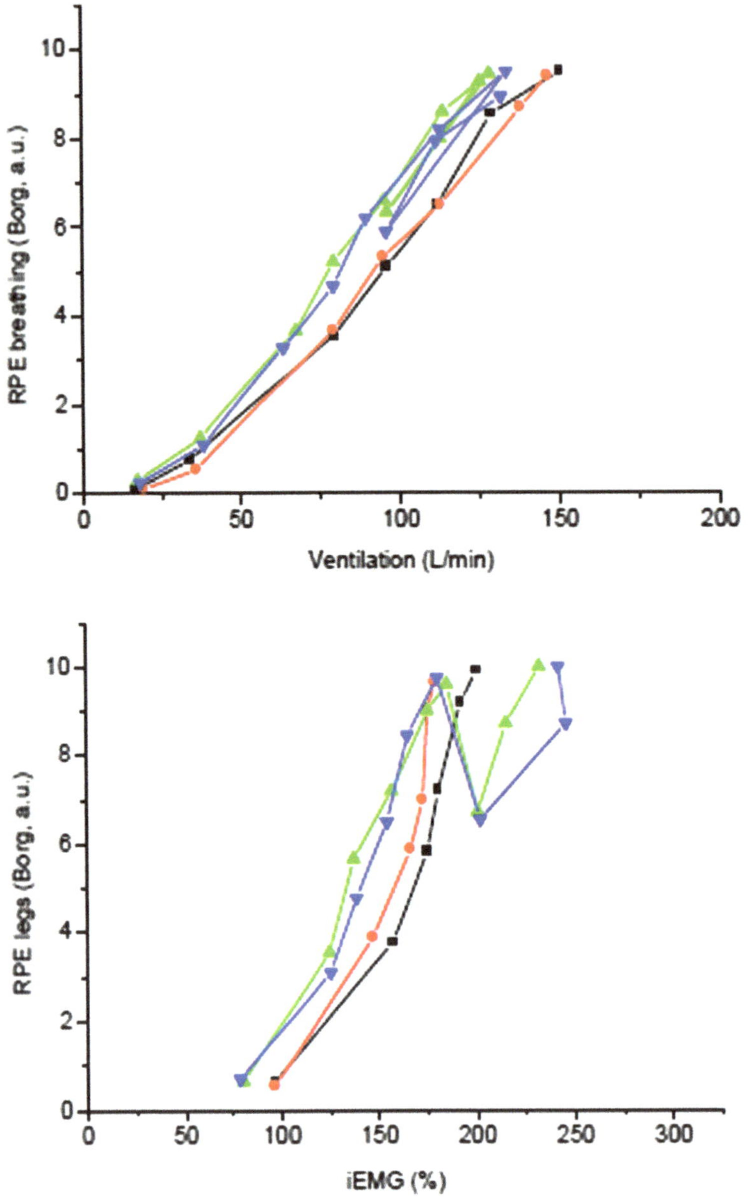

Figure 4 The *top panel* shows RPE breathing vs. total ventilation. The *bottom panel* shows RPE legs vs. iEMG.

affective component of the sensation of breathing was influenced by hypoxia and/or naloxone in our study, this did not have an effect on performance.

Ventilatory response to exercise

Anatomical and pharmacological evidence suggests that endogenous opioids play a role in the control of breathing. Mu (μ), delta (δ) and kappa (κ) opioid receptors are present in brainstem areas involved in respiration, and endogenous opioids like endorphins, enkephalins, dynorphins and endomorphins are found in medullary and pontine respiratory regions [6,31]. The depressant effects of exogenous opioids on ventilation are well known, and also, endogenous opioids are thought to be tonically active and have a depressant effect on ventilation [31]. Exogenous opioids also have a strong depressant effect on the hypoxic ventilatory response in animals and humans [32]. By contrast, on a local CNS level, endogenous opioids may exert an excitatory modulation of hypoxia-induced hyperventilation by acting on μ-receptors in the rostral medullary raphe at least in a rat model [33], illustrating that the overall systemic effects of exogenous opioids are not necessarily indicative of the role of endogenous opioids at specific sites in the CNS. Akiyama et al. [34] injected healthy subjects with naloxone hydrochloride and found an increase of both ventilatory (V'_E) and mouth pressure (Pm) responses to hypoxic progressive hypercapnia with inspiratory flow-resistive loading. Ward and Nitti [35] injected the opioid agonist sufentanil in trained athletes during exercise and found that the ventilatory response to exercise was reduced. We expected that the injection of 30 mg of naloxone would increase the ventilatory response to exercise. Our results indicate no effect of a general blockade of opioid receptors on the ventilatory response to incremental exercise in normoxia and hypoxia. It follows that it is unlikely that endogenous opioids play any important role in the ventilatory response to an incremental exercise challenge in normoxia and its increase in hypoxia, at least in healthy, young trained male subjects.

Central effects

Humans frequently report positive feelings during and after endurance efforts ('runner's high') that include both central effects (improved affect, sense of well-being, anxiety reduction, post-exercise calm) and peripheral effects (reduced pain sensation) [21]. Imaging studies provided evidence of endogenous opioid release in fronto-limbic brain regions after physical exercise correlated to perceived euphoria [21]. Endocannabinoids are also thought to play a role in runner's high [36]. Paulev et al. [37] compared naloxone (0.8 mg i.v.) to placebo during a Cooper test (running the longest possible distance within 12 min) in trained subjects. Performance was not influenced by naloxone, but perception of muscle pain was enhanced with naloxone. Sgherza et al. [9] compared incremental exercise capacity in 18 subjects under naloxone and placebo and reported a significant reduction with naloxone. They concluded that after naloxone administration, in laboratory conditions, endurance trained subjects stop exercise at lower levels than those under placebo, suggesting that peak exercise capacity was limited by the individual's perception of exertion, exacerbated by a lack of effect from endogenous opioids, rather than by physiological fatigue. Even though several subjects in our study reported feeling 'bland' after exercise under naloxone, we did not see the reduction in exercise capacity reported by Sgherza et al. [9] in normoxia. Their results were based on 18 subjects, and earlier studies with fewer subjects and lower dosage of naloxone had failed to find significant effects. We therefore cannot exclude that our results, obtained in ten subjects, are limited by type-II error, but given the absence of any change in the variables monitored, it seems quite unlikely that in hypoxia an effect of opioid blockade plays any important role.

Leg afferents

Apart from their involvement in noxious signalling, spinal cord level opioid receptors may play a role in the exercise pressor response. Amann et al. [38-40] used lumbar intrathecal fentanyl to block central projection of μ-opioid-receptor-sensitive group III/IV muscle afferents from the lower limbs during different exercises: single-leg mild to moderate intensity knee extensor exercise, 5-km cycling time trial exercise, incremental cycling exercise and constant load exercise to exhaustion. Afferent blockade had no effect on central and peripheral haemodynamics or ventilation at rest, but during exercise cardiac output, mean arterial pressure and femoral blood flow were attenuated in the knee extensor exercise, pacing during the time trial was severely perturbed, and heart rate, blood pressure and ventilation were impeded during cycling at 80% of aerobic maximum. These findings suggest an important role of group III/IV muscle afferents in the regulation of the cardiorespiratory response to rhythmic exercise. In rats, Tsuchimochi et al. [41] found that stimulation of peripheral μ-opioid receptors attenuated the exercise pressor reflex and that this effect could be blocked with naloxone. These findings in humans and animals would suggest that endogenous opioids play a role in the regulation of muscle afferent traffic, but from our results, it appears that in healthy, young, physically active subjects doing a 20- to 30-min incremental exercise challenge in normoxia or severe hypoxia, endogenous opioids are not attenuating the normal cardiovascular response to exercise through the stimulation of type III/IV afferent μ-receptors at the spinal level, leaving the question on their role and significance open.

Acute normoxia switch

The limitation of exercise performance in severe hypoxia is still not well understood [11-13]. Lack of oxygen is the reason, but it remains unclear what mechanism in hypoxia leads to an earlier disengagement from an exercise challenge as compared to normoxia. Verges et al. [13] argue that because biochemical, electromyographic and mechanical signs of muscle fatigue at exhaustion are reduced in severe hypoxia compared with normoxia, muscle metabolic fatigue is not the main factor responsible for impaired whole body exercise performance, as proposed before [12,15]. Our subjects were able to continue cycling after reaching their maximum in hypoxia when switched to normoxia. iEMG, an indicator of locomotor muscle drive, increased upon the normoxia switch, a finding arguing in favour of supraspinal limitation of exercise performance in hypoxia by a rapidly reversible withdrawal of motor drive. Amann et al. [42] found that the degree of hypoxia influences the relative role of muscle fatigue in the cessation of dynamic exercise with large muscle groups. Those authors proposed a threshold of SaO_2 for a switch from a predominant effect of peripheral fatigue to a predominant effect of CNS hypoxia on central motor output and exercise performance. They found similar levels of muscle fatigue in task failure from constant load exercise to exhaustion when SaO_2 averaged 94%, 82% or 76% (FIO_2 0.21–0.12), but not at a SaO_2 of 67% (FIO_2 0.10). They suggest the dominance of CNS hypoxia over peripheral muscle fatigue in influencing central motor output below SaO_2 levels of 70%–75%. Our results of early exhaustion in hypoxia with SaO_2 below 70% and rapid restoration of exercise capacity upon the normoxia switch are in accordance with those contentions.

Limits of performance in severe hypoxia

The origins of the signals leading to the cessation of the central motor drive at exhaustion during heavy large muscle group exercise in severe hypoxia thus remain unclear. Possible candidates controlling the signal to stop exercise include arterial oxygen (O_2) desaturation with exercise causing marked central nervous system hypoxia, other factors acting on the respiratory and/or other higher nervous centres, with or without contribution of fatigued respiratory muscles, or the effects of pulmonary hypertension and right ventricular overload [4,12,43,44]. Millet et al. [45] showed in a biceps brachii repeated isometric contraction model that in pronounced hypoxia (9% O_2, SaO_2 75%), central drive is diminished independently of afferent feedback and peripheral fatigue and concluded that submaximal performance in severe hypoxia is related directly to brain oxygenation, results corroborating those of Goodall et al. [46] who also showed that peripheral mechanisms of fatigue contribute relatively more to the reduction in force-generating capacity of the knee extensors following submaximal intermittent isometric contractions in normoxia and mild to moderate hypoxia, whereas supraspinal fatigue plays a greater role in more pronounced degrees of hypoxia.

Study limitations

Our results pertain to a limited sample size of healthy, young, trained male subjects and cannot be generalised. Further limitations to our study design are acknowledged. Prolonged hypoxia leads to ventilatory acclimatisation changing ventilation at rest and during exercise. We performed our experiments in acute normobaric hypoxia, and it is possible that in chronic hypobaric hypoxia, findings would differ. It therefore remains to be described what the effects of opioids or opioid receptor antagonists on breathing sensation and exercise performance in conditions of prolonged hypobaric hypoxia would be. Finally, we used a short incremental exercise protocol to exhaustion. It remains an open question if more prolonged submaximal time trial like exercise would be influenced by opioid receptor blockade.

Conclusions

We compared incremental cycling exercise capacity in conditions of normoxia and hypoxia after injection of the opioid antagonist naloxone, in comparison with placebo. Since naloxone had no effect on the ventilatory response to exercise nor on the sensation of exertion, neither in normoxia nor in hypoxia, it follows that endogenous xopioid receptors do not play a role in the perceived exertion and the regulation of maximal aerobic exercise performance in conditions of severe hypoxia.

Competing interests

The authors declare that they have no competing interests.

Authors' contributions

BK and LK designed the experiment and collected data. LK did the data analysis under the supervision of BK. Both authors wrote the manuscript. BK is the guarantor. Both authors read and approved the final manuscript.

Acknowledgements

The authors thank Maximilien Jung, Edmund Biason, Mireille Wenger and Benoît Delapierre for their excellent technical help in setting up and performing the experiments, and the subjects for their dedication and time.

Author details

[1]Sports Medicine Unit, La Tour Hospital, Meyrin 1217, Switzerland. [2]Institute of Movement Sciences and Sports Medicine, Faculty of medicine, University of Geneva, 10, rue du Conseil Général, Genève 4 1205, Switzerland.

References

1. Stendardi L, Grazzini M, Gigliotti F, Lotti P, Scano G: **Dyspnea and leg effort during exercise.** *Respir Med* 2005, **99:**933–942.
2. Borg E, Borg G, Larsson K, Letzter M, Sundblad B-M: **An index for breathlessness and leg fatigue.** *Scand J Med Sci Sports* 2010, **20:**644–650.
3. Jones NL, Killian KJ: **Exercise limitation in health and disease.** *N Engl J Med* 2000, **343:**632–641.
4. Kayser B: **Exercise starts and ends in the brain.** *Eur J Appl Physiol* 2003, **90:**411–419.
5. Parshall MB, Schwartzstein RM, Adams L, Banzett RB, Manning HL, Bourbeau J, Calverley PM, Gift AG, Harver A, Lareau SC, Mahler DA, Meek PM, O'Donnell DE, ATS Committee on Dyspnea: **An official American Thoracic Society statement: update on the mechanisms, assessment, and management of dyspnea.** *Am J Resp Crit Care* 2012, **185:**435–452.
6. Mahler DA: **Understanding mechanisms and documenting plausibility of palliative interventions for dyspnea.** *Curr Opin Support Palliat Care* 2011, **5:**71–76.
7. Jensen D, Alsuhail A, Viola R, Dudgeon DJ, Webb KA, O'Donnell DE: **Inhaled fentanyl citrate improves exercise endurance during high-intensity constant work rate cycle exercise in chronic obstructive pulmonary disease.** *J Pain and Symptom Manage* 2012, **43:**706–719.
8. Jennings A-L: **A systematic review of the use of opioids in the management of dyspnoea.** *Thorax* 2002, **57:**939–944.
9. Sgherza AL, Axen K, Fain R, Hoffman RS, Dunbar CC, Haas F: **Effect of naloxone on perceived exertion and exercise capacity during maximal cycle ergometry.** *J Appl Physiol* 2002, **93:**2023–2028.
10. Aliverti A, Kayser B, Mauro AL, Quaranta M, Pompilio P, Dellacà RL, Ora J, Biasco L, Cavalleri L, Pomidori L, Cogo A, Pellegrino R, Miserocchi G: **Respiratory and leg muscles perceived exertion during exercise at altitude.** *Respir Physiol Neurobiol* 2011, **177:**162–168.
11. Amann M, Kayser B: **Nervous system function during exercise in hypoxia.** *High Alt Med Biol* 2009, **10:**149–164.
12. Kayser B: **Why is endurance performance decreased at high altitude?** *Schweizerische Zeitschrift für Sportmedizin und Sporttraumatologie* 2005, **53:**54–60.

13. Verges S, Rupp T, Jubeau M, Wuyam B, Esteve F, Levy P, Perrey S, Millet GY: **Cerebral perturbations during exercise in hypoxia.** *Am J Physiol Regul Integr Comp Physiol* 2012, **302:**R903–R916.
14. Ngai SH, Berkowitz BA, Yang JC, Hempstead J, Spector S: **Pharmacokinetics of naloxone in rats and in man: basis for its potency and short duration of action.** *Anesthesiology* 1976, **44:**398–401.
15. Kayser B, Narici M, Binzoni T, Grassi B, Cerretelli P: **Fatigue and exhaustion in chronic hypobaric hypoxia: influence of exercising muscle mass.** *J Appl Physiol* 1994, **76:**634–640.
16. Clarke SFJ, Dargan PI, Jones AL: **Naloxone in opioid poisoning: walking the tightrope.** *Emerg Med J* 2005, **22**(9):612–616.
17. Suzuki T, Ohmuro A, Miyata M, Furuishi T, Hidaka S, Kugawa F, Fukami T, Tomono K: **Involvement of an influx transporter in the blood–brain barrier transport of naloxone.** *Biopharm Drug Dispos* 2010, **31**(4):243–252.
18. Melichar JK, Nutt DJ, Malizia AL: **Naloxone displacement at opioid receptor sites measured in vivo in the human brain.** *Eur J Pharmacol* 2003, **459:**217–219.
19. Santiago TV, Edelman NH: **Opioids and breathing.** *J Appl Physiol* 1985, **59:**1675–1685.
20. Janal MN, Colt EWD, Clark WC, Glusman M: **Pain sensitivity, mood and plasma endocrine levels in man following long-distance running: effects of naloxone.** *Pain* 1984, **19:**13–25.
21. Boecker H, Sprenger T, Spilker ME, Henriksen G, Koppenhoefer M, Wagner KJ, Valet M, Berthele A, Tolle TR: **The runner's high: opioidergic mechanisms in the human brain.** *Cereb Cortex* 2008, **18:**2523–2531.
22. Bellofiore S, Di Maria GU, Privitera S, Sapienza S, Milic-Emili J, Mistretta A: **Endogenous opioids modulate the increase in ventilatory output and dyspnea during severe acute bronchoconstriction.** *Am Rev Respir Dis* 1990, **142:**812–816.
23. Mahler DA, Murray JA, Waterman LA, Ward J, Kraemer WJ, Zhang X, Baird JC: **Endogenous opioids modify dyspnoea during treadmill exercise in patients with COPD.** *Eur Resp J* 2009, **33:**771–777.
24. Coyne PJ, Viswanathan R, Smith TJ: **Nebulized fentanyl citrate improves patients' perception of breathing, respiratory rate, and oxygen saturation in dyspnea.** *J Pain and Symptom Manage* 2002, **23:**157–160.
25. Banzett RB, Adams L, O'Donnell CR, Gilman SA, Lansing RW, Schwartzstein RM: **Using laboratory models to test treatment: morphine reduces dyspnea and hypercapnic ventilatory response.** *Am J Resp Crit Care* 2011, **184:**920–927.
26. American Thoracic Society: **Dyspnea. Mechanisms, assessment, and management: a consensus statement. American Thoracic Society.** *Am J Respir Crit Care Med* 1999, **159:**321–340.
27. Wan L, Stans L, Bogaerts K, Decramer M, Van den Bergh O: **Sensitization in medically unexplained dyspnea: differential effects on intensity and unpleasantness.** *Chest* 2012, **141:**989–995.
28. Macklem PT: **Exercise in COPD: damned if you do and damned if you don't.** *Thorax* 2005, **60:**887–888.
29. Mansoor JK, Eldridge MW, Yoneda KY, Schelegle ES, Wood SC: **Role of airway receptors in altitude-induced dyspnea.** *Med Sci Sports Exerc* 2001, **33:**1449–1455.
30. Smirmaul BDPC: **Sense of effort and other unpleasant sensations during exercise: clarifying concepts and mechanisms.** *Br J Sports Med* 2012, **46:**308–311.
31. Lalley PM: **Opioidergic and dopaminergic modulation of respiration.** *Respir Physiol Neurobiol* 2008, **164:**160–167.
32. Zhang Z, Zhuang J, Zhang C, Xu F: **Activation of opioid μ-receptors in the commissural subdivision of the nucleus tractus solitarius abolishes the ventilatory response to hypoxia in anesthetized rats.** *Anesthesiology* 2011, **115:**353–363.
33. Dias MB, Nucci TB, Branco LGS, Gargaglioni LH: **Opioid μ-receptors in the rostral medullary raphe modulate hypoxia-induced hyperpnea in unanesthetized rats.** *Acta Physiol* 2011, **204:**435–442.
34. Akiyama Y, Nishimura M, Kobayashi S, Yoshioka A, Yamamoto M, Miyamoto K, Kawakami Y: **Effects of naloxone on the sensation of dyspnea during acute respiratory stress in normal adults.** *J Appl Physiol* 1993, **74:**590–595.
35. Ward DS, Nitti GJ: **The effects of sufentanil on the hemodynamic and respiratory response to exercise.** *Med Sci Sports Exerc* 1988, **20:**579–586.
36. Raichlen DA, Foster AD, Gerdeman GL, Seillier A, Giuffrida A: **Wired to run: exercise-induced endocannabinoid signaling in humans and cursorial mammals with implications for the 'runner's high'.** *J of Exp Biol* 2012, **215:**1331–1336.
37. Paulev PE, Thorbøll JE, Nielsen U, Kruse P, Jordal R, Bach FW, Fenger M, Pokorski M: **Opioid involvement in the perception of pain due to endurance exercise in trained man.** *Jpn J Physio* 1989, **39:**67–74.
38. Amann M, Proctor LT, Sebranek JJ, Pegelow DF, Dempsey JA: **Opioid-mediated muscle afferents inhibit central motor drive and limit peripheral muscle fatigue development in humans.** *J Physiol (Lond.)* 2009, **587:**271–283.
39. Amann M, Blain GM, Proctor LT, Sebranek JJ, Pegelow DF, Dempsey JA: **Group III and IV muscle afferents contribute to ventilatory and cardiovascular response to rhythmic exercise in humans.** *J Appl Physiol* 2010, **109:**966–976.
40. Amann M, Runnels S, Morgan DE, Trinity JD, Fjeldstad AS, Wray DW, Reese VR, Richardson RS: **On the contribution of group III and IV muscle afferents to the circulatory response to rhythmic exercise in humans.** *J Physiol (Lond)* 2011, **589:**3855–3866.
41. Tsuchimochi H, McCord JL, Kaufman MP: **Peripheral μ-opioid receptors attenuate the augmented exercise pressor reflex in rats with chronic femoral artery occlusion.** *Am J Physiol Heart Circ Physiol* 2010, **299**(2):H557–H565.
42. Amann M, Romer LM, Subudhi AW, Pegelow DF, Dempsey JA: **Severity of arterial hypoxaemia affects the relative contributions of peripheral muscle fatigue to exercise performance in healthy humans.** *J Physiol (Lond)* 2007, **581:**389–403.
43. Naeije R, Huez S, Lamotte M, Retailleau K, Neupane S, Abramowicz D, Faoro V: **Pulmonary artery pressure limits exercise capacity at high altitude.** *Eur Resp J* 2010, **36:**1049–1055.
44. Subudhi AW, Olin JT, Dimmen AC, Polaner DM, Kayser B, Roach RC: **Does cerebral oxygen delivery limit incremental exercise performance?** *J Appl Physiol* 2011, **111:**1727–1734.
45. Millet GY, Muthalib M, Jubeau M, Laursen PB, Nosaka K: **Severe hypoxia affects exercise performance independently of afferent feedback and peripheral fatigue.** *J Appl Physiol* 2012, **112:**1335–1344.
46. Goodall S, Ross EZ, Romer LM: **Effect of graded hypoxia on supraspinal contributions to fatigue with unilateral knee-extensor contractions.** *J Appl Physiol* 2010, **109:**1842–1851.

Permissions

All chapters in this book were first published in ASNEM, by BioMed Central; hereby published with permission under the Creative Commons Attribution License or equivalent. Every chapter published in this book has been scrutinized by our experts. Their significance has been extensively debated. The topics covered herein carry significant findings which will fuel the growth of the discipline. They may even be implemented as practical applications or may be referred to as a beginning point for another development.

The contributors of this book come from diverse backgrounds, making this book a truly international effort. This book will bring forth new frontiers with its revolutionizing research information and detailed analysis of the nascent developments around the world.

We would like to thank all the contributing authors for lending their expertise to make the book truly unique. They have played a crucial role in the development of this book. Without their invaluable contributions this book wouldn't have been possible. They have made vital efforts to compile up to date information on the varied aspects of this subject to make this book a valuable addition to the collection of many professionals and students.

This book was conceptualized with the vision of imparting up-to-date information and advanced data in this field. To ensure the same, a matchless editorial board was set up. Every individual on the board went through rigorous rounds of assessment to prove their worth. After which they invested a large part of their time researching and compiling the most relevant data for our readers.

The editorial board has been involved in producing this book since its inception. They have spent rigorous hours researching and exploring the diverse topics which have resulted in the successful publishing of this book. They have passed on their knowledge of decades through this book. To expedite this challenging task, the publisher supported the team at every step. A small team of assistant editors was also appointed to further simplify the editing procedure and attain best results for the readers.

Apart from the editorial board, the designing team has also invested a significant amount of their time in understanding the subject and creating the most relevant covers. They scrutinized every image to scout for the most suitable representation of the subject and create an appropriate cover for the book.

The publishing team has been an ardent support to the editorial, designing and production team. Their endless efforts to recruit the best for this project, has resulted in the accomplishment of this book. They are a veteran in the field of academics and their pool of knowledge is as vast as their experience in printing. Their expertise and guidance has proved useful at every step. Their uncompromising quality standards have made this book an exceptional effort. Their encouragement from time to time has been an inspiration for everyone.

The publisher and the editorial board hope that this book will prove to be a valuable piece of knowledge for researchers, students, practitioners and scholars across the globe.

List of Contributors

Douglas S Kalman, Samantha Feldman and Diane R Krieger
Miami Research Associates, Nutrition/Endocrinology Department, 6141 Sunset Drive, Suite 301, Miami, FL 33143

Richard J Bloomer
The University of Memphis, Cardiorespiratory/Metabolic Laboratory, Department of Health and Sport Sciences, 106 Roane Fieldhouse, Memphis, TN 38152

Bill Campbell
Exercise and Performance Nutrition Laboratory, Dept. of Physical Education and Exercise Science, University of South Florida, 4202 E. Fowler Avenue, PED 214, Tampa, FL 33620, USA

Colin Wilborn and Lem Taylor
Human Performance Laboratory, University of Mary Hardin-Baylor, Belton, TX 76513, USA

Paul La Bounty
Department of Health, Human Performance, and Recreation, Baylor University, Box 97313, Waco, TX 76798, USA

Mike T Nelson
Department of Health and Human Performance, University of St. Thomas, St. Paul, MN 55105, USA

Mike Greenwood and Richard B Kreider
Exercise & Sport Nutrition Lab, Department of Health & Kinesiology, Texas A&M University, College Station, Texas, TX 77843-4243, USA.

Tim N Ziegenfuss and Hector L Lopez
The Center for Applied Health Sciences, Stow, OH 44224, USA

Jay R Hoffman and Jeffrey R Stout
Institute of Exercise Physiology and Wellness, Department of Sport and Exercise Science, University of Central Florida, Orlando, FL 32816, USA

Stephen Schmitz
Medical Surveillance and Risk Management, Shire HGT, 300 Shire Way, Lexington, MA 02421, USA

Rick Collins
Collins, McDonald & Gann, PC, Mineola, NY, USA

Doug S Kalman
Miami Research Associates, Endocrinology & Nutrition Department, 6141 Sunset Drive - Suite 301, Miami, FL 33143, USA

Jose Antonio
Farquhar College of Arts and Sciences, Nova Southeastern University, Fort Lauderdale, FL, USA

Katherine Herman, Christian Barton, Peter Malliaras and Dylan Morrissey
Centre for Sports and Exercise Medicine, William Harvey Research Institute, Bart's and the London School of Medicine and Dentistry, Queen Mary University of London, Mile End Hospital, Bancroft road, London, E1 4DG, UK

J Luke Pryor
Department of Kinesiology, University of Connecticut, Storrs, CT 06269, U-1110, USA

Stuart AS Craig
DuPont Nutrition & Health, Tarrytown, NY, USA

Thomas Swensen
Ithaca College, Ithaca, NY, USA

Wolfgang Freund, Sonja Faust, Arthur P Wunderlich, Marguerite Müller, Christian Billich, Markus S Juchems and Uwe H Schütz
Department of Diagnostic and Interventional Radiology, University Hospitals Ulm, Albert-Einstein-Allee 23, 89081 Ulm, Germany

Frank Birklein
Department of Neurology, University Medical Centre Mainz, Langenbeckstraße 1/503, 55131 Mainz, Germany

Christian Gaser
Departments of Psychiatry and Neurology, Jena University Hospital, Jahnstraße 3, 07743 Jena, Germany

Bernd L Schmitz
Section Neuroradiology, University Hospitals Ulm, Albert- Einstein-Allee 23, 89081 Ulm, Germany

Georg Grön
Section Neuropsychology and Functional Imaging, University Hospitals Ulm, Leimgrubenweg 12-14, 89073 Ulm, Germany

Uwe H Schütz
Outpatient Rehabilitation Centre at University Hospitals Ulm, Pfarrer-Weiß-Weg 10, 89077 Ulm, Germany

Kåre Birger Hagen, Hanne Dagfinrud, Rikke Helene Moe, Nina Østerås, Ingvild Kjeken, Margreth Grotle and Geir Smedslund
National Resource Centre for Rehabilitation in Rheumatology, Department of Rheumatology, Diakonhjemmet Hospital, P.O. Box 23 Vinderen, 0319 Oslo, Norway

Paul R Jones, Christian Barton, Dylan Morrissey, Nicola Maffulli and Stephanie Hemmings
Centre for Sports and Exercise Medicine, William Harvey Research Institute, Bart's and the London School of Medicine and Dentistry, Queen Mary University of London, Mile End Hospital, Bancroft Road, London E1 4DG, UK

Paul R Jones
King's College London School of Medicine and Dentistry, King's College London, Guy's Campus, London SE1 9UL, UK

Uwe HW Schütz, Hans-Jürgen Brambs, Heike Wiedelbach, Martin Ehrhardt, Wolfgang Freund, Horst Brunner, Christian Billich
Department of Diagnostic and Interventional Radiology, University Hospital of Ulm, Germany

Uwe HW Schütz
Outpatient Rehabilitation Centre at University Hospital of Ulm, Germany

Arno Schmidt-Trucksäss
3Institute of Exercise and Health Sciences, Sports Medicine, University of Basel, Switzerland

Beat Knechtle
Health Center St. Gallen and Department of General Practice, University Hospital of Zürich, Switzerland

Jürgen Machann
Section on Experimental Radiology, Department of Diagnostic and Interventional Radiology, University Hospital of Tübingen, Germany

Stefan Gröninger
Siemens Healthcare, Magnetic Resonance, Stuttgart, Germany

Ingo Schulze
Main organizer and race director TransEurope FootRace 2009, Horb, Germany

Uwe HW Schütz
Department of Diagnostic and Interventional Radiology, University Hospital of Ulm, Albert-Einstein-Allee 23, 89081, Ulm, Germany
Outpatient Rehabilitation Centre at University Hospital of Ulm, Pfarrer-Weiß-Weg 10,89073, Ulm, Germany

Christian Billich, Hans-Jürgen Brambs and Heike Wiedelbach
Department of Diagnostic and Interventional Radiology, University Hospital of Ulm, Albert-Einstein-Allee 23, 89081, Ulm, Germany

Kathrin König and Christian Würslin
Section on Experimental Radiology, Department of Diagnostic and Interventional Radiology, University Hospital of Tübingen, Tübingen, Germany

Jürgen Machann
Section on Experimental Radiology, Department of Diagnostic and Interventional Radiology, University Hospital of Tübingen, Tübingen, Germany Institute for Diabetes Research and Metabolic Diseases (IDM), Metabolic Imaging - of the Helmholtz Center Munich at University of Tübingen (Paul Langerhaus Institute Tübingen), Tübingen, Germany

Hugo Olmedillas, José A Casajus, Alejandro González-Agüero and Germán Vicente-Rodríguez
GENUD 'Growth, Exercise, Nutrition and Development' Research Group, Universidad de Zaragoza, Zaragoza, Spain Faculty of Health and Sport Sciences (FCSD), Department of Physiatry and Nursing, Universidad de Zaragoza, Huesca, Spain

Luis A Moreno
GENUD 'Growth, Exercise, Nutrition and Development' Research Group, Universidad de Zaragoza, Zaragoza, Spain School of Health Science (EUCS), Universidad de Zaragoza, Zaragoza, Spain

Evan JH Lewis
Department of Nutritional Sciences, University of Toronto, 150 College Street, Toronto, ON M5S 3E2, Canada

Sarah J Fraser
Faculty of Life Sciences, McMaster University, 1280 Main Street West, Hamilton, ON L8S 4L8, Canada

Scott G Thomas
Faculty of Kinesiology and Physical Education, The University of Toronto, 55 HarbordStreet, Toronto, ON M5R 2W6, Canada

Greg D Wells
Faculty of Kinesiology and Physical Education, The University of Toronto, 55 HarbordStreet, Toronto, ON M5R 2W6, CanadaPhysiology and Experimental Medicine, The Hospital for Sick Children, 555 University Avenue, Toronto, ONM5G 1X8, Canada

Oluwatoyosi Babatunde Alex Owoeye, Ashiyat Kehinde Akodu, Bayonle Matt Oladokun and Sunday Rufus Akinwumi Akinbo
Department of Physiotherapy, College of Medicine, University of Lagos, Idi-Araba, Lagos, Nigeria

Mélanie L Beaulieu and Scott G McLean
School of Kinesiology, University of Michigan, Ann Arbor, MI, USA

Marianne JR Gittoes and Gareth Irwin
Cardiff School of Sport, Cardiff Metropolitan University, Cardiff, Cyncoed Road, Cardiff, UK, CF23 6XD

Maarten Hendrik Moen and Frank Backx
Rehabilitation and Sports Medicine Department, University Medical Center Utrecht, Utrecht, Holland

Leonoor Holtslag
Department of Orthopedic Surgery, Academic Medical Center Amsterdam, Amsterdam, Holland

Eric Bakker
Department of Clinical Epidemiology, Biostatistics and Bioinformatics, Academic Medical Center Amsterdam, Amsterdam, Holland

Carl Barten
Department of Physical Therapy, Academy of Physical Education, The Hague, Holland

Adam Weir and Johannes L Tol
Department of Sports Medicine, Medical Center Haaglanden, Leidschendam, Holland

Daniel S Moran
Heller Institute of Medical Research, Sheba Medical Center, Tel Hashomer, ISRAEL

Ariel University Center of Samaria, Ariel, ISRAEL

Yuval Heled, Yael Arbel and Ran Yanovich
Heller Institute of Medical Research, Sheba Medical Center, Tel Hashomer, ISRAEL

Eran Israeli
Division of Medicine, Department of Gastroenterology, Hebrew University-Hadassah Medical Center, Jerusalem, ISRAEL

Aharon S Finestone
Heller Institute of Medical Research, Sheba Medical Center, Tel Hashomer, ISRAELThe, Orthopaedic Department, Assaf Harofeh Medical Center, Zerifin and The Sackler School of Medicine, Tel Aviv University, Zerifin, Tel Aviv, ISRAEL

Rachel K Evans
Military Performance Division, U.S. Army Research Institute of Environmental Medicine, Natick, MA, USA

Michael D Kennedy
Faculty of Physical Education and Recreation, University of Alberta, Edmonton, AB, Canada

Robyn Fischer, Kristine Fairbanks, Lauren Lefaivre, Lauren Vickery and Janelle Molzan
Department of Physical Therapy, Faculty of Rehabilitation Medicine, University of Alberta, Edmonton, AB, Canada

Eric Parent
Department of Physical Therapy, Faculty of Rehabilitation Medicine, University of Alberta, Edmonton, AB, Canada Glenrose Rehabilitation Hospital, Alberta Health Services, Edmonton, AB,Canada

Beat Knechtle
Gesundheits zentrum St. Gallen, Vadianstrasse 26, St., Gallen 9011, SwitzerlandInstitute of General Practice and Health Services Research, University of Zurich, Rämistrasse 71, Zurich 8006, Switzerland

Patrizia Knechtle
Gesundheitszentrum St. Gallen, Vadianstrasse 26, St., Gallen 9011, Switzerland

Romuald Lepers
INSERM U1093, Faculty of Sport Sciences, University of Burgundy, Esplanade Erasme,Dijon 21000, France

Christoph Knoth
Department of Orthopaedics and Traumatology, Kantonsspital St. Gallen, St. Gallen, Switzerland

Christoph Alexander Rüst and Thomas Rosemann
Institute of General Practice and for Health Services Research, University of Zurich, Zurich, Switzerland

Romuald Lepers
INSERM U1093, Faculty of Sport Sciences, University of Burgundy, Dijon, France

Kyle J Hackney
Department of Exercise Science, Syracuse University, 820 Comstock Ave, Room 201Women's Building, Syracuse, NY 13244, USA Wyle Integrated Science and Engineering, Exercise Physiology and Countermeasures Project, Houston, TX 77058, USA

Summer B Cook
Department of Kinesiology, University of New Hampshire, 124 Main Street, Durham, NH 03824, USA

Timothy J Fairchild
School of Chiropractic and Sports Science, Murdoch University, 90 South Street, Murdoch, WA 6150, Australia

Lori L Ploutz-Snyder
Universities Space and Research Association, Exercise Physiology and Countermeasures Project, NASA Lyndon B Johnson Space Center, 2101 NASA Parkway, SK/261, Houston, TX 77058, USA

Dimirela Meili
Institute of General Practice and for Health Services Research, University of Zurich, Pestalozzistrasse 24, Zurich 8091, Switzerland

Beat Knechtle
Institute of General Practice and for Health Services Research, University of Zurich, Pestalozzistrasse 24, Zurich 8091, SwitzerlandFacharzt FMH für Allgemeinmedizin, Gesundheitszentrum St. Gallen, Vadianstrasse 26, St.Gallen 9001, Switzerland

Romuald Lepers
INSERM U1093, Faculty of Sport Sciences, University of Burgundy, UFR STAPS, BP 27877, Dijon Cedex 21078, France

Kristina da Fonseca-Engelhardt, Christoph Alexander Rüst, and Thomas Rosemann
Institute of General Practice and for Health Services Research, University of Zurich, Zurich 8091, Switzerland

Beat Knechtle
Gesundheitszentrum St. Gallen, St. Gallen 9000, Switzerland
Facharzt FMH für Allgemeinmedizin, Gesundheitszentrum St. Gallen, Vadianstrasse 26, St. Gallen 9001, Switzerland

Patrizia Knechtle
Gesundheitszentrum St. Gallen, St. Gallen 9000, Switzerland

Romuald Lepers
INSERM U1093, Faculty of Sport Sciences, University of Burgundy, Dijon 21078Cedex, France

Laurent Koglin
Sports Medicine Unit, La Tour Hospital, Meyrin 1217, Switzerland

Bengt Kayser
Institute of Movement Sciences and Sports Medicine, Faculty of medicine, University of Geneva, 10, rue du Conseil Général, Genève 4 1205, Switzerland